Two-Dimensional Optical Spectroscopy

Two-Dimensional Optical Spectroscopy

Minhaeng Cho

CRC Press
Taylor & Francis Group
Boca Raton London New York

CRC Press is an imprint of the
Taylor & Francis Group, an **informa** business

CRC Press
Taylor & Francis Group
6000 Broken Sound Parkway NW, Suite 300
Boca Raton, FL 33487-2742

First issued in paperback 2020

ISBN-13: 978-0-367-57732-2 (pbk)
ISBN-13: 978-1-4200-8429-0 (hbk)

Library of Congress Cataloging-in-Publication Data

Cho, Minhaeng, 1965-
Two-dimensional optical spectroscopy / Minhaeng Cho.
p. cm.
Includes bibliographical references and index.
ISBN 978-1-4200-8429-0 (hard back : alk. paper)
1. Optical spectroscopy. 2. Quantum optics. I. Title.

QC454.O66C46 2009
535.8'4--dc22 2009015407

Visit the Taylor & Francis Web site at
http://www.taylorandfrancis.com

and the CRC Press Web site at
http://www.crcpress.com

Table of Contents

Preface

The purpose of this book is twofold: It provides a detailed account of basic theory required for an understanding of the two-dimensional vibrational and electronic spectroscopy, and it also bridges the gap between the formal development of nonlinear optical spectroscopy and the application of the theory to the explanation of experimental results. The main emphasis is on principles rather than on practical aspects, though the reader may find sections where practical applications of the two-dimensional optical spectroscopy to complicated molecular systems, such as proteins and light-harvesting complexes, dominate.

It is assumed that the reader has the usual undergraduate background knowledge of quantum mechanics, electromagnetic theory, spectroscopy, statistical mechanics, and physical chemistry. This book is intended to serve as a monograph for researchers in this particular topic as well as a textbook for advanced graduate students. I hope that it helps to fulfill the needs of time-domain spectroscopists who wish to deepen their understanding of the basic features of nonlinear response function theory and intermolecular interaction-induced phenomena and who intend to apply the recently developed tools of vibrational and electronic spectroscopy in two dimensions.

The scope of the material is restricted in various ways, but most importantly, theoretical descriptions of two-dimensional spectroscopy of coupled two-level systems and anharmonic oscillators are generally valid and can be easily extended to account for the two-dimensional spectroscopy of coupled multi-chromophore systems.

About the Author

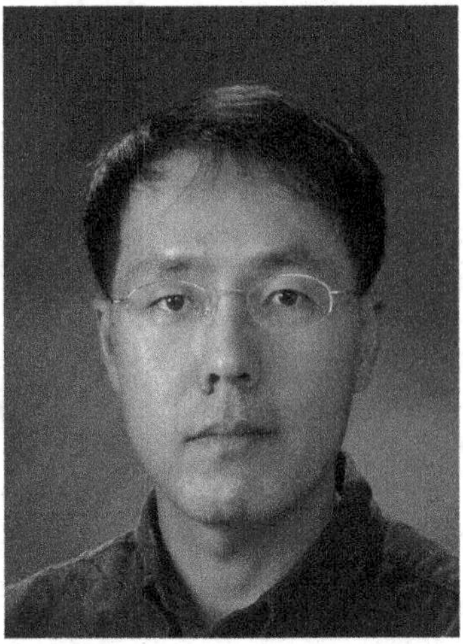

Minhaeng Cho was born in Seoul. He received a BS and an MS in chemistry from Seoul National University in 1987 and 1989, and a PhD from the University of Chicago in 1993 under the direction of Graham R. Fleming. After his post-doctoral training at Massachusetts Institute of Technology in Robert J. Silbey's group from 1994 to 1996, he joined the faculty of Korea University and has been there since March of 1996. He is currently director of the Center for Multidimensional Spectroscopy. His areas of research interest are in theoretical and computational chemistry and ultrafast nonlinear optical spectroscopy.

Acknowledgments

I am grateful to many friends, colleagues, collaborators, graduate students, and postdoctoral researchers, past and present. I am in debt to Jeffrey Cina and Jonggu Jeon for their critical readings of the manuscript, which resulted in many changes and corrections. I would like to express my deep gratitude to those who taught me about the fundamental principles of nonlinear optical spectroscopy, guided my interests toward time domain spectroscopy, corrected misconceptions, and carried out fruitful collaborations: Graham R. Fleming, Shaul Mukamel, Richard M. Stratt, Iwao Ohmine, Robert J. Silbey, Shinji Saito, Yoshitaka Tanimura, Mischa Bonn, Andrei Tokmakoff, John C. Wright, Michael D. Fayer, Hogyu Han, and Seung-Joon Jeon. I wish to thank many scientists around the world for stimulating discussions and clarifying concepts. Finally, I owe special thanks to the production editor, Tara Nieuwesteeg, and the CRC Press staff for their help and encouragement.

1 Introduction

Two-dimensional (2D) optical spectroscopy is an optical analog of 2D nuclear magnetic resonance (NMR) and utilizes multiple ultrashort laser pulses in infrared or UV-visible (vis) frequency range. It has been used to study protein structure and dynamics, hydrogen-bonding dynamics in solutions, femtosecond solvation dynamics, solute-solvent complexation, chemical reaction and exchange dynamics, excitation migration process in photosynthetic light-harvesting complexes, exciton dynamics in semiconductors, and coherence transfers in electronically coupled multi-chromophore systems.[1–19] Due to dramatic advancements of ultrafast laser technologies, femtosecond laser systems operating in infrared and visible frequency ranges have been commercially available so that we have seen a wide range of applications utilizing such ultrafast nonlinear optical spectroscopic techniques.

Most of the conventional linear spectroscopic methods, though they have been proven to be extremely useful for studying structural and dynamical properties of complex molecules in condensed phases, provide highly averaged information. Therefore, novel spectroscopic techniques capable of providing much higher information content have been sought and tested incessantly. In the research community of NMR spectroscopy, such efforts led to developing a variety of 2D NMR techniques such as NOESY (nuclear Overhauser enhancement spectroscopy) and COSY (correlation spectroscopy) methods among many others, and they have been extensively used to study structural and dynamical properties of proteins in solutions.[1, 2]

Although the 2D optical spectroscopy that has been considered to be an optical analog of 2D NMR does not provide atomic resolution structures of complex molecules, optical domain multidimensional spectroscopy has certain advantages because of the dramatic gain in time resolution (~ subpicosecond scale) possible and the ability to directly observe and quantify the couplings between quantum states involved in molecular dynamical processes.[19] An elementary and highly simplified schematic diagram in Figure 1.1 demonstrates that time-resolved 2D vibrational spectroscopic technique can provide detailed information on the 3D structure of a given complex molecule, that is, proteins.[20] A pair of vibrational chromophores, for example, amide I local modes in polypeptide backbone, are coupled to each other via hydrogen-bonding interaction, which results in cross-peaks in the 2D amide I infrared (IR) spectrum. As a molecule undergoes a structural transition along a certain reaction (folding or unfolding) coordinate, where hydrogen-bond breaking occurs, the cross-peaks will disappear in time.[21] Consequently, the transient 2D vibrational spectroscopy will provide information on the local conformational change of the target molecule in this case.

As theoretically and experimentally demonstrated over the last decade, the existence of cross-peaks is direct evidence on the vibrational couplings whose magnitudes depend on relative distances and orientations between vibrational chromophores

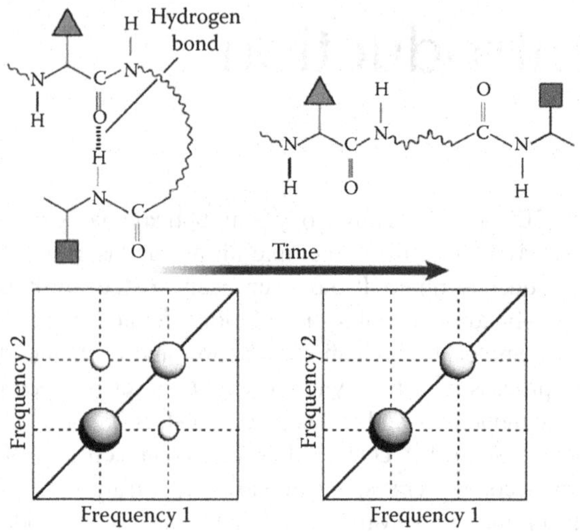

FIGURE 1.1 Two-dimensional spectroscopy of changes in molecular structure. The peaks on the diagonal line of this typical 2D infrared spectrum are associated with vibrations of the chemical groups in red and blue in the structures above (the square and the triangle represent amino acid side groups). The cross-peaks in green are produced by the coupling of these vibrations. As the molecule unfolds, the length of the hydrogen bond increases and the vibrational coupling decreases, so that the cross-peaks become less intense. The cross-peaks disappear when the hydrogen bond is broken. By examining the amplitudes of cross-peaks from a series of time-resolved spectra, the breaking of a hydrogen bond, and so the structural evolution of a small molecule, can be probed in time.

that are comparatively localized anharmonic oscillators.[10] Similarly, if two optical chromophores absorbing UV-vis lights are spatially close to each other, the electronic transition coupling between the two induces an electronic exciton formation and produces cross-peaks in the 2D electronic spectrum.[22] Therefore, experimental observation of cross-peaks in a measured 2D electronic spectrum and their transient behaviors in time provides invaluable information about electronic coupling strength between two chromophores and about exciton-exciton coherence and population transfers or even on structural changes.[9, 22, 23]

Ultrafast nonlinear optical spectroscopy utilizing IR and/or visible field has been a vital and incisive tool with a rich and long history, and an optical analog of NMR phase coherent multiple pulse spectroscopy was alluded before, where the acousto-optic modulation technique was used to generate an optical pulse sequence for a photon echo experiment.[3] Particularly, optical photon echo spectroscopy has been extensively used to study solvation dynamics and ultrafast inertial motions of bath degrees of freedom coupled to electronic transitions of chromophores in condensed phases.[24, 25] An IR photon echo experiment utilizing a free electron laser was performed in early 1990s.[26] Since the photon echo spectroscopy involves two either vibrational or electronic coherence evolutions during τ and t periods that are separated by another delay time T, the measured echo signal is expressed as $S(t,T,\tau)$.

The 2D spectrum $\tilde{S}(\omega_t, T, \omega_\tau)$ can therefore be obtained by carrying out double Fourier transformations of $S(t, T, \tau)$ with respect to τ and t. T is the so-called waiting time during which the system density matrix element is one of the diagonal elements (populations) or off-diagonal elements (coherences).

A typical 2D spectrum $\tilde{S}(\omega_t, T, \omega_\tau)$ thus obtained exhibits a variety of peaks. There are diagonal and off-diagonal peaks revealing different dynamics of the complex system of interest. For a two-level system, the 2D shape of a diagonal peak provides information on the relative contributions from the inhomogeneous and homogeneous dephasing processes.[27, 28] The extent of elongation along the diagonal and the slope of the elongation direction are often time-dependent, and their changes were found to be related to the transition frequency–frequency time–correlation function, which is in turn related to the associated solvation dynamics around the chromophore.[10, 28] For an anharmonic oscillator, which can be successfully modeled as a three-level system, the diagonal peak in the real part of the 2D photon echo spectrum is divided into two parts with positive and negative amplitudes, which reveals overtone anharmonicity. Here, it should be noted that the target oscillators should not be perfectly harmonic to make the associated nonlinear response function nonvanishing. Certain nonlinearities in nuclear and electronic motions are basic requirements. In a given 2D spectrum of anharmonic oscillator, the negative peak corresponds to the excited state absorption contribution to the signal and the positive peak to the sum of ground state bleaching and stimulated emission contributions. The cross-peaks can also be either antidiagonally or diagonally elongated, which corresponds to the cases when the two different transition frequencies are negatively or positively correlated in time. For a coupled homo- or hetero-dimer system, a negative correlation can be induced by modulation of the coupling constant, and a positive correlation results from modulation of the transition frequencies of the two monomers. The intensities of the cross-peaks can change in time, and their time-dependencies originate from various processes such as excitation transfers between two different excitonic or monomeric states, coherence transfers, chemical exchanges and reactions, population-dependent dephasing processes, conformation and chemical structural transitions, and so forth.[10] Thus, any 2D optical spectrum has undoubtedly high information content and uniquely provides underlying dynamics and mechanisms of chemical or physical processes considered.

By using femtosecond IR pulses and dispersive pump–probe spectroscopic technique, 2D IR spectroscopic measurements of proteins in solution were performed in 1998.[4] Also, interesting combinations of IR and visible beams together to carry out IR-vis four-wave-mixing experiments were theoretically suggested in the late 1990s and shown to be useful in studying electric and mechanical anharmonicity-induced couplings between two different vibrational modes in 1999 experimentally.[6, 8, 11, 29, 30] This is analogous to the heteronuclear NMR spectroscopy, since both vibrational (bosonic) and electronic (fermionic) degrees of freedom and their couplings were under investigation. Also, electronic photon echo signals from a dye molecule or a photosynthetic light-harvesting protein complex were experimentally measured by using a Fourier transform (FT) spectral interferometry employing the Mach–Zehnder interferometer.[7, 9] In the latter case, it was found that ultrafast excitation relaxations within the manifold of one-exciton states and coherence evolution in electronically coupled multi-chromophore systems could be studied by examining the time-dependent changes of the 2D photon echo spectrum and by measuring the cross-peak amplitude changes in time T.[22] A conditional probability of finding the system on a specific quantum state ψ_k at a later time when it was initially on a different state ψ_j was found to be the key factor determining the time-dependency of the associated cross-peak amplitude at $(\omega_t = \omega_k, \omega_\tau = \omega_j)$.[19] In addition, we have seen 2D IR spectroscopic studies of chemical exchange dynamics and hydrogen-bond network in water.[31–37] These works clearly demonstrated how such novel spectroscopic methods can be of use in studying fundamental solute-solvent interaction dynamics in real time with an unprecedented time resolution that cannot be reached by any other spectroscopic means. Technically, a femtosecond collinear phase-coherent 2D spectroscopy and a single-shot 2D pump–probe spectroscopy were experimentally demonstrated, which will speed up data collection times and extend applications of the technique to a wide variety of problems.[38–40] In parallel with these experimental efforts, numerous theoretical and computational methods combining molecular dynamics (MD) simulation, quantum chemistry calculation, quantum mechanical/molecular mechanical (QM/MM) simulation, and hybrid QM/MD simulation have been developed to accurately simulate the 2D vibrational and electronic spectra of complicated molecular systems such as proteins, nucleic acids, and light-harvesting complexes over the last decade.[10]

Before we close this chapter, it would be interesting to provide a viewpoint on how and why the 2D optical spectroscopy is a better tool for studying molecular structure and dynamics, in comparison with the other linear or quasi-linear spectroscopy. Note that the time-resolved spectroscopy capable of recording 1D spectra with respect to time is considered to be quasi-linear spectroscopy because quantitative information on couplings still cannot be directly provided. The discussion on this begins with comparing the hierarchy of protein structures with that of spectroscopic properties. Linear spectroscopy such as IR absorption and Raman scattering can provide critical information on the distribution of vibrational modes in a given polyatomic molecule. There are a variety of marker bands in an IR absorption spectrum of polyatomic molecule. Analysis of IR absorption spectrum of an unknown molecule can thus provide information on the constituent chemical groups and bonds included in the molecule. However, if these vibrational chromophores interact or couple to produce delocalized vibrational states, the linear absorption spectrum provides limited information on such coupling strengths that are however keenly dependent on the 3D structure such as inter-chromophore distances and orientations. Thus, the 2D vibrational spectroscopy capable of measuring such small quantities can be an incisive tool to shed light on the detailed structure and its structural change in time.

In Figure 1.2, there is an interesting analogy between various levels of spectroscopic properties and hierarchical protein structures.[10, 18, 20] The primary structure of protein is nothing but a sequence of amino acids encoded in the corresponding gene. The relevant energy associated with the primary protein structure formation is the covalent bond energy, that is, peptide bond, of which magnitude is about 100 kJ/mol. The secondary protein structures such as α-helix, β-sheet, β-hairpin, and so forth are mainly determined by the relatively weak hydrogen bonds with energy of about 10 kJ/mol. The protein tertiary (domain) structure formation involves a

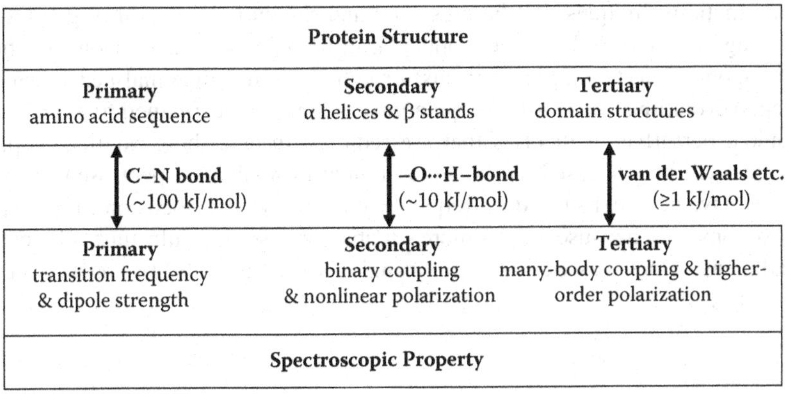

FIGURE 1.2 Analogy between hierarchies of spectroscopic properties and protein structures.

variety of interactions such as electrostatic, hydrophobic, van der Waals, disulfide bond interactions and the like. Thus, the protein structure hierarchy can be viewed as a descending order of interaction energy. Similarly, one can develop the same hierarchical concept for spectroscopically measurable properties. The primary spectroscopic properties are fundamental transition frequencies and transition dipole strengths that are principal quantities extracted from an analysis of 1D spectrum, and such primary spectroscopic properties are largely determined by the nature of covalent bonds involved in a given vibrational (or electronic) chromophore, (e.g., C=O stretch, C-H stretch and bend). Most of the 1D spectroscopic means are consequently very useful in delineating the distribution of individual chromophore in the target molecule, and thus they can be considered to be a *one-body* spectroscopy identifying each single chromophore. On the other hand, the coupling between two different chromophores (electronic or vibrational oscillators) within a molecule is associated with comparatively weak inter-chromophore interactions such as hydrogen bond. Consequently, the secondary spectroscopic properties (e.g., vibrational or electronic couplings, nonlinear optical strengths, anharmonic couplings) require nonzero two-body interactions between different chromophores and thus are very sensitive to the detailed configuration, that is, 3D structure, of the constituent chromophores in the molecule. As has been shown over the last decade, the coherent 2D optical spectroscopy based on a variety of nonlinear optical spectroscopic techniques is superior to the 1D method in extracting such quantitatively small secondary spectroscopic properties of complicated molecules like proteins and molecular aggregates via measuring the two-body interaction terms. Thus, the 2D spectroscopy can be considered as *two-body* spectroscopy. Extending this analogy further, one can envisage the 3D (*three-body*) spectroscopy, which is likely to be of use in measuring the tertiary spectroscopic properties such as three-body (three-chromophore) couplings and higher-order nonlinear optical strengths, as a technique that enables determination of higher-order hierarchical molecular structure.

In this book, we will provide detailed discussions on the underlying physics and interpretation methods of a variety of 2D optical spectroscopic methods. Novel diagrammatic techniques will be presented and shown to be useful in graphically describing the associated nonlinear optical transition pathways and involved population (diagonal density matrix elements) or coherence (off-diagonal density matrix elements) evolutions. The basics of quantum dynamics are explained first, and time-dependent perturbation theories that are required in describing nonlinear optical processes will be discussed. Although a number of nonlinear spectroscopic investigations have been performed in frequency domain, we will focus on time-domain spectroscopy only because it is far more suitable for describing ultrafast coherent 2D optical measurements as well as directly analogous to the 2D NMR spectroscopy in many ways.

REFERENCES

1. Ernst, R. R.; Bodenhausen, G.; Wokaun, A., *Nuclear magnetic resonance in one and two dimensions*. Oxford University Press: Oxford, 1987.
2. Wüthrich, K., *NMR of proteins and nucleic acids*. John Wiley & Sons: New York, 1986.
3. Warren, W. S.; Zewail, A. H., Optical analogs of NMR phase coherent multiple pulse spectroscopy. *Journal of Chemical Physics* 1981, 75, 5956–5958.
4. Hamm, P.; Lim, M. H.; Hochstrasser, R. M., Structure of the amide I band of peptides measured by femtosecond nonlinear infrared spectroscopy. *Journal of Physical Chemistry B* 1998, 102, 6123–6138.
5. Tanimura, Y.; Mukamel, S., Two-dimensional femtosecond vibrational spectroscopy of liquids. *Journal of Chemical Physics* 1993, 99, 9496–9511.
6. Park, K.; Cho, M., Time- and frequency-resolved coherent two-dimensional IR spectroscopy: Its complementary relationship with the coherent two-dimensional Raman scattering spectroscopy. *Journal of Chemical Physics* 1998, 109, 10559–10569.
7. Hybl, J. D.; Albrecht, A. W.; Gallagher Faeder, S. M.; et al., Two-dimensional electronic spectroscopy. *Chem. Phys. Lett.* 1998, 297, 307–313.
8. Zhao, W.; Wright, J. C., Measurement of $\chi^{(3)}$ for doubly vibrationally enhanced four wave mixing spectroscopy. *Physical Review Letters* 1999, 83, 1950–1953.
9. Brixner, T.; Stenger, J.; Vaswani, H. M.; et al., Two-dimensional spectroscopy of electronic couplings in photosynthesis. *Nature* 2005, 434, 625–628.
10. Cho, M., Coherent two-dimensional optical spectroscopy. *Chemical Reviews* 2008, 108, 1331–1418.
11. Cho, M., Two-dimensional vibrational spectroscopy. In *Advances in multi-photon processes and spectroscopy*, Lin, S. H., Villaeys, A. A., Fujimura, Y., (Eds.) World Scientific Publishing Co.: Singapore, 1999; Vol. 12, pp 229–300.
12. Mukamel, S., Multidimensional femtosecond correlation spectroscopies of electronic and vibrational excitations. *Annual Review of Physical Chemistry* 2000, 51, 691–729.
13. Khalil, M.; Demirdoven, N.; Tokmakoff, A., Coherent 2D IR spectroscopy: Molecular structure and dynamics in solution. *Journal of Physical Chemistry A* 2003, 107, 5258–5279.
14. Woutersen, S.; Hamm, P., Nonlinear two-dimensional vibrational spectroscopy of peptides. *Journal of Physics-Condensed Matter* 2002, 14, R1035–R1062.
15. Jonas, D. M., Two-dimensional femtosecond spectroscopy. *Annual Review of Physical Chemistry* 2003, 54, 425–463.

16. Cho, M., Ultrafast vibrational spectroscopy in condensed phases. *PhysChemComm* 2002, 40–58.
17. Ge, N. H.; Hochstrasser, R. M., Femtosecond two-dimensional infrared spectroscopy: IR-COSY and THIRSTY. *PhysChemComm* 2002, 17–26.
18. Cho, M., Coherent two-dimensional optical spectroscopy. *Bull. Kor. Chem. Soc* 2006, 27, 1940–1960.
19. Cho, M.; Brixner, T.; Stiopkin, I.; et al., Two-dimensional electronic spectroscopy of molecular complexes. *Journal of the Chinese Chemical Society* 2006, 53, (1), 15–24.
20. Cho, M., Spectroscopy: Molecular motion pictures. *Nature* 2006, 444, 431.
21. Kolano, C.; Helbing, J.; Kozinski, M.; et al., Watching hydrogen-bond dynamics in a β-turn by transient two-dimensional infrared spectroscopy. *Nature* 2006, 444, 469–472.
22. Cho, M.; Vaswani, H. M.; Brixner, T.; et al., Exciton analysis in 2D electronic spectroscopy. *Journal of Physical Chemistry B* 2005, 109, 10542–10556.
23. Engel, G. S.; Calhoun, T. R.; Read, E. L.; et al., Evidence for wavelike energy transfer through quantum coherence in photosynthetic systems. *Nature* 2007, 446, 782–786.
24. Fleming, G. R.; Cho, M., Chromophore-solvent dynamics. *Annual Review of Physical Chemistry* 1996, 47, 109–134.
25. De Boeij, W. P.; Pshenichnikov, M. S.; Wiersma, D. A., Ultrafast solvation dynamics explored by femtosecond photon echo spectroscopies. *Annual Review of Physical Chemistry* 1998, 49, 99–123.
26. Zimdars, D.; Tokmakoff, A.; Chen, S.; et al., Picosecond infrared vibrational echoes in a liquid and glass using a free electron laser. *Physical Review Letters* 1993, 70, 2718–2721.
27. Tokmakoff, A., Two-dimensional line shapes derived from coherent third-order nonlinear spectroscopy. *Journal of Physical Chemistry A.* 2000, 104, 4247–4255.
28. Kwac, K.; Cho, M., Two-color pump–probe spectroscopies of two- and three-level systems: 2-dimensional line shapes and solvation dynamics. *Journal of Physical Chemistry A* 2003, 107, 5903–5912.
29. Park, K.; Cho, M. H.; Hahn, S.; et al., Two-dimensional vibrational spectroscopy. II. Ab initio calculation of the coherent 2D infrared response function of $CHCl_3$ and comparison with the 2D Raman response function. *Journal of Chemical Physics* 1999, 111, 4131–4139.
30. Zhao, W.; Wright, J. C., Spectral simplification in vibrational spectroscopy using doubly vibrationally enhanced infrared four wave mixing. *Journal of the American Chemical Society* 1999, 121, 10994–10998.
31. Woutersen, S.; Mu, Y.; Stock, G.; et al., Hydrogen-bond lifetime measured by time-resolved 2D–IR spectroscopy: N-methylacetamide in methanol. *Chemical Physics* 2001, 266, 137–147.
32. Kwac, K.; Lee, H.; Cho, M., Non-Gaussian statistics of amide I mode frequency fluctuation of N-methylacetamide in methanol solution: Linear and nonlinear vibrational spectra. *Journal of Chemical Physical* 2004, 120, 1477.
33. Kim, Y. S.; Hochstrasser, R. M., Chemical exchange 2D IR of hydrogen-bond making and breaking. *Proceeding of the National Academy of Sciences of the United States of America* 2005, 102, 11185–11190.
34. Zheng, J.; Kwak, K.; Asbury, J. B.; et al., Ultrafast dynamics of solute-solvent complexation observed at thermal equilibrium in real time. *Science* 2005, 309, 1338–1343.
35. Cowan, M. L.; Bruner, B. D.; Huse, N.; et al., Ultrafast memory loss and energy redistribution in the hydrogen bond network of liquid H_2O. *Nature* 2005, 434, 199–202.

36. Asbury, J. B.; Steinel, T.; Stromberg, C.; et al., Water dynamics: Vibrational echo correlation spectroscopy and comparison to molecular dynamics simulations. *Journal of Physical Chemistry A* 2004, 108, 1107–1119.
37. Eaves, J. D.; Loparo, J. J.; Fecko, C. J.; et al., Hydrogen bonds in liquid water are broken only fleetingly. *Proceeding of the National Academy of Sciences of the United States of America* 2005, 102, 13019–13022.
38. Tian, P.; Keusters, D.; Suzaki, Y.; et al., Femtosecond phase–coherent two-dimensional spectroscopy. *Science* 2003, 300, 1553–1555.
39. DeCamp, M. F.; DeFlores, L. P.; Jones, K. C.; et al., Single-shot two-dimensional infrared spectroscopy. *Optics Express* 2007, 15, 233–241.
40. DeCamp, M. F.; Tokmakoff, A., Single-shot two-dimensional spectrometer. *Optics Letters* 2006, 31, 113–115.

2 Quantum Dynamics

A principal goal of spectroscopic investigation is to study electronic or magnetic properties of materials by measuring radiation–matter interaction-induced changes of radiation states in frequency and/or time domains.[1–4] Since the electromagnetic field amplitude oscillates and the temporal envelope of laser pulse used changes in time,[5] the radiation–matter interaction Hamiltonian is intrinsically time-dependent, and the time evolutions of the matter states might be fully determined by the time-dependent Schrödinger equation,

$$\frac{\partial}{\partial t} | \psi(t) > = -\frac{i}{\hbar} \hat{H}(t) | \psi(t) > \tag{2.1}$$

Here, $| \psi(t) >$ is the Dirac *ket* state. The corresponding *bra* state is denoted as $< \psi(t) |$. The time-dependent Schrödinger equation (2.1) is one of the most fundamental and important postulates in quantum mechanics.[6–8] In this chapter, we introduce the concept of linear vector (wavefunction) and matrix (density operator) spaces to describe the quantum dynamics of matters interacting with external radiations.

2.1 TIME EVOLUTION IN HILBERT SPACE

Hilbert space is a linear vector space of functions. In quantum mechanics, a vector in the Hilbert space is wavefunction $\psi(t)$ and the complete and orthonormal basis set used to define the quantum mechanical Hilbert space consists of eigenvectors of the time-independent Schrödinger equation, that is,

$$\hat{H} | \phi_n > = E_n | \phi_n > . \tag{2.2}$$

From the orthonormalization condition of unit vectors in the Hilbert space, we have

$$< \phi_n | \phi_m > = \delta_{nm} . \tag{2.3}$$

From the completeness condition, the identity operator is defined as

$$\sum_m | \phi_m >< \phi_m | = 1. \tag{2.4}$$

With the Dirac's bra-ket notation, the inner product of any given pair of vectors (wavefunctions) is defined as

$$< \psi_j(t) | \psi_k(t) > \equiv \int_V \psi_j^*(\mathbf{r},t) \psi_k(\mathbf{r},t) d\mathbf{r}, \tag{2.5}$$

where V is the quantization volume.

Any vector, wavefunction in this Hilbert space can therefore be expanded as

$$|\psi(t)> = \sum_n c_n(t)|\phi_n> \tag{2.6}$$

where the expansion coefficient is the projection of the vector onto each unit vector,

$$c_n(t) \equiv <\phi_n|\psi(t)>. \tag{2.7}$$

EXERCISE 2.1

Consider a two-level system. Assume that the system at time t_0 is a superposition state of the two eigenvectors, that is, $|\psi(t_0)> = \frac{1}{\sqrt{2}}(|\phi_1> + |\phi_2>)$, and that the Hamiltonian is given as $\hat{H} = \Delta(|\phi_1><\phi_2| + |\phi_2><\phi_1|)$. Calculate the ket function $|\psi(t)>$ at time t.

In the case when the Hamiltonian is time-independent, the formal solution of the time-dependent Schrödinger equation is given as

$$|\psi(t)> = \exp\left(-\frac{i}{\hbar}\hat{H}(t-t_0)\right)|\psi(t_0)> = u(t,t_0)|\psi(t_0)> \tag{2.8}$$

where $u(t,t_0)$ represents the forward time evolution operator when $t > t_0$:

$$u(t,t_0) \equiv \exp\left(-\frac{i}{\hbar}\hat{H}(t-t_0)\right). \tag{2.9}$$

The backward time evolution operator is then defined as

$$u^\dagger(t,t_0) \equiv \exp\left(\frac{i}{\hbar}\hat{H}(t-t_0)\right). \tag{2.10}$$

It is noted that the Hamiltonian operator is Hermitian. The time evolution operator $u(t,t_0)$ ($u^\dagger(t,t_0)$) describes the forward (backward) time evolution of the ket (bra) vector, whereas the same operator does backward (forward) time evolution of the bra (ket) vector. The Hilbert space for a ket vector is nothing but a mirror image of that for a bra vector. The two spaces are related to each other via Hermitian conjugate relationship. Note that the quantum mechanical Hilbert space is a complex space where a vector can have both real and imaginary parts. If one needs to calculate any real observable at time t, one should consider the ket and bra vectors at t simultaneously. However, since the time evolution of the ket vector is just a mirror image of (Hermitian conjugate relationship to) that of the corresponding bra vector, it is enough to consider one of the two time-evolved vectors in a given Hilbert space.

EXERCISE 2.2

Prove that $u(t,t_0)u^\dagger(t,t_0) = u^\dagger(t,t_0)u(t,t_0) = 1$. (Hint: use $\exp(x) = 1 + \Sigma_n (1/n!)x^n$ and the Baker-Haudorf lemma, $e^{\hat{A}}e^{\hat{B}} = e^{\hat{A}+\hat{B}}e^{(1/2)[\hat{A},\hat{B}]}$).[9]

In the Schrödinger picture, where the wavefunction is time-dependent whereas an operator $\hat{A}$ corresponding to the observable A is not, the expectation value may be calculated as, on the basis of one of the quantum mechanical postulates,

$$\bar{A}(t) = <\psi(t)|\hat{A}|\psi(t)> = <\psi(t_0)|u^\dagger(t,t_0)\hat{A}u(t,t_0)|\psi(t_0)>. \tag{2.11}$$

The physical meaning of the right-hand side of Equation 2.11 is that when the initial wavefunction is known at time t_0, the ket vector $|\psi(t_0)>$ evolves in the forward direction in time from t_0 to t by the $u(t,t_0)$ operator, and the bra vector $<\psi(t_0)|$ also does from t_0 to t by the $u^\dagger(t,t_0)$ operator. Then, the expectation value of $\hat{A}$ over the wavefunction at time t provides the value of $\bar{A}(t)$.

Defining the time-dependent operator $\hat{A}(t)$ as

$$\hat{A}_H(t) = u^\dagger(t,t_0)\hat{A}u(t,t_0) = \exp\left(\frac{i}{\hbar}\hat{H}(t-t_0)\right)\hat{A}\exp\left(-\frac{i}{\hbar}\hat{H}(t-t_0)\right), \tag{2.12}$$

the expectation value of $\hat{A}$ at time t can be rewritten as

$$\bar{A}(t) = <\psi(t_0)|\hat{A}_H(t)|\psi(t_0)>. \tag{2.13}$$

This route to the calculation of any expectation value has been known to be the Heisenberg picture.

EXERCISE 2.3

Show that the time-dependent operator defined in Equation 2.12 obeys the Heisenberg equation, i.e., $\frac{\partial}{\partial t}\hat{A}_H(t) = \frac{i}{\hbar}[\hat{H},\hat{A}_H(t)]$. Here, it is assumed that the operator $\hat{A}$ does not depend on time explicitly.

In spectroscopy, the radiation–matter interaction Hamiltonian is time-dependent so that the time evolution of the wavefunction needs to be described differently from the case of time-independent Hamiltonian. The total Hamiltonian of the composite system consisting of matter and radiation may be written as

$$\hat{H}(t) = \hat{H}_{mat} + \hat{H}_{rad} + \hat{H}_{rad-mat}(t). \tag{2.14}$$

From the time-dependent Schrödinger equation (2.1), let us assume that the formal solution of the wavefunction of the ket vector is given as

$$|\psi(t)> = U(t,t_0)|\psi(t_0)>. \tag{2.15}$$

To determine the time evolution operator, $U(t,t_0)$, in Equation 2.15, one can substitute Equation 2.15 into 2.1 and find that

$$\frac{\partial}{\partial t}U(t,t_0) = -\frac{i}{\hbar}\hat{H}(t)\,U(t,t_0). \tag{2.16}$$

Carrying out the integration of Equation 2.16 with respect to t, we have

$$\underline{U(t,t_0)} = 1 - \frac{i}{\hbar}\int_{t_0}^{t} d\tau \hat{H}(\tau)\underline{U(\tau,t_0)}. \tag{2.17}$$

By repeatedly inserting the right-hand side of Equation 2.17 into the $U(\tau,t_0)$ term in the integrand, one can formally derive the following series solution for the time evolution operator, $U(t,t_0)$, when the Hamiltonian is explicitly time-dependent, as

$$U(t,t_0) = 1 + \sum_{n=1}^{\infty}\left(-\frac{i}{\hbar}\right)^n \int_{t_0}^{t} d\tau_n \int_{t_0}^{\tau_n} d\tau_{n-1} \cdots \int_{t_0}^{\tau_2} d\tau_1\, \hat{H}(\tau_n)\hat{H}(\tau_{n-1}) \cdots \hat{H}(\tau_1). \tag{2.18}$$

Note that the above series expansion is not identical to the Taylor expansion of the exponential function and that the integration time variables have the following order, $\tau_n \geq \tau_{n-1} \geq \cdots \geq \tau_1$. For the sake of notational simplicity of the forward time evolution operator $U(t,t_0)$, the positive time-ordering exponential operator is defined as

$$U(t,t_0) = \exp_+\left(-\frac{i}{\hbar}\int_{t_0}^{t} d\tau\, \hat{H}(\tau)\right). \tag{2.19}$$

EXERCISE 2.4

Show that the forward time evolution operator $U(t,t_0)$ defined in Equation 2.19 with 2.18 becomes $u(t,t_0)$ when the Hamiltonian is time-independent.

Then, the backward time evolution operator, which is the Hermitian conjugate of $U(t,t_0)$, is found to be

$$U^{\dagger}(t,t_0) = \exp_-\left(\frac{i}{\hbar}\int_{t_0}^{t} d\tau\, \hat{H}(\tau)\right)$$

$$= 1 + \sum_{n=1}^{\infty}\left(\frac{i}{\hbar}\right)^n \int_{t_0}^{t} d\tau_n \int_{t_0}^{\tau_n} d\tau_{n-1} \cdots \int_{t_0}^{\tau_2} d\tau_1\, \hat{H}(\tau_1)\hat{H}(\tau_2) \cdots \hat{H}(\tau_n). \tag{2.20}$$

EXERCISE 2.5

Show that $U(t,t_0)U^{\dagger}(t,t_0) = U^{\dagger}(t,t_0)U(t,t_0) = 1$.

2.2 TIME-DEPENDENT PERTURBATION THEORY IN HILBERT SPACE

Although the time evolution operators in Equations 2.18 and 2.20 are exact for describing the quantum dynamics of composite system consisting of materials, bath, and radiation, the corresponding time-dependent Schrödinger equation cannot be directly solved to calculate any expectation values, quantum transition amplitudes and probabilities, and matter's electronic and magnetic properties. That is not only because the series summation requires an infinite number of terms but also because the eigenvalue equation such as $\hat{H}(\tau_1)|\psi> = E|\psi>$ cannot be easily solved for the Hamiltonian describing optical chromophores interacting with both surrounding bath degrees of freedom and external radiations. Therefore, it is inevitable to develop a proper time-dependent perturbation theory, and the total Hamiltonian is divided into two parts as

$$\hat{H}(t) = \hat{H}_0(t) + \hat{H}'(t), \tag{2.21}$$

where the zero-order Hamiltonian $\hat{H}_0(t)$ serves as the reference and the second term $\hat{H}'(t)$ is treated as perturbation Hamiltonian. In spectroscopy, the system, bath, and radiation Hamiltonians constitute the zero-order Hamiltonian, and the field-matter interaction is considered to be the perturbation Hamiltonian. The perturbation theory can thus provide quantitatively reliable information when $\hat{H}'(t)$ is properly chosen so that the perturbation series successfully converges.

It turns out that the interaction picture instead of the Schrödinger or Heisenberg picture discussed above is quite useful for a development of time-dependent perturbation theory. In the interaction picture, the time evolutions of the wavefunction is fully described by the zero-order Hamiltonian $\hat{H}_0(t)$, not by the total Hamiltonian $\hat{H}(t)$. In addition, the perturbation Hamiltonian $\hat{H}'(t)$ also evolves in time in the Heisenberg picture determined by $\hat{H}_0(t)$. Thus, the interaction picture can be viewed as a hybrid of both Schrödinger and Heisenberg pictures. We assume that the forward time evolution operator $U(t,t_0)$ can be written as a product of two operators as

$$U(t,t_0) = U_0(t,t_0)U_I(t,t_0), \tag{2.22}$$

where

$$U_0(t,t_0) = \exp_+\left(-\frac{i}{\hbar}\int_{t_0}^{t} d\tau\,\hat{H}_0(\tau)\right) \tag{2.23}$$

$$U_I(t,t_0) = \exp_+\left(-\frac{i}{\hbar}\int_{t_0}^{t} d\tau\,\hat{H}'_I(\tau)\right). \tag{2.24}$$

Here, the time-dependent perturbation Hamiltonian operator in the Heisenberg picture described by the zero-order Hamiltonian, $\hat{H}_0(t)$, is defined as

$$\hat{H}'_I(t) = U_0^\dagger(t,t_0)\hat{H}'(t)U_0(t,t_0). \tag{2.25}$$

In this interaction picture, the expectation value of the time-dependent operator $\hat{A}(t)$ is given as

$$\begin{aligned}\bar{A}(t) &= <\psi(t_0)|U_I^\dagger(t,t_0)U_0^\dagger(t,t_0)\hat{A}(t)U_0(t,t_0)U_I(t,t_0)|\psi(t_0)> \\ &= <\psi_I(t)|\hat{A}_I(t)|\psi_I(t)>,\end{aligned} \tag{2.26}$$

where

$$\hat{A}_I(t) \equiv U_0^\dagger(t,t_0)\hat{A}(t)U_0(t,t_0). \tag{2.27}$$

$$|\psi_I(t)> \equiv U_I(t,t_0)|\psi(t_0)>. \tag{2.28}$$

Note that, in the interaction picture, both the wavefunction and operator evolve in time.

EXERCISE 2.6
Show that $|\psi(t)> = U_0(t,t_0)U_I(t,t_0)|\psi(t_0)>$ indeed obeys the time-dependent Schrödinger equation.

In order to develop a time-dependent perturbation theory, one can expand $U_I(t,t_0)$ given in Equation 2.24 as a power series of the time-evolved perturbation Hamiltonian $\hat{H}_I'(\tau)$ and find that the forward time evolution operator can be expanded as

$$\begin{aligned} U(t,t_0) &= U_0(t,t_0) + \left(-\frac{i}{\hbar}\right)\int_{t_0}^{t} d\tau_1 U_0(t,\tau_1)\hat{H}'(\tau_1)U_0(\tau_1,t_0) \\ &+ \left(-\frac{i}{\hbar}\right)^2 \int_{t_0}^{t} d\tau_2 \int_{t_0}^{\tau_2} d\tau_1 U_0(t,\tau_2)\hat{H}'(\tau_2)U_0(\tau_2,\tau_1)\hat{H}'(\tau_1)U_0(\tau_1,t_0) + \cdots \\ &= \sum_{n=0}^{\infty} U_n(t,t_0), \end{aligned} \tag{2.29}$$

where the nth-order perturbation term, $U_n(t,t_0)$, is defined as

$$\begin{aligned} U_n(t,t_0) \equiv \left(-\frac{i}{\hbar}\right)^n \int_{t_0}^{t} d\tau_n \int_{t_0}^{\tau_n} d\tau_{n-1} \cdots \int_{t_0}^{\tau_2} d\tau_1 U_0(t,\tau_n)\hat{H}'(\tau_n)U_0(\tau_n,\tau_{n-1}) \times \cdots \\ \times U_0(\tau_2,\tau_1)\hat{H}'(\tau_1)U_0(\tau_1,t_0). \end{aligned} \tag{2.30}$$

Similarly, the backward time evolution operator in the interaction picture can be written as

$$U^\dagger(t,t_0) = U_I^\dagger(t,t_0)U_0^\dagger(t,t_0) = \sum_{n=0}^{\infty} U_n^\dagger(t,t_0) \tag{2.31}$$

where

$$\begin{aligned} U_n^\dagger(t,t_0) \equiv \left(\frac{i}{\hbar}\right)^n \int_{t_0}^{t} d\tau_n \int_{t_0}^{\tau_n} d\tau_{n-1} \cdots \int_{t_0}^{\tau_2} d\tau_1 U_0^\dagger(\tau_1,t_0)\hat{H}'(\tau_1)U_0^\dagger(\tau_2,\tau_1) \times \cdots \\ \times U_0^\dagger(\tau_n,\tau_{n-1})\hat{H}'(\tau_n)U_0^\dagger(t,\tau_n). \end{aligned} \tag{2.32}$$

EXERCISE 2.7

To obtain Equations 2.30 and 2.32, the following operator equalities, $U_0(t,t_0)U_0^\dagger(\tau,t_0)=U_0(t,\tau)$ and $U_0(\tau,t_0)U_0^\dagger(t,t_0)=U_0^\dagger(t,\tau)$, were used. Prove these two equalities.

2.3 DIAGRAM REPRESENTATION OF THE TIME-DEPENDENT PERTURBATION THEORY IN HILBERT SPACE

Formal expressions and results on the time evolution operators and expectation values in terms of perturbation series were presented and discussed above, but it has always been found to be useful to represent each term in terms of graphical diagrams. In this regard, the Feynman diagram representation of the perturbation theory has been considered to be one of the simplest pictures and allows one to understand the time evolution of the system when a certain number of perturbation actions to the zero-order wavefunction occur in time. Here, we will introduce a modified Feynman diagram technique for the perturbation theory. The complete time evolution operator $U(t,t_0)$ was given as a series of perturbation terms as

$$U(t,t_0)=U_0(t,t_0)+U_1(t,t_0)+U_2(t,t_0)+\cdots \tag{2.33}$$

It will be assumed that the diagrams corresponding to each term in Equation 2.33 are defined as

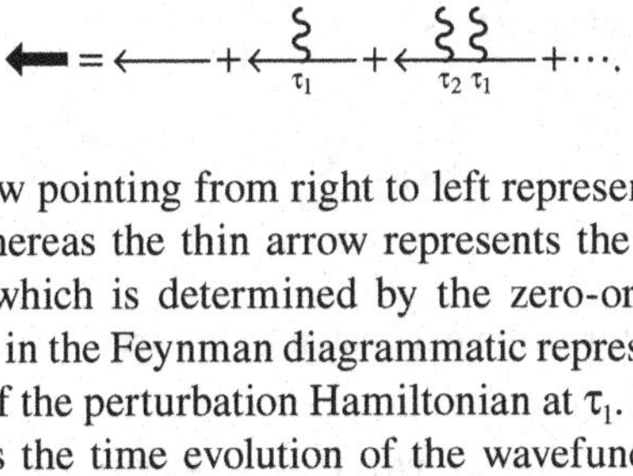

(2.34)

The thick, solid arrow pointing from right to left represents the total time evolution operator $U(t,t_0)$, whereas the thin arrow represents the zero-order time evolution operator, $U_0(\tau,t_0)$, which is determined by the zero-order Hamiltonian $\hat{H}_0(t)$. The wavy line symbol $\wr$ in the Feynman diagrammatic representation of $U_1(t,t_0)$ corresponds to the action of the perturbation Hamiltonian at τ_1. Note that the first-order term, $U_1(t,t_0)$, describes the time evolution of the wavefunction from t_0 to t when there is a single perturbation by $\hat{H}'(\tau_1)$ at time τ_1 ($t\geq\tau_1\geq t_0$). Since the perturbation action occurs at any time from t_0 to t, one should take into consideration all possibilities so that the integration over τ_1 in the range from t_0 to t should be performed. From Equation 2.15, the first time-derivative of $\Leftarrow$ is given as

$$\frac{\partial}{\partial t}\Leftarrow=-\frac{i}{\hbar}\hat{H}(t)\Leftarrow. \tag{2.35}$$

Similarly, the backward time evolution operator given as a series of the perturbation terms is

$$U^\dagger(t,t_0)=U_0^\dagger(t,t_0)+U_1^\dagger(t,t_0)+U_2^\dagger(t,t_0)+\cdots \tag{2.36}$$

and the corresponding diagram representation is

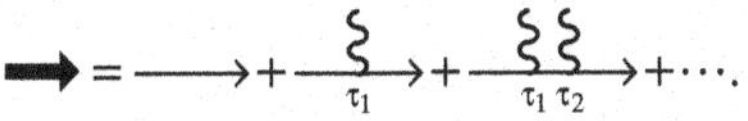

(2.37)

Note that the directions of the arrows are the opposite of those in the forward time evolution operators, indicating that the time runs from left to right. The first derivative of $\boldsymbol{\Rightarrow}$ satisfies the following differential equation:

$$\frac{\partial}{\partial t}\boldsymbol{\Rightarrow} = \boldsymbol{\Rightarrow}\frac{i}{\hbar}\hat{H}(t). \tag{2.38}$$

Using the diagrams introduced above, the time-evolved ket and bra vectors can be diagrammatically represented as

$$|\psi(t)\rangle = \longleftarrow|\psi(t_0)\rangle + \overset{\wr}{\longleftarrow}|\psi(t_0)\rangle + \overset{\wr\wr}{\longleftarrow}|\psi(t_0)\rangle + \cdots \tag{2.39}$$

$$\langle\psi(t)| = \langle\psi(t_0)|\longrightarrow + \langle\psi(t_0)|\overset{\wr}{\longrightarrow} + \langle\psi(t_0)|\overset{\wr\wr}{\longrightarrow} + \cdots. \tag{2.40}$$

Therefore, the expectation value of an operator $\hat{A}(t)$ is, in the diagram representation, simply given as

$$\overline{A}(t) = \langle\psi(t_0)|\boldsymbol{\Rightarrow}\hat{A}(t)\boldsymbol{\Leftarrow}|\psi(t_0)\rangle. \tag{2.41}$$

Then, the series expansion of $\overline{A}(t)$ is

$$\overline{A}(t) = \sum_{n=0}^{\infty}\overline{A}^{(n)}(t), \tag{2.42}$$

where the first three perturbation expansion terms are

$$\overline{A}^{(0)}(t) = \langle\psi(t_0)|\rightarrow\hat{A}\leftarrow|\psi(t_0)\rangle$$

$$\overline{A}^{(1)}(t) = \langle\psi(t_0)|\rightarrow\hat{A}\overset{\wr}{\leftarrow}|\psi(t_0)\rangle + \langle\psi(t_0)|\overset{\wr}{\rightarrow}\hat{A}\leftarrow|\psi(t_0)\rangle$$

$$\overline{A}^{(2)}(t) = \langle\psi(t_0)|\rightarrow\hat{A}\overset{\wr\wr}{\leftarrow}|\psi(t_0)\rangle + \langle\psi(t_0)|\overset{\wr}{\rightarrow}\hat{A}\overset{\wr}{\leftarrow}|\psi(t_0)\rangle + \langle\psi(t_0)|\rightarrow\hat{A}\overset{\wr\wr}{\leftarrow}|\psi(t_0)\rangle. \tag{2.43}$$

Instead of considering the perturbation expansion of the wavefunction, one can equally calculate the same expectation value in the Heisenberg picture as

$$\overline{A}(t) = \langle\psi(t_0)|\hat{A}_H(t)|\psi(t_0)\rangle = \langle\psi(t_0)|\sum_{n=0}^{\infty}\hat{A}_H^{(n)}(t)|\psi(t_0)\rangle \tag{2.44}$$

where, in the diagram representation, the perturbationally expanded time-evolved Heisenberg operators of $\hat{A}(t)$ are

$$\hat{A}_H(t) = \boldsymbol{\longrightarrow}\ \hat{A}(t)\ \boldsymbol{\longleftarrow}$$

$$\hat{A}_H^{(0)}(t) = \longrightarrow \hat{A}(t) \longleftarrow$$

$$\hat{A}_H^{(1)}(t) = \overset{\wr}{\longrightarrow} \hat{A}(t) \longleftarrow + \longrightarrow \hat{A}(t) \overset{\wr}{\longleftarrow}$$

$$\hat{A}_H^{(2)}(t) = \overset{\wr\wr}{\longrightarrow} \hat{A}(t) \longleftarrow + \overset{\wr}{\longrightarrow} \hat{A}(t) \overset{\wr}{\longleftarrow} + \longrightarrow \hat{A}(t) \overset{\wr\wr}{\longleftarrow} \qquad (2.45)$$

EXERCISE 2.8

Show that $\hat{A}_H(t)$ defined in Equation 2.45 is identical to $U^{\dagger}(t,t_0)\hat{A}U(t,t_0)$ and that its time evolution is determined by the Heisenberg equation (see Exercise 2.3).

2.4 TRANSITION AMPLITUDE AND PROBABILITY IN HILBERT SPACE

Most of spectroscopic observables require calculations of the amplitude or probability of the transition from a specific initial state $|m>$ at t_0 to a final state $|n>$ at a later time t, when such a transition is induced by the perturbation Hamiltonian $\hat{H}'(t)$. By definition, the transition amplitude in this case is calculated by

$$TA_{nm}(t) \equiv <n\,|\,U(t,t_0)\,|\,m> = <n\,|\,U_0(t,t_0)U_I(t,t_0)\,|\,m>. \qquad (2.46)$$

We shall assume that the initial and final states are eigenvectors (stationary states) of the zero-order Hamiltonian, i.e., $H_0\,|\,m>= E_m\,|\,m>$ and $H_0\,|\,n> = E_n\,|\,n>$. Then, the first-order perturbation theory provides us the first-order transition amplitude as

$$TA_{nm}^{(1)}(t) \equiv <n\,|\,U_1(t,t_0)|\,m> = \left(-\frac{i}{\hbar}\right)\int_{t_0}^{t} d\tau_1 <n\,|\,U_0(t,\tau_1)\hat{H}'(\tau_1)U_0(\tau_1,t_0)\,|\,m>. \qquad (2.47)$$

This can be re-expressed as, in terms of the corresponding Feynman diagram,

$$TA_{nm}^{(1)}(t) = <n\,|\overset{\wr}{\longleftarrow}|\,m>. \qquad (2.48)$$

However, what is experimentally measured is not the transition amplitude but the corresponding transition probability that is defined as the square of the transition amplitude as

$$TP_{nm}(t) \equiv |TA_{nm}(t)|^2. \qquad (2.49)$$

We find that the second-order transition probability of being in state $|n\rangle$ at time t is

$$TP_{nm}^{(2)}(t) = \langle n | \overleftarrow{\S} | m \rangle\langle m | \overrightarrow{\S} | n \rangle. \tag{2.50}$$

This expression can be written as a double integral as

$$TP_{nm}^{(2)}(t) = \left(\frac{1}{\hbar^2}\right)\int_{t_0}^{t} d\tau_1 \int_{t_0}^{t} d\tau_2 \langle n | U_0(t,\tau_1)\hat{H}'(\tau_1)U_0(\tau_1,t_0) | m \rangle$$

$$\times \langle m | U_0^{\dagger}(\tau_2,t_0)\hat{H}'(\tau_2)U_0^{\dagger}(t,\tau_2) | n \rangle. \tag{2.51}$$

For the sake of simplicity, let us consider the case that the zero-order Hamiltonian does not explicitly depend on time. Then, Equation 2.51 can be simplified as

$$TP_{nm}^{(2)}(t) = \frac{1}{\hbar^2}\left|\int_{t_0}^{t} d\tau e^{i\omega_{nm}\tau} H'_{nm}(\tau)\right|^2 \tag{2.52}$$

where $\omega_m \equiv E_m/\hbar$, $\omega_{nm} \equiv \omega_n - \omega_m$, and

$$H'_{nm}(\tau) \equiv \langle n | \hat{H}'(\tau) | m \rangle. \tag{2.53}$$

If the initial time t_0 is $-\infty$, the transition probability evaluated at $t = \infty$ is

$$TP_{nm}^{(2)}(t=\infty) = \frac{1}{\hbar^2} |\tilde{H}'_{nm}(\omega_{nm})|^2 \tag{2.54}$$

where $\tilde{H}'_{nm}(\omega_{nm})$ is the Fourier transform of $H'_{nm}(t)$ at $\omega = \omega_{nm}$. Throughout this book, the Fourier and inverse Fourier transforms are defined as

$$\tilde{f}(\omega) = \int_{-\infty}^{\infty} dt\, f(t)e^{i\omega t} \tag{2.55}$$

$$f(t) = \frac{1}{2\pi}\int_{-\infty}^{\infty} dt \tilde{f}(\omega)e^{-i\omega t}. \tag{2.56}$$

EXERCISE 2.9

One can derive the well-known Fermi's Golden Rule (FGR) expression for a rate of transition, $w = \frac{2\pi}{\hbar}\rho(E_n)|H'_{nm}|^2$, where the perturbation Hamiltonian is time-independent so that H'_{nm} is a constant. To obtain the FGR expression given above, it was assumed (1) that the final states are closely spaced in energy so that they form a continuum with density of states $\rho(E_n)$, (2) that only the long-time behavior is considered, (3) that H'_{nm} and $\rho(E_n)$ do not strongly depend on n, and (4) that the above second-order expression for $TP_{nm}^{(2)}(t)$ is valid.

In order to obtain the result in Equation 2.54, it was assumed that the initial state at t_0 is a pure state on $|m>$. However, if the initial state is a mixed state such as a canonical ensemble, one should take an ensemble average over the thermal distribution of the initial states. Suppose that the probability of being in state $|m>$ is $P_m(T)$ at temperature T. Then, the transition probability of finding the system being in state $|n>$ is given by a sum over all $|m>$ with distribution $P_m(T)$ as

$$\begin{aligned} TP_n^{(2)}(t) &= \sum_m P_m(T) \times TP_{nm}^{(2)}(t) \\ &= \sum_m < n \,|\overset{\wr}{\longleftarrow} |\, m > P_m(T) < m \,|\overset{\wr}{\longrightarrow} |\, n >. \end{aligned} \tag{2.57}$$

If one introduces an operator $\rho(t_0)$ in a matrix form and if the diagonal matrix elements, which are still operator, are given as $\rho_{mm}(t_0) = |\, m > P_m(T) < m\,|$, the transition probability in Equation 2.57 can be rewritten as

$$\begin{aligned} TP_n^{(2)}(t) &= \sum_m < n \,|\overset{\wr}{\longleftarrow} \rho_{mm}(t_0) \overset{\wr}{\longrightarrow} |\, n > \\ &= < n \,|\overset{\wr}{\longleftarrow} \mathrm{Tr}[\rho(t_0)] \overset{\wr}{\longrightarrow} |\, n >. \end{aligned} \tag{2.58}$$

Now, the second-order time-evolved density operator $\rho^{(2)}(t)$ is graphically represented as

$$\rho^{(2)}(t) = \overset{\wr}{\longleftarrow} \mathrm{Tr}[\rho(t_0)] \overset{\wr}{\longrightarrow} \tag{2.59}$$

so that we have

$$TP_n^{(2)}(t) = \rho_{nn}^{(2)}(t) \equiv < n \,|\, \rho^{(2)}(t) \,|\, n >. \tag{2.60}$$

Using the description of the time evolution of wavefunction in Hilbert space in terms of the time evolution operators, one can calculate the transition amplitude but not probability directly. As shown above from Equations 2.57 to 2.60, the transition probability calculation requires a few more steps of derivations and additional ensemble averaging calculation when the system is initially in a thermal equilibrium state at finite temperature T. However, by directly considering the time evolution operator in a matrix form instead of a vectorial form, one can easily perform such multistep calculations. In addition, an ensemble averaging calculation is straightforward since the initial density operator contains information on the mixed state. Furthermore, for developing a higher-order time-dependent perturbation theory, the density operator representation has been found to be useful for bookkeeping quite a number of nonlinear optical transition pathways contributing to the transition probability or measured signal of interest.

2.5 TIME EVOLUTION IN LIOUVILLE SPACE

In the Hilbert space spanned by the eigenvectors of the time-independent Schrodinger equation, wavefunction is a vector and its time evolution is determined by the time-dependent Schrodinger equation. However, if one has to deal with a statistically mixed state such as systems in a canonical ensemble, transition probability calculation is often easier and conceptually simpler if the dynamics of the system are described in a Liouville (density matrix) space.[2, 10, 11] In addition, time evolutions of quantum coherence and population can be easily described by using the density operator formalism.[12] In the previous section, it was already shown that the second-order perturbation theory for calculating transition probability can be expressed in terms of density operator.

The conventional definition of density operator is

$$\rho(t) = |\psi(t)\rangle\langle\psi(t)|. \tag{2.61}$$

Using the diagrammatic representations of the forward and backward time evolution operators $U(t,t_0)$ and $U^{\dagger}(t,t_0)$, one can re-express Equation 2.61 as

$$\rho(t) = \longleftarrow \; \rho(t_0) \; \longrightarrow \tag{2.62}$$

with $\rho(t_0) = |\psi(t_0)\rangle\langle\psi(t_0)|$. In comparison to the Hilbert space where wavefunction is a linear vector, the corresponding vector in Liouville space is density operator. One can prove that the density operator defined above obeys the following differential equation:

$$\frac{\partial}{\partial t}\rho(t) = -\frac{i}{\hbar}[\hat{H}(t),\rho(t)], \tag{2.63}$$

which is the quantum Liouville equation. Equation 2.63 can be obtained by using Equations 2.35 and 2.38 and taking the first derivative of Equation 2.62, that is,

$$\frac{\partial}{\partial t}\rho(t) = \left(\frac{\partial}{\partial t}\longleftarrow\right)\rho(t_0)\longrightarrow + \longleftarrow\rho(t_0)\left(\frac{\partial}{\partial t}\longrightarrow\right). \tag{2.64}$$

We now search for a simple diagrammatic representation of the time evolution operator in the Liouville space. In the case of the time evolution of a wavefunction in a Hilbert space, a single arrow $\longleftarrow$ was enough, since the time evolution of either ket or bra vector is all we need. On the other hand, since the density operator is a product of ket and bra vectors, one should take into consideration of time evolutions of ket and bra sides altogether. Therefore, we introduce another type of arrow representing the time evolution of the density operator as

$$\rho(t) = \Longleftarrow\!\!=\!\rho(t_0). \tag{2.65}$$

Introducing the Liouville operator, L, defined as

$$L(t)\hat{A}(t) = [\hat{H}(t), \hat{A}(t)], \tag{2.66}$$

the quantum Liouville equation in 2.63 can be rewritten as

$$\frac{\partial}{\partial t}\rho(t) = -\frac{i}{\hbar}L(t)\rho(t). \tag{2.67}$$

Then, one can find that the time evolution operator in the Liouville space is given as

$$V(t,t_0) = \exp_+\left(-\frac{i}{\hbar}\int_{t_0}^{t} d\tau L(\tau)\right), \tag{2.68}$$

which corresponds to $\Leftarrow$, that is,

$$V(t,t_0) = \Longleftarrow. \tag{2.69}$$

The Hermitian conjugate of $V(t,t_0)$ is then

$$V^{\dagger}(t,t_0) = \exp_-\left(\frac{i}{\hbar}\int_{t_0}^{t} d\tau L(\tau)\right) \tag{2.70}$$

so that we have

$$V^{\dagger}(t,t_0) = \Longrightarrow. \tag{2.71}$$

Now, from the definition of the expectation value in Equation 2.41 and using the completeness condition in Equation 2.3, we can rewrite the expectation value as

$$\begin{aligned}
\bar{A}(t) &= \sum_{m,n} < \psi(t_0) | \rightarrow | m > A_{mn}(t) < n | \leftarrow | \psi(t_0) > . \\
&= \sum_{m,n} A_{mn}(t) < n | \leftarrow | \psi(t_0) >< \psi(t_0) | \rightarrow | m > \\
&= \sum_{m,n} A_{mn}(t)\rho_{nm}(t) \\
&= Tr[\hat{A}(t)\rho(t)] \\
&= < \hat{A}(t)\rho(t) > .
\end{aligned} \tag{2.72}$$

Here, the angle bracket $<\hat{O}>$ without bra-ket notation means taking the trace of $\hat{O}$ in matrix representation. Using the diagrammatic technique, the expectation value can be simply represented as

$$\bar{A}(t) = < \hat{A}(t) \Longleftarrow \rho(t_0) > . \tag{2.73}$$

2.6 TIME-DEPENDENT PERTURBATION THEORY IN LIOUVILLE SPACE

When the total Hamiltonian is divided into the zero-order reference Hamiltonian and the perturbation Hamiltonian as Equation 2.21, the Liouville operator can also be written as

$$L(t) = L_0(t) + L'(t). \tag{2.74}$$

Then, in the interaction representation, the time evolution operator in the Liouville space is found to be

$$V(t,t_0) = V_0(t,t_0)V_I(t,t_0) \tag{2.75}$$

where

$$V_0(t,t_0) = \exp_+\left(-\frac{i}{\hbar}\int_{t_0}^{t} d\tau L_0(\tau)\right) \tag{2.76}$$

$$V_I(t,t_0) = \exp_+\left(-\frac{i}{\hbar}\int_{t_0}^{t} d\tau L_I'(\tau)\right). \tag{2.77}$$

Here, the time-dependent operator $L_I'(t)$ in the interaction representation is defined as

$$L_I'(t) = V_0^\dagger(t,t_0)L'(t)V_0(t,t_0). \tag{2.78}$$

Following the same procedure used to derive the time-ordered expansion expression for $U(t,t_0)$ with respect to $H'(t)$, one can expand the Liouville space time-evolution operator $V(t,t_0)$ as

$$\begin{aligned} V(t,t_0) &= V_0(t,t_0) + \left(-\frac{i}{\hbar}\right)\int_{t_0}^{t} d\tau_1\, V_0(t,\tau_1)L'(\tau_1)V_0(\tau_1,t_0) \\ &\quad + \left(-\frac{i}{\hbar}\right)^2 \int_{t_0}^{t} d\tau_2 \int_{t_0}^{\tau_2} d\tau_1 V_0(t,\tau_2)L'(\tau_2)V_0(\tau_2,\tau_1)L'(\tau_1)V_0(\tau_1,t_0) + \cdots \\ &= \sum_{n=0}^{\infty} V_n(t,t_0), \end{aligned} \tag{2.79}$$

where the nth-order perturbation expansion term, $V_n(t,t_0)$, is defined as

$$V_n(t,t_0) \equiv \left(-\frac{i}{\hbar}\right)^n \int_{t_0}^{t} d\tau_n \int_{t_0}^{\tau_n} d\tau_{n-1} \cdots \int_{t_0}^{\tau_2} d\tau_1\, V_0(t,\tau_n)L'(\tau_n)V_0(\tau_n,\tau_{n-1})\times\cdots$$
$$\times V_0(\tau_2,\tau_1)L'(\tau_1)V_0(\tau_1,t_0). \quad (2.80)$$

Similarly, the backward time evolution operator in the interaction picture can be written as

$$V^\dagger(t,t_0) = V_I^\dagger(t,t_0)V_0^\dagger(t,t_0) = \sum_{n=0}^{\infty} V_n^\dagger(t,t_0) \quad (2.81)$$

where

$$V_n^\dagger(t,t_0) \equiv \left(\frac{i}{\hbar}\right)^n \int_{t_0}^{t} d\tau_n \int_{t_0}^{\tau_n} d\tau_{n-1} \cdots \int_{t_0}^{\tau_2} d\tau_1\, V_0^\dagger(\tau_1,t_0)L'(\tau_1)V_0^\dagger(\tau_2,\tau_1)\times\cdots$$
$$\times V_0^\dagger(\tau_n,\tau_{n-1})L'(\tau_n)V_0^\dagger(t,\tau_n). \quad (2.82)$$

The time evolution operators in the Liouville space are directly analogous to those in the Hilbert space, except that the vector in the Liouville space is the density operator instead of wavefunction. Since the time evolution operator, which is a commutator instead of a normal linear operator, describes propagation of both ket and bra vectors in time, the corresponding diagrams in the Liouville space should be different from those in the Hilbert space. The first few terms in the perturbation expansion of $V(t,t_0)$ in Equation 2.79 are now graphically represented as

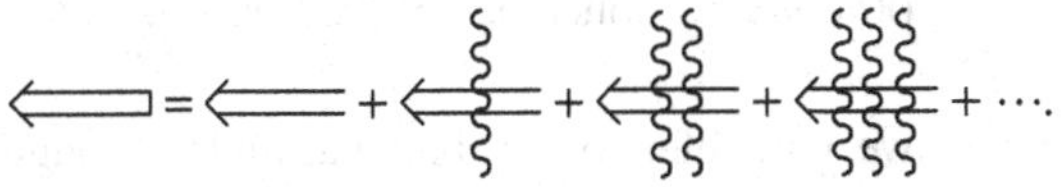
(2.83)

The Hermitian conjugate of $V(t,t_0)$ is then

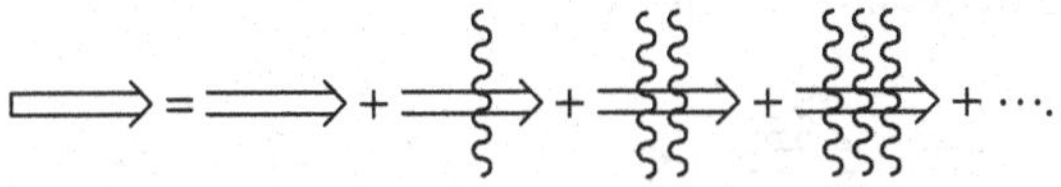
(2.84)

Although the corresponding diagram in the Hilbert space (see Equation 2.34) is identical to a single integral expression, that in the Liouville space is given as a sum of 2^n distinctively different terms for the nth-order perturbation expansion term.

Graphically, the upper (lower) horizontal line in ⇐ therefore describes the time evolution of the ket (bra) state by the time evolution operator ←. In the first-order perturbation theory, $V_1(t,t_0)$ equals to the sum of two terms as

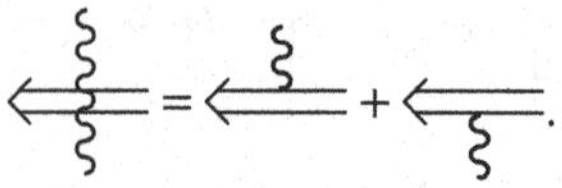

(2.85)

Note that the first term on the right-hand side of Equation 2.85 describes the time evolution of the initial ket vector with a single perturbation in between t_0 and t as well as the time evolution of the initial bra vector without any perturbation. The second term in Equation 2.85 describes the other case. For instance, if the initial density operator is $|m><n|$, one can find the analogy between the two perturbation-expanded time evolution operators in the Liouville and Hilbert spaces,

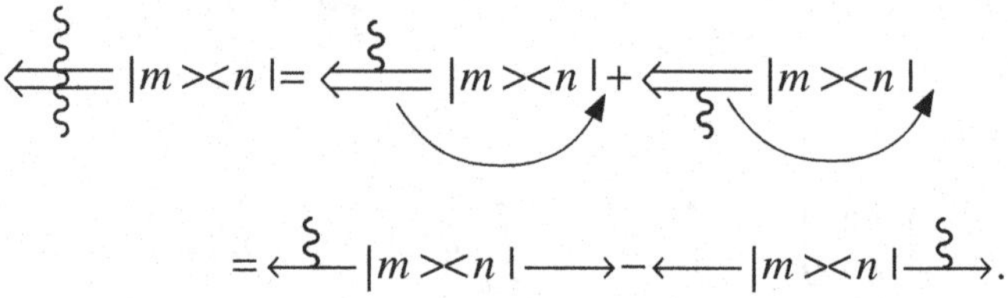

(2.86)

Since the perturbation operator, $L'(t)$, in Liouville space is a commutator, that is, $L'(t)\hat{A} = [\hat{H}'(t), \hat{A}]$, the second term in Equation 2.85 or 2.86 acquires a negative sign because it involves $-\hat{A}\hat{H}'(t)$ term in the expansion form of the commutator, $[\hat{H}'(t), \hat{A}] = \hat{H}'(t)\hat{A} - \hat{A}\hat{H}'(t)$. Here, we now introduce the definitions of population and coherence in Liouville space. The population corresponds to one of the diagonal matrix elements of the total density operator, whereas the coherence corresponds to an off-diagonal matrix element, that is,

$$\rho_{mm}(t) \equiv < m \,|\, \rho(t) \,|\, m >: \quad \text{population of the state } | m > \tag{2.87}$$

$$\rho_{nm}(t) \equiv < n \,|\, \rho(t) \,|\, m >: \quad \text{coherence of the states } | n > \text{and } | m >. \tag{2.88}$$

Throughout this book, we will refer to the diagonal and off-diagonal elements of density matrix as the population and coherence, respectively.

Now, the second-order perturbation expansion term, $V_2(t,t_0)$, in Equation 2.83 is given as a sum of four contributions as

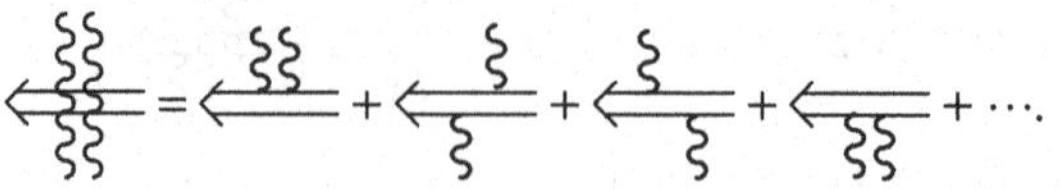

(2.89)

Here, it is noted that the four terms in this equation involve two perturbations, and they are time ordered as $t \geq \tau_2 \geq \tau_1 \geq t_0$.

EXERCISE 2.10

Prove that the operator 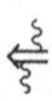 () is complex conjugate of  ().

For the numerical calculations of any arbitrary expectation values within the second-order perturbation theory, the four terms contributing to $V_2(t,t_0)|m\rangle\langle n|$ should be written as double integrals over τ_1 and τ_2,

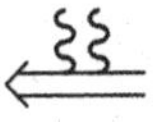 $|m\rangle\langle n|$

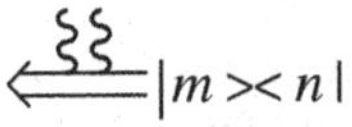

$$=\left(-\frac{i}{\hbar}\right)^2\int_{t_0}^{t}d\tau_2\int_{t_0}^{\tau_2}d\tau_1\,U_0(t,\tau_2)\hat{H}'(\tau_2)U_0(\tau_2,\tau_1)\hat{H}'(\tau_1)U_0(\tau_1,t_0)|m\rangle\langle n|U_0^\dagger(t,t_0)$$

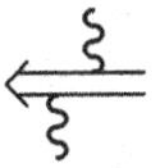 $|m\rangle\langle n|$

$$=-\left(-\frac{i}{\hbar}\right)^2\int_{t_0}^{t}d\tau_2\int_{t_0}^{\tau_2}d\tau_1\,U_0(t,\tau_1)\hat{H}'(\tau_1)U_0(\tau_1,t_0)|m\rangle\langle n|U_0^\dagger(\tau_2,t_0)\hat{H}'(\tau_2)U_0^\dagger(t,\tau_2)$$

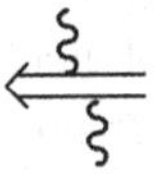 $|m\rangle\langle n|$

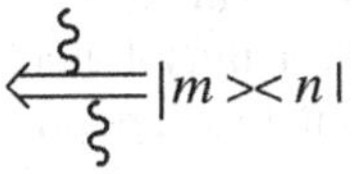

$$=-\left(-\frac{i}{\hbar}\right)^2\int_{t_0}^{t}d\tau_2\int_{t_0}^{\tau_2}d\tau_1\,U_0(t,\tau_2)\hat{H}'(\tau_2)U_0(\tau_2,t_0)|m\rangle\langle n|U_0^\dagger(\tau_1,t_0)\hat{H}'(\tau_1)U_0^\dagger(t,\tau_1)$$

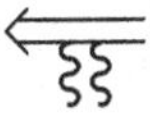 $|m\rangle\langle n|$

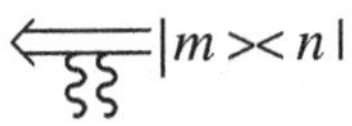

$$=\left(-\frac{i}{\hbar}\right)^2\int_{t_0}^{t}d\tau_2\int_{t_0}^{\tau_2}d\tau_1 U_0(t,t_0)|m\rangle\langle n|U_0^\dagger(\tau_1,t_0)\hat{H}'(\tau_1)U_0^\dagger(\tau_2,\tau_1)\hat{H}'(\tau_2)U_0^\dagger(t,\tau_2).$$

(2.90)

Note that we always have $\tau_2 \ge \tau_1$ and that the second and third terms that involve one wavy line connected to the lower horizontal line in  and  have the negative sign factor in the integral expression because they involve one perturbation operator acting on the bra side. Now, the third-order expansion term, $V_3(t,t_0)$, is given as a sum of eight terms as

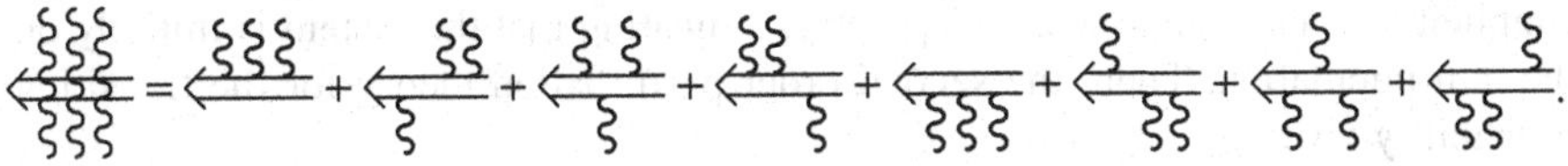

(2.91)

Using the diagrammatic expansion of the Liouville space time evolution operator, one can find that the expectation value of $\hat{A}(t)$ is

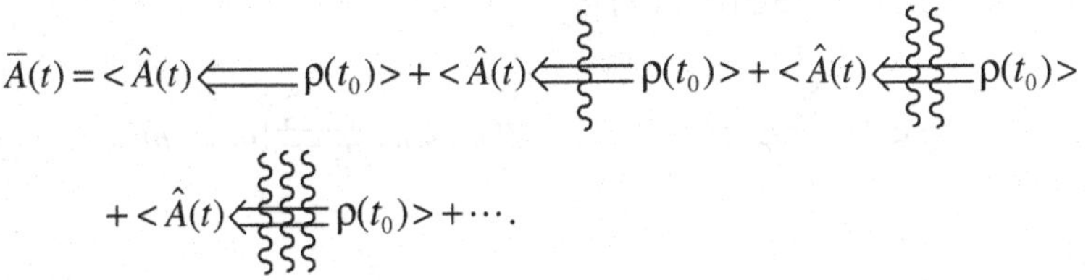

(2.92)

Noting that the perturbation-expanded forms of the time evolution operator are always given as a sum of terms that are complex conjugate to each other, one can easily show that the expectation value of any arbitrary Hermitian operator, $\hat{A}(t)$, is real, as expected.

Later in this book, we will consider the third-order perturbation expression for the expectation value of electric dipole operator, which is responsible for generating third-order signal electric field. The third-order dipole response function that is associated with a variety of four-wave-mixing spectroscopies probing all-electric–dipole-allowed transitions corresponds to the third-order perturbation expansion term of the expectation value of electric dipole operator as

$$P^{(3)}(t) = N < \hat{\mu} \overset{\wr\wr\wr}{\underset{\wr\wr\wr}{\Longleftarrow}} \rho(t_0) >, \tag{2.93}$$

where N is the number density of optical chromophores in the sample. Throughout this book, we will assume that the number density, N, is assumed to be a unity. Later, we will examine the result in Equation 2.93 in more detail for various nonlinear optical spectroscopic techniques.

2.7 TRANSITION PROBABILITY IN LIOUVILLE SPACE AND PATHWAYS

In this section we will consider a few examples on how to use the diagram methods to calculate the second-order transition probabilities.

2.7.1 Second-Order Transition between Two Populations

First of all, let us consider the state-to-state transition probability from one population to the other. Suppose that one is interested in population transfer from an initial population $\rho_{mm}(t_0)$ to a final population $|n><n|$ (for $m \neq n$), where $|m>$ and $|n>$ are ket states of the time-independent Schrödinger equation. For the sake of simplicity, let us assume that $\rho_{kk}(t_0) = \delta_{mk}$, indicating that the system is initially on the mth population. Then, the second-order perturbation theory for the transition probability gives

$$\begin{aligned} TP^{(2)}_{nn,mm}(t) &= Tr[|n><n| V_2(t,t_0) |m><m|] \\ &= <|n><n| \overset{\wr\wr}{\underset{\wr\wr}{\Longleftarrow}} |m><m|> \\ &= <|n><n| \overset{\wr}{\underset{\wr}{\Longleftarrow}} |m><m|> + <|n><n| \overset{\wr}{\underset{\wr}{\Longleftarrow}} |m><m|>. \end{aligned} \tag{2.94}$$

Two other diagrams in the perturbation expansion of $V_2(t,t_0)$ that are

$$<|n><n| \overset{\wr\wr}{\Longleftarrow} |m><m|> \tag{2.95}$$

and

$$<|n><n| \underset{\wr\wr}{\Longleftarrow} |m><m|> \tag{2.96}$$

vanish due to the orthorgonality condition of the eigenvectors, that is,

$$<m| \longrightarrow |n> = 0$$

$$<n| \longleftarrow |m> = 0. \tag{2.97}$$

One can rewrite the two terms on the right-hand side of Equation 2.94 as time-ordered integrals. Since $\overset{\wr}{\underset{\wr}{\Leftarrow}}$ is the complex conjugate of $\overset{\wr}{\underset{\wr}{\Leftarrow}}$, one can rewrite Equation 2.94 as

$$TP^{(2)}_{nn,mm}(t) = 2\,\mathrm{Re}\, <|n><n| \overset{\wr}{\underset{\wr}{\Longleftarrow}} |m><m|>$$

$$= \frac{2}{\hbar^2}\mathrm{Re}\int_{t_0}^{t} d\tau_2 \int_{t_0}^{\tau_2} d\tau_1 <|n><n|U_0(t,\tau_1)\hat{H}'(\tau_1)U_0(\tau_1,t_0)|m><m|U_0^\dagger(\tau_2,t_0)\hat{H}'(\tau_2)$$
$$U_0^\dagger(t,\tau_2)>$$

$$= \frac{2}{\hbar^2}\mathrm{Re}\int_{t_0}^{t} d\tau_2 \int_{t_0}^{\tau_2} d\tau_1 <n|U_0(t,\tau_1)\hat{H}'(\tau_1)U_0(\tau_1,t_0)|m><m|U_0^\dagger(\tau_2,t_0)\hat{H}'(\tau_2)$$
$$U_0^\dagger(t,\tau_2)|n>. \tag{2.98}$$

If the initial time t_0 is $-\infty$, the transition probability evaluated at $t = \infty$ is again found to be

$$TP^{(2)}_{nm}(t=\infty) = \frac{1}{\hbar^2}|\tilde{H}'_{nm}(\omega_{nm})|^2\,. \tag{2.99}$$

EXERCISE 2.10

Derive Equation 2.99 from 2.98.

2.7.2 Second-Order Transition between Two Coherences

If the initial state is prepared on a coherence, $\rho_{mn}(t_0)$ (for $m \neq n$) at t_0 and if the final coherence is ρ_{jk} (for $j \neq k$), the coherence-to-coherence transition probability is

$$TP^{(2)}_{jk,mn}(t) = Tr[|\, j><k \,|\, V_2(t,t_0) \,|\, m><n \,|]$$

$$= <|\, j><k \,|\underset{\wr\wr}{\overset{\wr\wr}{\Longleftarrow}}|m><n|>$$

$$= <|\, j><k \,|\overset{\wr\wr}{\Longleftarrow}|m><n|> + <|\, j><k \,|\underset{\wr\wr}{\Longleftarrow}|m><n|>$$

$$+ <|\, j><k \,|\underset{\wr}{\overset{\wr}{\Longleftarrow}}|m><n|> + <|\, j><k \,|\underset{\wr}{\overset{\wr}{\Longleftarrow}}|m><n|>. \quad (2.100)$$

Using the orthogonality conditions between two different eigenstates, one can verify that $j = n$ and $k = m$ in the first and second diagrams of Equation 2.100, respectively. In addition, during the time period between τ_2 and τ_1 the system can be in coherence or population depending on the intermediate quantum states during the second-order transition pathways. Thus, we have

$$TP^{(2)}_{jk,mn}(t) = <|\, n><k \,|\overset{\wr\wr}{\Longleftarrow}|m><n|>\delta_{jn} + <|\, j><m \,|\underset{\wr\wr}{\Longleftarrow}|m><n|>\delta_{km}$$

$$+ <|\, j><k \,|\underset{\wr}{\overset{\wr}{\Longleftarrow}}|m><n|> + <|\, j><k \,|\underset{\wr}{\overset{\wr}{\Longleftarrow}}|m><n|>. \quad (2.101)$$

The physical meanings of the four contributions in Equation 2.101 can be understood by considering each transition pathway in terms of coherence and population evolutions. The first term involves two perturbations to the ket vector $|m>$, whereas the bra vector $<n|$ remains unchanged. Using the completeness condition,that is, $\Sigma_l \,|\, l><l \,| = 1$,one can rewrite the first term on the right-hand side of Equation 2.101 as

$$<|\, n><k \,|\overset{\wr\wr}{\Longleftarrow}|m><n|> = \sum_l <|\, n><k \,|\overset{\wr\, l\, \wr}{\Longleftarrow}|m><n|> \quad (2.102)$$

where the summation over all possible intermediate states l should be performed. Considering the case when $l = n$ separately, we have

$$<|\, n><k \,|\overset{\wr\wr}{\Longleftarrow}|m><n|> = <|\, n><k \,|\overset{\wr\, n\, \wr}{\Longleftarrow}|m><n|>$$

$$+ \sum_{l \neq n} <|\, n><k \,|\overset{\wr\, l\, \wr}{\Longleftarrow}|m><n|>. \quad (2.103)$$

The first term on the right-hand side of Equation 2.103 involves population evolution during the time period between τ_1 and τ_2, whereas all the other terms in the summation $\Sigma_{l \neq n}$ involve coherence evolutions during $\tau_2 - \tau_1$ period, and they are oscillating with frequencies ω_{nl}. Therefore, if the time integrations are taken, they are likely to be small in comparison to the first term. Thus, within this approximation, we get

$$<|n><k| \overset{\wr\wr}{\Longleftarrow} |m><n|> = <|n><k| \overset{\wr n \wr}{\Longleftarrow} |m><n|>. \tag{2.104}$$

Similarly, ignoring the highly oscillating terms in the integrands for evaluating the time integrals, we have

$$<|j><m| \underset{\wr\wr}{\Longleftarrow} |m><n|> = <|j><m| \underset{\wr m \wr}{\Longleftarrow} |m><n|>$$

$$<|j><k| \overset{\wr}{\underset{\wr}{\Longleftarrow}} |m><n|> = <|j><n| \overset{n\wr}{\underset{\wr}{\Longleftarrow}} |m><n|> \delta_{kn}$$

$$<|j><k| \overset{\wr}{\underset{\wr}{\Longleftarrow}} |m><n|> = <|m><k| \overset{\wr}{\underset{m\wr}{\Longleftarrow}} |m><n|> \delta_{jm}. \tag{2.105}$$

Finally, using the above results, the transition probability of $TP^{(2)}_{jk,mn}(t)$ is given as the sum of four distinctively different contributions as

$$TP^{(2)}_{jk,mn}(t) = <|n><k| \overset{\wr n \wr}{\Longleftarrow} |m><n|> \delta_{jn} + <|j><m| \underset{\wr m \wr}{\Longleftarrow} |m><n|> \delta_{km}$$

$$+ <|j><n| \overset{n\wr}{\underset{\wr}{\Longleftarrow}} |m><n|> \delta_{kn} + <|m><k| \overset{\wr}{\underset{m\wr}{\Longleftarrow}} |m><n|> \delta_{jm}. \tag{2.106}$$

A detailed expression for $TP^{(2)}_{jk,mn}(t)$ requires proper system–bath interaction model as well as the perturbation Hamiltonian. Thus, we shall not provide any further discussion along this line here, but one can obtain theoretical expressions for these four terms when the system–bath interaction and perturbation Hamiltonians are specified for a given molecular system of interest.

2.7.3 First-Order Transition between Population and Coherence

Lastly, if the initial state is prepared on a coherence, $\rho_{mn}(t_0)$ (for $m \neq n$) at t_0, and if the final state is a population, ρ_{mm}, the coherence-to-population transition probability within the first-order perturbation theory is

$$TP^{(1)}_{mm,mn}(t) = Tr[|m><m| V_1(t,t_0) |m><n|]. \tag{2.107}$$

Note that the initial ket vector $|m>$ does not undergo any quantum transition so that we need to consider the first-order perturbation-induced $n \rightarrow m$ transition. Thus, Equation 2.107 can be diagrammatically represented as

$$TP^{(1)}_{mn,mn}(t) = <|m><m| \xLeftarrow[\xi]{} |m><n|>. \tag{2.108}$$

Only when the above expectation value of the population operator $|m><m|$ does not vanish, the transition from the coherence $\rho_{mn}(t_0)$ to the population on the mth state becomes allowed and finite. One can obtain the similar expression for the transition probability associated with transition from $\rho_{mn}(t_0)$ to ρ_{nn}. In addition, it is possible to obtain the diagram representations of the transition probabilities from a population to a coherence. These calculations again require specific system–bath interaction and perturbation Hamiltonians so that we will not provide any further discussions along this line.

REFERENCES

1. Shen, Y. R., *The principles of nonlinear optics*. John Wiley & Sons: New York, 1984.
2. Mukamel, S., *Principles of nonlinear optical spectroscopy*. Oxford University Press: Oxford, 1995.
3. Craig, D. P.; Thirunamachandran, T., *Molecular quantum electrodyanmics: An introduction to radiation molecule interactions*. Dover Publications, Inc.: New York, 1998.
4. Cohen-Tannoudji, C.; DuPont-Roc, I.; Grynberg, G., *Photons and atoms: Introduction to quantum electrodynamics*. Wiley: New York, 1989.
5. Loudon, R., *The quantum theory of light*. Clarendon Press: Oxford, 1983.
6. Dirac, P. A. M., *The principles of quantum mechanics*. 4th ed.; Oxford: London, 1976.
7. Schiff, L. I., *Quantum mechanics*. 3rd ed.; McGraw-Hill: New York, 1968.
8. Cohen-Tannoudji, C.; Diu, B.; Laloe, F., *Quantum mechanics*. Wiley: New York, 1977.
9. Louisell, W. H., *Quantum statistical properties of radiation*. Wiley: New York, 1973.
10. Fano, U., Description of states in quantum mechanics by density matrix and operator techniques. *Reviews of Modern Physics* 1957, 29, 74–93.
11. Blum, K., *Density matrix theory and applications*. Plenum Press: New York, 1981.
12. Ernst, R. R.; Bodenhausen, G.; Wokaun, A., *Nuclear magnetic resonance in one and two dimensions*. Oxford University Press: Oxford, 1987.

3 Linear Response Spectroscopy

The conventional definition of the linear spectroscopy is spectroscopy with an observable that is linearly proportional to the intensity of external field.[1–4] Then, the observable signal can be expressed in terms of the corresponding linear response function. However, there are cases in which this definition may not apply. For instance, the electronically nonresonant hyper-Raman scattering signal is proportional to squares of intensity of the incident electric field. Nevertheless, the hyper-Raman scattering can be described in terms of linear response function of the first hyperpolarizability.[5] Another example is the surface-specific electronically nonresonant IR-vis sum frequency generation (SFG) spectroscopy.[6] Although the measured signal is proportional to both IR and visible field intensities, it can be described in terms of dipole-polarizability linear response function.[7] Consequently, it is necessary to generalize the definition of linear spectroscopy in such a way that the linear spectroscopic observable is linearly proportional to a properly chosen *effective* radiation–matter interaction as well as that the linear spectroscopy is the one that can be fully characterized by properly defined linear response function.

There are a number of linear spectroscopic techniques that are capable of measuring distinctively different molecular properties, and they differ from one another by the nature of radiation–matter interactions involved. In this regard, we find it useful to introduce various radiation–matter interaction Hamiltonians, where each constitutes a conjugate pair of matter-operator-inducing quantum transitions and associated external field causing them. Throughout this book we will treat external electromagnetic field as a classical function. Generally, the radiation–matter interaction Hamiltonian can be written as a dot product of a vectorial matter or radiation-induced matter operator and an external field vector, that is,

$$H_{rad\text{-}mat}(t) = -\hat{\mathbf{V}} \cdot \mathbf{F}(\mathbf{r},t) \tag{3.1}$$

where $\mathbf{F}(\mathbf{r},t)$ is the external field and $\hat{\mathbf{V}}$ is its conjugate operator that induces quantum transitions between any two different quantum states. In this book, the following seven conjugate pairs are sufficient enough to describe most of the spectroscopic measurements considered here,

$\hat{\mathbf{V}}$		$\mathbf{F}(\mathbf{r},t)$
$\boldsymbol{\mu}$	$\leftrightarrow$	$\mathbf{E}(\mathbf{r},t)$
$\mathbf{m}$	$\leftrightarrow$	$\mathbf{B}(\mathbf{r},t)$
$\mathbf{Q}$	$\leftrightarrow$	$(1/2)\nabla\mathbf{E}(\mathbf{r},t)$
$\boldsymbol{\alpha}$	$\leftrightarrow$	$\mathbf{E}^2(\mathbf{r},t)$
$\mathbf{G}$ and $\bar{\mathbf{G}}$	$\leftrightarrow$	$\mathbf{E}(\mathbf{r},t)\mathbf{B}(\mathbf{r},t)$ and $\mathbf{E}(\mathbf{r},t)\mathbf{B}(\mathbf{r},t)$
$\mathbf{A}$ and $\bar{\mathbf{A}}$	$\leftrightarrow$	$(1/2)\mathbf{E}(\mathbf{r},t)\nabla\mathbf{E}(\mathbf{r},t)$ and $(1/2)\nabla\mathbf{E}(\mathbf{r},t)\mathbf{E}(\mathbf{r},t)$
$\boldsymbol{\beta}$	$\leftrightarrow$	$\mathbf{E}^3(\mathbf{r},t)$

SCHEME 3.1

Note that the first three conjugate pairs are linearly proportional to the electromagnetic field amplitude, whereas the second three pairs are second order. The last interaction is third order with resepct to $\mathbf{E}(\mathbf{r},t)$.

The first pair describes the interaction between electric dipole $\boldsymbol{\mu}$ and electric field $\mathbf{E}(\mathbf{r},t)$ and the corresponding radiation–matter interaction Hamiltonian $-\boldsymbol{\mu}\cdot\mathbf{E}(\mathbf{r},t)$ should be considered to describe electric-dipole-allowed linear and nonlinear optical processes. The second pair represents the interaction between magnetic dipole (m) and external magnetic field $\mathbf{B}(\mathbf{r},t)$. This is an important radiation–matter interaction for understanding various linear and nonlinear optical activity spectroscopy such as circular dichroism, optical rotatory dispersion, Raman optical activity, and so forth. This is the topic covered in Chapters 15 and 16. The third radiation–matter interaction describes the interaction between electric quadrupole $\mathbf{Q}$ and spatial gradient of electric field. In this list of conjugate pairs in Scheme 3.1, only the first three terms are essentially linearly dependent on the electric field because $\mathbf{B} = \hat{\mathbf{k}} \times \mathbf{E}$ and $\nabla\mathbf{E}^{\pm} = \pm i\mathbf{k}\mathbf{E}^{\pm}$ where $\mathbf{k}$ is the wavevector and $\mathbf{E}^{\pm}$ are the two counter-propagating components in $\mathbf{E}(\mathbf{r},t)$.

Now, the fourth radiation–matter interaction is between matter's polarizability and square of electric field, and that is responsible for Raman or Rayleigh scattering processes as well as the two-photon absorption, depending on detailed sequence of radiation–matter interactions considered.[8] As will be shown later, the measure of the light scattering amplitude depends on the magnitude of polarizability ($\boldsymbol{\alpha}$) matrix element of a given molecule on the electronic ground state.[9, 10] If the molecule undergoes a two-photon absorption, the transition matrix element of $\boldsymbol{\alpha}$ from the ground state to the two-photon-accessible excited state is an important quantity describing such a two-photon absorption probability.

The fifth pair describes the interaction energy between the so-called magnetic dipole-Raman optical activity (ROA) tensor and external electromagntic field, whereas the sixth does that between electric quadrupole-ROA tensor and external electromagnetic field.[11–13] The fifth and sixth interactions are crucial in theoretically describing the Raman optical activity and higher-order nonlinear optical activity spectroscopy in general. The fourth to sixth radiation–matter interactions are second-order with respect to the electric field amplitude. Finally, the seventh pair corresponds to the interaction of first hyperpolarizability $\boldsymbol{\beta}$ with external electric field $\mathbf{E}^3(\mathbf{r},t)$. Depending on the electric field frequencies, it describes hyper-Raman or hyper-Rayleigh scattering, three-photon absorption, and so forth.

These conjugate pairs provide a guideline for theoretically describing any one or multidimensional spectroscopy. All the spectroscopies require both preparation and detection steps. The preparation step involves single or multiple radiation–matter interactions. As will be discussed later, the multidimensional spectroscopy involves two or more effective radiation–matter interactions with matter to create electronic or vibrational coherences, and the corresponding oscillating nuclear or electronic dipoles, then radiate signal electric field. If those dipoles oscillate in phase, the constructive interference among the radiated fields produces a coherently generated electric field whose amplitude is linearly proportional to the number of interacting molecules. If the generated electric field amplitude **E** (or intensity $|\mathbf{E}|^2$) is detected experimentally, one should choose the first conjugate pair for theoretically describing the detection step because the emissive radiation–matter interaction is between the electric dipole operator and vaccum electric field. In this chapter, we will focus on the case when the preparation step involves just one of the effective radiation–matter interactions given in Scheme 3.1. Therefore, by definition, they are linear response spectroscopies.

3.1 LINEAR RESPONSE FUNCTION

Spectroscopic observable corresponds to the expectation value of particular operator $\hat{B}$. Now, suppose that the operator $\hat{A}$ is the conjugate operator of external field $F(t)$. Then, the total Hamiltonian is the sum of zero-order Hamiltonian and perturbation Hamiltonian, where the latter describes the interaction energy of the system with $F(t)$ as

$$\hat{H}(t) = \hat{H}_0(t) + \hat{H}'(t) = \hat{H}_0(t) - \hat{A}F(t). \tag{3.2}$$

Then, the expectation value of $\hat{B}$ at time t should be calculated to determine the spectroscopic observable. Using the time-dependent perturbation theory, we have

$$\bar{B}(t) = <\hat{B}\rho_A^{(1)}(t)>$$

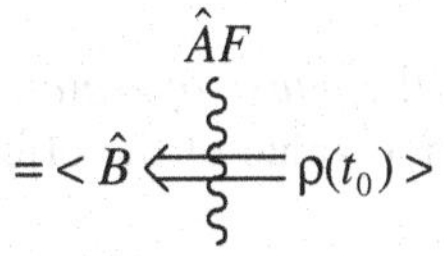

$$= -\frac{i}{\hbar}\int_{t_0}^{t} d\tau < \hat{B}V_0(t,\tau)L'(\tau)V_0(\tau,t_0)\rho(t_0) >$$

$$= \frac{i}{\hbar}\int_{t_0}^{t} d\tau < \hat{B}U_0(t,\tau)\hat{A}U_0(\tau,t_0)\rho(t_0)U_0^{\dagger}(t,t_0) > F(\tau)$$

$$-\frac{i}{\hbar}\int_{t_0}^{t} d\tau < \hat{B}U_0(t,t_0)\rho(t_0)U_0^{\dagger}(\tau,t_0)\hat{A}U_0^{\dagger}(t,\tau) > F(\tau)$$

$$= \frac{i}{\hbar}\int_{t_0}^{t} d\tau < [\hat{B}(t),\hat{A}(\tau)]\rho(t_0) > F(\tau). \tag{3.3}$$

Here, it was assumed that the external field $F(t)$ is a real function in time, and the time-evolved operators $\hat{A}(\tau)$ and $\hat{B}(t)$ are defined as, respectively,

$$\hat{A}(\tau) = U_0^\dagger(\tau,t_0)\hat{A}U_0(\tau,t_0)$$

$$\hat{B}(t) = U_0^\dagger(t,t_0)\hat{B}U_0(t,t_0). \tag{3.4}$$

Now, changing the integration variable and assuming $t_0 = -\infty$, we find that

$$\bar{B}(t) = \int_0^\infty d\tau \phi_{BA}(\tau)F(t-\tau) \tag{3.5}$$

or

$$\bar{B}(t) = \int_{-\infty}^t d\tau \phi_{BA}(t-\tau)F(\tau) \tag{3.6}$$

and the linear response function $\phi(\tau)$ is defined as

$$\phi_{BA}(\tau) \equiv \frac{i}{\hbar} < [\hat{B}(\tau), \hat{A}(0)]\rho(-\infty) > . \tag{3.7}$$

Although the integration range in Equation 3.5 is from 0 to infinity, one can replace the lower bound with $-\infty$ because of the causality condition. Since the cause must precede the effect, we will redefine the linear response function as

$$\phi_{BA}(\tau) \equiv \frac{i}{\hbar}\theta(\tau) < [\hat{B}(\tau), \hat{A}(0)]\rho(-\infty) > . \tag{3.8}$$

Throughout the book, the operator $\hat{A}$ is called the *cause operator*, and the operator $\hat{B}$ is the *effect operator.* Then, the expectation value of the effect operator $\hat{B}$ is given as

$$\bar{B}(t) = \int_{-\infty}^\infty d\tau \phi_{BA}(\tau)F(t-\tau). \tag{3.9}$$

In the frequency domain, from the definition of the susceptibility as

$$\tilde{\bar{B}}(\omega) = \chi_{BA}(\omega)\tilde{F}(\omega), \tag{3.10}$$

we have

$$\chi_{BA}(\omega) = \int_{-\infty}^\infty dt\, \phi_{BA}(t)e^{i\omega t} = \int_0^\infty dt\, \phi_{BA}(t)e^{i\omega t}. \tag{3.11}$$

Using the properties of Fourier transformation, one can rewrite Equation 3.9 as

$$\bar{B}(t) = \frac{1}{2\pi}\int_{-\infty}^{\infty} d\omega\, \chi_{BA}(\omega)\tilde{F}(\omega)e^{-i\omega t}. \tag{3.12}$$

where $\tilde{F}(\omega)$ is the Fourier transform of $F(t)$.

Denoting the real and imaginary parts of the susceptibility as $\chi'_{BA}(\omega)$ and $\chi''_{BA}(\omega)$, respectively, we have

$$\chi_{BA}(\omega) = \chi'_{BA}(\omega) + i\chi''_{BA}(\omega) \tag{3.13}$$

and

$$\chi'_{BA}(\omega) = \int_0^{\infty} dt\, \phi_{BA}(t)\cos\omega t \tag{3.14}$$

$$\chi''_{BA}(\omega) = \int_0^{\infty} dt\, \phi_{BA}(t)\sin\omega t. \tag{3.15}$$

From these relationships, one can obtain the Kramers–Kronig relations:

$$\chi'_{BA}(\omega) = \frac{1}{\pi} PP \int d\omega' \frac{\chi''_{BA}(\omega')}{\omega' - \omega} \tag{3.16}$$

and

$$\chi''_{BA}(\omega) = -\frac{1}{\pi} PP \int d\omega' \frac{\chi'_{BA}(\omega')}{\omega' - \omega}, \tag{3.17}$$

where *PP* stands for the principal part of the integral.

EXERCISE 3.1

Derive the Kramers–Kronig relations given in Equations 3.16 and 3.17.

Complete information on the linear response of molecular system against the external perturbation by $\hat{H}'(t)(= -\hat{A}F(t))$ is included in either the linear response function in time domain or the linear susceptibility in frequency domain. Experimentally, one can measure one of the two functions either using an ultrafast laser pulse with time-resolved measurement of free-induction-decay or using a continuous wave with frequency scanning measurement of frequency-resolved observable. In the former case, the temporal envelop of the external field is assumed to be close to a Dirac delta function, that is,

$$F(t) = F_0\,\delta(t)e^{-i\omega t}. \tag{3.18}$$

In this impulsive limit, we have

$$\bar{B}(t) \propto F_0\phi_{BA}(t). \tag{3.19}$$

Note that the measured expectation value $\bar{B}(t)$ is linearly proportional to the linear response function directly.

Next, let us consider the other limiting case when the temporal envelope function of the external field is constant as

$$F(t) = 2F_0 \sin\omega_0 t = iF_0(e^{-i\omega_0 t} - e^{i\omega_0 t}) \quad (3.20)$$

which gives

$$\tilde{F}(\omega) = 2\pi i F_0\{\delta(\omega - \omega_0) - \delta(\omega + \omega_0)\}. \quad (3.21)$$

Then, for such a frequency-domain measurement, we have

$$\bar{B}(t) = iF_0\left[\chi_{BA}(\omega_0)e^{-i\omega_0 t} - \chi_{BA}(-\omega_0)e^{i\omega_0 t}\right]. \quad (3.22)$$

This result shows that the expectation value $\bar{B}(t)$ also oscillates with frequency of ω_0. One can rewrite Equation 3.22 as

$$\bar{B}(t) = 2F_0[\chi'_{BA}(\omega_0)\sin(\omega_0 t) - \chi''_{BA}(\omega_0)\cos(\omega_0 t)]. \quad (3.23)$$

The first term on the right-hand side of Equation 3.23 is in phase with the external field, and the coefficient is determined by the real part of the susceptibility. On the other hand, the second term, whose magnitude is determined by the imaginary (dissipative) part of the susceptibility, is out of phase with the external field. This explains why the imaginary part of the susceptibility is related to the absorption of light by matter.

3.2 SYSTEM–BATH INTERACTION AND LINE BROADENING

In this book, we shall consider a few model systems to provide detailed descriptions of relationships between the linear and nonlinear spectroscopic observables and molecular properties. In this section, we focus on a two-level system (2LS), which is a good model for most of electronic chromophores or spin systems. The corresponding Hamiltonian is written as

$$\hat{H}_{2LS} = \hbar\omega_{eg}a^{\dagger}a. \quad (3.24)$$

Here, the creation and annihilation operators of the 2LS excited state are denoted as $a^{\dagger}$ and a, respectively. The energy gap between the excited state e and ground state g was denoted as

$$\hbar\omega_{eg} = E_e - E_g. \quad (3.25)$$

Two-level chromophores in solution interact with surrounding bath degrees of freedom, and such system–bath interactions are responsible for a number of interesting processes such as fluctuations of energies and coupling constants, dephasing, decoherence, excitation transfer between two internal states, spectral diffusion, fluorescence Stokes shift, dissipation, and the like.[4, 14] The total matter Hamiltonian is thus given as

$$\hat{H}_{mat} = \hat{H}_{2LS} + \hat{H}_B + \hat{H}_{SB}, \tag{3.26}$$

where $\hat{H}_B$ is the bath Hamiltonian. The system–bath (chromophore-bath) interaction Hamiltonian, denoted as $\hat{H}_{SB}$, is assumed to be diagonal with respect to the system eigenstates as

$$\hat{H}_{SB} = V_{eg}(\mathbf{q})a^{\dagger}a, \tag{3.27}$$

where the bath degrees of freedom are denoted as $\mathbf{q}$ and the potential energy difference between the excited and ground states is defined as

$$V_{eg}(\mathbf{q}) = V_e(\mathbf{q}) - V_g(\mathbf{q}). \tag{3.28}$$

Therefore, we have

$$\hat{H}_{mat} = \{\hbar\omega_{eg} + V_{eg}(\mathbf{q}) + H_B(\mathbf{q})\}a^{\dagger}a. \tag{3.29}$$

Here, the ground state adiabatic Hamiltonian $\hat{H}_g(\mathbf{q})$ is given as $\hat{H}_g(\mathbf{q}) = \hbar\omega_g + V_g(\mathbf{q}) + H_B(\mathbf{q})$ and will be treated as the reference Hamiltonian. Then, $\hat{H}_e(\mathbf{q})$ can be written as

$$\hat{H}_e(\mathbf{q}) = \hat{H}_g(\mathbf{q}) + \hbar\omega_{eg} + V_{eg}(\mathbf{q}). \tag{3.30}$$

Treating $\hat{H}_g(\mathbf{q})$ as the zero-order Hamiltonian $\hat{H}_0$ and taking the last two terms in Equation 3.30 altogether as $\hat{H}'$, we find that, in the interaction picture, the forward and backward time evolution operators by $\hat{H}_e(\mathbf{q})$ are

$$\exp\left(-\frac{i}{\hbar}\hat{H}_e t\right) = \exp(-i\bar{\omega}_{eg}t)\exp\left(-\frac{i}{\hbar}\hat{H}_g t\right)\exp_+\left(-\frac{i}{\hbar}\int_0^t d\tau U(\tau)\right) \tag{3.31}$$

$$\exp\left(\frac{i}{\hbar}\hat{H}_e t\right) = \exp\left(i\bar{\omega}_{eg}t\right)\exp_-\left(\frac{i}{\hbar}\int_0^t d\tau U(\tau)\right)\exp\left(\frac{i}{\hbar}\hat{H}_g t\right). \tag{3.32}$$

where

$$\bar{\omega}_{eg} = \omega_{eg} + < V_{eg}(\mathbf{q}) >$$

$$U \equiv V_{eg}(\mathbf{q}) - < V_{eg}(\mathbf{q}) >$$

$$U(t) = U(\mathbf{q}(t)) = \exp\left(\frac{i}{\hbar}\hat{H}_B t\right) U(\mathbf{q}) \exp\left(-\frac{i}{\hbar}\hat{H}_B t\right). \tag{3.33}$$

Here, $< V_{eg}(\mathbf{q}) >$ is the average value taken on the ground electronic state.

EXERCISE 3.2
Show the two operator equalities in Equations 3.31 and 3.32.

Hereafter it is assumed that the initial density operator may be written as a product of the system and bath density operators as

$$\rho(-\infty) = \rho_S(-\infty)\rho_B(-\infty). \tag{3.34}$$

In the case when the energy gap between the two states is much larger than the thermal energy, that is, $\hbar\omega_{eg} >> k_B T$, the system is in a thermal equilibrium state on its ground state and the initial density operator is simply given as

$$\rho(-\infty) = | g > \rho_B(\mathbf{q}) < g | = | g > \frac{e^{-\beta\hat{H}_B(\mathbf{q})}}{< e^{-\beta\hat{H}_B(\mathbf{q})} >_B} < g |. \tag{3.35}$$

where $< \cdots >_B$ is the trace operation and the basis set consists of bath eigenstates and $\beta = 1/k_B T$.

Now, to obtain an approximate expression for the $\hat{B} \leftarrow \hat{A}$ susceptibility, one should take into account the effects of the system–bath interaction on the corresponding linear response function $\phi_{BA}(\tau)$. For the above 2LS, using the operator identities in Equations 3.31 and 3.32, one can find that the linear response function is given as

$$\phi_{BA}(t) = \frac{i}{\hbar}\theta(t)\left\{ B_{ge}A_{eg}e^{-i\bar{\omega}_{eg}t} < \exp_+\left(-\frac{i}{\hbar}\int_0^t d\tau U(\tau)\right)\rho_B >_B \right.$$

$$\left. - B_{eg}A_{ge}e^{i\bar{\omega}_{eg}t} < \exp_-\left(\frac{i}{\hbar}\int_0^t d\tau U(\tau)\right)\rho_B >_B \right\}$$

$$= \frac{i}{\hbar}\theta(t)\left\{ B_{ge}A_{eg}e^{-i\bar{\omega}_{eg}t} < \exp_+\left(-\frac{i}{\hbar}\int_0^t d\tau U(\tau)\right)\rho_B >_B - c.c. \right\}. \tag{3.36}$$

The next step is to rewrite $\phi_{BA}(t)$ in terms of the time-correlation function of the difference potential operator $U(t)$ by using the cumulant expansion technique.[4] The expectation value of exponential operator should be expanded first. Then, take the averages of each expanded terms. Then, the expanded series is approximately written as an exponential function, where the second order cumulant expansion term is the exponent.

Thus, we have

$$
\begin{aligned}
&< \exp_+\left(-\frac{i}{\hbar}\int_0^t d\tau U(\tau)\right)\rho_B >_B \\
&= 1 - \frac{i}{\hbar}\int_0^t d\tau < U(\tau)\rho_B >_B + \left(-\frac{i}{\hbar}\right)^2 \int_0^t d\tau_2 \int_0^{\tau_2} d\tau_1 < U(\tau_2)U(\tau_1)\rho_B >_B + \cdots \\
&\cong \exp\left\{-\frac{1}{\hbar^2}\int_0^t d\tau_2 \int_0^{\tau_2} d\tau_1 < U(\tau_2)U(\tau_1)\rho_B >_B\right\} \\
&= \exp\{-g(t)\},
\end{aligned}
\tag{3.37}
$$

where $g(t)$ is the line-broadening function because its time-dependency determines the spectral line shape in general and it is defined as

$$
\begin{aligned}
g(t) &= \frac{1}{\hbar^2}\int_0^t d\tau_2 \int_0^{\tau_2} d\tau_1 < U(\tau_2)U(\tau_1)\rho_B >_B \\
&= \frac{1}{\hbar^2}\int_0^t d\tau_2 \int_0^{\tau_2} d\tau_1 < U(\tau_1)U(0)\rho_B >_B \\
&= \int_0^t d\tau_2 \int_0^{\tau_2} d\tau_1 C(\tau_1).
\end{aligned}
\tag{3.38}
$$

Here, the time-correlation function of the difference potential $U(t)$ was defined as

$$
C(t) \equiv \frac{1}{\hbar^2} < U(t)U(0)\rho_B >_B . \tag{3.39}
$$

which has been known as the fluctuating transition frequency-frequency correlation function (FFCF) since the system–bath interaction modulates the transition energy (or frequency) in time. Consequently, the general $\hat{B} \leftarrow \hat{A}$ linear response function is simplified as

$$
\begin{aligned}
\phi_{BA}(t) &= \frac{i}{\hbar}\theta(t)\left\{B_{ge}A_{eg}e^{-i\bar{\omega}_{eg}t-g(t)} - c.c.\right\} \\
&= -\frac{2}{\hbar}\theta(t)\,\mathrm{Im}\left[B_{ge}A_{eg}e^{-i\bar{\omega}_{eg}t-g(t)}\right].
\end{aligned}
\tag{3.40}
$$

To obtain the second equality in Equation 3.40, it is assumed that $A_{ge} = A_{eg}$ and $B_{ge} = B_{eg}$ and they are real. However, this is not a necessary assumption in general.

The linear response function component consists of three different parts:

$$\frac{i}{\hbar}\theta(t)B_{ge}A_{eg}\exp(-i\bar{\omega}_{eg}t)\exp(-g(t))$$

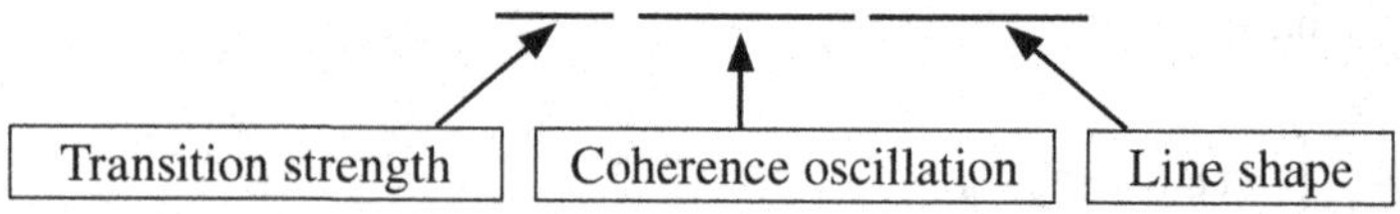

The transition strength term $B_{ge}A_{eg}$ determines the amplitude of the oscillatory linear response function, where the oscillating pattern is described by the coherence oscillation term $\exp(-i\bar{\omega}_{eg}t)$. The last term $\exp(-g(t))$ is the *line shape* function, and its decaying pattern determines the shape of the frequency-dependent susceptibility or spectral line shape.

The corresponding susceptibility is then

$$\chi_{BA}(\omega)=\frac{i}{\hbar}\int_0^{\infty} dt\left\{B_{ge}A_{eg}e^{-i(\bar{\omega}_{eg}-\omega)t-g(t)}-B_{eg}A_{ge}e^{i(\bar{\omega}_{eg}+\omega)t-g^*(t)}\right\}, \quad (3.41)$$

which is a complex function. When the external field frequency ω is close to the ensemble-averaged transition frequency $\bar{\omega}_{eg}$, the first integral in Equation 3.41 is much larger than the second integral (note that an integral of highly oscillating function is small). This is the resonance condition, and the first and second terms correspond to the resonant and nonresonant contributions to the frequency-dependent susceptibility when $\omega \cong \bar{\omega}_{eg}$. Typical line shapes of the real and imaginary parts of the linear susceptibility for a two-level system are shown in Figure 3.1.

If more than one excited states are to be considered, the time-domain response function in Equation 3.40 and the frequency-domain susceptibility in Equation 3.41

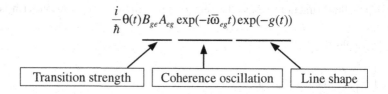

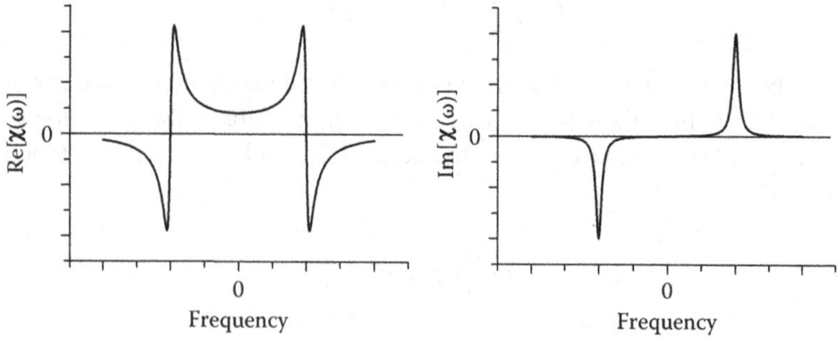

FIGURE 3.1 Real and imaginary parts of linear susceptibility of a two-level system.

should be written as summations over all optically allowed excited states, that is,

$$\phi_{BA}(t) = \frac{i}{\hbar}\theta(t)\sum_e \left\{ B_{ge}A_{eg}e^{-i\bar{\omega}_{eg}t - g_{ee}(t)} - B_{eg}A_{ge}e^{i\bar{\omega}_{eg}t - g_{ee}^*(t)} \right\}$$

$$\chi_{BA}(\omega) = \frac{i}{\hbar}\sum_e \int_0^\infty dt \left\{ B_{ge}A_{eg}e^{-i(\bar{\omega}_{eg}-\omega)t - g_{ee}(t)} - B_{eg}A_{ge}e^{i(\bar{\omega}_{eg}+\omega)t - g_{ee}^*(t)} \right\}. \tag{3.42}$$

EXERCISE 3.3

If the time-dependent fluctuating potential obeys Gaussian statistics, Equation 3.37 is exact. Why?

There are a few different models for the line-broadening function $g(t)$. It was shown that the time-correlation function $C(t)$ plays an important role and contains information on the strength of system–bath coupling as well as on the memory loss rate of the bath degrees of freedom that are coupled to the quantum transition $g \leftrightarrow e$. If the memory loss is extremely fast, such process is called Markovian. Using the Kubo's stochastic model,[15] one can assume that the time-correlation function $C(t)$ is an exponentially decaying function as

$$C(t) = C(0)\exp(-\Gamma t) \quad \text{and} \quad C(0) = \frac{1}{\hbar^2} < U^2\rho_B >_B . \tag{3.43}$$

The Markovian limit corresponds to the case when Γ is very large, and in this limit the line-broadening function is given as approximately

$$g(t) = \frac{C(0)}{\Gamma}t = \gamma t. \tag{3.44}$$

The amplitude of the oscillating linear response function, in this case, exponentially decays in time. From Equations 3.11 and 3.40, one can find that the susceptibility is

$$\chi_{BA}(\omega) = \frac{1}{\hbar}B_{ge}A_{eg}\left\{ \frac{1}{\bar{\omega}_{eg} - \omega - i\gamma} + \frac{1}{\bar{\omega}_{eg} + \omega + i\gamma} \right\}. \tag{3.45}$$

This is the well-known Lorentzian line shape.

As the opposite limit, if the coupled bath degrees of freedom have long memory, the FFCF is approximated as

$$C(t) = C(0). \tag{3.46}$$

Then, the line-broadening function is, in this inhomogeneous line-broadening limit,

$$g(t) = \frac{1}{2}C(0)t^2 = \frac{1}{2}\Omega^2 t^2. \tag{3.47}$$

Throughout this book, the square root of $C(0)$ of a 2LS, which is the root-mean-square of fluctuating transition frequency, will be especially denoted as Ω. The line shape function is then a Gaussian in time,

$$\exp\{-g(t)\} = \exp\left(-\frac{1}{2}\Omega^2 t^2\right). \tag{3.48}$$

Then, the half-life $t_{1/2}$, defined as $\exp(-\Omega^2 t_{1/2}^2/2) = 1/2$, is

$$t_{1/2} = \sqrt{\frac{2\ln 2}{\Omega^2}} = \sqrt{\frac{2\ln 2}{C(0)}}. \tag{3.49}$$

The complex susceptibility, when the line shape function is given as Equation 3.48, is then found to be

$$\chi_{BA}(\omega) = \frac{i\sqrt{\pi}}{\sqrt{2}\Omega\hbar}\left\{B_{ge}A_{eg}e^{-(\omega-\bar{\omega}_{eg})^2/2\Omega^2} erfc(-i(\omega-\bar{\omega}_{eg})/\sqrt{2}\Omega)\right.$$
$$\left. -B_{eg}A_{ge}e^{-(\omega+\bar{\omega}_{eg})^2/2\Omega^2} erfc(-i(\omega+\bar{\omega}_{eg})/\sqrt{2}\Omega)\right\}, \tag{3.50}$$

where *erfc* is the complementary error function. The imaginary part of $\chi_{BA}(\omega)$ is simply given as the sum of two Gaussian functions at $\omega = \bar{\omega}_{eg}$ and $\omega = -\bar{\omega}_{eg}$ as

$$\chi''_{BA}(\omega) = \frac{\sqrt{\pi}}{\sqrt{2}\hbar\Omega}\left\{B_{ge}A_{eg}e^{-(\omega-\bar{\omega}_{eg})^2/2\Omega^2} - B_{eg}A_{ge}e^{-(\omega+\bar{\omega}_{eg})^2/2\Omega^2}\right\}. \tag{3.51}$$

From the Kubo's exponential model for $C(t)$ given in Equation 3.43, one can obtain the line-broadening function $g(t)$ as

$$g(t) = \frac{C(0)}{\Gamma^2}\{\exp(-\Gamma t) + \Gamma t - 1\}. \tag{3.52}$$

It can be shown that the above Kubo model interpolates from the Markovian limit to the inhomogeneous line-broadening limit. However, the more general approach was developed by introducing the spectral density, which describes the frequency distribution of the system–bath coupling strengths. In general, the time-correlation function $C(t)$ is complex. Denoting the real and imaginary parts of $C(t)$ as $C_R(t)$ and $C_I(t)$, that is,

$$C(t) = C_R(t) + iC_I(t), \tag{3.53}$$

we have

$$C_R(t) = \frac{1}{2\hbar^2}\{< U(t)U(0)\rho_B > + < U(0)U(t)\rho_B >\}$$

$$C_I(t) = -\frac{i}{2\hbar^2}\{< U(t)U(0)\rho_B > - < U(0)U(t)\rho_B >\}. \tag{3.54}$$

These two parts are in fact related to each other via the fluctuation-dissipation theorem as[16]

$$C_I(t) = -\tan\left\{\frac{\beta\hbar}{2}\frac{\partial}{\partial t}\right\} C_R(t). \tag{3.55}$$

In the classical limit, as $\hbar \to 0$ or $T \to \infty$, we get

$$C_I(t) \cong -\frac{\beta\hbar}{2}\frac{\partial}{\partial t} C_R(t). \tag{3.56}$$

EXERCISE 3.4
Prove Equation 3.55.

From Equations 3.53 and 3.54, one can find that the time-correlation function has the property $C^*(t) = C(-t)$. Therefore, the Fourier transform of $C(t)$ is real. Furthermore, the corresponding Fourier transforms $\tilde{C}_R(\omega)$ and $\tilde{C}_I(\omega)$ of the real and imaginary parts of $C(t)$ are purely real and imaginary, respectively. Therefore, one can show that $\tilde{C}_R(\omega)$ and $\tilde{C}_I(\omega)$ are related to each other in frequency domain

$$\tilde{C}_R(\omega) = \coth(\beta\hbar\omega/2)\,\mathrm{Im}[\tilde{C}_I(\omega)]. \tag{3.57}$$

In the classical limit of $\hbar \to 0$, we get

$$\tilde{C}_R(\omega) = (2/\beta\hbar\omega)\,\mathrm{Im}[\tilde{C}_I(\omega)]. \tag{3.58}$$

The expressions in Equation 3.55 and 3.57 are useful for the calculation of the response function by using classical molecular dynamics simulation. From the classical molecular dynamics trajectories, one can calculate the classical time-correlation function, $C_{cl}(t) = \hbar^{-2} < U_{cl}(t)U_{cl}(0) >_{cl}$, where $U_{cl}(t)$ is the scalar quantity representing the system–bath interaction energy that causes transition frequency fluctuation. Then, assuming that

$$C_R(t) \cong C_{cl}(t), \tag{3.59}$$

one can directly obtain the response function $C_I(t)$ or one-sided quantum correlation function $C(t)$ as

$$C_I(t) \cong -\tan\left\{\frac{\beta\hbar}{2}\frac{\partial}{\partial t}\right\} C_{cl}(t)$$

$$C(t) \cong \left(1 - i\tan\left\{\frac{\beta\hbar}{2}\frac{\partial}{\partial t}\right\}\right) C_{cl}(t) \tag{3.60}$$

or equivalently

$$\mathrm{Im}[\tilde{C}_I(\omega)] = \tanh(\beta\hbar\omega/2)\tilde{C}_{cl}(\omega)$$

$$\tilde{C}(\omega) = \{1 - \tanh(\beta\hbar\omega/2)\}\tilde{C}_{cl}(\omega). \tag{3.61}$$

EXERCISE 3.5
Derive Equation 3.61 from 3.60.

Hereafter, defining the spectral density as

$$\rho(\omega) \equiv \frac{\mathrm{Im}[\tilde{C}_I(\omega)]}{\pi\omega^2}, \tag{3.62}$$

one can rewrite the real and imaginary parts of the FFCF as

$$C_R(t) = \int_0^\infty d\omega\,\rho(\omega)\coth(\hbar\omega\beta/2)\omega^2\cos\omega t$$

$$C_I(t) = -\int_0^\infty d\omega\,\rho(\omega)\omega^2\sin\omega t. \tag{3.63}$$

The line-broadening function can then be written as integrals over the spectral density as[14]

$$g(t) = -i\lambda t/\hbar + \int_0^\infty d\omega\,\rho(\omega)\coth(\hbar\omega\beta/2)(1-\cos\omega t) + i\int_0^\infty d\omega\,\rho(\omega)\sin\omega t. \tag{3.64}$$

Here, the solvent reorganization energy λ is defined as

$$\lambda \equiv \hbar\int_0^\infty d\omega\,\rho(\omega)\omega. \tag{3.65}$$

If the line-broadening function $g(t)$ is Taylor-expanded with respect to t up to the second order terms, the line shape function $\exp(-g(t))$ is simply a Gaussian. Then, one can find that the half-life $t_{1/2}$ can be obtained in terms of the spectral density. In the high-temperature (classical) limit, we get

$$t_{1/2} = \sqrt{\frac{\hbar^2 \ln 2}{\lambda k_B T}} = t_{decoherence}. \tag{3.66}$$

For typical electronic or vibrational chromophores, the solvent reorganization energy varies from 10 to 1000 cm^{-1}. Then, the half-life $t_{1/2}$, which is approximately the time scale of decoherence (or dephasing of coherence), is on the order of 10 to

100 femtoseconds. Throughout this book, $t_{decoherence}$ in Equation 3.66 will be referred to as the approximate decoherence time. Now, inserting Equation 3.64 for $g(t)$ into Equation 3.42 and numerically carrying out the integration over time, one can obtain the $\hat{B} \leftarrow \hat{A}$ susceptibility for any arbitrary operators $\hat{A}$ and $\hat{B}$. In the following sections, we shall consider a few specific cases.

Before we close this section, it is necessary to provide a discussion on the lifetime broadening effect. Since the system–bath interaction Hamiltonian considered here with Equation 3.27 cannot describe the intrinsic lifetime broadening process, the lifetime broadening is often taken into account by using an *ad hoc* approximation as

$$g(t) \to g(t) + t/2T_e \tag{3.67}$$

where T_e is the lifetime of the excited state. Throughout this book, the lifetime broadening effects on multidimensional spectra will be included by using this approximate description, when it is necessary.

3.3 ROTATIONAL AVERAGING OF TENSORS

Linear and nonlinear spectroscopic observables are conveniently expressed in terms of the corresponding response functions. Since they involve vectorial or tensorial properties of molecules such as transition dipoles and polarizabilities, the linear and nonlinear response functions are nth-rank tensors $\mathrm{T}^{(n)}$. Properly controlling the beam polarization states, one can selectively measure one specific tensor element $T^{(n)}_{l_1l_2l_3\cdots l_n}$ or sometimes a combination of multiple tensor elements. Here, l_k is one of the three Cartesian coordinates in a laboratory-fixed frame.

If molecules have the same orientation in space, macroscopically measured signal electric field amplitude, when the constituent molecules are independent and do not interact with each other, is simply given as N times of electric field generated by a single molecule. However, when the optical chromophores (molecules) are dissolved in an isotropic medium such as solution, the orientation of each individual molecule is random without any long-range orientation correlation. In this case, the measured signal field should be the rotational average so that the corresponding tensorial response function should be rotationally averaged over the randomly oriented molecules. If the tensor $\mathbf{t}^{(n)}$ in a molecule-fixed frame is known, the averaged $\mathbf{T}^{(n)}$ tensor in a laboratory-fixed frame is related to $\mathbf{t}^{(n)}$ as

$$\widehat{T}^{(n)}_{l_1l_2l_3\cdots l_n} = I^{(n)}_{l_1l_2l_3\cdots l_n;m_1m_2m_3\cdots m_n} t^{(n)}_{m_1m_2m_3\cdots m_n} \tag{3.68}$$

where m_k is one of the three Cartesian axes in the molecule-fixed frame. The molecular properties $t^{(n)}_{m_1m_2m_3\cdots m_n}$ in a given molecule-fixed frame can be calculated by using various methods such as *ab initio* calculations, molecular dynamics simulations, quantum mechanical/molecular mechanical simulations, *ab initio* molecular dynamics simulations, and so forth. $I^{(n)}_{l_1l_2l_3\cdots l_n;m_1m_2m_3\cdots m_n}$ plays a crucial role in connecting the tensorial molecular properties in a molecule-fixed frame to those in a laboratory-fixed frame, and detailed expressions for $I^{(n)}_{l_1l_2l_3\cdots l_n;m_1m_2m_3\cdots m_n}$ have been well known.[17] In the present section, we will just summarize the results for the sake of completeness.

For $n = 2$, the only rotationally invariant tensor is the Kronecker delta function, so that we have

$$I^{(2)} = \frac{1}{3}\delta_{l_1l_2}\delta_{m_1m_2}. \tag{3.69}$$

Here, $\delta_{xx} = \delta_{yy} = \delta_{zz} = 1$ and $\delta_{jk} = 0$ for $j \neq k$. For example, the ZZ tensor element of $\mathbf{T}^{(2)}$ is given as

$$\widehat{T}_{ZZ}^{(2)} = \frac{1}{3}\delta_{ZZ}\sum_{m_1,m_2}\delta_{m_1m_2}t_{m_1m_2}^{(2)} = \frac{1}{3}\sum_{m}t_{mm}^{(2)} = \frac{1}{3}\left(t_{xx}^{(2)} + t_{yy}^{(2)} + t_{zz}^{(2)}\right). \tag{3.70}$$

Throughout this book, the notation $\widehat{T}^{(n)}$ means that it is the rotational average over the randomly oriented molecules in an isotropic medium such as solution. The x, y, and z are the three Cartesian coordinates in a molecule-fixed frame, whereas X, Y, and Z are those in a laboratory-fixed frame.

For $n = 3$, the Levi–Civita epsilon is the only isomer that is rotationally invariant. Therefore, we have

$$I^{(3)} = \frac{1}{6}\varepsilon_{l_1l_2l_3}\varepsilon_{m_1m_2m_3}, \tag{3.71}$$

where the Levi–Civita epsilon tensor elements are $\varepsilon_{XYZ} = \varepsilon_{YZX} = \varepsilon_{ZXY} = -\varepsilon_{XZY} = -\varepsilon_{YXZ} = -\varepsilon_{ZYX} = 1$ and $\varepsilon_{ijk} = 0$ (for all the other cases). As an example, consider the XYZ tensor element of $\mathbf{T}^{(3)}$. Its rotationally averaged element is

$$\widehat{T}_{XYZ}^{(3)} = \frac{1}{6}\varepsilon_{XYZ}\sum_{m_1,m_2,m_3}\varepsilon_{m_1m_2m_3}t_{m_1m_2m_3}^{(3)} = \frac{1}{6}\left\{t_{xyz}^{(3)} + t_{yzx}^{(3)} + t_{zxy}^{(3)} - t_{xzy}^{(3)} - t_{yxz}^{(3)} - t_{zyx}^{(3)}\right\}. \tag{3.72}$$

For $n = 4$, we have

$$I^{(4)} = \frac{1}{30}\left(\delta_{l_1l_2}\delta_{l_3l_4} \quad \delta_{l_1l_3}\delta_{l_2l_4} \quad \delta_{l_1l_4}\delta_{l_2l_3}\right)\begin{pmatrix} 4 & -1 & -1 \\ -1 & 4 & -1 \\ -1 & -1 & 4 \end{pmatrix}\begin{pmatrix} \delta_{m_1m_2}\delta_{m_3m_4} \\ \delta_{m_1m_3}\delta_{m_2m_4} \\ \delta_{m_1m_4}\delta_{m_2m_3} \end{pmatrix}. \tag{3.73}$$

For $n = 5$, we have

$$\begin{aligned} I^{(5)} = \frac{1}{30}(&\varepsilon_{l_1l_2l_3}\delta_{l_4l_5}\varepsilon_{m_1m_2m_3}\delta_{m_4m_5} + \varepsilon_{l_1l_2l_4}\delta_{l_3l_5}\varepsilon_{m_1m_2m_4}\delta_{m_3m_5} + \varepsilon_{l_1l_2l_5}\delta_{l_3l_4}\varepsilon_{m_1m_2m_5}\delta_{m_3m_4} \\ &+ \varepsilon_{l_1l_3l_4}\delta_{l_2l_5}\varepsilon_{m_1m_3m_4}\delta_{m_2m_5} + \varepsilon_{l_1l_3l_5}\delta_{l_2l_4}\varepsilon_{m_1m_3m_5}\delta_{m_2m_4} + \varepsilon_{l_1l_4l_5}\delta_{l_2l_3}\varepsilon_{m_1m_4m_5}\delta_{m_2m_3} \\ &+ \varepsilon_{l_2l_3l_4}\delta_{l_1l_5}\varepsilon_{m_2m_3m_4}\delta_{m_1m_5} + \varepsilon_{l_2l_3l_5}\delta_{l_1l_4}\varepsilon_{m_2m_3m_5}\delta_{m_1m_4} + \varepsilon_{l_2l_4l_5}\delta_{l_1l_3}\varepsilon_{m_2m_4m_5}\delta_{m_1m_3} \\ &+ \varepsilon_{l_3l_4l_5}\delta_{l_1l_2}\varepsilon_{m_3m_4m_5}\delta_{m_1m_2}). \end{aligned} \tag{3.74}$$

One can find the corresponding expressions for higher-order tensors in literatures, but they are not needed in this book.

3.4 LINEAR ABSORPTION SPECTROSCOPY

The linear absorption spectroscopy within the electric dipole approximation (or long-wavelength limit) is fully described by the expectation value of time-evolved electric dipole operator when the radiation–matter interaction Hamiltonian is given as

$$H_{rad\text{-}mat}(t) = -\boldsymbol{\mu} \cdot \mathbf{E}(\mathbf{r},t) = -\mu_j E_j(\mathbf{r},t), \tag{3.75}$$

where the Einstein summation convention was used and the electric field is

$$\mathbf{E}(\mathbf{r},t) = \mathbf{E}^{+}(\mathbf{r},t) + \mathbf{E}^{-}(\mathbf{r},t) = \mathbf{e}E(t)e^{i\mathbf{k}_1\cdot\mathbf{r}-i\omega_1 t} + \mathbf{e}^{*}E^{*}(t)e^{-i\mathbf{k}_1\cdot\mathbf{r}+i\omega_1 t}. \tag{3.76}$$

The unit vector along the direction of the electric field polarization is denoted as **e**. In general, the unit vector **e** can be complex when the beam polarization state is not linearly polarized, for example, circularly or elliptically polarized beams. However, except for the cases when one is interested in linear and nonlinear optical activity measurements, which will be discussed in Chapters 15 and 16, we will consider the cases when the incident beams are linearly polarized. Thus, the $\mathbf{e}^{*}$ in the second term on the right-hand side of Equation 3.76 can be replaced with **e**. Nevertheless, one should not forget about the general complex nature of **e** when the incident beam polarization state is circularly or elliptically polarized.

In the case of the light absorption, the cause operator, its conjugate external field, and effect operator are given as

$$\hat{A} = \boldsymbol{\mu}, \quad F = \mathbf{E}(\mathbf{r},t), \quad \text{and} \quad \hat{B} = \boldsymbol{\mu}. \tag{3.77}$$

From the linear response theory, the expectation value of $\boldsymbol{\mu}$ at time t, which is the linear polarization, is given as[4]

$$\begin{aligned} \mathbf{P}^{(1)}(\mathbf{r},t) &= \boldsymbol{\mu}^{(1)}(\mathbf{r},t) = \left\langle \hat{\boldsymbol{\mu}} \overset{\boldsymbol{\mu}\mathbf{E}}{\Longleftarrow} \rho(t_0) \right\rangle \\ &= \int_0^{\infty} d\tau\, \phi_{\mu\mu}(\tau) \cdot \mathbf{E}(\mathbf{r},t-\tau) \end{aligned} \tag{3.78}$$

where the dipole-dipole linear response function, which is a second-rank tensor, is

$$\phi_{\mu\mu}(\tau) \equiv \frac{i}{\hbar}\theta(\tau) < [\boldsymbol{\mu}(\tau), \boldsymbol{\mu}(0)]\rho(-\infty) >. \tag{3.79}$$

Because it was assumed that the number density of the optical chromophore is a unity, $\mathbf{P}^{(1)}(t) = \bar{\boldsymbol{\mu}}^{(1)}(t)$. Ignoring the nonlinear polarization, from the Maxwell's field equation for a transverse field, we have

$$\nabla^2 \mathbf{E}(\mathbf{r},t) - \frac{1}{c^2}\frac{\partial^2}{\partial t^2}\mathbf{E}(\mathbf{r},t) = \frac{4\pi}{c^2}\frac{\partial^2}{\partial t^2}\mathbf{P}^{(1)}(\mathbf{r},t). \tag{3.80}$$

Defining the time-dependent dielectric function as

$$\boldsymbol{\varepsilon}(t) \equiv \delta(t)\mathbf{I} + 4\pi\phi_{\mu\mu}(t), \tag{3.81}$$

one can rewrite Equation 3.80 as

$$\nabla^2 \mathbf{E}(\mathbf{r},t) - \frac{1}{c^2}\frac{\partial^2}{\partial t^2}\left[\int_{-\infty}^{t} d\tau\, \boldsymbol{\varepsilon}(t-\tau)\cdot \mathbf{E}(\mathbf{r},\tau)\right] = 0. \tag{3.82}$$

I is the 3 by 3 identity matrix. Hereafter, we will use the following notation for the product of an nth-rank tensor $\mathbf{T}^{(n)}$ and n-1 vectors, $\mathbf{v}_1 - \mathbf{v}_{n-1}$, to obtain a new vector **V**:

$$\mathbf{V} = \mathbf{T}^{(n)} \otimes \mathbf{v}_1\mathbf{v}_2\cdots\mathbf{v}_{n-1} \tag{3.83}$$

where the jth element of **V** is, when $v_k^{m_1}$ denotes the m_ith element of the $\mathbf{v}_k$ vector,

$$V_j = \sum_{m_1,m_2,\cdots m_{n-1}=x,y,z} T^{(n)}_{jm_1m_2\cdots m_{n-1}} v_1^{m_1} v_2^{m_2} \cdots v_{n-1}^{m_{n-1}}. \tag{3.84}$$

For instance, $(\boldsymbol{\varepsilon}\cdot\mathbf{E})_X = \varepsilon_{XX}E_X + \varepsilon_{XY}E_Y + \varepsilon_{XZ}E_Z$.

Now, let us consider the simple optical measurement of absorption of a weak stationary plane wave propagating along the Z direction in a linear and isotropic medium. The incident electric field is assumed to be linearly polarized along the X-direction, that is, $\mathbf{e} = \hat{X}$. Within the electric-dipole approximation, the XX tensor element of the dielectric function is the only one required, and its Fourier transform will be denoted as $\varepsilon(\omega)$, which is related to the complex susceptibility as

$$\varepsilon(\omega) = 1 + 4\pi\chi(\omega). \tag{3.85}$$

Then, assuming that the solution of the above field equation in Equation 3.82 is given as

$$\mathbf{E}(Z,t) = E_0\hat{X}\exp(ikZ - i\omega t), \tag{3.86}$$

inserting Equation 3.86 into 3.82 and taking the Fourier transform of the resultant equation, one can find the dispersion relationship

$$\frac{kc}{\omega} = \sqrt{\varepsilon(\omega)} \equiv n(\omega) + i\kappa(\omega). \tag{3.87}$$

Here $n(\omega)$ and $\kappa(\omega)$ are the index of refraction and the extinction coefficient, respectively. Therefore, the electric field at Z in the optical medium is

$$\mathbf{E}(Z,t) = E_0\hat{X}\exp(ik'(\omega)Z - i\omega t - \kappa_a(\omega)Z/2), \tag{3.89}$$

where k' is the wavevector of the electric field in the medium, and $\kappa_a(\omega)$ is the absorption coefficient. These two frequency-dependent functions are given as

$$k'(\omega) \equiv k_0 n(\omega) \tag{3.90}$$

$$\kappa_a(\omega) \equiv 2k_0\kappa(\omega). \tag{3.91}$$

Here, the vacuum wavevector ω/c is denoted as k_0. Note that the field intensity, which is the square of the electric field amplitude, exponentially decays with the decaying constant of $\kappa_a(\omega)$ as it propagates through the absorptive (lossy) medium. From the definition of the time-dependent dielectric function, $\varepsilon(t)$, and the definition of the susceptibility in Equation 3.85, we have

$$\sqrt{1 + 4\pi\chi'(\omega) + 4\pi i\chi''(\omega)} = n(\omega) + i\kappa(\omega). \tag{3.92}$$

For $1 + 4\pi\chi'(\omega) >> 4\pi\chi''(\omega)$, we obtain

$$n(\omega) = \sqrt{1 + 4\pi\chi'(\omega)} \tag{3.93}$$

$$\kappa(\omega) = \frac{2\pi\chi''(\omega)}{n(\omega)}. \tag{3.94}$$

The absorption coefficient $\kappa_a(\omega)$ is thus related to the imaginary part of the susceptibility as

$$\kappa_a(\omega) = \frac{4\pi\omega}{n(\omega)c}\chi''(\omega) = \frac{4\pi\omega}{n(\omega)c}\int_0^\infty dt\,\hat{\phi}_{\mu\mu}(t)\sin\omega t, \tag{3.95}$$

where the XX tensor element of the rotationally averaged linear response function $\hat{\boldsymbol{\phi}}_{\mu\mu}(t)$ was denoted as $\hat{\phi}_{\mu\mu}(t)$.

The absorption coefficient can be determined by properly calculating the dipole-dipole linear response function $\phi_{\mu\mu}(t)$. Using the line-broadening function, we obtained the linear response function in Equation 3.42. In the present case of the electric-dipole-allowed light absorption process for a two-level system, after rotational averaging of the dipole-dipole response function we have

$$\hat{\phi}_{\mu\mu}(t) = \frac{i}{3\hbar}\theta(t)\,|\boldsymbol{\mu}_{ge}|^2\,\{e^{-i\bar{\omega}_{eg}t - g(t)} - e^{i\bar{\omega}_{eg}t - g^*(t)}\}. \tag{3.96}$$

Since the above linear response function is the rotationally averaged one, the factor 1/3 appears on the right-hand side of Equation 3.96. Here, the transition electric dipole matrix element was defined as $\boldsymbol{\mu}_{ge} \equiv \langle g|\hat{\mu}|e\rangle$. The absorption coefficient is

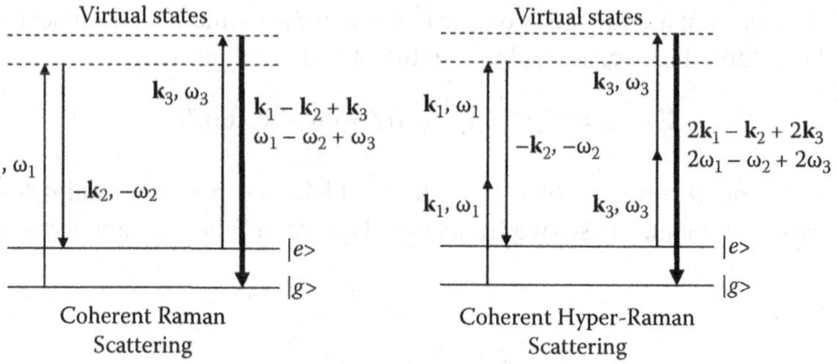

FIGURE 3.2 Time-resolved coherent Raman and hyper-Raman scatterings.

therefore given as

$$\kappa_a(\omega) = -\frac{8\pi\omega}{n(\omega)\hbar c} |\mu_{ge}|^2 \int_0^\infty dt \, \mathrm{Im}[e^{-i\bar{\omega}_{eg}t - g(t)}] \sin \omega t. \quad (3.97)$$

Using a few models for $g(t)$ discussed in Section 3.2, one can directly obtain the corresponding analytical expressions for the absorption line shape determined by the frequency-dependent absorption coefficient.

3.5 RAMAN SCATTERING

Rayleigh and Raman scatterings are two-photon processes with one-photon absorption and one-photon emission.[9] In the Raman scattering, the final state of the molecule is different from the initial state, and usually the two states are vibrational eigenstates (See Figure 3.2). Instead of spontaneous Raman scattering in frequency domain, we shall focus on the coherent Raman scattering (CRS) in time domain.[18–21] Furthermore, the electromagnetic field frequency is assumed to be nonresonant with any electronic transitions so that the ground state vibrational dynamics can only be probed. Later, the connection between the optically heterodyne-detected CRS and the spontaneous Raman scattering will be discussed.

The effective radiation–matter interaction Hamiltonian for the light scattering is

$$H_{rad-mat} = -\boldsymbol{\mu}_{ind}(\mathbf{r},t) \cdot \mathbf{E}(\mathbf{r},t), \quad (3.98)$$

where the induced dipole is given as

$$\boldsymbol{\mu}_{ind}(\mathbf{r},t) = \sum_{n=1} \boldsymbol{\mu}_{ind}^{(n)}(\mathbf{r},t) = \boldsymbol{\alpha} \cdot \mathbf{E}(\mathbf{r},t) + \boldsymbol{\beta} : \mathbf{E}^2(\mathbf{r},t) + \boldsymbol{\gamma} \vdots \mathbf{E}^3(\mathbf{r},t) + \cdots. \quad (3.99)$$

The expansion coefficients in this equation are polarizability, hyperpolarizability, and second hyperpolarizability, respectively, for the first three terms.[3] In the cases of the Raman and Rayleigh scatterings, the first term in Equation 3.99 is responsible for such a two-photon scattering process. Consequently, the effective radiation–matter interaction Hamiltonian is given as

$$H_{rad-mat} = -\boldsymbol{\alpha} : \mathbf{E}^2(\mathbf{r},t). \tag{3.100}$$

This is the second conjugate pair in Scheme 3.1. The electronic ground state polarizability operator is defined as

$$\boldsymbol{\alpha}(\omega) \equiv \frac{1}{\hbar}\sum_{e \neq g} \frac{\boldsymbol{\mu}\,|\,e\rangle\langle e\,|\,\boldsymbol{\mu}}{\omega_{eg} - \omega} + \frac{\boldsymbol{\mu}\,|\,e\rangle\langle e\,|\,\boldsymbol{\mu}}{\omega_{eg} + \omega}, \tag{3.101}$$

where the summation is over all possible quantum states except for the ground state.

Coherent Raman scattering measurement has been carried out by employing one of the transient grating configurations.[22] Two pump pulses with center frequencies ω_1 and ω_2 and wavevectors $\mathbf{k}_1$ and $\mathbf{k}_2$ are used to create transient grating with wavevector $\mathbf{k}_1 - \mathbf{k}_2$ in the sample, and the transient grating oscillates in time with frequency $\omega_1 - \omega_2$. After a finite delay time T, a third pulse with frequency ω_3 and wavevector $\mathbf{k}_3$ is injected into the sample to stimulate a scattering process. The scattering signal field with wavevector $\mathbf{k}_1 - \mathbf{k}_2 + \mathbf{k}_3$ is then detected. From the linear response theory, the two pump pulse-matter interactions can be treated with a single effective radiation–matter interaction Hamiltonian in Equation 3.100. The interaction between the ω_1-field propagating in the direction of $\mathbf{k}_1$ and molecular polarizability creates an induced dipole, which then interacts with the ω_2-field propagating toward $-\mathbf{k}_2$ direction. Since the two pump pulses overlap in time, there is no time-ordering of these two radiation–matter interactions. However, due to the phase-matching condition, one can selectively measure a specific signal field emitting toward the specific direction of $\mathbf{k}_1 - \mathbf{k}_2 + \mathbf{k}_3$. Now, the third pulse field component propagating in the direction of $\mathbf{k}_3$ again creates an oscillating induced dipole. In this case of the CRS spectroscopy, the cause operator, its conjugate external field, and effect operator are given as

$$\hat{A} = \boldsymbol{\alpha} \cdot \mathbf{E}_1(\mathbf{r},t), \quad F = \mathbf{E}_2(\mathbf{r},t) \quad \text{and} \quad \hat{B} = \boldsymbol{\alpha} \cdot \mathbf{E}_3(\mathbf{r},t). \tag{3.102}$$

Therefore, the coherent light-scattering process is to measure the expectation value of the electric dipole induced by the third field when the molecule effectively interacts with the first two external fields via Equation 3.100.

The electric field in a CRS experiment consists of three modes,

$$\mathbf{E}(\mathbf{r},t) = \mathbf{e}_1 E_1(t+T)\,e^{i\mathbf{k}_1\cdot\mathbf{r} - i\omega_1 t} + \mathbf{e}_2 E_2(t+T)\,e^{i\mathbf{k}_2\cdot\mathbf{r} - i\omega_2 t} + \mathbf{e}_3 E_3(t)\,e^{i\mathbf{k}_3\cdot\mathbf{r} - i\omega_3 t} + c.c.. \tag{3.103}$$

The effective radiation–matter interaction Hamiltonian that creates Raman-active vibrational coherences in the optical sample is

$$H_{rad-mat} = -\boldsymbol{\alpha} : \mathbf{E}_2^*(t+T)\mathbf{E}_1(t+T)\,e^{i(\mathbf{k}_1-\mathbf{k}_2)\cdot\mathbf{r} - i(\omega_1-\omega_2)t}. \tag{3.104}$$

The induced dipole that is responsible for the creation of scattering field is then

$$\boldsymbol{\mu}_{ind}(\mathbf{r},t) = \boldsymbol{\alpha} \cdot \mathbf{E}_3(t)\, e^{i\mathbf{k}_3\cdot\mathbf{r} - i\omega_3 t}. \tag{3.105}$$

From the linear response theory, one can find that the expectation value of the above induced dipole operator at time t is

$$\bar{\boldsymbol{\mu}}_{ind}(\mathbf{r},t) = <\boldsymbol{\alpha}\cdot\mathbf{E}_3 \overset{\boldsymbol{\alpha}\mathbf{E}_2^*\mathbf{E}_1}{\Longleftarrow} \rho(t_0)>$$

$$= e^{i(\mathbf{k}_1-\mathbf{k}_2+\mathbf{k}_3)\cdot\mathbf{r} - i(\omega_1-\omega_2+\omega_3)t} E_3(t)\int_0^\infty d\tau\, \phi_{\alpha\alpha}(\tau) \vdots \mathbf{e}_3\mathbf{e}_2\mathbf{e}_1 E_2^*(t+T-\tau)E_1(t+T-\tau)\, e^{i(\omega_1-\omega_2)\tau}. \tag{3.106}$$

Here, the polarizability–polarizability response function, which is a fourth-rank tensor, is defined as

$$\phi_{\alpha\alpha}(\tau) \equiv \frac{i}{\hbar}\theta(\tau) < [\boldsymbol{\alpha}(\tau), \boldsymbol{\alpha}(0)]\rho(-\infty) >$$

$$= \frac{i}{\hbar}\theta(\tau)\boldsymbol{\alpha}_{ge}\boldsymbol{\alpha}_{eg}\{e^{-i\bar{\omega}_{eg}\tau - g(\tau)} - e^{i\bar{\omega}_{eg}\tau - g^*(\tau)}\}. \tag{3.107}$$

It is noted that the expectation value of $\boldsymbol{\mu}_{ind}(\mathbf{r},t)$ is linearly proportional to each of the three electric field amplitudes. Therefore, the CRS process shown here is a third-order nonlinear optical spectroscopy with respect to the external electric field amplitude. However, since the timescale of the electronic coherence evolution is extremely short in comparison with the nuclear dynamics in the electronic ground state, it was possible to reduce the third-order nonlinear optical process to a linear response optical process. The CRS polarization, $\mathbf{P}_{CRS}(\mathbf{r},t) = \bar{\boldsymbol{\mu}}_{ind}(\mathbf{r},t)$, given in Equation 3.106 is then written as

$$\mathbf{P}_{CRS}(\mathbf{r},t) = \mathbf{P}_{CRS}(t)\, e^{i(\mathbf{k}_1-\mathbf{k}_2+\mathbf{k}_3)\cdot\mathbf{r} - i(\omega_1-\omega_2+\omega_3)t}, \tag{3.108}$$

where the temporal envelope of the CRS polarization is given as

$$\mathbf{P}_{CRS}(t) = E_3(t)\int_0^\infty d\tau\, \phi_{\alpha\alpha}(\tau) \vdots \mathbf{e}_3\mathbf{e}_2^*\mathbf{e}_1 E_2^*(t+T-\tau)E_1(t+T-\tau)\, e^{i(\omega_1-\omega_2)\tau}. \tag{3.109}$$

Now, the above third-order polarization acts like a source for generating an electric field. From Maxwell's equations, one can obtain the relationship between the nonlinear polarization and thus generated electric field. Detailed derivation along this line is presented in the Appendix. From Equation A.3.6, we find that the CRS electric field is given as

$$\mathbf{E}_{CRS}(t) \propto i\omega_s E_3(t)\int_0^\infty d\tau\, \phi_{\alpha\alpha}(\tau) \vdots \mathbf{e}_3\mathbf{e}_2^*\mathbf{e}_1 E_2^*(t+T-\tau)E_1(t+T-\tau)\, e^{i(\omega_1-\omega_2)\tau}. \tag{3.110}$$

Depending on the detection method, either homodyne or heterodyne, the intensity ($|\mathbf{E}_{CRS}(t)|^2$) or amplitude ($\mathbf{E}_{CRS}(t)$) can be measured experimentally. In the frequency domain, the CRS is induced by temporally broad fields so that the pulse envelop functions are assumed to be almost constant in comparison to the time scale of Raman response function at least. In this case, the frequency-domain CRS field intensity is found to be

$$S_{CRS}(\omega_1 - \omega_2) \propto \left| \int_0^\infty d\tau \phi_{\alpha\alpha}(\tau) \vdots \mathbf{e}_3 \mathbf{e}_2^* \mathbf{e}_1 \, e^{i(\omega_1-\omega_2)\tau} \right|^2 . \tag{3.111}$$

For the sake of comparison, we provide an expression for the spontaneous Raman scattering:

$$\mathbf{S}_{SRS}(\omega_1 - \omega_2) \propto \int_{-\infty}^{\infty} d\tau < \boldsymbol{\alpha}(\tau)\boldsymbol{\alpha}(0)\rho(-\infty) > e^{i(\omega_1-\omega_2)\tau}, \tag{3.112}$$

which is a fourth-rank tensor.

EXERCISE 3.6

The Kramers-Heisenberg equation for light scattering is well known and can be found in many literatures. Show that the Kramers-Heisenberg theory is consistent with the Fourier transform expression of the spontaneous Raman scattering in Equation 3.112.

Using the results in Section 3.3, one can perform the rotational averaging of the fourth-rank tensorial polarizability-polarizability response function and find the relationship between a specific tensor element in a laboratory-fixed frame to those in a molecule-fixed frame. The conventional depolarized Raman signal corresponds to the *YZYZ* tensor element of $\mathbf{S}_{SRS}$ in Equation 3.112, and the spectrum $S_{SRS}^{YZYZ}(\omega = \omega_1 - \omega_2)$ peaks when the frequency ω becomes identical to a molecular vibrational frequency. Using the fluctuation-dissipation theorem, one can obtain the relationship between the *YZYZ* tensor element of the CRS susceptibility and the depolarized Raman spectrum $S_{SRS}^{YZYZ}(\omega_1 - \omega_2)$ as[20]

$$\chi_{CRS}^{YZYZ}(\omega) \propto (1 - e^{-\hbar\omega/k_B T})^{-1} \, \mathrm{Im}\left[\chi_{SRS}^{YZYZ}(\omega)\right] \tag{3.113}$$

where

$$\chi_{CRS}^{YZYZ}(\omega) = \int_0^\infty d\tau \hat{\phi}_{\alpha\alpha}^{YZYZ}(\tau) e^{i\omega\tau} . \tag{3.114}$$

Here, $\hat{\phi}_{\alpha\alpha}^{YZYZ}$ represents the *YZYZ* tensor element of the rotationally averaged polarizability-polarizability response function of molecules in an isotropic medium.

EXERCISE 3.7

What are the Raman selection rules? For a solution sample, what are the rotationally invariant CRS susceptibility tensor elements?

3.6 HYPER-RAMAN SCATTERING

Hyper-Raman scattering spectroscopy in frequency domain has been found to be useful for measuring the transition probability involving a three-photon process. Two photons are absorbed by molecules, and one photon with twice the energy of the absorbed photon is emitted. If the difference between the emitted field frequency and twice the absorbed field frequency is close to the frequency of a hyper-Raman-active mode, the hyper-Raman scattering is resonantly enhanced. In this case, the second-order induced dipole should be used to describe the effective radiation–matter interaction, and the induced dipole is

$$\boldsymbol{\mu}_{ind}^{(2)}(\mathbf{r},t) \cong \boldsymbol{\beta} : \mathbf{E}^2(\mathbf{r},t), \tag{3.115}$$

and the effective radiation–matter interaction is described as

$$H_{rad-mat} = -\boldsymbol{\beta} \vdots \mathbf{E}^3(\mathbf{r},t). \tag{3.116}$$

Depending on the definition of the first hyperpolarizability $\boldsymbol{\beta}$, there appears a constant factor 1/2 or 1/6 in literatures—note that it depends on whether the Taylor expansion of radiation–matter interaction energy or of electric field-induced dipole with respect to electric field is considered. However, such a constant factor will be omitted in the following description of the hyper-Raman scattering spectroscopy in the present section.

We will specifically consider the coherent hyper-Raman scattering (CHRS) experiment based on a transient grating configuration (See Figure 3.2). Two pump pulses with center frequencies ω_1 and ω_2 ($\approx 2\omega_1$) and wavevectors $\mathbf{k}_1$ and $\mathbf{k}_2$ are used to create vibrational transient grating with wavevector $2\mathbf{k}_1 - \mathbf{k}_2$ in the sample, and thus generated transient grating oscillates in time with frequency $2\omega_1 - \omega_2$. In this particular case, the frequency-dependent hyperpolarizability operator is defined as[5]

$$\begin{aligned}\boldsymbol{\beta}(\omega_1,\omega_2) \equiv \frac{1}{\hbar^2}\sum_{e\neq g}\sum_{f\neq g} \boldsymbol{\mu}|e\rangle\langle e|\boldsymbol{\mu}|f\rangle\langle f|\boldsymbol{\mu}\Bigg(&\frac{1}{(\omega_{fg}-\omega_1)(\omega_{eg}-\omega_2)} \\ &+\frac{1}{(\omega_{fg}-\omega_2)(\omega_{eg}-\omega_1)}+\frac{1}{(\omega_{fg}-\omega_1)(\omega_{eg}+\omega_1)}+\frac{1}{(\omega_{fg}+\omega_1)(\omega_{eg}-\omega_1)} \\ &+\frac{1}{(\omega_{fg}+\omega_2)(\omega_{eg}+\omega_1)}+\frac{1}{(\omega_{fg}+\omega_1)(\omega_{eg}+\omega_2)}\Bigg).\end{aligned} \tag{3.117}$$

It should be noted that the $\mathbf{k}_1$ field interacts twice with the molecule, and that the frequency of the ω_2-field is close to $2\omega_1$ but not exactly $2\omega_1$. After a finite delay time T, a third pulse with frequency ω_3 ($\approx \omega_1$) and wavevector $\mathbf{k}_3$ is injected into the sample to stimulate the CHRS process. The intensity or amplitude of the signal field with wavevector $2\mathbf{k}_1 - \mathbf{k}_2 + 2\mathbf{k}_3$ is detected. The first three radiation–matter interactions are therefore treated with the effective radiation–matter Hamiltonian in Equation 3.116.

That is to say, the two interactions between the ω_1-field and molecular hyperpolarizability create an induced dipole, which then interacts with the ω_2-field. Now, the third ($\mathbf{k}_3$-) pulse again creates an induced dipole by two interactions with the same molecule, and thus the induced dipole radiates the scattering field whose frequency is $2\omega_1 - \omega_2 + 2\omega_3$. In this case of the CHRS spectroscopy, the cause operator, its conjugate external field, and effect operator are given as

$$\hat{A} = \boldsymbol{\beta} : \mathbf{E}_1^2(\mathbf{r},t), \quad F = \mathbf{E}_2(\mathbf{r},t), \quad \text{and} \quad \hat{B} = \boldsymbol{\beta} : \mathbf{E}_3^2(\mathbf{r},t). \tag{3.118}$$

The electric field used for such a CHRS experiment is

$$\mathbf{E}(\mathrm{r},t) = \mathbf{e}_1 E_1(t+T)\,\mathrm{e}^{i\mathbf{k}_1\cdot\mathbf{r}-i\omega_1 t} + \mathbf{e}_2 E_2(t+T)\,\mathrm{e}^{i\mathbf{k}_2\cdot\mathbf{r}-i\omega_2 t} + \mathbf{e}_3 E_3(t)\,\mathrm{e}^{i\mathbf{k}_3\cdot\mathbf{r}-i\omega_3 t} + c.c.. \tag{3.119}$$

The effective radiation–matter interaction Hamiltonian that creates hyper-Raman-active vibrational coherences in the optical sample is

$$H_{rad-mat} = -\boldsymbol{\beta} \vdots \mathbf{e}_2^*\mathbf{e}_1\mathbf{e}_1 E_2^*(t+T) E_1^2(t+T)\,\mathrm{e}^{i(2\mathbf{k}_1-\mathbf{k}_2)\cdot\mathbf{r}-i(2\omega_1-\omega_2)t}. \tag{3.120}$$

The induced dipole that is responsible for the creation of CHRS field is then

$$\boldsymbol{\mu}_{ind}(\mathbf{r},t) = \boldsymbol{\beta} : \mathbf{e}_3\mathbf{e}_3 E_3^2(t)\,\mathrm{e}^{2i\mathbf{k}_3\cdot\mathbf{r}-2i\omega_3 t}. \tag{3.121}$$

From the linear response theory, one can find that the expectation value of the above induce dipole at time t is given by

$$\begin{aligned}\bar{\boldsymbol{\mu}}_{ind}(\mathbf{r},t) &= \left\langle \boldsymbol{\beta}\mathbf{E}_3^2 \overset{\boldsymbol{\beta}\mathbf{E}_2^*\mathbf{E}_1^2}{\Longleftarrow\!\!\!\wr\!\!\!=} \rho(t_0) \right\rangle \\ &= \mathrm{e}^{i(2\mathbf{k}_1-\mathbf{k}_2+2\mathbf{k}_3)\cdot\mathbf{r}-i(2\omega_1-\omega_2+2\omega_3)t}\, E_3^2(t)\int_0^\infty d\tau\,\phi_{\beta\beta}(\tau) \vdots \mathbf{e}_3\mathbf{e}_3\mathbf{e}_2^*\mathbf{e}_1\mathbf{e}_1 \\ &\quad \times E_2^*(t+T-\tau)E_1^2(t+T-\tau)\,\mathrm{e}^{i(2\omega_1-\omega_2)\tau}. \end{aligned} \tag{3.122}$$

Here, the hyperpolarizability–hyperpolarizability response function, which is a sixth-rank tensor, is defined as

$$\phi_{\beta\beta}(\tau) \equiv \frac{i}{\hbar}\theta(\tau) < [\boldsymbol{\beta}(\tau),\boldsymbol{\beta}(0)]\rho(-\infty) > = \frac{i}{\hbar}\theta(\tau)\boldsymbol{\beta}_{ge}\boldsymbol{\beta}_{eg}\{e^{-i\bar{\omega}_{eg}\tau-g(\tau)} - e^{i\bar{\omega}_{eg}\tau-g^*(\tau)}\}. \tag{3.123}$$

From Equation 3.122, one can find that the CHRS process is a fifth-order nonlinear optical spectroscopy with respect to external electric field amplitude. The coherent hyper-Raman polarization, $\mathbf{P}_{CHRS}(\mathbf{r},t) = \bar{\boldsymbol{\mu}}_{ind}(\mathbf{r},t)$, given in Equation 3.122 is then written as

$$\mathbf{P}_{CHRS}(\mathbf{r},t) = \mathrm{P}_{CHRS}(t)\,\mathrm{e}^{i(2\mathbf{k}_1-\mathbf{k}_2+2\mathbf{k}_3)\cdot\mathbf{r}-i(2\omega_1-\omega_2+2\omega_3)t} \tag{3.124}$$

where the temporal envelope of the CHRS polarization is given as

$$\mathbf{P}_{CHRS}(t) = E_3^2(t)\int_0^{\infty} d\tau \widehat{\phi}_{\beta\beta}(\tau) \otimes \mathbf{e}_3\mathbf{e}_3\mathbf{e}_2^*\mathbf{e}_1\mathbf{e}_1 E_2^*(t+T-\tau)E_1^2(t+T-\tau)e^{i(2\omega_1-\omega_2)\tau}. \tag{3.125}$$

Solving the corresponding Maxwell equation with the above CHRS polarization treated as a source term, the CHRS electric field generated is given as

$$\mathbf{E}_{CHRS}(t) \propto i\omega_s \mathbf{P}_{CHRS}(t). \tag{3.126}$$

In frequency domain, the CHRS is induced by temporally broad fields so that the pulse envelope functions are assumed to be constant in comparison to the time scales of hyper-Raman nuclear motions. The frequency-domain CRS field intensity is then found to be

$$S_{CHRS}(2\omega_1 - \omega_2) \propto \left| \int_0^{\infty} d\tau \widehat{\phi}_{\beta\beta}(\tau) \otimes \mathbf{e}_3\mathbf{e}_3\mathbf{e}_2^*\mathbf{e}_1\mathbf{e}_1\, e^{i(2\omega_1-\omega_2)\tau} \right|^2. \tag{3.127}$$

The spontaneous hyper-Raman scattering signal, which is a sixth-rank tensor, is expressed as

$$S_{SHRS}(\omega_1 - \omega_2) \propto \int_{-\infty}^{\infty} d\tau < \beta(\tau)\beta(0)\rho(-\infty) > e^{i(2\omega_1-\omega_2)\tau}. \tag{3.128}$$

Using the fluctuation-dissipation theorem, one can find the relationship between the spontaneous hyper-Raman scattering spectrum and the Fourier-transformed CHRS signal.

EXERCISE 3.8

What are the hyper-Raman selection rules? Compare them with those of IR absorption and Raman scattering.

3.7 IR-RAMAN SURFACE VIBRATIONAL SPECTROSCOPY

The IR-vis sum frequency generation (IV-SFG) is a three-wave-mixing process, and it has been found to be a useful surface vibrational spectroscopy.[6, 23] An IR beam that is tuned to be in resonance with a certain vibrational mode of molecules adsorbed on surface or at interface is used to create a vibrational coherence. Then, an electronically nonresonant visible beam interacts with the molecule again, and thus created electronic coherence or generated induced dipole radiates IR-vis sum frequency field. Therefore, the IV-SFG can be viewed as an IR excitation–Raman detection technique. Thus, it will be referred to as IR-Raman vibrational spectroscopy. In another section we will consider the other case of the so-called Raman-IR surface vibrational spectroscopy, where a vibrational coherence is created by a Raman process and then the radiated IR signal field is detected.

The IV-SFG has been known as one of the second-order optical processes, because the IV-SFG signal field amplitude is proportional to both IR and visible field amplitudes. However, still it can be considered as a linear response spectroscopy, since it probes the linear response of the molecular system with respect to the incident IR beam. Note that the difference between this and conventional IR spectroscopy is that the probing of vibrational coherence dynamics is performed by using a stimulated Raman measurement. In this section, we will mainly consider the time-domain coherent IV-SFG measurement.[7] We assume that the IR pulse precedes the visible pulse by a finite delay time T. The first radiation–matter interaction Hamiltonian is as usual given as

$$H_{rad\text{-}mat}(t) = -\boldsymbol{\mu}\cdot\mathbf{E}_{IR}(\mathbf{r},t), \tag{3.129}$$

where

$$\mathbf{E}_{IR}(\mathbf{r},t) = \mathbf{e}_{IR}E_{IR}(t+T)e^{i\mathbf{k}_{IR}\cdot\mathbf{r}-i\omega_{IR}t} + c.c. \tag{3.130}$$

The IV-SFG polarization is the expectation value of the induced dipole at time t, where the visible beam-induced dipole operator is

$$\boldsymbol{\mu}_{ind}(\mathbf{r},t) = \boldsymbol{\alpha}\cdot\mathbf{E}_{vis}(t)e^{i\mathbf{k}_{vis}\cdot\mathbf{r}-i\omega_{vis}t}. \tag{3.131}$$

Here, the $\mathbf{E}^{+}_{vis}(\mathbf{r},t)$ component is only considered, since the corresponding radiation–matter interaction is an absorptive process. For this surface IR-Raman spectroscopy, the cause operator, its conjugate external field, and effect operator are thus given as

$$\hat{A} = \boldsymbol{\mu}, \quad F = \mathbf{E}_{IR}(\mathbf{r},t), \quad \text{and} \quad \hat{B} = \boldsymbol{\alpha}\cdot\mathbf{E}^{+}_{vis}(\mathbf{r},t). \tag{3.132}$$

The expectation value of the above induced dipole in Equation 3.131 is then found to be

$$\mathbf{P}_{IR\text{-}Raman}(\mathbf{r},t) = \langle \boldsymbol{\alpha}\mathbf{E}_{vis} \overset{\boldsymbol{\mu}\mathbf{E}_{IR}}{\Longleftarrow} \rho(t_0)\rangle$$

$$= e^{i(\mathbf{k}_{IR}+\mathbf{k}_{vis})\cdot\mathbf{r}-i(\omega_{IR}+\omega_{vis})t}E_{vis}(t)\int_0^\infty d\tau\,\phi_{\alpha\mu}(\tau):\mathbf{e}_{vis}\mathbf{e}_{IR}E_{IR}(t+T-\tau)e^{i\omega_{IR}\tau}. \tag{3.133}$$

Note that the phase-matching condition suggests that the IV-SFG field radiated by the above polarization propagates in the direction of $\mathbf{k}_{IR}+\mathbf{k}_{vis}$ and oscillates with frequency $\omega_{IR}+\omega_{vis}$. Here, the dipole-polarizability response function, which is a third-rank tensor, is defined as

$$\phi_{\alpha\mu}(\tau) \equiv \frac{i}{\hbar}\theta(\tau) < [\alpha(\tau), \mu(0)]\rho(-\infty) > . \tag{3.134}$$

For a two-level system, we have

$$\phi_{\alpha\mu}(\tau) = \frac{i}{\hbar}\theta(\tau)\alpha_{ge}\mu_{eg}\{e^{-i\bar{\omega}_{eg}\tau - g(\tau)} - e^{i\bar{\omega}_{eg}\tau - g^*(\tau)}\}. \tag{3.135}$$

This result shows that the IV-SFG-active vibrational mode should be both Raman- and IR-active, which is a critical selection rule for the IV-SFG.

From Equation 3.133, the temporal envelop of the IV-SFG polarization is given as

$$\mathbf{P}_{IR-Raman}(t) = E_{vis}(t)\int_0^\infty d\tau\,\phi_{\alpha\mu}(\tau) : \mathbf{e}_{vis}\mathbf{e}_{IR}E_{IR}(t+T-\tau)e^{i\omega_{IR}\tau}. \tag{3.136}$$

The signal field amplitude is, with the phase-matching geometry,

$$\mathbf{E}_{IR-Raman}(t) \propto i\omega_s E_{vis}(t)\int_0^\infty d\tau\,\phi_{\alpha\mu}(\tau) : \mathbf{e}_{vis}\mathbf{e}_{IR}E_{IR}(t+T-\tau)e^{i\omega_{IR}\tau}. \tag{3.137}$$

Note that the signal field amplitude depends on the delay time T. If the IR pulse width is much smaller than the time scales of nuclear vibrations, one can assume that $E_{IR}(t+T-\tau) = E_{IR}\delta(t+T-\tau)$. Then, the signal field amplitude becomes simplified as

$$\mathbf{E}_{IR-Raman}(t) \propto i\omega_s E_{vis}(t)\phi_{\alpha\mu}(t+T) : \mathbf{e}_{vis}\mathbf{e}_{IR}. \tag{3.138}$$

If the temporal envelope of the incident visible pulse is short enough to replace that with a Dirac's delta function, the measured signal field amplitude with respect to the delay time T is just linearly proportional to the dipole-polarizability response function, $\phi_{\alpha\mu}(T) : \mathbf{e}_{vis}\mathbf{e}_{IR}$. One can easily obtain the IV-SFG susceptibility by using Equations 3.41 and 3.135 so that we won't provide any further discussion on the frequency-domain IV-SFG. Before this section is closed, it should be mentioned that the dipole-polarizability response function for molecules adsorbed on surface or at interface should be averaged over all possible orientations of adsorbed molecules. Let us denote the orientation distribution function as $P(\theta, \phi)$. Then, the averaged signal field that is directly related to experimental observable is given as

$$\hat{\mathbf{E}}_{IR-Raman}(t) = \frac{1}{4\pi}\int d\theta \sin\theta \int d\phi\, \mathbf{E}^{(2)}_{IR-Raman}(t;\theta,\phi)P(\theta,\phi). \tag{3.139}$$

Thus, the surface-specific vibrational spectra via IV-SFG measurements can provide detailed information on the orientation distribution of adsorbed molecules on surface.

3.8 RAMAN-IR SURFACE VIBRATIONAL SPECTROSCOPY

The IV-SFG spectroscopy discussed earlier is to measure the vibrational coherence created by the interaction between an IR field and a resonant vibrational mode. Instead, it is possible to use two (or one impulsive) electronically nonresonant beams to create vibrational coherences of Raman-active modes and then to detect coherently radiated IR signal field. The energy-level diagram for such a Raman-IR (surface difference frequency generation) experiment is shown in Figure 3.3. In this case, the effective radiation–matter interaction Hamiltonian is

$$H_{rad-mat} = -\boldsymbol{\alpha} : \mathbf{E}^2(\mathbf{r},t). \tag{3.140}$$

Particularly, let us consider the case when two pump pulses with center frequencies ω_1 and ω_2 and wavevectors $\mathbf{k}_1$ and $\mathbf{k}_2$ are used to create transient grating with wavevector $\mathbf{k}_1 - \mathbf{k}_2$ in the sample on surface or at interface. Then, the coherently radiated field toward the direction of $\mathbf{k}_1 - \mathbf{k}_2$ with frequency $\omega_1 - \omega_2$ is detected. The interaction between the ω_1-field propagating in the $\mathbf{k}_1$ direction and molecular polarizability creates an induced dipole, which then interacts with the ω_2-field propagating in the $-\mathbf{k}_2$ direction. Since the two pump pulses overlap in time, there is no time-ordering of these two radiation–matter interactions. However, due to the phase-matching condition, the signal field emitting in the specific direction of $\mathbf{k}_1 - \mathbf{k}_2$ can be selectively measured.

For this surface Raman-IR spectroscopy, the cause operator, its conjugate external field, and effect operator are given as

$$\hat{A} = \boldsymbol{\alpha} \cdot \mathbf{E}_1(\mathbf{r},t), \quad F = \mathbf{E}_2(\mathbf{r},t), \quad \text{and} \quad \hat{B} = \boldsymbol{\mu}. \tag{3.141}$$

Here, the total electric field used for this CRS experiment is given as

$$\mathbf{E}(\mathrm{r},t) = \mathbf{e}_1 E_1(t) e^{i\mathbf{k}_1\cdot\mathbf{r}-i\omega_1 t} + \mathbf{e}_2 E_2(t) e^{i\mathbf{k}_2\cdot\mathbf{r}-i\omega_2 t} + c.c.. \tag{3.142}$$

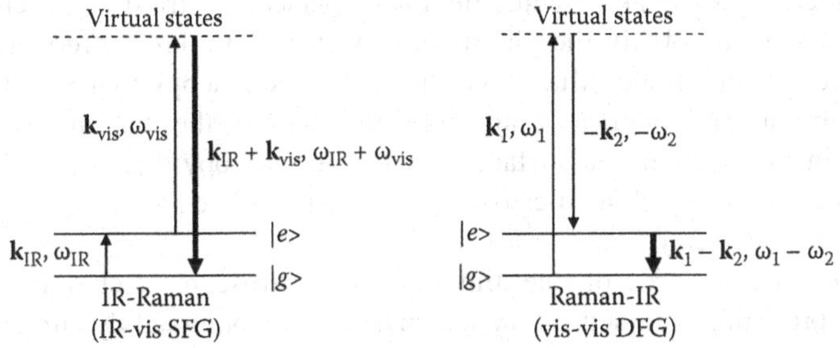

FIGURE 3.3 Time-resolved IR-Raman (IR-vis sum frequency generation) and Raman-IR (vis–vis difference frequency generation) spectroscopy.

Since the effective radiation–matter interaction Hamiltonian that creates Raman-active vibrational coherences in the optical sample is

$$H_{rad-mat} = -\boldsymbol{\alpha} : \mathbf{e}_2^* \mathbf{e}_1 E_2^*(t) E_1(t) e^{i(\mathbf{k}_1-\mathbf{k}_2)\cdot\mathbf{r}-i(\omega_1-\omega_2)t} \tag{3.143}$$

the Raman-IR polarization, from the linear response theory, is found to be

$$\mathbf{P}_{Raman-IR}^{(2)}(\mathbf{r},t)$$

$$= <\boldsymbol{\mu} \overset{\alpha \mathbf{E}_2^* \mathbf{E}_1}{\Longleftarrow} \rho(t_0)>$$

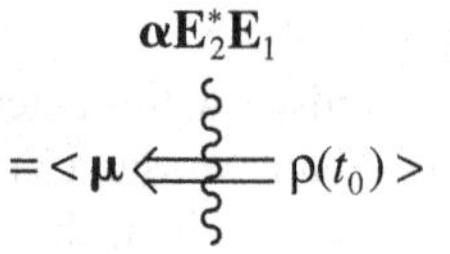

$$= e^{i(\mathbf{k}_1+\mathbf{k}_2)\cdot\mathbf{r}-i(\omega_1+\omega_2)t} \int_0^\infty d\tau\, \phi_{\mu\alpha}(\tau) : \mathbf{e}_2^* \mathbf{e}_1 E_2^*(t-\tau) E_1(t-\tau) e^{i(\omega_1-\omega_2)\tau}. \tag{3.144}$$

Here, the polarizability-dipole response function, which is a third-rank tensor, is defined as

$$\phi_{\mu\alpha}(\tau) \equiv \frac{i}{\hbar}\theta(\tau) < [\boldsymbol{\mu}(\tau),\boldsymbol{\alpha}(0)]\rho(-\infty)>. \tag{3.145}$$

Note that the selection rule of this Raman-IR spectroscopy is that the vibrational degrees of freedom should be both IR- and Raman-active, which is identical to that of the IR-Raman spectroscopy discussed earlier.

The present Raman-IR spectroscopy is surface-specfic Raman spectroscopy. Therefore, noting that the IR-Raman spectroscopy is a surface-specific IR spectroscopy, the Raman-IR spectroscopy can provide complementary information on the Raman-active modes of molecules on surface or at interface. In addition, by using a femtosecond laser pulse to create a spectrally wide range of vibrational coherences and by detecting the dispersed spectrum of the emitted IR signal field, one can obtain the vibrational spectrum in a broad frequency range in femtosecond time scale. Much like the CRS spectroscopy that has been used to study vibrational dynamics of molecules in solutions, the Raman-IR technique discussed in this section is a surface Raman spectroscopy that should be of use for studying vibrational dynamics of molecules on surface and at interface with a broken centrosymmetry.

We thus have a series of one-dimensional spectroscopic techniques that are capable of providing complementary information on vibrational dynamics. The IR absorption and Raman scattering are useful vibrational spectroscopic methods for molecules in an isotropic medium. On the other hand, the IR-Raman and Raman-IR three-wave-mixing spectroscopic methods discussed above are surface vibrational spectroscopy and form complementary tools.

APPENDIX: NONLINEAR POLARIZATION AND GENERATED SIGNAL ELECTRIC FIELD

In this appendix, a theoretical description of the relationship between the nonlinear polarization and signal electric field generated is presented. Let us consider the case when the nonlinear polarization created in the optical medium is given as

$$\mathbf{P}^{(n)}(\mathbf{r},t) = \mathbf{P}^{(n)}(t)\exp(i\mathbf{k}_s \cdot \mathbf{r} - i\omega_s t), \tag{A.3.1}$$

where $\mathbf{k}_s$ and ω_s are the wavevector and frequency of the material polarization. Let us assume that the direction of $\mathbf{k}_s$ vector is taken to be along the Z-axis and that the optical sample thickness is L. The above nonlinear polarization is then the source for generating a new electric field. In the limiting case when the signal field is weakly absorbed by the optical medium, the linear susceptibility is purely real and the Maxwell equation for the electric field is

$$\nabla \times \nabla \times \mathbf{E}(\mathbf{r},t) + \frac{n^2}{c^2}\frac{\partial^2}{\partial t^2}\mathbf{E}(\mathbf{r},t) = -\frac{4\pi}{c^2}\frac{\partial^2}{\partial t^2}\mathbf{P}^{(n)}(\mathbf{r},t). \tag{A.3.2}$$

Note that the refractive index n is related to the real part of the linear susceptibility as Equation 3.93. For the nonlinear polarization given in Equation A.3.1, we look for a solution for $\mathbf{E}(\mathbf{r},t)$ of the form:

$$\mathbf{E}^{(n)}(\mathbf{r},t) = \mathbf{E}^{(n)}(t)\exp(i\mathbf{k}'_s \cdot \mathbf{r} - i\omega_s t) + c.c.. \tag{A.3.3}$$

In general, due to the frequency dependency of the refractive index $n(\omega)$, the wavevector of the newly generated electric field, $\mathbf{k}'_s$, can be slightly different from $\mathbf{k}_s$. Now, assuming that the temporal envelopes of $\mathbf{P}^{(n)}(\mathbf{r},t)$ and $\mathbf{E}^{(n)}(\mathbf{r},t)$, which were denoted as $\mathbf{P}^{(n)}(t)$ and $\mathbf{E}^{(n)}(t)$, respectively, are slowly varying functions in time in comparison with the optical period, we get

$$ik'_s \frac{\partial}{\partial z}\mathbf{E}^{(n)}(t) = -\frac{2\pi\omega_s^2}{c^2}\mathbf{P}^{(n)}(t)\exp\{i\Delta k_s z\}, \tag{A.3.4}$$

where $\Delta k_s = |\mathbf{k}_s - \mathbf{k}'_s|$. The electric field amplitude at the rear boundary at $z = L$, is obtained by taking integration of Equation A.3.4 from 0 to L, and we get

$$\mathbf{E}^{(n)}(t) = \frac{2\pi i\omega_s L}{n(\omega_s)c}\mathbf{P}^{(n)}(t)\exp(i\Delta k_s L/2)\frac{\sin(\Delta k_s L/2)}{\Delta k_s L/2}. \tag{A.3.5}$$

The phase-matching condition is the case when $\sin(\Delta k_s L/2)/(\Delta k_s L/2)$ can be approximated as a Dirac delta function. In this ideally phase-matched case, we have

$$\mathbf{E}^{(n)}(t) \propto i\omega_s \mathbf{P}^{(n)}(t). \tag{A.3.6}$$

Note that the signal electric field amplitude is linearly proportional to the nonlinear polarization amplitude.

REFERENCES

1. Bloembergen, N., *Nonlinear optics*. W. A. Benjamin, Inc.: Reading, MA, 1965.
2. Butcher, P. N.; Cotter, D., *The elements of nonlinear optics*. Cambridge University Press: Cambridge, 1990.
3. Shen, Y. R., *The principles of nonlinear optics*. John Wiley & Sons: New York, 1984.
4. Mukamel, S., *Principles of nonlinear optical spectroscopy*. Oxford University Press: Oxford, 1995.
5. Cho, M., Off-resonant coherent hyper-Raman scattering spectroscopy. *Journal of Chemical Physics* 1997, 106, 7550–7557.
6. Shen, Y. R., Surface-properties probed by 2nd-harmonic and sum frequency generation. *Nature* 1989, 337, 519–525.
7. Cho, M., Time-resolved vibrational optical activity measurement by the infrared-visible sum frequency-generation with circularly polarized infrared light. *Journal of Chemical Physics* 2002, 116, 1562–1570.
8. Schatz, G. C., Ratner, M. A., *Quantum mechanics in chemistry*. Prentice-Hall: Englewood Cliffs, 1993.
9. McQuarrie, D. A., *Statistical mechanics*. Harper & Row: New York, 1976.
10. Berne, B. J.; Pecora, R., *Dynamic light scattering*. J. Wiley: New York, 1976.
11. Barron, L. D.; Bogaard, M. P.; Buckingham, A. D., Raman scattering of circularly polarized light by optically-active molecules. *Journal of the American Chemical Society* 1973, 95, 603–605.
12. Barron, L. D.; Hecht, L.; Blanch, E. W.; Bell, A. F., Solution structure and dynamics of biomolecules from Raman optical activity. *Progress in Biophysics and Molecular Biology* 2000, 73, 1–49.
13. Nafie, L. A., Theory of Raman scattering and Raman optical activity: Near resonance theory and levels of approximation. *Theoretical Chemistry Accounts* 2008, 119, 39–55.
14. Fleming, G. R.; Cho, M., Chromophore-solvent dynamics. *Annual Review of Physical Chemistry* 1996, 47, 109–134.
15. Kubo, R., A stochastic theory of line-shape and relaxation. In *Fluctuation, Relaxation and Resonance in Magnetic Systems*, Ter Haar, D., Ed., Oliver and Boyd: London, 1961.
16. Schofield, P., Space-time correlation function formalism for slow neutron scattering. *Physical Review Letters* 1960, 4, 239–240.
17. Craig, D. P.; Thirunamachandran, T., *Molecular quantum electrodyanmics: An introduction to radiation molecule interactions*. Dover Publications, Inc.: New York, 1998.
18. Lotshaw, W. T.; Mcmorrow, D.; Kalpouzos, C.; Kenney-Wallace, G. A., Femtosecond dynamics of the optical Kerr effect in liquid nitrobenzene and chlorobenzene. *Chemical Physics Letters* 1987, 136, 323–328.
19. Ruhman, S.; Joly, A. G.; Nelson, K. A., Time-resolved observations of coherent molecular vibrational motion and the general occurrence of impulsive stimulated scattering. *Journal of Chemical Physics* 1987, 86, 6563–6565.
20. Cho, M.; Du, M.; Scherer, N. F.; Fleming, G. R.; Mukamel, S., Off-resonant transient birefringence in liquids. *Journal of Chemical Physics* 1993, 99, 2410–2428.
21. Yan, Y. J.; Mukamel, S., Pulse shaping and coherent Raman-spectroscopy in condensed phases. *Journal of Chemical Physics* 1991, 94, 997–1005.
22. Fayer, M. D., Dynamics of molecules in condensed phases: Picosecond holographic grating experiments. *Annual Review of Physical Chemistry* 1982, 33, 63–87.
23. Zhu, X. D.; Suhr, H.; Shen, Y. R., Surface vibrational spectroscopy by infrared-visible sum frequency generation. *Physical Review B* 1987, 35, 3047–3050.

4 Second-Order Response Spectroscopy

If a spectroscopic observable is linearly proportional to an effective radiation–matter interaction and is fully described by the corresponding linear response function, it was considered to be a linear response spectroscopic technique. In the chapter entitled "Linear Response Spectroscopy," a few different linear spectroscopic methods were discussed in detail. In time-domain experiments, one can measure the linear response of the optical sample as a function of time T. In principle, the same molecular responses and spectroscopic properties are included in the linear susceptibility in frequency domain, because the frequency-dependent susceptibility is related to the time-domain response function via Fourier-Laplace transformation.

Now, two-dimensional (2D) spectroscopy is defined as a method that the spectroscopic observable is a function of two different time variables or conjugate frequency variables that are experimentally controlled.[1–5] There are numerous 2D spectroscopic methods differing from one another by the sequence of radiation–matter interactions inducing multiple optical transitions between matter's quantum states.[1, 6] Depending on the number of effective field-matter interactions, one can classify those multidimensional spectroscopic methods as second-, third-, or even higher-order nonlinear spectroscopy.

One of the interesting 2D spectroscopies is doubly resonant SFG, where two different incident field frequencies ω_1 and ω_2 are tuned to be in resonances with two different electronic or vibrational transitions. Then, the measured SFG signal field amplitude or intensity becomes a function of the two frequencies ω_1 and ω_2. For instance, if ω_1 and ω_2 are close to two vibrational transition frequencies ω_a and ω_b, the SFG spectrum in a two-dimensionally displayed frequency space would exhibit a peak at $\omega_1 = \omega_a$ and $\omega_2 = \omega_b$. It was shown that such a cross-peak when $\omega_a \neq \omega_b$ results from mechanical and/or electric anharmonicity-induced couplings, which are critically dependent on the structure and dynamics of molecules in general. This will be discussed in a later chapter. The SFG spectroscopy involves two radiation–matter interactions. However, there are many different types of 2D spectroscopic methods, much like the cases of various linear spectroscopic methods that are different from one another by the involved effective radiation–matter interactions chosen from the list in Scheme 3.1.

In this book, the second-order response spectroscopy refers to the case when a spectroscopic observable is second order with respect to the *effective* radiation-matter interaction Hamiltonians listed in Scheme 3.1. Then, the corresponding second-order response in time is a function of two time variables, t_1 and t_2. The second-order susceptibility is thus a 2D function of the conjugate Fourier frequencies ω_1 and ω_2. Here, it should be mentioned that the second-order response spectroscopy does not refer to those whose signal intensity is proportional to the square of incident electric field intensity. Bearing this in mind, let us consider the radiation–matter interaction Hamiltonian associated with the second-order response spectroscopy,

$$H_{rad\text{-}mat}(t) = -\hat{\mathbf{V}}_1 \cdot \mathbf{F}_1(\mathbf{r},t) - \hat{\mathbf{V}}_2 \cdot \mathbf{F}_2(\mathbf{r},t) \tag{4.1}$$

where seven possible conjugate pairs of $\hat{\mathbf{V}}$ and $\mathbf{F}(\mathbf{r},t)$ were discussed in Chapter 3 (see Scheme 3.1). From the definition of the second-order response spectroscopy above, the signal amplitude (intensity) is then linearly proportional to external field amplitudes $\mathbf{F}_1$ and $\mathbf{F}_2$ (intensities $|\mathbf{F}_1|^2$ and $|\mathbf{F}_2|^2$). Here, the external field $\mathbf{F}(\mathbf{r},t)$ can be $\mathbf{E}(\mathbf{r},t)$, $\mathbf{B}(\mathbf{r},t)$, $\nabla\mathbf{E}(\mathbf{r},t)$, $\mathbf{E}^2(\mathbf{r},t)$, $\mathbf{E}(\mathbf{r},t)\,\mathbf{B}(\mathbf{r},t)$, $\mathbf{B}(\mathbf{r},t)\,\mathbf{E}(\mathbf{r},t)$, $\mathbf{E}(\mathbf{r},t)\nabla\mathbf{E}(\mathbf{r},t)$, $(\nabla\mathbf{E}(\mathbf{r},t))\,\mathbf{E}(\mathbf{r},t)$, or $\mathbf{E}^3(\mathbf{r},t)$, depending on the effective radiation–matter interaction Hamiltonian that is relevant to specific experiment of interest.

Although one particular type of 2D spectroscopic techniques, which was based on the second-order response measurement, was mentioned above (e.g., SFG), there is another type of 2D spectroscopy that has been extensively used. Two representative examples are 2D pump–probe and photon echo methods, and they are based on a four-wave-mixing scheme.[1–4, 7] Using three laser pulses to create two electronic or vibrational coherences separated in time T, one can measure the correlation amplitude of the two coherences in time. This is known as photon echo.[8–10] The 2D photon echo spectrum have been obtained by taking double Fourier-Laplace transformations of the time-resolved photon echo signal.[2, 3, 11] However, in this case the spectroscopic observable, for example, heterodyne-detected photon echo spectrum, is produced by three radiation–matter (electric dipole-electric field) interactions. We shall classify such type of 2D spectroscopy as a third-order response measurement method, because it involves three radiation–matter interactions even though its 2D representation in the frequency domain has been reported for the sake of simplicity in presenting the complicated four-dimensional data, that is, signal amplitude versus three conjugate Fourier frequencies.

In this chapter, we shall focus on the second-order response spectroscopy. Depending on the choice of the two effective radiation–matter interaction energy operators in Equation 4.1, there are a number of different second-order response spectroscopic methods in general. Among them, only a few simple cases will be discussed in detail, but the other possibilities can be easily explored by using the general theoretical framework presented in this chapter.

4.1 SECOND-ORDER RESPONSE FUNCTION

The observable in a second-order response spectroscopy is assumed to be represented by an effect operator $\hat{B}$. The second-order response spectroscopy involves two actions of cause operators that could be identical to or different from each other. The two cause operators are denoted as $\hat{A}_1$ and $\hat{A}_2$ and the conjugate external fields are $F_1(t)$ and $F_2(t)$, respectively. The cause operators can induce quantum transitions between the system's two different stationary states. Then, the total Hamiltonian can be written as

$$\hat{H}(t) = \hat{H}_0(t) + \hat{H}'(t) = \hat{H}_0(t) - \hat{A}_1 F_1(t) - \hat{A}_2 F_2(t). \tag{4.2}$$

The expectation value of $\hat{B}$ is measured at time t, when the matter interacted with both $F_1(t)$ and $F_2(t)$. We now look for the convolution expression for the expectation value of the effect-operator $\hat{B}$ at time t, that is, $\overline{B}(t)$, in terms of the second-order response function and external fields. In particular, we will consider the case when $\overline{B}(t)$ is linearly proportional to both $F_1(t)$ and $F_2(t)$. Without loss of generality, we shall assume that the radiation–matter interaction $F_1(t)$ field precedes that with $F_2(t)$ field. In frequency domain, one should include all possible permutations of radiation–matter interaction sequences.

From the second-order time-dependent perturbation theory (see Equations 2.80 and 2.92), we have

$$\overline{B}(t) = <\hat{B}\rho^{(2)}_{A_2A_1}(t)>$$

$$= <\hat{B}$$ 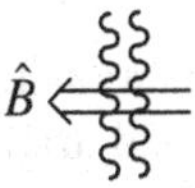 $$\rho(t_0)>$$

$$= \left(\frac{i}{\hbar}\right)^2 \int_{t_0}^{t} d\tau_2 \int_{t_0}^{\tau_2} d\tau_1 <\hat{B}V_0(t,\tau_2)L'(\tau_2)V_0(\tau_2,\tau_1)L'(\tau_1)V_0(\tau_1,t_0)\rho(t_0)>$$

$$= \left(\frac{i}{\hbar}\right)^2 \int_{t_0}^{t} d\tau_2 \int_{t_0}^{\tau_2} d\tau_1 <[[\hat{B}(t),\hat{A}_2(\tau_2)],\hat{A}_1(\tau_1)]\rho(t_0)> F_2(\tau_2)F_1(\tau_1). \tag{4.3}$$

Now, changing the integration variables and assuming $t_0 = -\infty$, we find that

$$\overline{B}(t) = \int_0^\infty dt_2 \int_0^\infty dt_1 \phi_{BA_2A_1}(t_2,t_1)F_2(t-t_2)F_1(t-t_2-t_1). \tag{4.4}$$

The second-order response function is defined as

$$\phi_{BA_2A_1}(t_2,t_1) = \left(\frac{i}{\hbar}\right)^2 \theta(t_2)\theta(t_1) <[[\hat{B}(t_2+t_1),\hat{A}_2(t_1)],\hat{A}_1(0)]\rho(-\infty)>. \tag{4.5}$$

Due to the causality condition, two heavy-side step functions are included in Equation 4.5. Expanding the two commutators in Equation 4.5, one can rewrite it as

$$\begin{aligned}\phi_{BA_2A_1}(t_2,t_1) = \left(\frac{i}{\hbar}\right)^2 \theta(t_2)\theta(t_1)\{&<\hat{B}(t_2+t_1)\hat{A}_2(t_1)\hat{A}_1(0)\rho(-\infty)> \\ &-<\hat{A}_2(t_1)\hat{B}(t_2+t_1)\hat{A}_1(0)\rho(-\infty)> \\ &-<\hat{A}_1(0)\hat{B}(t_2+t_1)\hat{A}_2(t_1)\rho(-\infty)> \\ &+<\hat{A}_1(0)\hat{A}_2(t_1)\hat{B}(t_2+t_1)\rho(-\infty)>\}.\end{aligned} \tag{4.6}$$

Inserting Equation 4.6 into Equation 4.4 for $\bar{B}(t)$ gives four different terms and the corresponding diagrams are

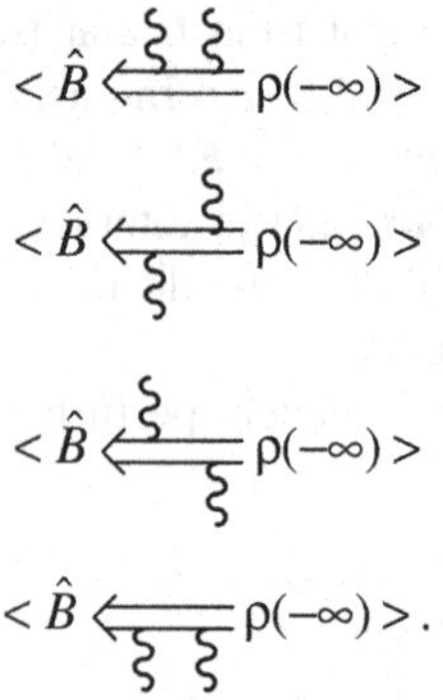

(4.7)

The physical meaning of the second-order response function in Equation 4.4 can be understood by considering the limiting case when the first pulsed field arrives at the optical sample first at $t = -T$ and the second pulse does at $t = 0$. Then, the external fields are approximately written as

$$F_1(t) = F_1\delta(t+T)e^{-i\omega_1 t}$$

$$F_2(t) = F_2\delta(t)e^{-i\omega_2 t}. \tag{4.8}$$

In this impulsive limit, we have

$$\bar{B}(t) = F_1F_2\phi_{BA_2A_1}(t,T)\exp(i\omega_1 T). \tag{4.9}$$

This shows that the second-order response function describes the average B value of matter that has experienced two time-separated external perturbations by F_1 and F_2 at $t = 0$ and $t = T$. Since there are two controllable time delays between the first and second pulsed fields and between the second pulsed field and the measurement time t, the observable $\bar{B}(t)$ is a function of two time variables, that is, $\bar{B}(t,T)$. Then, two-dimensional Fourier transformation of $\bar{B}(t,T)$ with respect to t and T gives the 2D spectrum $\tilde{\bar{B}}(\omega_t,\omega_T)$. This is why the second-order response spectroscopy is a 2D technique that is capable of providing critical information on nonlinear optical properties as well as on structure and dynamics of molecules under investigation. In a later chapter we will show that the second-order response spectroscopy can be of use to delineate hidden secondary spectroscopic properties such as electric and mechanical anharmonicity-induced couplings between two different vibrational modes.

Now, because of the causality conditions, one can rewrite Equation 4.4 as

$$\bar{B}(t) = \int_{-\infty}^{\infty} dt_2 \int_{-\infty}^{\infty} dt_1 \phi_{BA_2A_1}(t_2,t_1)F_2(t-t_2)F_1(t-t_2-t_1). \tag{4.10}$$

Considering the Fourier transforms of the two external fields and of the second-order response function,

$$\tilde{F}_1(\omega) = \int_{-\infty}^{\infty} dt\, F_1(t) e^{i\omega t}$$

$$\tilde{F}_2(\omega) = \int_{-\infty}^{\infty} dt F_2(t) e^{i\omega t}$$

$$\chi_{BA_2A_1}(\omega_2,\omega_1) = \int_{-\infty}^{\infty} dt_2 \int_{-\infty}^{\infty} dt_1 \phi_{BA_2A_1}(t_2,t_1) e^{i\omega_2 t_2 + i\omega_1 t_1}, \tag{4.11}$$

one can rewrite the expectation value of the effect operator $\hat{B}$ as

$$\bar{B}(t) = \left(\frac{1}{2\pi}\right)^2 \int_{-\infty}^{\infty} d\omega_2 \int_{-\infty}^{\infty} d\omega_1 \chi_{BA_2A_1}(\omega_2+\omega_1,\omega_1)\tilde{F}_2(\omega_2)\tilde{F}_1(\omega_1)e^{-i(\omega_2+\omega_1)t}. \tag{4.12}$$

In the case when the measured value is detected in frequency domain, the spectrum of $\bar{B}(t)$ can be directly measured and it is given as

$$\tilde{\bar{B}}(\omega) = \left(\frac{1}{2\pi}\right) \int_{-\infty}^{\infty} d\omega_2 \int_{-\infty}^{\infty} d\omega_1\, \chi_{BA_2A_1}(\omega_2+\omega_1,\omega_1)\tilde{F}_2(\omega_2)\tilde{F}_1(\omega_1)\delta(\omega-\omega_2-\omega_1)$$

$$= \left(\frac{1}{2\pi}\right) \int_{-\infty}^{\infty} d\omega_1 \chi_{BA_2A_1}(\omega,\omega_1)\tilde{F}_2(\omega-\omega_1)\tilde{F}_1(\omega_1). \tag{4.13}$$

Complete information on the second-order response of molecular system against the external perturbation $\hat{H}'(t)(= -\hat{A}_1F_1(t) - \hat{A}_2F_2(t))$ is thus included in either the second-order response function $\phi_{BA_2A_1}(t_2,t_1)$ in time domain or the 2D susceptibility $\chi_{BA_2A_1}(\omega_2,\omega_1)$ in frequency domain. Since the impulsive limit of the second-order response spectroscopy was already discussed above, let us consider the other limiting case that the temporal envelope functions of the external fields are constant in time. Assuming that the two field frequencies are denoted as Ω_1 and Ω_2, we have

$$\tilde{F}_1(\omega) = 2\pi i F_1\{\delta(\omega-\Omega_1) - \delta(\omega+\Omega_1)\}$$

$$\tilde{F}_2(\omega) = 2\pi i F_2\{\delta(\omega-\Omega_2) - \delta(\omega+\Omega_2)\}. \tag{4.14}$$

Then,

$$\bar{B}(t) = F_1F_2\left\{\chi_{BA_2A_1}(-\Omega_2+\Omega_1,\Omega_1)e^{i(\Omega_2-\Omega_1)t} + \chi_{BA_2A_1}(\Omega_2-\Omega_1,-\Omega_1)e^{-i(\Omega_2-\Omega_1)t}\right.$$

$$\left. - \chi_{BA_2A_1}(\Omega_2+\Omega_1,\Omega_1)e^{-i(\Omega_2+\Omega_1)t} - \chi_{BA_2A_1}(-\Omega_2-\Omega_1,-\Omega_1)e^{i(\Omega_2+\Omega_1)t}\right\}. \tag{4.15}$$

Using a specific experimental scheme, one can measure one of the four terms separately. In particular, the first and second terms describe difference frequency generation (DFG) processes because its oscillation frequency is identical to the difference of the two external field frequencies. On the other hand, the third and fourth terms are related to SFGs.

4.2 THREE-LEVEL SYSTEM AND LINE-BROADENING FUNCTION

The linear response spectroscopy discussed in a previous chapter has been found to be useful to probe a single quantum transition between two stationary states of matter. However, the second-order response requires at least two radiation–matter interaction-induced transitions so that a three-level system (3LS) can be the simplest but useful model to be considered. The 3LS Hamiltonian is written as

$$\hat{H}_{3LS} = |e> \hbar\omega_{eg} <e| + |f> \hbar\omega_{fg} <f|. \tag{4.16}$$

Here, in addition to the ground and excited states, $|g>$ and $|e>$, the ket vector of the third state denoted as $|f>$ is needed.

For example, doubly resonant SFG involves a sequence of transition from g to e to f state, where the third state is one of the high-lying excited states that is accessible from e as well as from g via electric-dipole-induced optical transitions. The above 3LS is also a good model for vibrational states of an anharmonic oscillator. Most of 2D vibrational spectroscopy of anharmonic oscillators involves vibrational transitions up to the second excited state, which is either overtone or combination state. For a single anharmonic oscillator, the fundamental transition frequency is $\omega_{eg} = \omega_e - \omega_g$. The frequency difference between the second excited (overtone) state and the first excited state, $\omega_{fe} = \omega_f - \omega_e$, is slightly different from ω_{eg} due to the overtone anharmonicity of the potential function.

When three-level chromophores are dissolved in solution, system–bath interactions cause fluctuations of transition frequencies, dephasing, relaxation, spectral diffusion, and so on. The matter Hamiltonian therefore consists of three terms,

$$\hat{H}_{mat} = \hat{H}_{3LS} + \hat{H}_B + \hat{H}_{SB}. \tag{4.17}$$

The system–bath (chromophore–bath) interaction Hamiltonian, denoted as $\hat{H}_{SB}$, is assumed to be diagonal with respect to the system eigenstates as

$$\hat{H}_{SB} = V_{eg}(\mathbf{q})|e><e| + V_{fg}(\mathbf{q})|f><f|, \tag{4.18}$$

where the bath degrees of freedom are denoted as $\mathbf{q}$ and the potential energy differences between a pair of system states are defined as

$$\begin{aligned} V_{eg}(\mathbf{q}) &= V_e(\mathbf{q}) - V_g(\mathbf{q}) \\ V_{fg}(\mathbf{q}) &= V_f(\mathbf{q}) - V_g(\mathbf{q}) \\ V_{fe}(\mathbf{q}) &= V_f(\mathbf{q}) - V_e(\mathbf{q}). \end{aligned} \tag{4.19}$$

Therefore, we have

$$\hat{H}_{mat} = \sum_{m=g,e,f} \{\hbar\omega_m + V_m(\mathbf{q}) + H_B(\mathbf{q})\} | m >< m | = \hat{H}_0 + \hat{H}' \tag{4.20}$$

where

$$\hat{H}_0 = \{\hbar\omega_g + V_g(\mathbf{q}) + H_B(\mathbf{q})\} \sum_{m=g,e,f} | m >< m |$$

$$\hat{H}' = \sum_{m=g,e,f} \{\hbar\omega_{mg} + V_{mg}(\mathbf{q})\} | m >< m | . \tag{4.21}$$

We will consider the ground-state adiabatic Hamiltonian $\hat{H}_g(\mathbf{q})$, which is defined as $\hat{H}_g(\mathbf{q}) = \hbar\omega_g + V_g(\mathbf{q}) + H_B(\mathbf{q})$, as the reference Hamiltonian. Then, $\hat{H}_e(\mathbf{q})$ and $\hat{H}_f(\mathbf{q})$ can be written as

$$\hat{H}_e(\mathbf{q}) = \hat{H}_g(\mathbf{q}) + \hbar\omega_{eg} + V_{eg}(\mathbf{q})$$

$$\hat{H}_f(\mathbf{q}) = \hat{H}_g(\mathbf{q}) + \hbar\omega_{fg} + V_{fg}(\mathbf{q}). \tag{4.22}$$

Treating $\hat{H}_g(\mathbf{q})$ as the zero-order Hamiltonian and taking the last two terms on the right-hand side of Equation 4.22 as the perturbation Hamiltonian, we find that in the interaction picture, the forward and backward time evolution operators determined by $\hat{H}_e(\mathbf{q})$ and $\hat{H}_f(\mathbf{q})$ are

$$\exp\left(-\frac{i}{\hbar}\hat{H}_e t\right) = \exp(-i\bar{\omega}_{eg}t)\exp\left(-\frac{i}{\hbar}\hat{H}_g t\right)\exp_+\left(-\frac{i}{\hbar}\int_0^t d\tau U_{eg}(\tau)\right)$$

$$\exp\left(\frac{i}{\hbar}\hat{H}_e t\right) = \exp(i\bar{\omega}_{eg}t)\exp_-\left(\frac{i}{\hbar}\int_0^t d\tau U_{eg}(\tau)\right)\exp\left(\frac{i}{\hbar}\hat{H}_g t\right)$$

$$\exp\left(-\frac{i}{\hbar}\hat{H}_f t\right) = \exp(-i\bar{\omega}_{fg}t)\exp\left(-\frac{i}{\hbar}\hat{H}_g t\right)\exp_+\left(-\frac{i}{\hbar}\int_0^t d\tau U_{fg}(\tau)\right)$$

$$\exp\left(\frac{i}{\hbar}\hat{H}_f t\right) = \exp(i\bar{\omega}_{fg}t)\exp_-\left(\frac{i}{\hbar}\int_0^t d\tau U_{fg}(\tau)\right)\exp\left(\frac{i}{\hbar}\hat{H}_g t\right), \tag{4.23}$$

where, for $j = e$ and f,

$$\bar{\omega}_{jg} = \omega_{jg} + < V_{jg}(\mathbf{q}) > / \hbar$$

$$U_{jg} \equiv V_{jg}(\mathbf{q}) - < V_{jg}(\mathbf{q}) >$$

$$U_{jg}(t) = U_{jg}(\mathbf{q}(t)) = \exp\left(\frac{i}{\hbar}\hat{H}_B t\right) U_{jg}(\mathbf{q}) \exp\left(-\frac{i}{\hbar}\hat{H}_B t\right). \tag{4.24}$$

Here, $< V_{eg}(\mathbf{q}) >$ and $< V_{fg}(\mathbf{q}) >$ are the average values over the ensemble, when the system is on the ground state.

The initial density operator may be written as a product of the system and bath density operators as

$$\rho(-\infty) = \rho_S(-\infty)\rho_B(-\infty). \tag{4.25}$$

For the sake of simplicity, we will assume that $\hbar\omega_{eg} >> k_B T$ and $\hbar\omega_{fg} >> k_B T$. Thus, the populations of the two excited states at thermal equilibrium state will be ignored. Therefore, the initial density operator is

$$\begin{aligned} \rho(-\infty) &= | g > \rho_B(\mathbf{q}) < g | \\ &= | g > \frac{e^{-\beta \hat{H}_B(\mathbf{q})}}{< e^{-\beta \hat{H}_B(\mathbf{q})} >_B} < g |. \end{aligned} \tag{4.26}$$

Using the operator identities in Equation 4.23 and using the cumulant expansion method briefly outlined earlier, one can find that the second-order response function is given as the sum of four different terms,

$$\begin{aligned} \phi_{BA_2A_1}(t_2,t_1) = \left(\frac{i}{\hbar}\right)^2 \theta(t_2)\theta(t_1) \sum_{e,f} \Big\{ & [B]_{gf}[A_2]_{fe}[A_1]_{eg} e^{-i\bar{\omega}_{fg}t_2 - i\bar{\omega}_{eg}t_1} G_1(t_2,t_1) \\ & - [A_2]_{gf}[B]_{fe}[A_1]_{eg} e^{-i\bar{\omega}_{ef}t_2 - i\bar{\omega}_{eg}t_1} G_2(t_2,t_1) \Big\} + c.c. \end{aligned} \tag{4.27}$$

where the two line-shape functions associated with different second-order transition pathways are

$$\begin{aligned} G_1(t_2,t_1) &= < \exp_+\left[-\frac{i}{\hbar}\int_0^{t_2} d\tau U_{fg}(\tau) \right] \exp_-\left[-\frac{i}{\hbar}\int_0^{t_1} d\tau U_{eg}(-\tau) \right] >_B \\ G_2(t_2,t_1) &= < \exp_+\left[\frac{i}{\hbar}\int_0^{t_2} d\tau U_{fg}(-\tau) \right] \exp_-\left[-\frac{i}{\hbar}\int_0^{t_1+t_2} d\tau U_{eg}(-\tau) \right] >_B . \end{aligned} \tag{4.28}$$

Note that each term in Equation 4.27 is written as a product of transition strength, coherence oscillation term, and line-shape function, that is,

$$\left(\frac{i}{\hbar}\right)^2 \theta(t_2)\theta(t_1) \underbrace{[B]_{gf}[A_2]_{fe}[A_1]_{eg}}_{\text{Transition strength}} \underbrace{\exp(-i\bar{\omega}_{fg}t_2 - i\bar{\omega}_{eg}t_1)}_{\text{Coherence oscillation}} \underbrace{G_1(t_2,t_1)}_{\text{Line shape}}$$

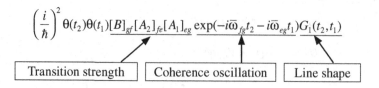

The first two terms on the right-hand side of Equation 4.27 correspond to the following two time-correlation functions (see Equation 4.6),

$$\left(\frac{i}{\hbar}\right)^2 \theta(t_2)\theta(t_1) < \hat{B}(t_2+t_1)\hat{A}_2(t_1)\hat{A}_1(0)\rho(-\infty) >$$

$$\left(\frac{i}{\hbar}\right)^2 \theta(t_2)\theta(t_1) < \hat{A}_2(t_1)\hat{B}(t_2+t_1)\hat{A}_1(0)\rho(-\infty) > . \quad (4.29)$$

Furthermore, they can be represented by the following two diagrams:

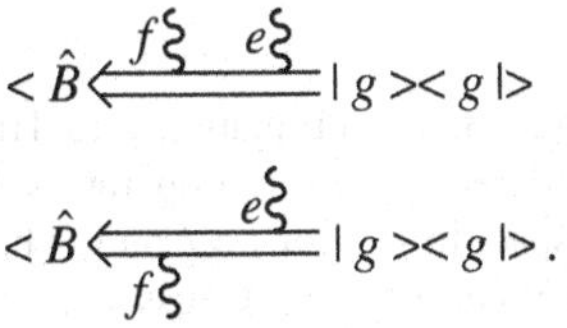

(4.30)

In the first diagram, the system is on the coherence $\rho_{eg}^{(1)}$ during the first t_1 period. Then, after an additional radiation–matter interaction, it is promoted to another coherence $\rho_{fg}^{(2)}$ during the t_2 period. Thus, the expectation value from the first diagram is an oscillating function $(\approx \exp(-i\bar{\omega}_{fg}t_2))$ with frequency $\bar{\omega}_{fg}$. On the other hand, the second diagram, even though the first coherence is identical to that of the first diagram, shows that the system is on the coherence $\rho_{ef}^{(2)}$ during the t_2 period. Therefore, the $\bar{B}(t)$ from the second diagram oscillates differently as $\exp(-i\bar{\omega}_{ef}t_2)$. Thus, these two contributions to $\bar{B}(t)$ are distinctively different from each other in their oscillating patterns.

The second-order cumulant expansion method can be used to obtain the two lineshape functions in Equation 4.28 and the resultant expressions are found to be[1, 12, 13]

$$G_1(t_2,t_1) = \exp\left\{-\left[\int_0^{t_2} d\tau_1 \int_0^{\tau_1} d\tau_2 C_{ff}(\tau_1-\tau_2) + \int_0^{t_1} d\tau_1 \int_0^{\tau_1} d\tau_2 C_{ee}(\tau_1-\tau_2) + \int_0^{t_2} d\tau_1 \int_0^{t_1} d\tau_2 C_{fe}(\tau_1+\tau_2)\right]\right\} \quad (4.31)$$

$$G_2(t_2,t_1) = \exp\left\{-\left[\int_0^{t_2} d\tau_1 \int_0^{\tau_1} d\tau_2 C_{ff}^*(\tau_1-\tau_2) + \int_0^{t_1+t_2} d\tau_1 \int_0^{\tau_1} d\tau_2 C_{ee}(\tau_1-\tau_2) - \int_0^{t_2} d\tau_1 \int_0^{t_1+t_2} d\tau_2 C_{fe}(\tau_2-\tau_1)\right]\right\}, \quad (4.32)$$

where

$$C_{ff}(t) = \frac{1}{\hbar^2} < U_{fg}(t) U_{fg}(0) \rho_B >_B$$

$$C_{ee}(t) = \frac{1}{\hbar^2} < U_{eg}(t) U_{eg}(0) \rho_B >_B$$

$$C_{fe}(t) = \frac{1}{\hbar^2} < U_{fg}(t) U_{eg}(0) \rho_B >_B . \tag{4.33}$$

EXERCISE 4.1

Derive Equations 4.31 and 4.32 from Equation 4.28. Hints: (1) Expand the positive and negative time-ordered exponential operators. (2) Ignore the first-order expansion terms with respect to U_{jg} (for $j = e$ and f) because they vanish when the fluctuating difference potentials obey Gaussian statistics. (3) Consider terms that are second-order with respect to U_{jg} (for $j = e$ and f). (4) Rewrite the series as normal exponential functions as an approximation.

The third frequency–frequency correlation function $C_{fe}(t)$ in Equation 4.33 describes how strongly the fluctuating transition frequency between g and f correlates with that between g and e. If such a cross-correlation amplitude is small in comparison to $C_{ff}(0)$ and $C_{ee}(0)$, that is,

$$C_{ff}(0) \approx C_{ee}(0) \gg C_{fe}(0), \tag{4.34}$$

the line-shape functions in Equations 4.31 and 4.32 are simplified as

$$G_1(t_2, t_1) = \exp\{-g_{ff}(t_2) - g_{ee}(t_1)\}$$

$$G_2(t_2, t_1) = \exp\{-g^*_{ff}(t_2) - g_{ee}(t_1 + t_2)\}. \tag{4.35}$$

Here, the line-broadening functions, associated with time-correlations $U_{fg}(t)$ and $U_{eg}(t)$, are defined as

$$g_{ff}(t) = \int_0^t d\tau_2 \int_0^{\tau_2} d\tau_1 C_{ff}(\tau_1)$$

$$g_{ee}(t) = \int_0^t d\tau_2 \int_0^{\tau_2} d\tau_1 C_{ee}(\tau_1). \tag{4.36}$$

The approximation in Equation 4.34 will be called the *uncorrelated frequency fluctuation* (UFF) approximation.[14]

The line-shape functions discussed above ignored the lifetime-broadening effects. By denoting the lifetimes of e and f states as T_e and T_f, respectively, the line-shape functions should be corrected as (for $j = 1$ and 2)

$$G_j(t_2,t_1) \to G_j(t_2,t_1)\exp(-t_2/2T_f - t_1/2T_e). \tag{4.37}$$

The lifetime-broadening process, which is induced by radiative, nonradiative, intramolecular vibrational energy relaxation and so forth, is an important factor in describing detailed spectral line shape. However, throughout this book, we will take it into account in an *ad hoc* manner as shown above, and unless it is necessary, such an exponentially decaying factor will be omitted for the sake of simplicity. It is also noted that the pure dephasing timescale is quite often much shorter than lifetimes of excited states. Thus, the entire line-broadening function associated with the second-order response spectroscopy such as SFG is usually determined by the system–bath interaction-induced dephasing that is described in Equations 4.31 and 4.32.

In the Markovian limit, one can replace the time correlation functions in Equation 4.33 with very quickly decaying exponential functions as, with large Γ_{ff} and Γ_{ee},

$$C_{ff}(t) = C_{ff}(0)\exp(-\Gamma_{ff}t) \quad \text{and} \quad C_{ee}(t) = C_{ee}(0)\exp(-\Gamma_{ee}t). \tag{4.38}$$

Using the UFF approximation in Equation 4.34, one finds that the two line-shape functions $G_1(t_2,t_1)$ and $G_2(t_2,t_1)$ are simplified as

$$G_1(t_2,t_1) = \exp\{-\gamma_{ff}t_2 - \gamma_{ee}t_1\}$$

$$G_2(t_1,t_2) = \exp\{-[\gamma_{ff} + \gamma_{ee}]t_2 - \gamma_{ee}t_1\}, \tag{4.39}$$

where the dephasing constants are defined as $\gamma_{ff} = C_{ff}(0)/\Gamma_{ff}$ and $\gamma_{ee} = C_{ee}(0)/\Gamma_{ee}$. In this simple case, the two-dimensional Fourier-Laplace transform of $G_j(t_2,t_1)$, which is defined as

$$\breve{G}_j(\omega_2,\omega_1) = \int_0^\infty dt_2 \int_0^\infty dt_1\ G_j(t_2,t_1)e^{i\omega_2 t_2 + i\omega_1 t_1}, \tag{4.40}$$

is

$$\breve{G}_1(\omega_2,\omega_1) = -\frac{1}{(\omega_2 + i\gamma_{ff})(\omega_1 + i\gamma_{ee})} \tag{4.41}$$

$$\breve{G}_2(\omega_2,\omega_1) = -\frac{1}{(\omega_2 + i[\gamma_{ff}(1-2\delta_{fe}) + \gamma_{ee}])(\omega_1 + i\gamma_{ee})}. \tag{4.42}$$

From these results, the second-order susceptibility in 2D frequency space is

$$\chi_{BA_2A_1}(\omega_2,\omega_1) = \left(\frac{i}{\hbar}\right)^2 \sum_{e,f} \{[B]_{gf}[A_2]_{fe}[A_1]_{eg}\breve{G}_1(\omega_2-\bar{\omega}_{fg},\omega_1-\bar{\omega}_{eg})$$

$$-[A_2]_{gf}[B]_{fe}[A_1]_{eg}\breve{G}_2(\omega_2-\bar{\omega}_{ef},\omega_1-\bar{\omega}_{eg})$$

$$+[A_1]_{ge}[A_2]_{ef}[B]_{fg}\breve{G}_1^*(-\omega_2-\bar{\omega}_{fg},-\omega_1-\bar{\omega}_{eg})$$

$$-[A_1]_{ge}[B]_{ef}[A_2]_{fg}\breve{G}_2^*(-\omega_2-\bar{\omega}_{ef},-\omega_1-\bar{\omega}_{eg})\}. \tag{4.43}$$

As will be shown later in this chapter, the first term on the right-hand side of Equation 4.43 is directly related to the SFG in the case when $\bar{\omega}_{fg} > \bar{\omega}_{eg}$ and the generated field frequency is the sum of the two incident beam frequencies.

In the inhomogeneous broadening limit, the two line shape functions in Equation 4.35 can be written as

$$G_1(t_2,t_1) = \exp\left\{-\frac{1}{2}\Delta_{ff}^2 t_2^2 - \frac{1}{2}\Delta_{ee}^2 t_1^2\right\}$$

$$G_2(t_2,t_1) = \exp\left\{-\frac{1}{2}\left[\Delta_{ff}^2(1-2\delta_{fe})+\Delta_{ee}^2\right]t_2^2 - \frac{1}{2}\Delta_{ee}^2 t_1^2\right\}. \tag{4.44}$$

Then, 2D Fourier-Laplace transformation of the second-order response function in this case can be performed to obtain the corresponding susceptibility.

EXERCISE 4.2

Obtain the expression for the second-order susceptibility in this inhomogenous broadening limit.

Despite that the two line-broadening cases were discussed previously, a more general approach is to use the spectral density representation of the system–bath interaction, which was already discussed and applied to the linear response function in a previous chapter. We shall not provide any further discussion along this line, but the following exercise deals with such an extension.

EXERCISE 4.3

The three time-correlation functions in Equation 4.33 can be expressed as integrals of spectral densities $\rho_{ff}(\omega)$, $\rho_{ee}(\omega)$, and $\rho_{fe}(\omega)$, respectively. In the limiting case when there is no cross-correlation between two different fluctuating difference potentials, that is, $C_{fe}(t) = 0$ for $f \neq e$, what are the expressions for $G_1(t_2,t_1)$ and $G_2(t_1,t_2)$ in terms of the two spectral densities, $\rho_{ff}(\omega)$ and $\rho_{ee}(\omega)$?

4.3 SUM FREQUENCY GENERATION

One of the most widely used second-order response measurement methods is the sum frequency generation (SFG) spectroscopy. The first interaction of matter with $\mathbf{E}_1$ electric field component ($\mathbf{E}_1^+(\mathbf{r},t)$) propagating in the direction of $\mathbf{k}_1$ induces an absorptive transition from g to e, and the second one with $\mathbf{E}_2$ electric field component ($\mathbf{E}_2^+(\mathbf{r},t)$) propagating along the $\mathbf{k}_2$ direction subsequently induces another absorptive transition from e to f. Then, thus created coherence $\rho_{fg}^{(2)}$ radiates electric field whose frequency is the sum of the $\mathbf{E}_1$ and $\mathbf{E}_2$ field frequencies (see Figure 4.1). Since all three radiation–matter interactions including the last spontaneous emission process are between electric dipole and electric fields, the two cause operators, their conjugate fields, and effect operator are

$$\hat{A}_1 F_1(t) = \boldsymbol{\mu}\cdot\mathbf{e}_1 E_1(t)e^{i\mathbf{k}_1\cdot\mathbf{r}-i\omega_1 t}$$

$$\hat{A}_2 F_2(t) = \boldsymbol{\mu}\cdot\mathbf{e}_2 E_2(t)e^{i\mathbf{k}_2\cdot\mathbf{r}-i\omega_2 t}$$

$$B = \boldsymbol{\mu}. \tag{4.45}$$

Using the second-order response function theory in Section 4.1, one finds that the expectation value of the effect-operator, which is the second-order SFG polarization, is given as

$$\mathbf{P}_{SFG}(\mathbf{r},t) = e^{i(\mathbf{k}_1+\mathbf{k}_2)\cdot\mathbf{r}-i(\omega_1+\omega_2)t}\int_0^\infty dt_2\int_0^\infty dt_1 \phi_{\mu\mu\mu}(t_2,t_1):\mathbf{e}_2\mathbf{e}_1 E_2(t-t_2)E_1(t-t_2-t_1)$$
$$\times e^{i(\omega_1+\omega_2)t_2+i\omega_1 t_1}, \tag{4.46}$$

where the third-rank tensorial all-electric-dipole second-order response function is defined as

$$\phi_{\mu\mu\mu}(t_2,t_1) = \left(\frac{i}{\hbar}\right)^2 \theta(t_2)\theta(t_1) < [[\boldsymbol{\mu}(t_2+t_1),\boldsymbol{\mu}(t_1)],\boldsymbol{\mu}(0)]\rho(-\infty) >. \tag{4.47}$$

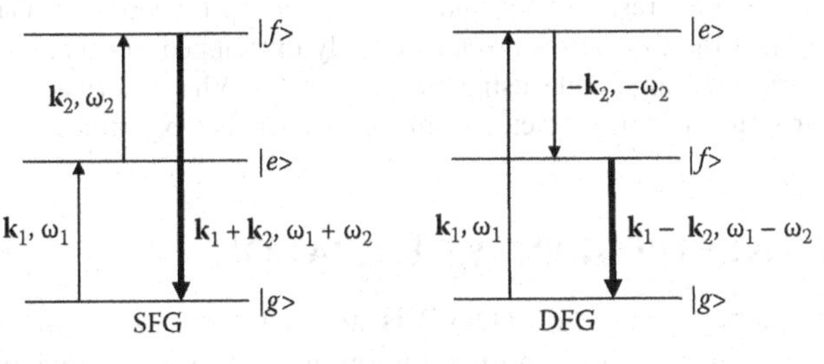

FIGURE 4.1 Energy level diagrams of SFG and DFG. Thin arrows represent the radiation–matter interaction-induced transitions. The thick arrow is the radiative transition.

Using Equation A.3.6, we find that the rotationally averaged signal field amplitude is, with the phase-matching geometry of $\mathbf{k}_s = \mathbf{k}_1 + \mathbf{k}_2$,

$$\hat{\mathbf{E}}_{SFG}(t) = i\omega_s \int_0^\infty dt_2 \int_0^\infty dt_1\ \hat{\phi}_{\mu\mu\mu}(t_2,t_1) : \mathbf{e}_2\mathbf{e}_1 E_2(t-t_2)E_1(t-t_2-t_1)e^{i(\omega_1+\omega_2)t_2+i\omega_1 t_1}. \tag{4.48}$$

If molecules under investigation are adsorbed on a metal surface with anisotropic orientational distribution, the rotationally averaged second-order response function becomes nonzero even within the electric dipole approximation. This is the main reason why the SFG spectroscopy has been extensively used to study surface-specific electronic or vibrational dynamics of molecules on surface or at interface.

The IV-SFG spectroscopy discussed in another chapter is one of the SFG techniques.[15] However, since the visible beam used in the IV-SFG is electronically nonresonant, it was classified as one of the linear response measurement methods. Another important application of SFG is to generate a second-harmonic beam by injecting an electronically nonresonant beam to nonlinear optical material.[16] Although the second-harmonic generation (or SFG in general) is useful in a number of spectroscopic applications, we will not consider them here. Instead, we will specifically consider the case when the two excited states $|e>$ and $|f>$ are real eigenstates of the matter Hamiltonian. Therefore, the SFG considered here is a doubly resonant process. When $E_f > E_e > E_g$, $\omega_1 + \omega_2 \simeq \bar{\omega}_{fg}$, and $\omega_1 \simeq \bar{\omega}_{eg}$, only the first term in Equation 4.27 is important due to the double-resonance condition. Then, we get

$$\hat{\mathbf{E}}_{SFG}(t) = -\frac{i\omega_s}{\hbar^2}\boldsymbol{\mu}_{gf}\boldsymbol{\mu}_{fe}\boldsymbol{\mu}_{eg} : \mathbf{e}_2\mathbf{e}_1 \int_0^\infty dt_2 \int_0^\infty dt_1\, G_1(t_2,t_1)$$
$$\times E_2(t-t_2)E_1(t-t_2-t_1)e^{i(\omega_1+\omega_2-\bar{\omega}_{fg})t_2+i(\omega_1-\bar{\omega}_{eg})t_1}. \tag{4.49}$$

In a later chapter, this result will be used to show that the doubly resonant SFG is a 2D second-order spectroscopy for studying chiral molecules in solutions.

EXERCISE 4.4

In the Markovian limit, the line-shape function $G_1(t_2, t_1)$ is given as an exponentially decaying function with respect to t_1 and t_2 (see Equation 4.39). Suppose that the temporal envelope functions of the two incident pulses peak at $t = 0$ and $t = T$ for E_1 and E_2, respectively, and that the envelop functions are Gaussian. Assuming that the two pulses are not strongly overlapped in time, obtain the SFG electric field amplitude using Equation 4.49. What information on the molecular system can be extracted from the T-dependent experiment?

4.4 DIFFERENCE FREQUENCY GENERATION

Difference frequency generation (DFG) is another three-wave-mixing spectroscopy involving two radiation–matter interactions between molecules' electric dipole and external electric field. Similar to the SFG, the first interaction of matter with $\mathbf{E}_1^+(\mathbf{r},t)$ propagating in the $\mathbf{k}_1$ direction induces an absorptive transition from g to e state, and the second one with $\mathbf{E}_2^-(\mathrm{r},t)$ propagating in the direction of $-\mathbf{k}_2$ induces a stimulated emissive transition from e to f—note that $E_e > E_f > E_g$. Then, thus created coherence $\rho_{fg}^{(2)}$ radiates electric field whose frequency is the difference of the $\mathbf{E}_1$ and $\mathbf{E}_2$ field frequencies (see Figure 4.1). The effective radiation–matter interactions and the effect operator are, in this case,

$$\hat{A}_1 F_1(t) = \boldsymbol{\mu}\cdot\mathbf{e}_1 E_1(t)\,e^{i\mathbf{k}_1\cdot\mathbf{r}-i\omega_1 t}$$

$$\hat{A}_2 F_2(t) = \boldsymbol{\mu}\cdot\mathbf{e}_2^* E_2^*(t)\,e^{-i\mathbf{k}_2\cdot\mathbf{r}+i\omega_2 t}$$

$$\hat{B} = \boldsymbol{\mu}. \tag{4.50}$$

Using the second-order response function theory in Section 4.1 with the above cause and effect operators with conjugate external fields, one can find that the second-order DFG polarization is given as

$$\mathbf{P}_{DFG}(\mathbf{r},t) = e^{i(\mathbf{k}_1-\mathbf{k}_2)\cdot\mathbf{r}-i(\omega_1-\omega_2)t}\int_0^\infty dt_2\int_0^\infty dt_1\,\phi_{\mu\mu\mu}(t_2,t_1):\mathbf{e}_2^*\mathbf{e}_1$$
$$\times E_2^*(t-t_2)E_1(t-t_2-t_1)\,e^{i(\omega_1-\omega_2)t_2+i\omega_1 t_1}, \tag{4.51}$$

where the third-rank tensorial all-electric-dipole response function is identical to that used to describe the SFG. Note that the second-order DFG polarization propagates in the direction of $\mathbf{k}_1$-$\mathbf{k}_2$ vector and oscillates with frequency of $\omega_1-\omega_2$. Thus, the DFG signal field amplitude is given as

$$\hat{\mathbf{E}}_{DFG}(t) = i\omega_s\int_0^\infty dt_2\int_0^\infty dt_1\,\hat{\phi}_{\mu\mu\mu}(t_2,t_1):\mathbf{e}_2^*\mathbf{e}_1 E_2^*(t-t_2)E_1(t-t_2-t_1)\,e^{i(\omega_1-\omega_2)t_2+i\omega_1 t_1}. \tag{4.52}$$

Since the DFG is a three-wave mixing, it can be applied to molecular systems with broken centrosymmetry, such as adsorbed molecules on surface or at interface.

The electronically nonresonant DFG has been widely used to obtain radiation with frequency smaller than that of commercially available laser. However, if the two excited states f and e are eigenstates of the molecular Hamiltonian, the doubly resonant DFG can be considered to be a 2D spectroscopy. In this case, the two optical transitions in the following sequence g → e → f are enhanced by resonance conditions, and the DFG signal electric field amplitude is given as

$$\hat{\mathbf{E}}_{DFG}(t) = -\frac{i\omega_s}{\hbar^2}\boldsymbol{\mu}_{gf}\boldsymbol{\mu}_{fe}\boldsymbol{\mu}_{eg}:\mathbf{e}_2^*\mathbf{e}_1\int_0^\infty dt_2\int_0^\infty dt_1\,G_1(t_2,t_1)$$
$$\times E_2^*(t-t_2)E_1(t-t_2-t_1)\,e^{i(\omega_1-\omega_2-\bar{\omega}_{fg})t_2+i(\omega_1-\bar{\omega}_{eg})t_1}. \tag{4.53}$$

The doubly resonant DFG has not been used as a 2D second-order spectroscopy for molecular systems on surface nor for chiral molecules in an isotropic medium. The latter possibility will be discussed in detail in another chapter.

4.5 IR–IR-VIS FOUR-WAVE MIXING

The SFG and DFG are potentially useful 2D optical spectroscopic techniques. As an example, two IR beams can be used to generate sum frequency field from adsorbed molecules on a surface, and then the measured spectrum as a function of the two IR-beam frequencies can provide information on the overtone and combination band frequencies and anharmonicity-induced mode-mode couplings. Nevertheless, most of the SFG and DFG experiments have focused on studying structures and dynamics of molecular systems on surface only.

However, the IR–IR-vis (IIV) SFG or DFG, where the visible field is electronically nonresonant, was shown to be a useful 2D vibrational spectroscopy for molecules in *solutions*.[1, 5, 17–20] The first two IR beams induce doubly resonant-enhanced transitions between vibrational states on the electronic ground state. Then, the last electronically nonresonant visible beam is used to stimulate a Raman scattering process to generate the coherent IIV four-wave-mixing signal field. In this particular case, the two cause-operators are electric dipole operator, and the effect-operator is the induced dipole that is produced by the radiation–matter interaction with the electronically nonresonant visible electric field. The energy level diagrams for two IIV four-wave-mixing processes are shown in Figure 4.2.

For the IIV SFG, we have

$$\hat{A}_1 F_1(t) = \boldsymbol{\mu} \cdot \mathbf{e}_{IR1} E_{IR1}(t) e^{i\mathbf{k}_{IR1}\cdot\mathbf{r} - i\omega_{IR1}t}$$

$$\hat{A}_2 F_2(t) = \boldsymbol{\mu} \cdot \mathbf{e}_{IR2} E_{IR2}(t) e^{i\mathbf{k}_{IR2}\cdot\mathbf{r} - i\omega_{IR2}t}$$

$$\hat{B} = \boldsymbol{\mu}_{ind}(\mathrm{r}, t) = \boldsymbol{\alpha} \cdot \mathbf{E}_{vis}(t) e^{i\mathbf{k}_{vis}\cdot\mathbf{r} - i\omega_{vis}t}. \quad (4.54)$$

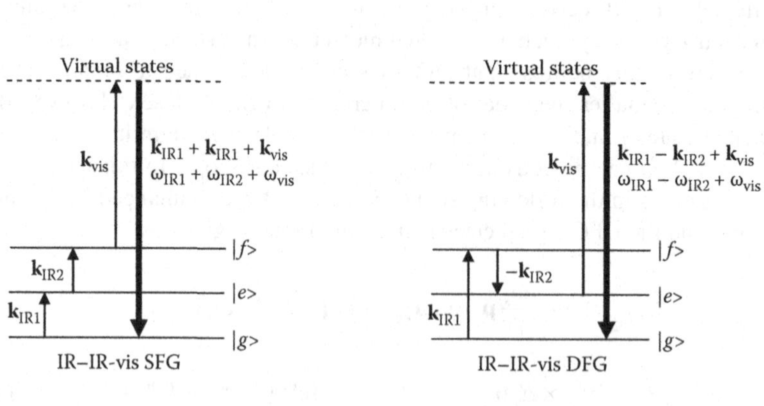

FIGURE 4.2 Energy-level diagrams of infrared–infrared visible SFG and DFG.

On the other hand, for the IIV DFG scheme in Figure 4.2, the corresponding interaction Hamiltonians and effect operator are

$$\hat{A}_1 F_1(t) = \boldsymbol{\mu} \cdot \mathbf{e}_{IR1} E_{IR1}(t) e^{i\mathbf{k}_{IR1}\cdot\mathbf{r} - i\omega_{IR1}t}$$

$$\hat{A}_2 F_2(t) = \boldsymbol{\mu} \cdot \mathbf{e}^*_{IR2} E^*_{IR2}(t) e^{-i\mathbf{k}_{IR2}\cdot\mathbf{r} + i\omega_{IR2}t}$$

$$\hat{B} = \boldsymbol{\mu}_{ind}(\mathrm{r}, t) = \boldsymbol{\alpha} \cdot \mathbf{e}_{vis} E_{vis}(t) e^{i\mathbf{k}_{vis}\cdot\mathbf{r} - i\omega_{vis}t}. \quad (4.55)$$

Since the theoretical result for the IIV DFG is essentially identical to that for the IIV SFG except that $\mathbf{k}_{IR2} \to -\mathbf{k}_{IR2}$ and $\omega_{IR2} \to -\omega_{IR2}$, the IIV SFG will be mainly discussed hereafter.

The second-order response function theory is used to obtain the IIV-SFG polarization,

$$\mathbf{P}_{IIV-SFG}(\mathbf{r}, t) = e^{i(\mathbf{k}_{IR1}+\mathbf{k}_{IR2}+\mathbf{k}_{vis})\cdot\mathbf{r} - i(\omega_{IR1}+\omega_{IR2}+\omega_{vis})t}$$

$$\times E_{vis}(t) \int_0^\infty dt_2 \int_0^\infty dt_1 \phi_{\alpha\mu\mu}(t_2, t_1) \vdots \mathbf{e}_{vis} \mathbf{e}_{IR2} \mathbf{e}_{IR1} E_{IR2}(t - t_2) E_{IR1}(t - t_2 - t_1) e^{i(\omega_{IR1}+\omega_{IR2})t_2 + i\omega_{IR1}t_1}. \quad (4.56)$$

Here, the second-order response function $\phi_{\alpha\mu\mu}(t_2, t_1)$ is

$$\phi_{\alpha\mu\mu}(t_2, t_1) = \left(\frac{i}{\hbar}\right)^2 \theta(t_2)\theta(t_1) < [[\boldsymbol{\alpha}(t_2 + t_1), \boldsymbol{\mu}(t_1)], \boldsymbol{\mu}(0)]\rho(-\infty) >. \quad (4.57)$$

When $E_f > E_e > E_g$, $\omega_{IR1} + \omega_{IR2} \cong \bar{\omega}_{fg}$, and $\omega_{IR1} \cong \bar{\omega}_{eg}$, only the first term in Equation 4.7 for the second-order response function is important due to the double-resonance condition. Then, one can find that the generated signal electric field amplitude is given as

$$\mathbf{E}_{IIV-SFG}(t) = -\frac{i\omega_s}{\hbar^2} \boldsymbol{\alpha}_{gf} \boldsymbol{\mu}_{fe} \boldsymbol{\mu}_{eg} \vdots \mathbf{e}_{vis} \mathbf{e}_{IR2} \mathbf{e}_{IR1}$$

$$\times E_{vis}(t) \int_0^\infty dt_2 \int_0^\infty dt_1 G_1(t_2, t_1) E_{IR2}(t - t_2) E_{IR1}(t - t_2 - t_1) e^{i(\omega_{IR1}+\omega_{IR2}-\bar{\omega}_{fg})t_2 + i(\omega_{IR1}-\bar{\omega}_{eg})t_1}. \quad (4.58)$$

The IIV SFG is a four-wave-mixing 2D vibrational spectroscopy, and its selection rule can be deduced from the above result in Equation 4.58. That is to say, the vibrational modes involved in the first two transitions should be IR-active. The transition from f to g should be Raman-allowed. Unlike the three-wave-mixing SFG and DFG, the IIV SFG spectroscopy is applicable to isotropic solution samples because the associated response function is a fourth-rank tensor. By using the results in Section 3.3, the rotational average of $\mathbf{E}_{IIV-SFG}(t)$ for randomly oriented molecules in an isotropic medium can be easily obtained. For instance, consider the case when the three incident beams are all linearly polarized along the X-axis in a laboratory-fixed frame. Also, the X-component of $\mathbf{E}_{IIV-SFG}(t)$ is assumed to be measured. Then, we have

$$[\hat{\mathbf{E}}_{IIV-SFG}(t)]_X = -\frac{i\omega_s}{\hbar^2}[\boldsymbol{\alpha}_{gf}\boldsymbol{\mu}_{fe}\boldsymbol{\mu}_{eg}]_{XXXX}$$

$$\times E_{vis}(t)\int_0^\infty dt_2\int_0^\infty dt_1\, G_1(t_2,t_1)E_{IR2}(t-t_2)E_{IR1}(t-t_2-t_1)e^{i(\omega_{IR1}+\omega_{IR2}-\bar{\omega}_{fg})t_2+i(\omega_{IR1}-\bar{\omega}_{eg})t_1}. \quad (4.59)$$

This result is quite general, but it is necessary to fully understand how the transition strength $\boldsymbol{\alpha}_{gf}\boldsymbol{\mu}_{fe}\boldsymbol{\mu}_{eg}$ can be quantitatively calculated for a specific molecular system. This will be discussed in a later chapter.

In the present section, we provided a theoretical description of IIV four-wave-mixing process by using the second-order response function theory. Since it is possible to experimentally control the delay times among the three pulses, that is, two time-separated IR pulses and a delayed visible pulse, the measured IIV four-wave-mixing signal is naturally a 2D function with respect to these two delay times. Then, its 2D Fourier-Laplace transform is 2D IIV SFG or IIV DFG spectrum. In particular, if two vibrational modes are coupled to each other and they are resonantly excited by the two IR pulses, the measured 2D IIV four-wave-mixing spectrum can provide critical information on mechanical and/or electrical anharmonicity-induced couplings between the two modes. For a coupled multi-chromophore system, this method can be of use in estimating couplings, which are in turn used to study mode-to-mode intramolecular vibrational energy relaxation pathways as well as to determine its 3D structure and absolute configuration.

REFERENCES

1. Cho, M., Coherent two-dimensional optical spectroscopy. *Chemical Reviews* 2008, 108, 1331–1418.
2. Mukamel, S., Multidimensional femtosecond correlation spectroscopies of electronic and vibrational excitations. *Annual Review of Physical Chemistry* 2000, 51, 691–729.
3. Jonas, D. M., Two-dimensional femtosecond spectroscopy. *Annual Review of Physical Chemistry* 2003, 54, 425–463.
4. Khalil, M.; Demirdoven, N.; Tokmakoff, A., Coherent 2D IR spectroscopy: Molecular structure and dynamics in solution. *Journal of Physical Chemistry A* 2003, 107, 5258–5279.
5. Wright, J. C., Coherent multidimensional vibrational spectroscopy. *International Reviews in Physical Chemistry* 2002, 21, 185–255.
6. Cho, M., Ultrafast vibrational spectroscopy in condensed phases. *PhysChemComm* 2002, 40–58.
7. Hamm, P.; Lim, M.; Hochstrasser, R. M., Structure of the amide I band of peptides measured by femtosecond nonlinear infrared spectroscopy. *Journal of Physical Chemistry B* 1998, 102, 6123–6138.

8. Fleming, G. R.; Cho, M., Chromophore-solvent dynamics. *Annual Review of Physical Chemistry* 1996, 47, 109–134.
9. Mukamel, S., *Principles of Nonlinear Optical Spectroscopy*. Oxford University Press: Oxford, 1995.
10. de Boeij, W. P.; Pshenichnikov, M. S.; Wiersma, D. A., Ultrafast solvation dynamics explored by femtosecond photon echo spectroscopies *Annual Review of Physical Chemistry* 1998, 49, 99–123.
11. Zanni, M. T.; Hochstrasser, R. M., Two-dimensional infrared spectroscopy: A promising new method for the time resolution of structures. *Current Opinion in Structural Biology* 2001, 11, 516–522.
12. Sung, J. Y.; Cho, M., Calculation of the two-dimensional vibrational response function. *Journal of Chemical Physics* 2000, 113, 7072–7083.
13. Sung, J. Y.; Silbey, R. J.; Cho, M., Effects of temperature on the nonlinear response function for two-dimensional vibrational spectroscopy. *Journal of Chemical Physics* 2001, 115, 1422–1428.
14. Cho, M.; Vaswani, H. M.; Brixner, T.; et al., Exciton analysis in 2D electronic spectroscopy. *Journal of Physical Chemistry B* 2005, 109, 10542–10556.
15. Zhu, X. D.; Suhr, H.; Shen, Y. R., Surface vibrational spectroscopy by infrared-visible sum frequency generation. *Physical Review B* 1987, 35, 3047–3050.
16. Shen, Y. R., *The Principles of Nonlinear Optics*. John Wiley & Sons: New York, 1984.
17. Park, K.; Cho, M., Time- and frequency-resolved coherent two-dimensional IR spectroscopy: Its complementary relationship with the coherent two-dimensional Raman scattering spectroscopy. *Journal of Chemical Physics* 1998, 109, 10559–10569.
18. Cho, M., Theoretical description of two-dimensional vibrational spectroscopy by infrared-infrared-visible sum frequency generation. *Physical Review A* 2000, 6102, 023406.
19. Zhao, W.; Wright, J. C., Measurement of $\chi^{(3)}$ for doubly vibrationally enhanced four wave mixing spectroscopy. *Physical Review Letters* 1999, 83, 1950–1953.
20. Zhao, W.; Wright, J. C., Doubly vibrationally enhanced four wave mixing: The optical analog to 2D NMR. *Physical Review Letters* 2000, 84, 1411–1414.

5 Third-Order Response Spectroscopy

Third-order response spectroscopy is usually based on a four-wave-mixing process within the electric dipole approximation.[1] Photon echo spectroscopy is one of the most extensively used techniques.[2, 3] The stimulated photon echo method utilizes three pulses to create the third-order polarization, which is then the source of the echo signal field. In this case of the photon echo, the three radiation–matter interactions are all electric dipole–electric field interactions.[3] Experimentally, one can measure the echo signal electric field amplitude as a function of two delay times during which the system evolves on a coherence.[4–6] Then, its 2D Fourier transformation gives 2D photon echo spectrum, which contains vital information on the electronic or vibrational couplings between two different quantum transitions.[7]

The radiation–matter interaction Hamiltonian associated with any arbitrary third-order response spectroscopy is therefore given as

$$H_{rad\text{-}mat}(t) = -\hat{\mathbf{V}}_1 \cdot \mathbf{F}_1(\mathbf{r},t) - \hat{\mathbf{V}}_2 \cdot \mathbf{F}_2(\mathbf{r},t) - \hat{\mathbf{V}}_3 \cdot \mathbf{F}_3(\mathbf{r},t). \tag{5.1}$$

From the definition of the generalized third-order response spectroscopy, the signal field amplitude (intensity) should be linearly proportional to each external field amplitude $\mathbf{F}_j$ (intensity $|\mathbf{F}_j|^2$). Depending on the choice of the three effective radiation–matter interaction Hamiltonians, there are a number of different third-order multidimensional spectroscopic methods in general. Among them, only a few simple cases will be discussed in detail in this chapter, but the other methods probing third-order molecular responses can be easily explored by using the general theoretical framework presented in this chapter.

5.1 THIRD-ORDER RESPONSE FUNCTION

The third-order response spectroscopy involves three actions of cause operators that could be identical to or different from one another. The three cause operators will be denoted as $\hat{A}_1$, $\hat{A}_2$, and $\hat{A}_3$ and the corresponding conjugate external fields are $F_1(t)$, $F_2(t)$, and $F_3(t)$, respectively. Then, the total Hamiltonian for third-order nonlinear optical processes can be written as

$$\hat{H}(t) = \hat{H}_0(t) + \hat{H}'(t) = \hat{H}_0(t) - \hat{A}_1 F_1(t) - \hat{A}_2 F_2(t) - \hat{A}_3 F_3(t). \tag{5.2}$$

The observable is then the expectation value of the effect operator $\hat{B}$ at time t. That can be written as a triple convolution of the third-order response function with three conjugate external fields. Without loss of generality, we shall assume that the radiation–matter interactions are time-ordered and the first interaction of the molecular system is with $F_1(t)$ and so on. In the frequency domain experiment, one should include all possible permutations of radiation–matter interaction sequences because there is no time-ordering among the three radiation–matter interactions.

From the third-order time-dependent perturbation theory, we have

$$\bar{B}(t) = <\hat{B}\rho^{(3)}_{A_3A_2A_1}(t)>$$

$= <\hat{B}$ 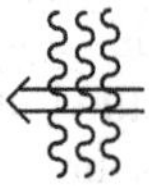 $\rho(t_0)>$

$$= \left(\frac{i}{\hbar}\right)^3 \int_{t_0}^{t} d\tau_3 \int_{t_0}^{\tau_3} d\tau_2 \int_{t_0}^{\tau_2} d\tau_1 <\hat{B}V_0(t,\tau_3)L'(\tau_3)V_0(\tau_3,\tau_2)L'(\tau_2)V_0(\tau_2,\tau_1)L'(\tau_1)$$

$$\times V_0(\tau_1,t_0)\rho(t_0)>$$

$$= \left(\frac{i}{\hbar}\right)^3 \int_{t_0}^{t} d\tau_3 \int_{t_0}^{\tau_3} d\tau_2 \int_{t_0}^{\tau_2} d\tau_1 <[[[\hat{B}(t),\hat{A}_3(\tau_3)],\hat{A}_2(\tau_2)],\hat{A}_1(\tau_1)]\rho(t_0)>$$

$$\times F_3(\tau_3)F_2(\tau_2)F_1(\tau_1). \tag{5.3}$$

EXERCISE 5.1

Derive Equation 5.3. The third-order time-dependent perturbation theory was discussed in Section 2.6, where the third-order time evolution operator in the second line of Equation 5.3 was shown to consist of eight different contributions. They correspond to the eight time-correlation functions obtained by taking expansion of the three commutators in the last line of Equation 5.3. Which diagram among the eight in Equation 2.91 corresponds to which time-correlation function?

Now, changing the integration variables and assuming $t_0 = -\infty$, we find that

$$\bar{B}(t) = \int_0^{\infty} dt_3 \int_0^{\infty} dt_2 \int_0^{\infty} dt_1\, \phi_{BA_3A_2A_1}(t_3,t_2,t_1)F_3(t-t_3)F_2(t-t_3-t_2)F_1(t-t_3-t_2-t_1). \tag{5.4}$$

The third-order response function is defined as

$$\phi_{BA_3A_2A_1}(t_3,t_2,t_1) = \left(\frac{i}{\hbar}\right)^3 \theta(t_3)\theta(t_2)\theta(t_1) <[[[\hat{B}(t_3+t_2+t_1),\hat{A}_3(t_2+t_1)],\hat{A}_2(t_1)],$$
$$\hat{A}_1(0)]\rho(-\infty)>. \tag{5.5}$$

The third-order response function describes the average B value of molecules at $t = t_1 + t_2 + t_3$, which have experienced time-separated three external perturbations by F_1, F_2, and F_3 at $t = 0$, t_1, and $t_1 + t_2$.

Due to the causality condition, one can rewrite Equation 5.4 as

$$\bar{B}(t)=\int_{-\infty}^{\infty}dt_3\int_{-\infty}^{\infty}dt_2\int_{-\infty}^{\infty}dt_1\phi_{BA_3A_2A_1}(t_3,t_2,t_1)F_3(t-t_3)F_2(t-t_3-t_2)F_1(t-t_3-t_2-t_1). \tag{5.6}$$

Defining the Fourier transforms of the external fields and the nonlinear response function as

$$\tilde{F}_j(\omega)=\int_{-\infty}^{\infty}dt\,F_j(t)e^{i\omega t}\quad (\text{for } j=1\sim 3) \tag{5.7}$$

$$\chi_{BA_3A_2A_1}(\omega_3,\omega_2,\omega_1)=\int_{-\infty}^{\infty}dt_3\int_{-\infty}^{\infty}dt_2\int_{-\infty}^{\infty}dt_1\;\phi_{BA_3A_2A_1}(t_3,t_2,t_1)e^{i\omega_3t_3+i\omega_2t_2+i\omega_1t_1}, \tag{5.8}$$

it is possible to rewrite the expectation value of the effect operator $\hat{B}$ as frequency integrals,

$$\bar{B}(t)=\left(\frac{1}{2\pi}\right)^3\int_{-\infty}^{\infty}d\omega_3\int_{-\infty}^{\infty}d\omega_2\int_{-\infty}^{\infty}d\omega_1\,\chi_{BA_3A_2A_1}(\omega_3+\omega_2+\omega_1,\omega_2+\omega_1,\omega_1)$$
$$\times\tilde{F}_3(\omega_3)\tilde{F}_2(\omega_2)\tilde{F}_1(\omega_1)e^{-i(\omega_3+\omega_2+\omega_1)t}. \tag{5.9}$$

If $\bar{B}(t)$ is detected in frequency domain, the spectrum of $\bar{B}(t)$ can be directly measured, and it is given as

$$\tilde{\bar{B}}(\omega)=\left(\frac{1}{2\pi}\right)^2\int_{-\infty}^{\infty}d\omega_3\int_{-\infty}^{\infty}d\omega_2\int_{-\infty}^{\infty}d\omega_1\,\chi_{BA_3A_2A_1}(\omega_3+\omega_2+\omega_1,\omega_2+\omega_1,\omega_1)$$
$$\times\tilde{F}_3(\omega_3)\tilde{F}_2(\omega_2)\tilde{F}_1(\omega_1)\delta(\omega-\omega_3-\omega_2-\omega_1) \tag{5.10}$$

$$=\left(\frac{1}{2\pi}\right)^2\int_{-\infty}^{\infty}d\omega_2\int_{-\infty}^{\infty}d\omega_1\chi_{BA_3A_2A_1}(\omega,\omega_2+\omega_1,\omega_1)\tilde{F}_3(\omega-\omega_2-\omega_1)\tilde{F}_2(\omega_2)\tilde{F}_1(\omega_1). \tag{5.11}$$

The third-order response function $\phi_{BA_3A_2A_1}(t_3,t_2,t_1)$ in time domain or the corresponding susceptibility $\chi_{BA_3A_2A_1}(\omega_3,\omega_2,\omega_1)$ in frequency domain contains complete information on the third-order response of the molecular system against the external perturbation $\hat{H}'(t)\;(=-\hat{A}_1F_1(t)-\hat{A}_2F_2(t)-\hat{A}_3F_3(t))$. In the impulsive limit, the three pulsed fields are approximately written as

$$F_1(t)=F_1\delta(t+T_2+T_1)e^{-i\omega_1t}$$
$$F_2(t)=F_2\delta(t+T_2)e^{-i\omega_2t}$$
$$F_3(t)=F_3\delta(t)e^{-i\omega_3t}. \tag{5.12}$$

Then, the expectation value is just linearly proportional to the third-order response function as

$$\bar{B}(t) = F_1 F_2 F_3\, \phi_{BA_3A_2A_1}(t, T_2, T_1)\exp\{i\omega_2 T_2 + i\omega_1(T_2 + T_1)\}. \tag{5.13}$$

Thus, $\phi_{BA_3A_2A_1}(t_3,t_2,t_1)$ is, as expected, the response of the molecular system when it interacts with three impulsive fields that are separated in time by T_1 and T_2.

In the case of the frequency-domain measurement with three continuous waves, we have

$$\tilde{F}_1(\omega) = 2\pi i F_1\{\delta(\omega - \Omega_1) - \delta(\omega + \Omega_1)\}$$

$$\tilde{F}_2(\omega) = 2\pi i F_2\{\delta(\omega - \Omega_2) - \delta(\omega + \Omega_2)\}$$

$$\tilde{F}_3(\omega) = 2\pi i F_3\{\delta(\omega - \Omega_3) - \delta(\omega + \Omega_3)\}. \tag{5.14}$$

Then, we get

$$\begin{aligned}\bar{B}(t) = (-i)F_1F_2F_3\big\{&\chi_{BA_3A_2A_1}(\Omega_3+\Omega_2+\Omega_1,\Omega_2+\Omega_1,\Omega_1)e^{-i(\Omega_3+\Omega_2+\Omega_1)t}\\ &-\chi_{BA_3A_2A_1}(\Omega_3+\Omega_2-\Omega_1,\Omega_2-\Omega_1,-\Omega_1)e^{-i(\Omega_3+\Omega_2-\Omega_1)t}\\ &-\chi_{BA_3A_2A_1}(\Omega_3-\Omega_2+\Omega_1,-\Omega_2+\Omega_1,\Omega_1)e^{-i(\Omega_3-\Omega_2+\Omega_1)t}\\ &-\chi_{BA_3A_2A_1}(-\Omega_3+\Omega_2+\Omega_1,\Omega_2+\Omega_1,\Omega_1)e^{-i(-\Omega_3+\Omega_2+\Omega_1)t}\\ &+\chi_{BA_3A_2A_1}(\Omega_3-\Omega_2-\Omega_1,-\Omega_2-\Omega_1,-\Omega_1)e^{-i(\Omega_3-\Omega_2-\Omega_1)t}\\ &+\chi_{BA_3A_2A_1}(-\Omega_3+\Omega_2-\Omega_1,\Omega_2-\Omega_1,-\Omega_1)e^{-i(-\Omega_3+\Omega_2-\Omega_1)t}\\ &+\chi_{BA_3A_2A_1}(-\Omega_3-\Omega_2+\Omega_1,-\Omega_2+\Omega_1,\Omega_1)e^{-i(-\Omega_3-\Omega_2+\Omega_1)t}\\ &-\chi_{BA_3A_2A_1}(-\Omega_3-\Omega_2-\Omega_1,-\Omega_2-\Omega_1,-\Omega_1)e^{i(\Omega_3+\Omega_2+\Omega_1)t}\big\}.\end{aligned} \tag{5.15}$$

Using different experimental methods, one can selectively measure one or just a few terms in Equation 5.15. For instance, the first term describes the third-harmonic generation if the three incident field frequencies are the same and the measured signal is the third-harmonic electric field.

EXERCISE 5.2

Degenerate four-wave-mixing spectroscopy involves three radiation–matter interactions with external electric fields having the same center frequency.[8] If such a degenerate four-wave-mixing experiment is performed in the frequency domain, how many possible combinations (permutations) are to be considered in Equation 5.15? In particular, what is the susceptibility associated with the third-harmonic generation?

5.2 FOUR-LEVEL SYSTEM AND LINE-BROADENING FUNCTION

In general, the three radiation–matter interactions can induce quantum transitions among four different stationary states including the initial ground state. We shall therefore consider a four-level system as a model for third-order response spectroscopy.[9, 10] The four-level-system Hamiltonian is

$$\hat{H}_{4LS} = |a> \hbar\omega_{ag} <a| + |b> \hbar\omega_{bg} <b| + |c> \hbar\omega_{cg} <c|. \tag{5.16}$$

Due to the system–bath interaction that is responsible for fluctuations of transition frequencies in the reduced density matrix representation, the total matter Hamiltonian is

$$\hat{H}_{mat} = \hat{H}_{4LS} + \hat{H}_B + \hat{H}_{SB}. \tag{5.17}$$

The system–bath (chromophore–bath) interaction Hamiltonian, denoted as $\hat{H}_{SB}$, is assumed to be diagonal with respect to the system eigenstates as

$$\hat{H}_{SB} = V_{ag}(\mathbf{q})|a><a| + V_{bg}(\mathbf{q})|b><b| + V_{cg}(\mathbf{q})|c><c| \tag{5.18}$$

where the bath degrees of freedom are denoted as $\mathbf{q}$ and the potential energy differences are defined as $V_{jg}(\mathbf{q}) = V_j(\mathbf{q}) - V_g(\mathbf{q})$ for $j = a$, b, and c.

Therefore, we have

$$\hat{H}_{mat} = \sum_{m=g,a,b,c} \{\hbar\omega_m + V_m(\mathbf{q}) + H_B(\mathbf{q})\}|m><m| = \hat{H}_0 + \hat{H}' \tag{5.19}$$

where

$$\hat{H}_0 = \{\hbar\omega_g + V_g(\mathbf{q}) + H_B(\mathbf{q})\} \sum_{m=g,a,b,c} |m><m|$$

$$\hat{H}' = \sum_{m=a,b,c} \{\hbar\omega_{mg} + V_{mg}(\mathbf{q})\}|m><m|. \tag{5.20}$$

The ground state adiabatic Hamiltonian $\hat{H}_g(\mathbf{q})$, which is defined as $\hat{H}_g(\mathbf{q}) = \hbar\omega_g + V_g(\mathbf{q}) + H_B(\mathbf{q})$, is considered to be the reference Hamiltonian. $\hat{H}_j(\mathbf{q})$ (for $j = a$, b, and c) can then be written as

$$\hat{H}_j(\mathbf{q}) = \hat{H}_g(\mathbf{q}) + \hbar\omega_{jg} + V_{jg}(\mathbf{q}). \tag{5.21}$$

Treating $\hat{H}_g(\mathbf{q})$ as the zero-order Hamiltonian and taking the last two terms on the right-hand side of Equation 5.21 as the perturbation Hamiltonian, we find that, in the interaction picture, the forward and backward time evolution operators described by $\hat{H}_j(\mathbf{q})$ (for $j = a$, b, and c) are

$$\exp\left(-\frac{i}{\hbar}\hat{H}_j t\right) = \exp(-i\bar{\omega}_{jg}t)\exp\left(-\frac{i}{\hbar}\hat{H}_g t\right)\exp_+\left(-\frac{i}{\hbar}\int_0^t d\tau U_{jg}(\tau)\right)$$

$$\exp\left(\frac{i}{\hbar}\hat{H}_j t\right) = \exp(i\bar{\omega}_{jg}t)\exp_-\left(\frac{i}{\hbar}\int_0^t d\tau U_{jg}(\tau)\right)\exp\left(\frac{i}{\hbar}\hat{H}_g t\right) \tag{5.22}$$

where

$$\bar{\omega}_{jg} = \omega_{jg} + \hbar^{-1} < V_{jg}(\mathbf{q}) >$$

$$U_{jg} \equiv V_{jg}(\mathbf{q}) - < V_{jg}(\mathbf{q}) >$$

$$U_{jg}(t) = U_{jg}(\mathbf{q}(t)) = \exp\left(\frac{i}{\hbar}\hat{H}_B t\right)U_{jg}(\mathbf{q})\exp\left(-\frac{i}{\hbar}\hat{H}_B t\right). \tag{5.23}$$

The initial density operator may be written as a product of the system, and bath density operators as $\rho(-\infty) = \rho_S(-\infty)\rho_B(-\infty)$. The energies of the excited states in comparison to the ground state energy are assumed to be large so that the populations of those excited states at thermal equilibrium will be ignored for the sake of simplicity. Expanding the three commutators in the definition of the third-order response function in Equation 5.5, one can show that $\phi_{BA_3A_2A_1}(t_3, t_2, t_1)$ is given by sum of eight different contributions as

$$\phi_{BA_3A_2A_1}(t_3, t_2, t_1) = \left(\frac{i}{\hbar}\right)^3 \theta(t_3)\theta(t_2)\theta(t_1)\sum_{\alpha=1}^{4}[R_\alpha(t_3, t_2, t_1) - R_\alpha^*(t_3, t_2, t_1)] \tag{5.24}$$

where

$$R_1(t_3, t_2, t_1) \equiv < \hat{A}_2(t_1)\hat{A}_3(t_1 + t_2)\hat{B}(t_1 + t_2 + t_3)\hat{A}_1(0)\rho(-\infty) >$$

$$R_2(t_3, t_2, t_1) \equiv < \hat{A}_1(0)\hat{A}_3(t_1 + t_2)\hat{B}(t_1 + t_2 + t_3)\hat{A}_2(t_1)\rho(-\infty) >$$

$$R_3(t_3, t_2, t_1) \equiv < \hat{A}_1(0)\hat{A}_2(t_1)\hat{B}(t_1 + t_2 + t_3)\hat{A}_3(t_1 + t_2)\rho(-\infty) >$$

$$R_4(t_3, t_2, t_1) \equiv < \hat{B}(t_1 + t_2 + t_3)\hat{A}_3(t_1 + t_2)\hat{A}_2(t_1)\hat{A}_1(0)\rho(-\infty) >. \tag{5.25}$$

Using the operator identities in Equation 5.22, one can rewrite the four terms in Equation 5.25 as

$$R_1(t_3,t_2,t_1)=\sum_{abc}[A_2]_{gc}[A_3]_{cb}[B]_{ba}[A_1]_{ag} < e^{iH_g t_1}\, e^{iH_c t_2}\, e^{iH_b t_3}\, e^{-iH_a(t_1+t_2+t_3)} >$$

$$=\sum_{abc}[A_2]_{gc}[A_3]_{cb}[B]_{ba}[A_1]_{ag}\exp\{-i\bar{\omega}_{ab}t_3-i\bar{\omega}_{ac}t_2-i\bar{\omega}_{ag}t_1\}F_1(t_3,t_2,t_1)$$

$$R_2(t_3,t_2,t_1)=\sum_{abc}[A_1]_{gc}[A_3]_{cb}[B]_{ba}[A_2]_{ag} < e^{iH_c(t_1+t_2)}\, e^{iH_b t_3}\, e^{-iH_a(t_2+t_3)}\, e^{-iH_g t_1} >$$

$$=\sum_{abc}[A_1]_{gc}[A_3]_{cb}[B]_{ba}[A_2]_{ag}\exp\{-i\bar{\omega}_{ab}t_3-i\bar{\omega}_{ac}t_2-i\bar{\omega}_{gc}t_1\}F_2(t_3,t_2,t_1)$$

$$R_3(t_3,t_2,t_1)=\sum_{abc}[A_1]_{gc}[A_2]_{cb}[B]_{ba}[A_3]_{ag} < e^{iH_c t_1}\, e^{iH_b(t_2+t_3)}\, e^{-iH_a t_3}\, e^{-iH_g(t_1+t_2)} >$$

$$=\sum_{abc}[A_1]_{gc}[A_2]_{cb}[B]_{ba}[A_3]_{ag}\exp\{-i\bar{\omega}_{ab}t_3-i\bar{\omega}_{gb}t_2-i\bar{\omega}_{gc}t_1\}F_3(t_3,t_2,t_1)$$

$$R_4(t_3,t_2,t_1)=\sum_{abc}[B]_{gc}[A_3]_{cb}[A_2]_{ba}[A_1]_{ag} < e^{iH_g(t_1+t_2+t_3)}e^{-iH_c t_3}e^{-iH_b t_2}e^{-iH_a t_1} >$$

$$=\sum_{abc}[B]_{gc}[A_3]_{cb}[A_2]_{ba}[A_1]_{ag}\exp\{-i\bar{\omega}_{cg}t_3-i\bar{\omega}_{bg}t_2-i\bar{\omega}_{ag}t_1\}F_4(t_3,t_2,t_1) \quad (5.26)$$

where the line-shape functions are

$$F_1(t_3,t_2,t_1)=< e_-^{i\int_{t_1}^{t_1+t_2}d\tau\, U_{cg}(\tau)}\; e_-^{i\int_{t_1+t_2}^{t_1+t_2+t_3}d\tau\, U_{bg}(\tau)}\; e_+^{-i\int_0^{t_1+t_2+t_3}U_{ag}(\tau)} >$$

$$F_2(t_3,t_2,t_1)=< e_-^{i\int_0^{t_1+t_2}d\tau\, U_{cg}}\; e_-^{i\int_{t_1+t_2}^{t_1+t_2+t_3}d\tau\, U_{bg}(\tau)}\; e_+^{-i\int_{t_1}^{t_1+t_2+t_3}d\tau\, U_{ag}(\tau)} >$$

$$F_3(t_3,t_2,t_1)=< e_-^{i\int_0^{t_1}d\tau\, U_{cg}(\tau)}\; e_-^{i\int_{t_1}^{t_1+t_2+t_3}d\tau\, U_{bg}(\tau)}\; e_+^{-i\int_{t_1+t_2}^{t_1+t_2+t_3}d\tau\, U_{ag}(\tau)} >$$

$$F_4(t_3,t_2,t_1)=< e_+^{-i\int_{t_1+t_2}^{t_1+t_2+t_3}d\tau U_{cg}(\tau)}\; e_+^{-i\int_{t_1}^{t_1+t_2}d\tau\, U_{bg}(\tau)}\; e_+^{-i\int_0^{t_1}d\tau\, U_{ag}(\tau)} >. \quad (5.27)$$

The four response function components, R_j (for $j = 1 \sim 4$), correspond to the following four diagrams representing specific transition pathways:

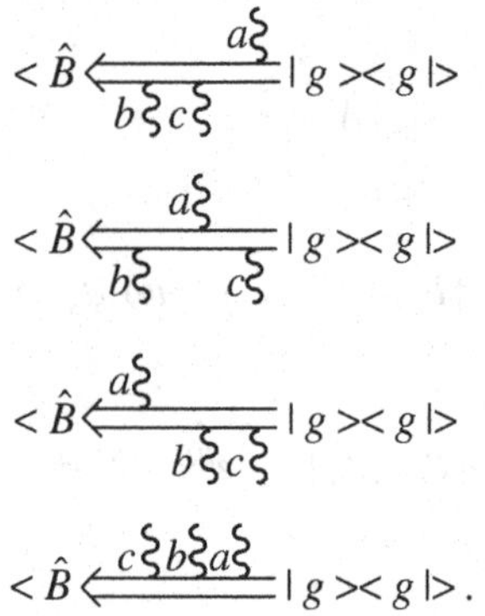

$$< \hat{B} \xleftarrow[b \zeta c \zeta]{a \zeta} | g >< g |>$$

$$< \hat{B} \xleftarrow[b \zeta \qquad c \zeta]{a \zeta} | g >< g |>$$

$$< \hat{B} \xleftarrow[b \zeta c \zeta]{a \zeta} | g >< g |>$$

$$< \hat{B} \xleftarrow{c \zeta b \zeta a \zeta} | g >< g |>. \qquad (5.28)$$

The physical meanings of these four different diagrams can be understood by following the same line of argument provided in Section 4.2 for the second-order response function.

Here, it is again noted that each third-order response function component consists of three parts, for example, for $R_1(t_3, t_2, t_1)$,

$$R_1(t_3, t_2, t_1) = \sum_{abc} [A_2]_{gc}[A_3]_{cb}[B]_{ba}[A_1]_{ag} \underbrace{\exp\{-i\bar{\omega}_{ab}t_3 - i\bar{\omega}_{ac}t_2 - i\bar{\omega}_{ag}t_1\}} F_1(t_3, t_2, t_1)$$

| Transition strength | Coherence oscillation | Line shape |

The first term is given as the product of four transition matrix elements, and it describes the amplitude of the specific nonlinear optical transition. The second term, which is a complex exponential function, describes the oscillations of involved coherences during the three time periods from t_1 to t_3 (see Figure 5.1). One can easily obtain the coherence oscillation term by simply examining the corresponding diagram shown in Equation 5.28. In the case of the $R_1(t_3, t_2, t_1)$ diagram in Figure 5.1, for example, we have

Coherence during t_1: $|a><g| \rightarrow$ coherence oscillation term: $\exp\{-i\bar{\omega}_{ag}t_1\}$
Coherence during t_2: $|a><c| \rightarrow$ coherence oscillation term: $\exp\{-i\bar{\omega}_{ac}t_2\}$
Coherence during t_3: $|a><b| \rightarrow$ coherence oscillation term: $\exp\{-i\bar{\omega}_{ab}t_3\}$.

Therefore the coherence oscillation term for $R_1(t_3, t_2, t_1)$ is $\exp\{-i\bar{\omega}_{ab}t_3 - i\bar{\omega}_{ac}t_2 - i\bar{\omega}_{ag}t_1\}$. Finally, the third term in each $R_j(t_3, t_2, t_1)$, which was denoted as $F_j(t_3, t_2, t_1)$, is a complex but decaying function. Essentially, the $(F_j(t_3, t_2, t_1))$ determines the line

$$<\hat{B} \xleftarrow[b \zeta \quad c \zeta]{a \zeta} |g><g|>$$

$$\underbrace{| \quad t_3 \quad | \quad t_2 \quad | \quad t_1 \quad |}$$

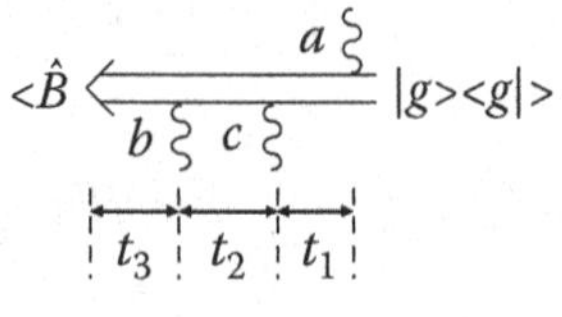

FIGURE 5.1 Time-ordered diagram representing the R_1 component.

shape of the third-order response function and spectrum. In order to develop a classical theory for the numerical calculations of the above nonlinear response function components, one can approximately replace the time-ordered exponential operators in Equation 5.27 with normal exponential functions with scalar difference potential energies instead of operators. This approximation strategy has been extensively used because one can obtain the trajectories of the difference potential energies by carrying out classical molecular dynamics simulations for any composite system consisting of a single solute molecule and hundreds to thousands of solvent molecules around it.

In order to obtain the approximate expressions for those line-shape functions, one can also use the cumulant expansion method to find the following results:

$$
\begin{aligned}
F_1(t_3,t_2,t_1) = \exp\{&-g^*_{cc}(t_2) - g^*_{bb}(t_3) - g_{aa}(t_1+t_2+t_3) - g^*_{cb}(t_2+t_3) + g^*_{cb}(t_2) + g^*_{cb}(t_3) \\
&+ g_{ca}(t_1+t_2) - g_{ca}(t_1) + g^*_{ca}(t_2+t_3) - g^*_{ca}(t_3) + g_{ba}(t_1+t_2+t_3) \\
&- g_{ba}(t_1+t_2) + g^*_{ba}(t_3)\} \\
F_2(t_3,t_2,t_1) = \exp\{&-g^*_{cc}(t_1+t_2) - g^*_{bb}(t_3) - g_{aa}(t_2+t_3) - g^*_{cb}(t_1+t_2+t_3) + g^*_{cb}(t_1+t_2) \\
&+ g^*_{cb}(t_3) + g_{ca}(t_2) + g^*_{ca}(t_1+t_2+t_3) - g^*_{ca}(t_1) - g^*_{ca}(t_3) + g_{ba}(t_2+t_3) \\
&- g_{ba}(t_2) + g^*_{ba}(t_3)\} \\
F_3(t_3,t_2,t_1) = \exp\{&-g^*_{cc}(t_1) - g^*_{bb}(t_2+t_3) - g_{aa}(t_3) - g^*_{cb}(t_1+t_2+t_3) + g^*_{cb}(t_1) + g^*_{cb}(t_2+t_3) \\
&+ g^*_{ca}(t_1+t_2+t_3) - g^*_{ca}(t_1+t_2) - g^*_{ca}(t_2+t_3) + g^*_{ca}(t_2) + g_{ba}(t_3) \\
&+ g^*_{ba}(t_2+t_3) - g^*_{ba}(t_2)\} \\
F_4(t_3,t_2,t_1) = \exp\{&-g_{cc}(t_3) - g_{bb}(t_2) - g_{aa}(t_1) - g_{cb}(t_2+t_3) + g_{cb}(t_2) + g_{cb}(t_3) \\
&- g_{ca}(t_1+t_2+t_3) + g_{ca}(t_1+t_2) + g_{ca}(t_2+t_3) - g_{ca}(t_2) - g_{ba}(t_1+t_2) \\
&+ g_{ba}(t_1) + g_{ba}(t_2)\}.
\end{aligned}
\tag{5.29}
$$

Here, the line-broadening function $g(t)$ was already defined before, and, for example,

$$g_{ba}(t) = \int_0^t d\tau_1 \int_0^{\tau_1} d\tau_2 C_{ba}(\tau_2) \tag{5.30}$$

where

$$C_{ba}(t) = \frac{1}{\hbar^2} < U_{bg}(t) U_{ag}(0) \rho_B >_B . \tag{5.31}$$

EXERCISE 5.3

Derive Equation 5.29. Hints: (1) Expand the positive and negative time-ordered exponential operators in Equation 5.27. (2) Ignore the first-order terms with respect to U_{jg} (for $j = a \sim f$) since the ensemble average of U_{jg} over Gaussian distributions vanishes. (3) Consider terms that are second-order with respect to U_{jg}. (4) Rewrite the series expansions as normal exponential functions as an approximation.

The fluctuation of the electronic transition frequency induces dephasing of the electronic coherence. One of the most widely used models for the electronic dephasing process is linear coupling model with harmonic oscillator bath, where the bath degrees of freedom are linearly coupled to the electronic transition. Thus, the fluctuating part of the electronic transition frequency is assumed to be given as $\delta\omega(t) = \sum_j h_j x_j(t)$, where x_j is the jth bath oscillator. This is essentially identical to the Brownian oscillator model, where the vibrational coordinates of the system are coupled to the bath degrees of freedom.[3, 11]

Although the effect of the general system–bath interaction on the third-order response function was properly taken into account by Equations 5.29, the Markovian limit will provide a conceptually simple picture about the dephasing effects on the third-order response function. The Markovian approximation to the fluctuating difference potential time-correlation functions means that

$$g_{xy}(t) \cong \gamma_{xy} t, \tag{5.32}$$

where γ_{xy} is the pure dephasing rate. Here, a caution should be taken when the physical meaning of γ_{xy} is examined. The off-diagonal element, such as γ_{ba}, is not the dephasing constant of the coherence, $\rho_{ba}(t)$. From the definition of $C_{ba}(t)$, γ_{ba} is related to the cross-correlation amplitude between the fluctuating difference potentials U_{bg} and U_{ag}. The usual dephasing rate of the coherence $\rho_{ag}(t)$ is represented by γ_{aa}. Typically, the amplitude of the cross-correlation between U_{xg} and U_{yg} for $x \neq y$ is likely to be smaller than that of the auto-correlation.[12] This was called the uncorrelated frequency fluctuation (UFF) approximation in Section 4.2.

Substituting the approximate expression Equation 5.32 into Equation 5.29, we have

$$\begin{aligned}
R_1(t_3,t_2,t_1) &= \sum_{abc} [A_2]_{gc}[A_3]_{cb}[B]_{ba}[A_1]_{ag} \exp\{-i\bar{\omega}_{ab}t_3 - i\bar{\omega}_{ac}t_2 - i\bar{\omega}_{ag}t_1\} \\
&\quad \times \exp(-\eta_{ba}t_3 - \eta_{ca}t_2 - \gamma_{aa}t_1) \\
R_2(t_3,t_2,t_1) &= \sum_{abc} [A_1]_{gc}[A_3]_{cb}[B]_{ba}[A_2]_{ag} \exp\{-i\bar{\omega}_{ab}t_3 - i\bar{\omega}_{ac}t_2 - i\bar{\omega}_{gc}t_1\} \\
&\quad \times \exp(-\eta_{ba}t_3 - \eta_{ca}t_2 - \gamma_{cc}t_1) \\
R_3(t_3,t_2,t_1) &= \sum_{abc} [A_1]_{gc}[A_2]_{cb}[B]_{ba}[A_3]_{ag} \exp\{-i\bar{\omega}_{ab}t_3 - i\bar{\omega}_{gb}t_2 - i\bar{\omega}_{gc}t_1\} \\
&\quad \times \exp(-\eta_{ba}t_3 - \gamma_{bb}t_2 - \gamma_{cc}t_1) \\
R_4(t_3,t_2,t_1) &= \sum_{abc} [B]_{gc}[A_3]_{cb}[A_2]_{ba}[A_1]_{ag} \exp\{-i\bar{\omega}_{cg}t_3 - i\bar{\omega}_{bg}t_2 - i\bar{\omega}_{ag}t_1\} \\
&\quad \times \exp\{-\gamma_{cc}t_3 - \gamma_{bb}t_2 - \gamma_{aa}t_1\},
\end{aligned} \tag{5.33}$$

where

$$\eta_{xy} \equiv (\gamma_{xx} + \gamma_{yy} - 2\gamma_{xy})(1 - \delta_{xy}) + \mathrm{T}_x \delta_{xy}. \tag{5.34}$$

Although the above results are based on the Markovian approximation to the energy gap (difference potential U_{jg}) fluctuation correlation, they provide a simple picture of each third-order response component. In Equation 5.34 are terms given as a combination of dephasing constants, for example, $\gamma_{cc} + \gamma_{bb} - 2\gamma_{cb}$. In order to fully calculate the response functions, the summations over all states *a*, *b*, and *c* should be performed, and then there is the case when $c = b$, for example. In this case, the diagonal density matrix evolution is involved in the nonlinear response of the molecular system. Therefore, the population relaxation process should be properly taken into account in the above third-order response function, and this can be achieved by introducing the inverse lifetime of the *x*-state as T_x in Equation 5.34. Such lifetime broadening effects on the third-order response function will be treated in an *ad hoc* manner by multiplying a proper exponentially decaying function to Equation 5.29 in this and following chapters. In the Markovian limit, the 3D Fourier-Laplace transforms of $F_j(t_3, t_2, t_1)$ can be easily performed to eventually get the 3D third-order susceptibility.

EXERCISE 5.4

Obtain the third-order susceptibility by taking triple Fourier-Laplace transformations of the third-order response function in Equation 5.33 in the Markovian limit.

The results presented in this chapter are quite general for any arbitrary four-level system. An early application of the third-order response spectroscopy was the degenerate four-wave-mixing technique such as pump–probe or photon echo spectroscopy of dye molecules in solutions. In that case, the optical chromophore was modeled as a two-level system instead of a four-level system. Then, the complicated line-broadening functions in Equation 5.29 are highly simplified so that the interpretation of four-wave-mixing signal was relatively straightforward. To show what information can be extracted from such a four-wave-mixing spectroscopic investigation, we shall consider the photon echo spectroscopy of a model two-level system later in this chapter.

5.3 SHORT-TIME APPROXIMATION TO THE THIRD-ORDER RESPONSE FUNCTION

The third-order response function in Equation 5.29 is exact in the case that the distribution of difference potential V_{jg} (or fluctuating part of the transition frequency U_{jg}) is a Gaussian. However, its implication to the calculation of the third-order signal electric field will require complicated convolution integrals that cannot be performed analytically. Although it is possible to carry out such numerical integrations without any difficulties, it is not always easy to understand the underlying physics nor to interpret the experimentally measured signal in terms of the usual dephasing constant, inhomogeneous width, dynamic correlation between two different transition frequency fluctuations in time, and so on. Furthermore, fitting the experimental data with properly modeled time-correlation functions $C_{xy}(t)$'s and with Equation 5.29 is not an easy task. Therefore, one may find it useful to consider an approximate expression for the third-order response function, which still contains most of the salient features of the third-order response by multilevel molecular systems. In this regard, the short-time approximation to the line shape functions, $F_j(t_3, t_2, t_1)$, has been found to be of use for such purposes.[12–15]

The short-time approximation is based on the fact that the system is in highly oscillating coherences during the first and third time periods, t_1 and t_3. Since the measured value, such as third-order polarization, is always given as triple convolutions over these time variables, only the short-time (slowly varying) parts of the third-order response during t_1 and t_3 are important and often sufficient to approximately describe the quantum decoherent processes.[13, 16] This is in priciple related to the stationary phase approximation or to the Laplace approximation for integration over highly oscillating functions. Nevertheless, it is necessary to take into consideration of the spectral diffusion and the correlation between the excitation and probing frequencies to describe a number of experimentally observed phenomena such as Stokes shift induced by solvation dynamics, photon echo peak shift, 2D peak shape changes, and so on. Then, one can achieve this goal by taking a 2D Taylor expansion of the exponents in Equations 5.29 with respect to t_1 and t_3.[12] We then find, for $j = 1$ - 4,

$$F_j(t_3, t_2, t_1) = \exp\left\{ f_j(t_2) - \frac{1}{2}\delta_j^2(t_2)t_1^2 - \frac{1}{2}\Delta_j^2(t_2)t_3^2 + H_j(t_2)t_1t_3 + iQ_j(t_2)t_3 \right\}. \quad (5.35)$$

Here, $f_j(t_2)$ describes the dephasing of the quantum coherences or populations during t_2 period, and for $j = 1$ - 4 they are

$$\begin{aligned} f_1(t_2) &= -g_{cc}^*(t_2) - g_{aa}(t_2) + 2\,\mathrm{Re}[g_{ca}(t_2)] \\ f_2(t_2) &= f_1(t_2) = -g_{cc}^*(t_2) - g_{aa}(t_2) + 2\,\mathrm{Re}[g_{ca}(t_2)] \\ f_3(t_2) &= -g_{bb}^*(t_2) \\ f_4(t_2) &= -g_{bb}(t_2). \end{aligned} \quad (5.36)$$

The expansion coefficients $\delta_j^2(t_2)$ in Equation 5.35 represent the mean square fluctuation amplitudes of the difference potentials (or transition frequency) that are associated with the off-diagonal density matrix evolutions during the first time period t_1. Note that, in the impulsive limit, $\delta_j^2(t_2)$ determines the spectral bandwidth of the corresponding 2D spectrum along the first frequency (ω_{t_1}) variable that is conjugate frequency of t_1. For $j = 1$ - 4, we have

$$\begin{aligned} \delta_1^2(t_2) &= C_{ca}(0) + \mathrm{Re}[C_{aa}(t_2) - C_{ca}(t_2)] \\ \delta_2^2(t_2) &= C_{ca}(0) - \mathrm{Re}[C_{ca}(t_2) - C_{cc}^*(t_2)] \\ \delta_3^2(t_2) &= C_{cc}(0) - C_{cb}(0) + \mathrm{Re}[C_{cb}(t_2)] \\ \delta_4^2(t_2) &= C_{aa}(0) - C_{ba}(0) + \mathrm{Re}[C_{ba}(t_2)]. \end{aligned} \quad (5.37)$$

Similarly, $\Delta_j^2(t_2)$ corresponds to the mean square frequency fluctuation amplitude of the coherence during the third time period, t_3, and they are

$$\Delta_1^2(t_2) = C_{bb}(0) - C_{cb}(0) - C_{ba}(0) + C_{ca}(0) + \mathrm{Re}[C_{aa}(t_2) + C_{cb}(t_2) - C_{ca}(t_2) - C_{ba}(t_2)]$$

$$\Delta_2^2(t_2) = C_{bb}(0) + C_{ca}(0) - C_{cb}(0) - C_{ba}(0) - \mathrm{Re}\,[C_{ca}(t_2) + C_{ba}(t_2) - C_{aa}(t_2) - C_{cb}(t_2)]$$

$$\Delta_3^2(t_2) = C_{aa}(0) - C_{ba}(0) + \mathrm{Re}[C_{bb}(t_2) - C_{ba}(t_2)]$$

$$\Delta_4^2(t_2) = C_{cc}(0) - C_{cb}(0) + \mathrm{Re}[C_{cb}(t_2)]. \tag{5.38}$$

The fourth term, $H_j(t_2)$, in Equation 5.35 describes how the two transition frequencies at t_1 and t_3 separated by t_2 are correlated with each other. In the limit that $H_j(t_2) = 0$, the transition frequency associated with the coherence created by the first field-matter interaction is completely uncorrelated with that induced by the third field-matter interaction. It turned out that this term is critical in understanding the photon echo peak shift, 2D spectral peak shape change in time, and so on. As will be shown later in this book, if the molecular system has large static inhomogeneity such as the cases of impurities in glass or polymer matrix, $H_j(t_2)$ doesn't decay to zero at least in the timescale of experimental measurements, which makes the photon echo peak shift value finite even at long time. A more detailed discussion along this line will be presented later in this chapter. Now, for j = 1 - 4, we have

$$H_1(t_2) = \mathrm{Re}[C_{ba}(t_2) - C_{aa}(t_2)]$$

$$H_2(t_2) = -\,\mathrm{Re}[C_{cb}(t_2) - C_{ca}(t_2)]$$

$$H_3(t_2) = -\,\mathrm{Re}[C_{cb}(t_2) - C_{ca}(t_2)]$$

$$H_4(t_2) = -\,\mathrm{Re}[C_{ca}(t_2)]. \tag{5.39}$$

The last term $Q_j(t_2)$ in Equation 5.35 describes the spectral diffusion, which is related to the fluorescence Stokes shift, during the second time period t_2:

$$Q_1(t_2) = \mathrm{Im}[\bar{C}_{aa}(0) - \bar{C}_{aa}(t_2) - \bar{C}_{cb}(0) + \bar{C}_{cb}(-t_2) + \bar{C}_{ca}(0) - \bar{C}_{ca}(-t_2) - \bar{C}_{ba}(0) + \bar{C}_{ba}(t_2)]$$

$$Q_2(t_2) = \mathrm{Im}[\bar{C}_{aa}(0) - \bar{C}_{aa}(t_2) - \bar{C}_{cb}(0) + \bar{C}_{cb}(-t_2) + \bar{C}_{ca}(0) - \bar{C}_{ca}(-t_2) - \bar{C}_{ba}(0) + \bar{C}_{ba}(t_2)]$$

$$Q_3(t_2) = \mathrm{Im}[\bar{C}^*_{bb}(0) - \bar{C}^*_{bb}(t_2) + \bar{C}_{ba}(0) - \bar{C}_{ba}(-t_2)]$$

$$Q_4(t_2) = \mathrm{Im}[\bar{C}_{cb}(0) - \bar{C}_{cb}(t_2)], \tag{5.40}$$

where

$$\bar{C}_{xy}(t) = \int_0^t d\tau\, C_{xy}(\tau). \tag{5.41}$$

It should be noted that the short-time expansion coefficients in Equation 5.35 were all described in terms of the linear *U-U* time-correlation functions, $C_{xy}(t)$'s. Within this short-time approximation, the line-shape functions, $F_j(t_3, t_2, t_1)$, are Gaussian functions with respect to t_1 and t_3. Consequently, if the temporal envelope functions of the external fields are Gaussian in time, one can perform the convolution integrations mathematically.

5.4 THIRD-ORDER RESPONSE FUNCTION OF A TWO-LEVEL SYSTEM

For a two-level system (2LS) consisting of the ground and excited states, the third-order response function components in Equation 5.26 with 5.29 are simplified as

$$\begin{aligned}
R_1(t_3,t_2,t_1) &= [A_2]_{ge}[A_3]_{eg}[B]_{ge}[A_1]_{eg}\exp(-i\bar{\omega}_{eg}t_3 - i\bar{\omega}_{eg}t_1)\\
&\quad\times\exp\{-g^*(t_3) - g(t_1) - f_+(t_3,t_2,t_1)\}\\
R_2(t_3,t_2,t_1) &= [A_1]_{ge}[A_3]_{eg}[B]_{ge}[A_2]_{eg}\exp(-i\bar{\omega}_{eg}t_3 + i\bar{\omega}_{eg}t_1)\\
&\quad\times\exp\{-g^*(t_3) - g^*(t_1) + f_+^*(t_3,t_2,t_1)\}\\
R_3(t_3,t_2,t_1) &= [A_1]_{ge}[A_2]_{eg}[B]_{ge}[A_3]_{eg}\exp(-i\bar{\omega}_{eg}t_3 + i\bar{\omega}_{eg}t_1)\\
&\quad\times\exp\{-g(t_3) - g^*(t_1) + f_-^*(t_3,t_2,t_1)\}\\
R_4(t_3,t_2,t_1) &= [B]_{ge}[A_3]_{eg}[A_2]_{ge}[A_1]_{eg}\exp(-i\bar{\omega}_{eg}t_3 - i\bar{\omega}_{eg}t_1)\\
&\quad\times\exp\{-g(t_3) - g(t_1) - f_-(t_3,t_2,t_1)\},
\end{aligned} \tag{5.42}$$

where the two auxiliary functions are defined as

$$\begin{aligned}
f_+(t_3,t_2,t_1) &= g^*(t_2) - g^*(t_2+t_3) - g(t_1+t_2) + g(t_1+t_2+t_3)\\
f_-(t_3,t_2,t_1) &= g(t_2) - g(t_2+t_3) - g(t_1+t_2) + g(t_1+t_2+t_3).
\end{aligned} \tag{5.43}$$

Here, the linear line-broadening function $g(t)$ for a 2LS was already discussed in detail in Section 3.2. The four response function components, R_j (for $j = 1 - 4$), in Equation 5.42 correspond to the following four diagrams representing specific transition pathways, respectively:

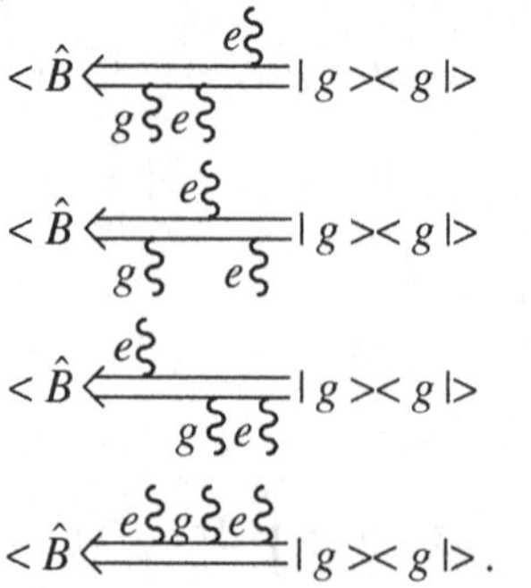

(5.44)

The first and fourth diagrams are called the nonrephasing diagrams. In these cases, the oscillating pattern of the coherence $\rho_{eg}^{(1)}$ during the first time period t_1 is identical to that during the third time period t_3. On the other hand, the rephasing diagrams are the second and third ones in Equation 5.42 or 5.44. In these cases, the first coherence during t_1 is $\rho_{ge}^{(1)}$ with oscillation frequency $\bar{\omega}_{ge}$, whereas that during t_3 is $\rho_{eg}^{(3)}$ with oscillation frequency $\bar{\omega}_{eg}$. Consequently, in the inhomogeneous broadening situation, the optical phase acquired during the first time period t_1 is reversed during t_3 so that the macroscopic optical coherence is rephased. This will be discussed more in detail in this chapter.

The first two diagrams R_1 and R_2 involve population evolutions on the excited state during t_2, whereas the last two diagrams associated with R_3 and R_4 involve population evolutions on the ground state during t_2. Therefore, in the language of pump–probe spectroscopy, the former two pathways (R_1 and R_2) are called stimulated emission (SE) terms because the third radiation–matter interaction stimulates an emissive process from the excited state molecule. On the other hand, the latter two pathways (R_3 and R_4) are known as the ground-state bleaching (GB). Thus, the four diagrams are usually grouped as

$$\begin{aligned} \text{Rephasing pathways: } & R_2(t_3,t_2,t_1) \quad \text{and} \quad R_3(t_3,t_2,t_1) \\ \text{Nonrephasing pathways: } & R_1(t_3,t_2,t_1) \quad \text{and} \quad R_4(t_3,t_2,t_1) \\ \text{SE pathways: } & R_1(t_3,t_2,t_1) \quad \text{and} \quad R_2(t_3,t_2,t_1) \\ \text{GB pathways: } & R_3(t_3,t_2,t_1) \quad \text{and} \quad R_4(t_3,t_2,t_1). \end{aligned} \tag{5.45}$$

The line-shape functions that are the last exponential parts in Equation 5.42 are determined by the pure dephasing processes originating from the fluctuating chromophore–bath interactions. However, there are additional contributions to the line broadening, which originate from the finite lifetimes of the excited states. For the four third-order response function components, by examining the corresponding diagrams, one can take account of the lifetime-broadening effects by multiplying the following exponentially decaying function to all R_j's

$$\exp(-t_3/2T_e - t_2/T_e - t_1/2T_e). \tag{5.46}$$

The SE pathways $R_1(t_3,t_2,t_1)$ and $R_2(t_3,t_2,t_1)$ involve excited-state population evolution during t_2 period so that the corresponding lifetime-broadening factor is $\exp(-t_2/T_e)$, where T_e is the excited-state lifetime. On the other hand, the GB pathways $R_3(t_3,t_2,t_1)$ and $R_4(t_3,t_2,t_1)$ involve ground-state population evolution during t_2 period. If the ground-state (bleaching) hole is filled by the population relaxation from the excited state to the ground state during t_2 and if there are no other intermediate states that act like excitation acceptors, the timescale of the ground-state hole filling is identical to the excited-state lifetime. That is why the two GB terms $R_3(t_3,t_2,t_1)$ and $R_4(t_3,t_2,t_1)$ should also be lifetime-broadened by the same factor of $\exp(-t_2/T_e)$. However, if the excited-state population is allowed to be transferred to other intermediate states, which is not the ground state, the disappearance timescale of the GB term is likely to be long, and the t_2-dependency of the GB terms $R_3(t_3,t_2,t_1)$ and $R_4(t_3,t_2,t_1)$ would be notably different from that of the SE terms $R_1(t_3,t_2,t_1)$ and $R_2(t_3,t_2,t_1)$. Although the lifetime-broadening processes are important in many spectroscopic phenomena, they will be omitted throughout this chapter not only because they are not the main concern of this book but also because one can always include such contributions to the multidimensional spectrum when it is necessary.

Although the general expression for the third-order response function has been used to interpret a number of four-wave-mixing processes of a 2LS, one may find it useful to consider its short-time approximated expression for further understanding of the detailed line shape.[15] Noting that the relaxation times of the off-diagonal (coherence) density matrix elements during t_1 and t_3 periods are very fast, it is generally acceptable to assume that $t_1 + t_2 \cong t_2$. Then, from Equation 5.42, the four response function components can be approximately written as

$$R_1(t_3,t_2,t_1) = [A_2]_{ge}[A_3]_{eg}[B]_{ge}[A_1]_{eg} \exp(-i\bar{\omega}_{eg}t_1 - i\{\bar{\omega}_{eg} + 2Q(t_2)\}t_3)$$
$$\times \exp\left\{-\frac{1}{2}\Omega^2 t_1^2 - \frac{1}{2}\Omega^2 t_3^2 - H(t_2)t_1t_3\right\}$$

$$R_2(t_3,t_2,t_1) = [A_1]_{ge}[A_3]_{eg}[B]_{ge}[A_2]_{eg} \exp(i\bar{\omega}_{eg}t_1 - i\{\bar{\omega}_{eg} + 2Q(t_2)\}t_3)$$
$$\times \exp\left\{-\frac{1}{2}\Omega^2 t_1^2 - \frac{1}{2}\Omega^2 t_3^2 + H(t_2)t_1t_3\right\}$$

$$R_3(t_3,t_2,t_1) = [A_1]_{ge}[A_2]_{eg}[B]_{ge}[A_3]_{eg} \exp(i\bar{\omega}_{eg}t_1 - i\bar{\omega}_{eg}t_3)$$
$$\times \exp\left\{-\frac{1}{2}\Omega^2 t_1^2 - \frac{1}{2}\Omega^2 t_3^2 + H(t_2)t_1t_3\right\}$$

$$R_4(t_3,t_2,t_1) = [B]_{ge}[A_3]_{eg}[A_2]_{ge}[A_1]_{eg} \exp(-i\bar{\omega}_{eg}t_1 - i\bar{\omega}_{eg}t_3)$$
$$\times \exp\left\{-\frac{1}{2}\Omega^2 t_1^2 - \frac{1}{2}\Omega^2 t_3^2 - H(t_2)t_1t_3\right\}. \quad (5.47)$$

Here, the mean square fluctuation amplitude of the difference potential (transition frequency) is defined as, in terms of the spectral density (see Section 3.2),

$$\Omega^2 \equiv \int d\omega\, \rho(\omega)\omega^2 \coth\frac{\hbar\omega\beta}{2}. \quad (5.48)$$

The spectral diffusion process is described by $Q(t)$, which is defined as

$$Q(t) \equiv \left(S(t) - \frac{\lambda}{\hbar} \right) \tag{5.49}$$

$$S(t) \equiv \int_0^\infty d\omega \, \rho(\omega)\omega \cos \omega t. \tag{5.50}$$

The fluorescence Stokes shift reflecting solvation dynamics is, within the linear response approximation, directly proportional to $S(t)$.[2]

The system–bath interaction-induced correlation between the transition frequency of the system during t_1 and that during t_3 is represented by $H(t)$ function that is defined as

$$H(t) \equiv \int_0^\infty d\omega \, \rho(\omega) \coth\left[\frac{\hbar\omega\beta}{2} \right] \omega^2 \cos \omega t. \tag{5.51}$$

From the definition of the time-correlation function of the difference potential, one can identify that

$$H(t) = \mathrm{Re}[C(t)] = \frac{1}{\hbar^2} \mathrm{Re}[< U(t)U(0)\rho_B >_B]. \tag{5.52}$$

Note that in the high-temperature limit (or classical limit), $H(t)$ is directly related to $S(t)$ by

$$H(t) \cong \frac{2}{\hbar\beta} \int_0^\infty d\omega \, \rho(\omega)\omega \cos \omega t = \frac{2}{\hbar\beta} S(t). \tag{5.53}$$

The line-shape functions in Equation 5.47, which are the last exponential functions, are two-dimensional Gaussians and the ellipticity of the 2D shape is determined by $H(t)$ or the real part of the time-correlation function $C(t)$. In the case when there is no truly static inhomogeneity, $H(t_2)$ decays in time and approaches zero so that the 2D peak shape becomes a 2D Gaussian with zero ellipticity at long time t_2. Due to the spectral diffusion function, $Q(t_2)$, the transition frequency of the system during t_3 changes from $\bar{\omega}_{eg}$ at $t_2 = 0$ to $\bar{\omega}_{eg} - 2\lambda/\hbar$ at $t_2 = \infty$ in the cases of the first two response function components. In Chapters 6 and 7, we will use these short-time approximation results in Equation 5.47 to present a discussion on the 2D peak shape of pump–probe and photon echo spectra of a 2LS, respectively.

5.5 PUMP–PROBE SPECTROSCOPY OF A TWO-LEVEL SYSTEM

Pump–probe spectroscopy has been extensively used to investigate the excited-state lifetime, vibrational wavepacket propagations on the electronically excited and ground states, chemical reaction dynamics in gas or condensed phases, and so on. Depending on the pulse configuration and detection method, a number of different types of pump–probe spectroscopies exist, which are still based on a four-wave-mixing scheme.[17] For example, transient grating (TG) spectroscopy has been used to study wavepacket (particle and hole) evolutions on the excited and ground states. By injecting two simultaneously propagating laser pulses with different wavevectors, vibrational coherences are created on the ground and excited states. A probe laser pulse delayed from the pump pulses is used to create a third-order polarization in the optical sample. Then, radiated signal field intensity (not amplitude) is measured in this case of the TG experiment. For a two-electronic-level system, the population relaxation and the electronic dephasing process induced by fluctuating chromophore-solvent interaction energy can therefore be studied with this TG method. Other methods to study the time evolution of the same third-order polarization are transient dichroism (TD) and transient birefringence (TB) measurements.[18] Instead of detecting the signal field *intensity*, it is possible to control the phase of the local oscillator to measure either the real or imaginary part of the third-order signal electric field. These correspond to the TD and TB experiments. These three (TG, TD, and TB) different spectroscopies can all be referred to as pump–probe spectroscopic methods in general.

The conventional transient grating measurement utilizes two pulses with wavevectors of $\mathbf{k}_1$ and $\mathbf{k}_2$. Then, the third ($\mathbf{k}_3$) pulse, which is delayed in time from the $\mathbf{k}_2$ pulse, is injected, and the scattered signal field intensity in the direction of $-\mathbf{k}_1+\mathbf{k}_2+\mathbf{k}_3$ is detected (homodyne detection). The self-heterodyned pump–probe spectroscopy, on the other hand, uses a single-pump pulse with wavevector of $\mathbf{k}_{pu}$; the $\mathbf{k}_{pr}$ probe pulse delayed in time is injected to create the corresponding third-order polarization, and the interference of the signal electric field generated by the third-order polarization with the probe field itself is measured (see Figure 5.2).[3] Therefore, the pump–probe signal in this case is linearly proportional to the third-order polarization, particularly

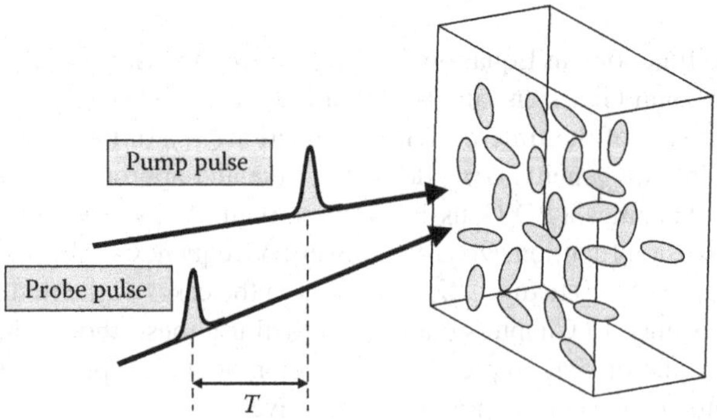

FIGURE 5.2 Experimental beam configuration of pump–probe spectroscopy.

the imaginary part of the polarization. If the phase of a local oscillator field could further be controlled, one could measure either the real or imaginary parts of the polarization separately, which correspond to TB and TD, respectively.

In the case of the two-pulse pump–probe spectroscopy in Figure 5.2, one needs to consider the following two cases together, since there are two time-nonordered radiation–matter interactions involved with the pump pulse:

Case 1)

$$\hat{A}_1F_1(t) = \boldsymbol{\mu}\cdot\mathbf{e}_{pu}E_{pu}(t+T)\,\mathrm{e}^{i\mathbf{k}_{pu}\cdot\mathbf{r}-i\omega_{pu}t}$$

$$\hat{A}_2F_2(t) = \boldsymbol{\mu}\cdot\mathbf{e}^*_{pu}E^*_{pu}(t+T)\,\mathrm{e}^{-i\mathbf{k}_{pu}\cdot\mathbf{r}+i\omega_{pu}t}$$

$$\hat{A}_3F_3(t) = \boldsymbol{\mu}\cdot\mathbf{e}_{pr}E_{pr}(t)\,\mathrm{e}^{i\mathbf{k}_{pr}\cdot\mathbf{r}-i\omega_{pr}t}$$

$$\hat{B} = \boldsymbol{\mu} \tag{5.54}$$

Case 2)

$$\hat{A}_1F_1(t) = \boldsymbol{\mu}\cdot\mathbf{e}^*_{pu}E^*_{pu}(t+T)\,\mathrm{e}^{-i\mathbf{k}_{pu}\cdot\mathbf{r}+i\omega_{pu}t}$$

$$\hat{A}_2F_2(t) = \boldsymbol{\mu}\cdot\mathbf{e}_{pu}E_{pu}(t+T)\,\mathrm{e}^{i\mathbf{k}_{pu}\cdot\mathbf{r}-i\omega_{pu}t}$$

$$\hat{A}_3F_3(t) = \boldsymbol{\mu}\cdot\mathbf{e}_{pr}E_{pr}(t)\,\mathrm{e}^{i\mathbf{k}_{pr}\cdot\mathbf{r}-i\omega_{pr}t}$$

$$\hat{B} = \boldsymbol{\mu}. \tag{5.55}$$

Here, the pump pulse is assumed to precede the probe pulse by a finite delay time T. Then, the third-order pump–probe polarization, which is the expectation value of the electric dipole operator, is

$$\begin{aligned}\mathbf{P}_{PP}(\mathrm{r},t) = \mathrm{e}^{i\mathbf{k}_{pr}\cdot\mathbf{r}-i\omega_{pr}t}\int_0^\infty dt_1\int_0^\infty dt_2\int_0^\infty dt_3\,\{&\phi_{\mu\mu\mu\mu}\,\vdots\,\mathbf{e}_{pr}\mathbf{e}^*_{pu}\mathbf{e}_{pu}E_{pr}(t-t_3)E^*_{pu}(t+T-t_3-t_2)\\ &\times E_{pu}(t+T-t_3-t_2-t_1)\exp(i\omega_{pr}t_3+i\omega_{pu}t_1)\\ &+\phi_{\mu\mu\mu\mu}\,\vdots\,\mathbf{e}_{pr}\mathbf{e}_{pu}\mathbf{e}^*_{pu}E_{pr}(t-t_3)E_{pu}(t+T-t_3-t_2)\\ &\times E^*_{pu}(t+T-t_3-t_2-t_1)\exp(i\omega_{pr}t_3-i\omega_{pu}t_1)\}.\end{aligned} \tag{5.56}$$

In order to simplify the above expression, we need to consider the resonant conditions. The third-order response function consists of eight different contributions as shown in Equation 5.24. However, their oscillating patterns in time or coherence oscillation terms are different from one another. For instance, the coherence oscillation term of $R_1(t_3,t_2,t_1)$ is $\exp(-i\bar{\omega}_{eg}t_1 - i\bar{\omega}_{eg}t_3)$. Therefore, this contribution can be resonantly enhanced with the electric field component oscillating as $\exp(i\omega_{pr}t_3 + i\omega_{pu}t_1)$ when $\omega_{pu} = \omega_{pr} = \bar{\omega}_{eg}$. In Equation 5.56, the first term in the integrand contains such term so that among eight different response function components (R_j (for $j = 1 - 4$) and their complex conjugates) only $R_1(t_3,t_2,t_1)$ and $R_4(t_3,t_2,t_1)$, which were classified to be the nonrephasing pathways are in resonance with the electric field component $\exp(i\omega_{pr}t_3 + i\omega_{pu}t_1)$ in the integrand of Equation 5.56. Similarly, the two rephasing pathways $R_2(t_3,t_2,t_1)$ and $R_3(t_3,t_2,t_1)$ are important when the electric field component oscillates as $\exp(i\omega_{pr}t_3 - i\omega_{pu}t_1)$. Thus, considering these resonant conditions (or the so-called rotating wave approximation), Equation 5.56 can be rewritten as

$$\mathbf{P}_{PP}(\mathbf{r},t) = e^{i\mathbf{k}_{pr}\cdot\mathbf{r}-i\omega_{pr}t}\left(\frac{i}{\hbar}\right)^3 \int_0^\infty dt_1 \int_0^\infty dt_2 \int_0^\infty dt_3 [\{R_1 + R_4\} \vdots \mathbf{e}_{pr}\mathbf{e}^*_{pu}\mathbf{e}_{pu}E_{pr}(t-t_3)$$

$$\times E^*_{pu}(t+T-t_3-t_2)E_{pu}(t+T-t_3-t_2-t_1)\exp(i\omega_{pr}t_3 + i\omega_{pu}t_1)$$

$$+ \{R_2 + R_3\} \vdots \mathbf{e}_{pr}\mathbf{e}_{pu}\mathbf{e}^*_{pu}E_{pr}(t-t_3)E_{pu}(t+T-t_3-t_2)$$

$$\times E^*_{pu}(t+T-t_3-t_2-t_1)\exp(i\omega_{pr}t_3 - i\omega_{pu}t_1)]. \qquad (5.57)$$

Now, let us consider the transient grating with phase-matching condition $\mathbf{k}_s = -\mathbf{k}_1 + \mathbf{k}_2 + \mathbf{k}_3$. In this case, the effective radiation–matter interactions and the effect operator are

$$\hat{A}_1 F_1(t) = \boldsymbol{\mu}\cdot\mathbf{e}^*_1 E^*_1(t+T)e^{-i\mathbf{k}_1\cdot\mathbf{r}+i\omega_1 t}$$

$$\hat{A}_2 F_2(t) = \boldsymbol{\mu}\cdot\mathbf{e}_2 E_2(t+T)e^{i\mathbf{k}_2\cdot\mathbf{r}-i\omega_2 t}$$

$$\hat{A}_3 F_3(t) = \boldsymbol{\mu}\cdot\mathbf{e}_3 E_3(t)e^{i\mathbf{k}_3\cdot\mathbf{r}-i\omega_3 t}$$

$$\hat{B} = \boldsymbol{\mu}. \qquad (5.58)$$

Then, the TG polarization is given as

$$\mathbf{P}_{TG}(\mathbf{r},t) = e^{i(-\mathbf{k}_1+\mathbf{k}_2+\mathbf{k}_3)\cdot\mathbf{r}-i(-\omega_1+\omega_2+\omega_3)t}\int_0^\infty dt_1 \int_0^\infty dt_2 \int_0^\infty dt_3\, \phi_{\mu\mu\mu\mu} \vdots \mathbf{e}_3\mathbf{e}_2\mathbf{e}^*_1 E_3(t-t_3)$$

$$\times E_2(t+T-t_3-t_2)E^*_1(t+T-t_3-t_2-t_1)\exp\{i(-\omega_1+\omega_2+\omega_3)t_3 - i(\omega_1-\omega_2)t_2 - i\omega_1 t_1\}. \qquad (5.59)$$

In the case of degenerate transient grating experiment, where the three incident field frequencies are identical, that is, $\omega_1 = \omega_2 = \omega_3 = \omega$, we get

$$\mathbf{P}_{TG}(\mathbf{r},t) = e^{i(-\mathbf{k}_1+\mathbf{k}_2+\mathbf{k}_3)\cdot\mathbf{r}-i\omega t}\int_0^\infty dt_1\int_0^\infty dt_2\int_0^\infty dt_3\, \phi_{\mu\mu\mu\mu} \vdots \mathbf{e}_3\mathbf{e}_2\mathbf{e}_1^* E_3(t-t_3)E_2(t+T-t_3-t_2)$$

$$\times E_1^*(t+T-t_3-t_2-t_1)\exp\{i\omega t_3 - i\omega t_1\}. \quad (5.60)$$

Considering the resonance conditions, one can approximately rewrite Equation 5.60 as

$$\mathbf{P}_{TG}(\mathbf{r},t) = e^{i(-\mathbf{k}_1+\mathbf{k}_2+\mathbf{k}_3)\cdot\mathbf{r}-i\omega t}\left(\frac{i}{\hbar}\right)^3\int_0^\infty dt_1\int_0^\infty dt_2\int_0^\infty dt_3\{R_2+R_3\}\vdots \mathbf{e}_3\mathbf{e}_2\mathbf{e}_1^* E_3(t-t_3)$$

$$\times E_2(t+T-t_3-t_2)E_1^*(t+T-t_3-t_2-t_1)\exp\{i\omega t_3 - i\omega t_1\}. \quad (5.61)$$

Note that the two rephasing pathways are important in this particular measurement technique as long as the pump and probe pulses are well separated in time.

The homodyne-detected TG signal and the heterodyne-detected pump–probe signal are given as

$$S_{TG}(\omega_{pu},\omega_{pr};T) = \int_{-\infty}^\infty dt \left|\mathbf{P}^{(3)}(\mathbf{k}_s,t)\right|^2$$

$$S_{HD-PP}(\omega_{pu},\omega_{pr};T;\phi) = \mathrm{Im}\left[e^{i\phi}\int_{-\infty}^\infty dt\, \mathbf{E}_{LO}^*(\mathbf{k}_{LO},t)\cdot\mathbf{P}^{(3)}(\mathbf{k}_s,t)\right]. \quad (5.62)$$

The phase ϕ of the local oscillator (LO) can be controlled to be zero or $\pi/2$, and then $S_{HD-PP}(\omega_{pu},\omega_{pr};T;\phi=0)$ and $S_{HD-PP}(\omega_{pu},\omega_{pr};T;\phi=\pi/2)$ correspond to the TD and TB signals, respectively. In a later chapter the 2D pump–probe spectroscopy will be discussed in detail by using the results presented in this section.

5.6 REPHASING PHOTON ECHO SPECTROSCOPY OF A TWO-LEVEL SYSTEM

Photon echo spectroscopy is an optical analog of the NMR spin echo.[19, 20] This is one of the most widely used 2D spectroscopic techniques. Particularly, in the inhomogenous broadening limit, the photon echo method is useful to selectively measure the homogeneous dephasing rates since the echo signal is produced by

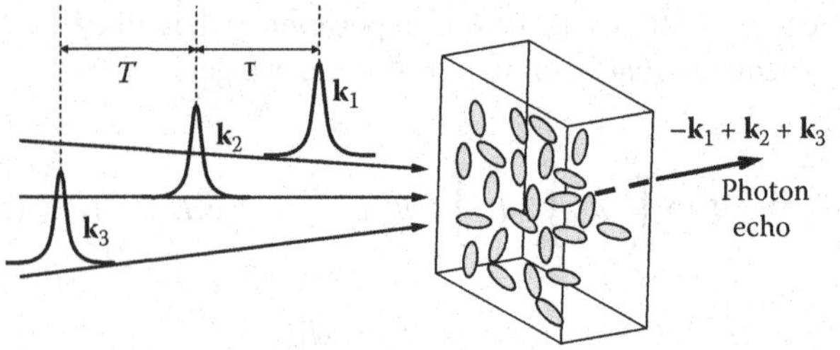

FIGURE 5.3 Experimental beam configuration of three-pulse photon echo spectroscopy.

a rephasing process. In this section, general three-pulse photon echo spectroscopy of a 2LS will be mainly discussed in detail (see Figure 5.3). The first pulse whose wavevector is $\mathbf{k}_1$ interacts with the optical sample and creates a distribution of coherences. Note that the coherences generated have the same phase at a short time. After a delay time τ, the second pulse with $\mathbf{k}_2$ propagation direction is injected to the optical sample. For a 2LS with only one excited state, the second radiation–matter interaction puts the molecular system onto populations on either the excited or ground state. However, if more than one excited state is accessible by the first two radiation–matter interactions, the coherence between two different electronically excited states or two different vibrational quantum states, which are responsible for quantum beats in the pump–probe signal or in the diagonal and cross-peak amplitudes in 2D photon echo spectrum, can be generated by the first two radiation–matter interactions with ultrashort pulses having broad spectral bandwidths. Now, the third pulse with $\mathbf{k}_3$ wavevector, which is delayed from the second pulse by T (waiting time) is used to put the molecules back into coherences between the ground and excited states. This final coherence oscillates in time, and its ensemble-averaged dipole moment is then the third-order photon echo polarization that radiates the signal electric field.

Using the third-order response function theory discussed in this chapter, one can formulate the photon echo polarization and signal electric field. Typical photon echo spectroscopy is to measure the echo signal field emitted in the direction of $-\mathbf{k}_1+\mathbf{k}_2+\mathbf{k}_3$ (see Figure 5.3) so that the three radiation–matter interaction terms and the effect-operator are, respectively,

$$\hat{A}_1 F_1(t) = \boldsymbol{\mu}\cdot\mathbf{e}_1^* E_1^*(t+\tau+T)e^{-i\mathbf{k}_1\cdot\mathbf{r}+i\omega_1 t}$$

$$\hat{A}_2 F_2(t) = \boldsymbol{\mu}\cdot\mathbf{e}_2 E_2(t+T)e^{i\mathbf{k}_2\cdot\mathbf{r}-i\omega_2 t}$$

$$\hat{A}_3 F_3(t) = \boldsymbol{\mu}\cdot\mathbf{e}_3 E_3(t)e^{i\mathbf{k}_3\cdot\mathbf{r}-i\omega_3 t}$$

$$\hat{B} = \boldsymbol{\mu}. \tag{5.63}$$

Note that temporal envelope functions include the delay time variables τ and T properly. Throughout this book, unless it is necessary to distinguish the rephasing photon echo from the nonrephasing photon echo, the rephasing ($-\mathbf{k}_1+\mathbf{k}_2+\mathbf{k}_3$) photon echo will be just referred to as the photon echo.

Now, the photon echo polarization is then given as

$$\mathbf{P}_{PE}(\mathbf{r},t) = e^{i(-\mathbf{k}_1+\mathbf{k}_2+\mathbf{k}_3)\cdot\mathbf{r}-i(-\omega_1+\omega_2+\omega_3)t}\int_0^\infty dt_1\int_0^\infty dt_2\int_0^\infty dt_3\,\phi_{\mu\mu\mu\mu}\,\vdots\,\mathbf{e}_3\mathbf{e}_2\mathbf{e}_1^* E_3(t-t_3)E_2(t+T$$

$$-t_3-t_2)E_1^*(t+\tau+T-t_3-t_2-t_1)\exp\{i(\omega_3+\omega_2-\omega_1)t_3+i(\omega_2-\omega_1)t_2-i\omega_1 t_1\}. \tag{5.64}$$

The above expression is fairly general for an arbitrary nondegenerate photon echo spectroscopy, where the three incident field frequencies can be different from one another. Furthermore, the photon echo is very similar to the TG geometry, except that the delay time between the first two pulses is experimentally controlled and scanned for the photon echo measurement, whereas the TG is essentially identical to the photon echo with $\tau = 0$. Usually, most of the photon echo experiments have been performed by using pulses with the same center frequency, that is, degenerate limit, so that the degenerate photon echo polarization is simplified as

$$\mathbf{P}_{PE}(\mathbf{r},t) = e^{i(-\mathbf{k}_1+\mathbf{k}_2+\mathbf{k}_3)\cdot\mathbf{r}-i\omega t}\int_0^\infty dt_1\int_0^\infty dt_2\int_0^\infty dt_3\,\phi_{\mu\mu\mu\mu}\,\vdots\,\mathbf{e}_3\mathbf{e}_2\mathbf{e}_1^* E_3(t-t_3)E_2(t+T-t_3-t_2)$$

$$\times E_1^*(t+\tau+T-t_3-t_2-t_1)\exp\{i\omega t_3-i\omega t_1\}$$

$$\cong e^{i(-\mathbf{k}_1+\mathbf{k}_2+\mathbf{k}_3)\cdot\mathbf{r}-i\omega t}\left(\frac{i}{\hbar}\right)^3\int_0^\infty dt_1\int_0^\infty dt_2\int_0^\infty dt_3\,\{R_2+R_3\}\,\vdots\,\mathbf{e}_3\mathbf{e}_2\mathbf{e}_1^* E_3(t-t_3)$$

$$\times E_2(t+T-t_3-t_2)E_1^*(t+\tau+T-t_3-t_2-t_1)\exp\{i\omega t_3-i\omega t_1\}. \tag{5.65}$$

The second approximate equality in Equation 5.65 was obtained by considering the relevant resonance conditions.

In the case of the degenerate photon echo spectroscopy in the well-separated pulse limit, during t_1 and t_3 periods the electric field components oscillating as $\exp(-i\omega t_1)$ and $\exp(i\omega t_3)$, respectively, are involved in the radiation–matter interactions. Therefore, among the eight response function components in $\phi_{\mu\mu\mu\mu}$ only two of them satisfy the resonance condition, and they are the two rephasing pathways,

$R_2(t_3,t_2,t_1)$ and $R_3(t_3,t_2,t_1)$, because their time-dependent parts include the coherence oscillation term, $\exp(i\omega_{eg}t_1 - i\omega_{eg}t_3)$. In Equation 5.65, they are

$$R_2(t_3,t_2,t_1) = \boldsymbol{\mu}_{ge}\boldsymbol{\mu}_{eg}\boldsymbol{\mu}_{ge}\boldsymbol{\mu}_{eg}\exp(i\bar{\omega}_{eg}t_1 - i\{\bar{\omega}_{eg} + 2Q(t_2)\}t_3)$$
$$\times \exp\left\{-\frac{1}{2}\Omega^2 t_1^2 - \frac{1}{2}\Omega^2 t_3^2 + H(t_2)t_1t_3\right\} \tag{5.66}$$

$$R_3(t_3,t_2,t_1) = \boldsymbol{\mu}_{ge}\boldsymbol{\mu}_{eg}\boldsymbol{\mu}_{ge}\boldsymbol{\mu}_{eg}\exp(i\bar{\omega}_{eg}t_1 - i\bar{\omega}_{eg}t_3)\exp\left\{-\frac{1}{2}\Omega^2 t_1^2 - \frac{1}{2}\Omega^2 t_3^2 + H(t_2)t_1t_3\right\}. \tag{5.67}$$

Using these results, one can understand the rephasing process observed in an ensemble having large static inhomogeneity. For the sake of simplicity, let us consider only the highly oscillating factor $\exp(i\bar{\omega}_{eg}t_1 - i\bar{\omega}_{eg}t_3)$ in Equations 5.66 and 5.67. In the inhomogeneous broadening limit, each individual molecule has a different transition frequency. Then, the transition frequency of the jth molecule can be written as

$$\omega_{eg}^j = \bar{\omega}_{eg} + \varepsilon_j. \tag{5.68}$$

Here, the ensemble-averaged transition frequency over all molecules is denoted as $\bar{\omega}_{eg}$, and ε_j is the deviation of the jth molecule's transition frequency from the average value. Note that the ε variable is broadly distributed if molecules have distinctively different local environments and if the timescale of transition from one local environment to the other is sufficiently slow. Then, the third-order response function should be averaged over the distribution of ε, where the distribution function of ε will be denoted as $I(\varepsilon)$. Thus, we have to consider the following average:

$$\int d\varepsilon\, I(\varepsilon)\exp\{i(\bar{\omega}_{eg}+\varepsilon)t_1 - i(\bar{\omega}_{eg}+\varepsilon)t_3\} = \exp\{i\bar{\omega}_{eg}t_1 - i\bar{\omega}_{eg}t_3\}\int d\varepsilon\, I(\varepsilon)\exp\{i\varepsilon(t_1-t_3)\}$$
$$= 2\pi\exp\{i\bar{\omega}_{eg}t_1 - i\bar{\omega}_{eg}t_3\}\tilde{I}(t_3-t_1), \tag{5.69}$$

where $\tilde{I}(t)$ is the inverse Fourier transform of $I(\varepsilon)$. If $I(\varepsilon)$ is broad, the corresponding inverse Fourier transform, $\tilde{I}(t)$, is narrow in time and so that $\tilde{I}(t_3-t_1)$ peaks at $t_1 = t_3$. In the case of the large inhomogeneous broadening limit, $\tilde{I}(t_3-t_1)$ can be approximately replaced with a Dirac delta function as

$$\tilde{I}(t_3-t_1) = \delta(t_3-t_1). \tag{5.70}$$

This clearly indicates the phase reversal in time domain, because the phase distribution of the coherences at t_1 is narrowed down to zero at $t_3 = t_1$. Furthermore, in the impulsive limit, the temporal envelope of the photon echo polarization is simplified as

$$\mathbf{P}_{PE}(t) \propto R_2(t_3=\tau, t_2=T, t_1=\tau) + R_3(t_3=\tau, t_2=T, t_1=\tau). \tag{5.71}$$

Note that the first two delay times τ and T are experimentally controlled variables. Equation 5.71 shows that the echo signal field amplitude (polarization) peaks after a finite delay time at $t = \tau$ from the third pulse. This is why the present spectroscopy has been called the photon *echo*. In solution, however, there is no truly static inhomogeneity so that the rephasing process is not perfect. Nevertheless, for a short time (< bath correlation time), the transition frequencies of optical chromophores are inhomogeneously distributed since the initial distribution of local environments around the solutes is still broad, and then the rephasing process plays a critical role in generating the echo signal field.

5.7 NONREPHASING PHOTON ECHO SPECTROSCOPY OF A TWO-LEVEL SYSTEM

In the previous section, the rephasing photon echo spectroscopy was discussed, where the echo signal field propagating in the direction of $-\mathbf{k}_1+\mathbf{k}_2+\mathbf{k}_3$ was measured. In that case, only two ($R_2(t_3,t_2,t_1)$ and $R_3(t_3,t_2,t_1)$) out of eight response function components in $\phi_{\mu\mu\mu\mu}$ satisfy the resonance condition because their time-dependent parts include the required coherence oscillation term, $\exp(i\omega_{eg}t_1 - i\omega_{eg}t_3)$. One can also selectively measure the nonrephasing terms that are $R_1(t_3,t_2,t_1)$ and $R_4(t_3,t_2,t_1)$ with coherence oscillation $\exp(-i\omega_{eg}t_1 - i\omega_{eg}t_3)$ by focusing on the emitted signal in the direction of $\mathbf{k}_1 - \mathbf{k}_2 + \mathbf{k}_3$ instead.[2] This has been called the nonrephasing photon echo (NR-PE) experiment. In this case, even in the limit of very large static inhomogeneity, the radiated field does not show any echo behavior so that it should not be called a photon echo, but traditionally it was developed within the context of photon echo spectroscopy so that it will be distinguished from the rephasing photon echo by calling it the NR-PE. Nevertheless, for this experimental beam configuration and detection, one can find that the three radiation–matter interaction terms and the effect operator are

$$\hat{A}_1F_1(t) = \boldsymbol{\mu}\cdot\mathbf{e}_1E_1(t+\tau+T)\,e^{i\mathbf{k}_1\cdot\mathbf{r}-i\omega_1 t}$$

$$\hat{A}_2F_2(t) = \boldsymbol{\mu}\cdot\mathbf{e}_2^*E_2^*(t+T)e^{-i\mathbf{k}_2\cdot\mathbf{r}+i\omega_2 t}$$

$$\hat{A}_3F_3(t) = \boldsymbol{\mu}\cdot\mathbf{e}_3E_3(t)\,e^{i\mathbf{k}_3\cdot\mathbf{r}-i\omega_3 t}$$

$$\hat{B} = \boldsymbol{\mu}. \tag{5.72}$$

It is again assumed that the delay times between the first and second pulses and between the second and third pulses are controlled to be τ and T, respectively. The NR-PE polarization is then given as

$$\mathbf{P}_{NR-PE}(\mathbf{r},t) = e^{i(\mathbf{k}_1-\mathbf{k}_2+\mathbf{k}_3)\cdot\mathbf{r}-i(\omega_1-\omega_2+\omega_3)t}\int_0^\infty dt_1\int_0^\infty dt_2\int_0^\infty dt_3\,\phi_{\mu\mu\mu\mu}\,\vdots\,\mathbf{e}_3\mathbf{e}_2^*\mathbf{e}_1E_3(t-t_3)E_2^*(t+T-t_3$$
$$-t_2)E_1(t+\tau+T-t_3-t_2-t_1)\exp\{i(\omega_3-\omega_2+\omega_1)t_3 - i(\omega_2-\omega_1)t_2 + i\omega_1t_1\}. \tag{5.73}$$

In the case of the degenerate NR-PE, its polarization is simplified as

$$\mathbf{P}_{NR-PE}(\mathbf{r},t) = e^{i(\mathbf{k}_1 - \mathbf{k}_2 + \mathbf{k}_3)\cdot\mathbf{r} - i\omega t}\int_0^\infty dt_1 \int_0^\infty dt_2 \int_0^\infty dt_3\, \phi_{\mu\mu\mu\mu} \vdots \mathbf{e}_3\mathbf{e}_2^*\mathbf{e}_1 E_3(t-t_3)E_2^*(t+T-t_3-t_2)$$

$$\times E_1(t+\tau+T-t_3-t_2-t_1)\exp\{i\omega t_3 + i\omega t_1\}$$

$$\cong e^{i(\mathbf{k}_1 - \mathbf{k}_2 + \mathbf{k}_3)\cdot\mathbf{r} - i\omega t}\left(\frac{i}{\hbar}\right)^3 \int_0^\infty dt_1 \int_0^\infty dt_2 \int_0^\infty dt_3 \{R_1 + R_4\} \vdots \mathbf{e}_3\mathbf{e}_2^*\mathbf{e}_1 E_3(t-t_3)$$

$$\times E_2^*(t+T-t_3-t_2)E_1(t+\tau+T-t_3-t_2-t_1)\exp\{i\omega t_3 + i\omega t_1\}. \quad (5.74)$$

Due to the resonance condition, only the two nonrephasing components $R_1(t_3,t_2,t_1)$ and $R_4(t_3,t_2,t_1)$ play an important role in this particular experimental configuration. Note that only these components have the coherence oscillation term $\exp(-i\omega_{eg}t_3 - i\omega_{eg}t_1)$.

Consequently, in the inhomogeneous broadening limit, the ensemble-averaged nonrephasing response function over the distribution of the inhomogeneity factor ε in Equation 5.68 is

$$\int d\varepsilon\, I(\varepsilon)\exp\{-i(\bar{\omega}_{eg}+\varepsilon)t_1 - i(\bar{\omega}_{eg}+\varepsilon)t_3\} = \exp\{-i\bar{\omega}_{eg}t_1 - i\bar{\omega}_{eg}t_3\}\int d\varepsilon\, I(\varepsilon)$$

$$\times \exp\{-i\varepsilon(t_1+t_3)\}$$

$$= 2\pi \exp\{-i\bar{\omega}_{eg}t_1 - i\bar{\omega}_{eg}t_3\}\tilde{I}(t_1+t_3). \quad (5.75)$$

Again, for a broad $I(\varepsilon)$, $\tilde{I}(t_1+t_3)$ should be a narrow function in time and peaks at $t_1 = -t_3$. This means that the emitted field polarization amplitude monotonically decreases in positive time t_3, and there won't be time-delayed echo after the final (third) pulse in this NR-PE experiment.

5.8 THREE-PULSE PHOTON ECHO PEAK SHIFT (PEPS)

The photon echo experiment has been performed by measuring the integrated intensity of the echo field after the last incident δ-function-like pulse. That is to say, the measured integrated echo signal is

$$I_{PE}(T,\tau) = \int_0^\infty dt\, |\mathbf{E}_{PE}(t,T,\tau)|^2. \quad (5.76)$$

Since the photon echo signal electric field is linearly proportional to the photon echo polarization, in the impulsive limit the integrated echo signal is approximately given as

$$I_{PE}(T,\tau) \propto \int_0^\infty dt \, | f(t,T,\tau)\{1+\exp(-2iQ(T)t)\} |^2 \tag{5.77}$$

where

$$f(t,T,\tau) \equiv \exp\left\{-\frac{1}{2}\Omega^2\tau^2 - \frac{1}{2}\Omega^2 t^2 + H(T)\tau t\right\}. \tag{5.78}$$

Here, it should be noted that the rephasing photon echo spectroscopy by measuring the echo signal field propagating toward the $-\mathbf{k}_1+\mathbf{k}_2+\mathbf{k}_3$ direction is only considered here. In practice, the PEPS was experimentally estimated by measuring the half of the peak-to-peak difference along the τ-dependent integrated signals of the rephasing ($-\mathbf{k}_1+\mathbf{k}_2+\mathbf{k}_3$) and nonrephasing ($\mathbf{k}_1-\mathbf{k}_2+\mathbf{k}_3$) photon echoes. Note that the corresponding integrated signal of the nonrephasing echo peaks at negative τ. Hereafter, we will assume that the PEPS is the maximum position of the integrated rephasing photon echo signal plotted as a function of τ.[2, 13, 21]

In order to perform the integration in Equation 5.77, let us ignore the spectral diffusion process during T, that is to say, $\exp(-2iQ(T)t) \approx 1$. Then, one can find that

$$I_{PE}(T,\tau) \sim \exp\left(-\frac{(\Omega^4 - H^2(T))\tau^2}{\Omega^2}\right)[1+erf\{H(T)\tau/\Omega\}], \tag{5.79}$$

where *erf* is the error function. Note that the first term in Equation 5.79 is a Gaussian-decay function with respect to τ, whereas the second term inside the square bracket increases in τ. Due to the incomplete rephasing process, the photon echo signal initially increases in τ, reaches a maximum value at τ^*, and decays to zero as τ further increases. Therefore, the PEPS τ^* is defined as the temporal shift of the maximum echo signal from $\tau = 0$. One can approximately obtain the PEPS τ^* by taking a Taylor expansion of the approximate photon echo signal in Equation 5.79 up to the second-order with respect to τ. From the quadratic equation, the PEPS τ^* as a function of T is found to be

$$\tau^*(T) = \frac{\Omega H(T)}{\sqrt{\pi}\{\Omega^4 - H^2(T)\}}. \tag{5.80}$$

Since $H(t)$ is the real part of the time-correlation function $C(t)$ in the case of a two-level system, that is, $H(t) = C_R(t)$, the PEPS in Equation 5.80 can be rewritten as

$$\tau^*(T) = \frac{\sqrt{C(0)}C_R(T)}{\sqrt{\pi}\{C^2(0) - C_R^2(T)\}}. \tag{5.81}$$

At $T = 0$, Equation 5.81 diverges, because $H(T = 0) = \Omega^2$. This unrealistic behavior originates from a few approximations invoked to obtain Equation 5.80, such as (1) short-time approximation to the third-order response function, (2) ignorance of finite pulse widths, and (3) ignorance of nonrephasing diagram contributions to the measured signal when the incident pulses are overlapped in time. Nevertheless, after a very short time T, the PEPS value becomes linearly proportional to $H(T)$, which is then related to the solvation correlation function, so that we have

$$\tau^*(T) \approx \frac{H(T)}{\sqrt{\pi}\Omega^3} \cong \frac{2}{\hbar\beta\sqrt{\pi}\Omega^3} S(T). \tag{5.82}$$

Thus, the long-time decaying part of the PEPS with respect to T provides critical information on the solvation dynamics.[2]

In order to demonstrate the general behaviors of integrated photon echo and PEPS, we shall consider a model system. For numerical simulation of the echo response function, it is necessary to have the spectral density and solvation reorganization energy that are key ingredients for the calculation of the line broadening function $g(t)$. Here, let us assume that the spectral density is an Ohmic form and the solvent reorganization energy λ is 500 cm^{-1}, that is,

$$\rho(\omega) \propto \frac{1}{\omega} \exp(-\omega/\omega_c). \tag{5.83}$$

The cutoff frequency ω_c is assumed to be 30 cm^{-1}. If the high-temperature approximation is invoked, the mean square fluctuation amplitude, Ω^2, of the electronic transition frequency is approximately calculated to be $\Omega^2 \cong 2\lambda k_B T = 2.07 \times 10^5$ cm^{-2}, which is close to the value $\Omega^2 = 2.08 \times 10^5$ cm^{-2} from Equation 5.48. The two auxiliary functions, $Q(T)$ and $H(T)$, that are needed for numerical calculations of rephasing photon echo response functions in Equations 5.77 and 5.78 are calculated and plotted in Figure 5.4. Note that the solvation correlation function is identical to $Q(T)$ except for the constant offset of $\lambda/\hbar$ (see Equation 5.49). The decaying pattern of $H(T)$ in this case is almost indistinguishable from $S(T)$, indicating that the high-temperature

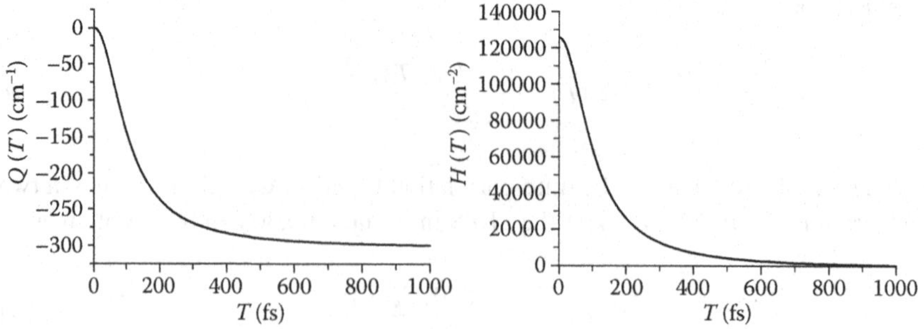

FIGURE 5.4 Calculated $Q(t)$ in cm^{-1} and $H(t)$ in cm^{-2} for the model 2LS discussed in the context.

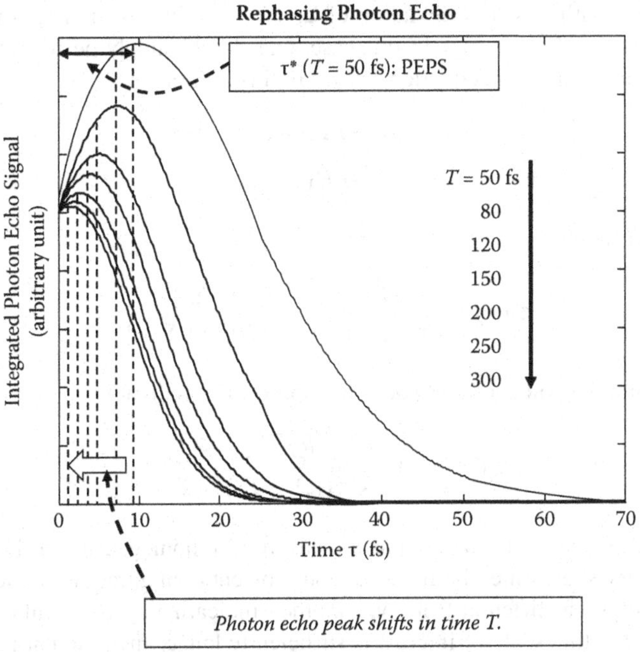

FIGURE 5.5 Integrated rephasing photon echo signals versus τ. The waiting time T varies from 50 to 300 fs. The peak position of the integrated echo signal shifts toward $\tau = 0$ as the waiting time T increases. This T-dependent behavior is called the three-pulse photon echo peak shift (PEPS).

approximation is quantitatively acceptable. In the literatures, the solvation correlation time has been defined as

$$\tau_{sol} \equiv \int_0^\infty dt\, S(t)/S(0). \tag{5.84}$$

With the spectral density given above, we find that τ_{sol} is about 235 fs.

By using the above parameters, the integrated rephasing photon echo signal is calculated as a function of τ and is plotted in Figure 5.5 for varying T from 50 to 300 fs. For instance, let us consider the integrated photon echo signal when $T = 50$ fs. The signal increases initially and then reaches its maximum value at around $\tau = 10$ fs. Then it decays rapidly down to zero in about a few tens of femtoseconds. One of the most notable features is that the peak position of $I_{PE}(T,\tau)$ vs. τ moves toward $\tau = 0$ as the waiting time T increases. This is the PEPS, and its time-dependent decaying pattern is, as predicted, given by Equation 5.80 approximately.

In the above, the static inhomogeneous contribution to line broadening has not been included in the description of PEPS. Although there is no truly static inhomogeneity in solution, chromophores in a glassy material or a polymer matrix could have sizable static inhomogeneous environments. If it is approximately given as a Gaussian with standard deviation of Σ, $\tilde{I}(t_3-t_1)$ in Equation 5.69 is given as $\tilde{I}(t_3-t_1) \propto \exp(-\frac{1}{2}\Sigma^2(t_3-t_1)^2)$. In this case, one should simply perform the following replacements in all the equations above in this section:

$$\Omega^2 \rightarrow \Omega^2 + \Sigma^2$$
$$H(T) \rightarrow H(T) + \Sigma^2. \tag{5.85}$$

Then, $\tau^*(T)$ is given as

$$\tau^*(T) = \frac{\sqrt{\Omega^2+\Sigma^2}\{H(T)+\Sigma^2\}}{\sqrt{\pi}\{(\Omega^2+\Sigma^2)^2-(H(T)+\Sigma^2)^2\}} \tag{5.86}$$

and the asymptotic value of $\tau^*(T)$ does not approach zero, that is,

$$\tau^*(T \rightarrow \infty) = \frac{\sqrt{\Omega^2+\Sigma^2}\Sigma^2}{\sqrt{\pi}\{(\Omega^2+\Sigma^2)^2-\Sigma^4\}}. \tag{5.87}$$

The PEPS $\tau^*(T)$ can be considered as a measure of inhomogeneity in the timescale of T. At a very short time, the instantaneous solvent configuration of each individual chromophore is different from one another, indicating a sizable inhomogeneity. However, if the timescale of interest is sufficiently longer than the bath correlation time, $T \gg \tau_{bath}$, and if the chromophores are dissolved in solution without truly static inhomogeneity, $H(T) \approx 0$ and $\tau^*(T) \approx 0$. This means that the chromophores see the solvent as a homogeneous medium in such a long timescale. Let us consider a chemical reaction dynamics in solution. If a reactive species undergoes a barrier crossing and the timescale of the barrier crossing of a single reactant is much shorter than the bath correlation time, the surrounding solvent configurations around the reactants would appear to be inhomogeneously distributed. However, if the bath correlation time is sufficiently faster than a given barrier-crossing process, the solvent molecules will rapidly follow the reaction along the reaction coordinate and the solvent can be treated as a homogeneous medium. From this, it should be clear that the PEPS measurement can provide information on not only the solvation timescale but also the extent of inhomogeneity within the timescale of T.

Despite that the general expressions of photon echo and pump–probe spectroscopic observables are presented in this chapter, due to the complicated triple convolution integrals it is not easy to extract critical information directly from the signal. Therefore, in the following chapters, the 2D pump–probe and photon echo spectroscopy will be discussed in detail by invoking the short-time approximation to the third-order response function and the well-separated pulse approximation for the triple integrations required in the calculation of third-order polarization.

REFERENCES

1. Shen, Y. R., *The principles of nonlinear optics*. John Wiley & Sons: New York, 1984.
2. Fleming, G. R.; Cho, M., Chromophore-solvent dynamics. *Annual Review of Physical Chemistry* 1996, 47, 109–134.

3. Mukamel, S., *Principles of nonlinear optical spectroscopy*. Oxford University Press: Oxford, 1995.
4. Jonas, D. M., Two-dimensional femtosecond spectroscopy. *Annual Review of Physical Chemistry* 2003, 54, 425–463.
5. Asplund, M. C.; Zanni, M. T.; Hochstrasser, R. M., Two-dimensional infrared spectroscopy of peptides by phase-controlled femtosecond vibrational photon echoes. *Proceedings of the National Academy of Sciences of the United States of America* 2000, 97, 8219–8224.
6. Khalil, M.; Demirdoven, N.; Tokmakoff, A., Coherent 2D IR spectroscopy: Molecular structure and dynamics in solution. *Journal of Physical Chemistry A*. 2003, 107, 5258–5279.
7. Cho, M., Coherent two-dimensional optical spectroscopy. *Chemical Reviews* 2008, 108, 1331–1418.
8. Bloembergen, N., *Nonlinear Optics*. W. A. Benjamin, Inc.: Reding, 1965.
9. Cho, M., Nonlinear response functions for the three-dimensional spectroscopies. *Journal of Chemical Physics* 2001, 115, 4424.
10. Sung, J. Y.; Silbey, R. J., Four wave mixing spectroscopy for a multilevel system. *Journal of Chemical Physics* 2001, 115, 9266–9287.
11. Cho, M.; Fleming, G. R., Electron transfer and solvent dynamics in two- and three-state systems. *Advances in Chemical Physics* 1999, 107, 311–370.
12. Cho, M.; Vaswani, H. M.; Brixner, T.; et al., Exciton analysis in 2D electronic spectroscopy. *Journal of Physical Chemistry B* 2005, 109, 10542–10556.
13. Cho, M.; Yu, J.-Y.; Joo, T.; et al., The integrated photon echo and solvation dynamics. *Journal of Physical Chemistry* 1996, 100, 11944–11953.
14. Cho, M.; Brixner, T.; Stiopkin, I.; et al., Two dimensional electronic spectroscopy of molecular complexes. *Journal of the Chinese Chemical Society* 2006, 53, 15–24.
15. Kwac, K.; Cho, M., Two-color pump–probe spectroscopies of two- and three-level systems: 2-dimensional line shapes and solvation dynamics. *Journal of Physical Chemistry A* 2003, 107, 5903–5912.
16. de Boeij, W.; Pshenichnikov, M. S.; Wiersma, D. A., On the relation between the echo peak shift and brownian oscillator correlation function. *Chemical Physics Letters* 1996, 253, 53–60.
17. Mukamel, S., Femtosecond optical spectroscopy: A direct look at elementary chemical events. *Annual Review of Physical Chemistry* 1990, 41, 647–681.
18. Cho, M.; Fleming, G. R.; Mukamel, S., Nonlinear response functions for birefringence and dichroism measurements in condensed phases. *Journal of Chemical Physics* 1993, 98, 5314–5326.
19. Warren, W. S.; Zewail, A. H., Optical analogs of NMR phase coherent multiple pulse spectroscopy. *Journal of Chemical Physics* 1981, 75, 5956–5958.
20. Weiner, A. M.; de Silvestri, S.; Ippen, E. P., Three-Pulse scattering for femtosecond dephasing studies: Theory and experiment. *Journal of the Optical Society of America B-Optical Physics* 1985, 2, 654–662.
21. Joo, T. H.; Jia, Y. W.; Yu, J. Y.; et al., Third-order nonlinear time domain probes of solvation dynamics. *Journal of Chemical Physics* 1996, 104, 6089–6108.

6 Two-Dimensional Pump–Probe Spectroscopy

As emphasized throughout this book and found in innumerable experiments, the two-level approximation is valid and useful for describing resonant electronic transition of a chromophore in solution when the incident radiation frequency is close to the transition frequency between the ground state and one particular excited state. Therefore, discussions on the 2D spectroscopy of a model 2LS will be presented first. Among a variety of 2D optical spectroscopic techniques, we will focus on the 2D peak shape of pump–probe spectrum.[1–4]

General results of pump–probe and photon echo spectroscopy for multi-level systems were presented previously. The pump–probe polarization, which is the expectation value of the electric dipole operator over the appropriate third-order perturbation-expanded density operator, was given as a triple convolution of the third-order response function with three interacting external fields.[5, 6] Therefore, any quantitative calculations of pump–probe signal require numerical integrations, and pump and probe pulses should be treated realistically. This is achievable, but the numerical calculation results cannot provide a conceptually clear picture on the 2D pump–probe spectroscopy in general. Consequently, in the present chapter, we will use a few approximations to perform the triple convolution integrations mathematically and present the resultant expressions for the frequency-scanning 2D pump–probe spectra of a model 2LS.

6.1 INTRODUCTION TO TWO-DIMENSIONAL PUMP–PROBE SPECTROSCOPY

A number of different coherent 2D optical spectroscopic methods can be devised by combining a sequence of optical excitation and probing processes, and one of the early 2D vibrational spectroscopic experiments was based on a pump–probe, that is, dynamic hole-burning spectroscopy.[4, 7] In a self-heterodyne-detected pump–probe measurement, the molecular system is subjected to two light pulses, that is, pump and probe, of which center frequencies are ω_{pu} and ω_{pr}, respectively. The incoming field is therefore given as

$$\mathbf{E}(\mathbf{r},t) = \mathbf{E}_{pu}(t+T)\exp(i\mathbf{k}_{pu}\cdot\mathbf{r} - i\omega_{pu}t) + \mathbf{E}_{pr}(t)\exp(i\mathbf{k}_{pr}\cdot\mathbf{r} - i\omega_{pr}t) + c.c., \tag{6.1}$$

where T is the delay time. Then, the probe difference absorption that is defined as the total probe absorption in the presence of the pump minus that in the absence of the pump is detected. In particular, the first two radiation–matter interactions are between a chromophore and pump pulse. The pump–probe signal field should satisfy the following phase-matching condition: $\mathbf{k}_s = \mathbf{k}_{pu} - \mathbf{k}_{pu} + \mathbf{k}_{pr} = \mathbf{k}_{pr}$. After the first two field-matter interactions with pump pulse, not only the ground-state hole but also excited-state population (particle) or vibronic coherence can be generated.[5] Note that the first two field-matter interactions occur within the temporal envelope of the pump pulse. After a finite delay time T, the incoming probe field stimulates light emission of the excited state particle, is absorbed by the excited-state particle, or is scattered by the ground-state hole. In between the first two field-matter interactions, the system is on a coherence oscillating with frequency of $\bar{\omega}_{eg}$. If one uses a very short pump pulse whose spectral bandwidth is sufficiently broad enough to cover the entire manifold of singly excited states of coupled multi-chromophore system, for example, light-harvesting complex consisting of a few to hundreds of chlorophylls, one can simultaneously create an ensemble of population and coherence on the electronically excited states. In this case of multilevel system, frequency-resolution of the excited states by using the present pump–probe method is not feasible, because the measured pump–probe signal has no dependency on the first coherence evolution time t_1 (note that the two radiation–matter interactions occur within the ultrashort pump–pulse envelope). This is in contrast with the photon echo technique that involves a τ-scanning in the experiment, and the τ-dependent signal contains information on the first coherence evolution during the first t_1 period. Nevertheless, the pump–probe signal can be dispersed by using a monochromator to detect the spectral distribution of the pump–probe signal field. This turned out to be analogous to taking the Fourier-transform of the pump–probe signal with respect to t, which is the last coherence evolution time. Therefore, for the ultrafast pump–ultrafast probe measurement, the signal can only be displayed as a function of the pump–probe delay time T and frequency ω_t, that is, $\tilde{S}_{PP}(\omega_t, T)$.

As a matter fact, to obtain the full 2D pump–probe spectrum, it was therefore necessary to perform a series of dynamic hole-burning experiments with a tunable and spectrally narrow band pump pulse of which bandwidth should be sufficiently narrow enough to frequency-resolve the one-quantum excited states or to selectively excite only a subset of the excited states. In addition to such a frequency-scanning, another requirement is that the temporal envelope of the narrow-band pump pulse should not be exceedingly broad in comparison to the lifetime of the excited states or any dynamical processes of interest to achieve time-resolution.[7]

In this case of the mixed frequency-time resolved pump–probe, the difference absorption signal is given as a function of the center frequency of the pump, the pump–probe delay time T, and the frequency ω_t that is the conjugate frequency of the electronic coherence time t, that is, $\tilde{S}_{PP}(\omega_t, T, \omega_\tau = \omega_{pu})$. To construct the full 2D pump–probe spectrum, one should therefore scan the pump frequency, ω_{pu}, and assemble the 1D transient difference spectra as a function of the peak frequency ω_{pu} of the pump pulse. Consequently, this method using a series of dynamic hole-burning experiments by tuning the frequency of spectrally narrow pump pulse is technically not directly analogous to the 2D NMR spectroscopy that utilizes temporally narrow radio frequency pulses and that requires double Fourier transformations to obtain the corresponding 2D NMR spectrum.

Often the frequency scanning of the spectrally narrow pump requires a large amount of data collection time to obtain a single 2D spectrum. One of the experimental breakthroughs was achieved by overcoming this low efficiency. An essential element of the experimental design is to maximally use a 2D array detector in the visible frequency ranges.[8, 9] Using spherically focusing mirrors, the two-dimensionally (X and Y space) spreaded pump–probe signal field is a direct image of the 2D spectrum spatially encoded in the sample, where spatial dimensions along the X- and Y-axes in the recorded image correspond to ω_τ and ω_t, respectively.

In the present chapter, we will present a theoretical description of 2D pump–probe spectroscopy of simple model systems such as 2LS and anharmonic oscillator. Detailed analyses of 2D peak shape of the pump–pump spectra are shown to be useful in understanding the underlying chromophore-solvent dynamics and sometimes intrinsic vibrational properties such as overtone anharmonic frequency shift.[1]

6.2 TWO-DIMENSIONAL PUMP–PROBE SPECTRUM OF A TWO-LEVEL SYSTEM

In the previous chapter, the pump–probe polarization was discussed and its temporal amplitude was found to be (see Equation 5.57)

$$\begin{aligned}\mathbf{P}_{PP}(t) = \left(\frac{i}{\hbar}\right)^3 \int_0^\infty dt_1 \int_0^\infty dt_2 \int_0^\infty dt_3 [\{R_1 + R_4\} \vdots \mathbf{e}_{pr}\mathbf{e}^*_{pu}\mathbf{e}_{pu} E_{pr}(t-t_3)E^*_{pu}(t+T-t_3-t_2)\\ \times E_{pu}(t+T-t_3-t_2-t_1)\exp(i\omega_{pr}t_3 + i\omega_{pu}t_1)\\ + \{R_2 + R_3\} \vdots \mathbf{e}_{pr}\mathbf{e}_{pu}\mathbf{e}^*_{pu} E_{pr}(t-t_3)E_{pu}(t+T-t_3-t_2)\\ \times E^*_{pu}(t+T-t_3-t_2-t_1)\exp(i\omega_{pr}t_3 - i\omega_{pu}t_1)].\end{aligned} \tag{6.2}$$

The four contributions from $R_1 - R_4$ to the pump–probe polarization are related to the following four diagrams:

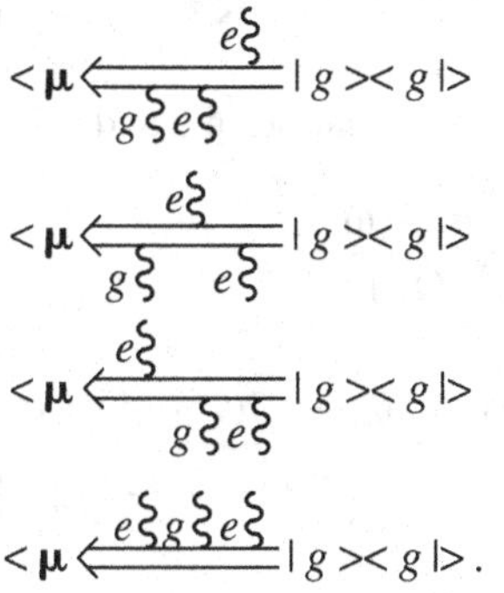

(6.3)

Introducing a new integration variable $t' = t + T - t_3 - t_2$ and assuming that the delay time T is sufficiently larger than the pulse widths, one can obtain the following approximate expression for the pump–probe polarization:

$$\begin{aligned}\mathbf{P}_{PP}(t) = \left(\frac{i}{\hbar}\right)^3 \int_0^\infty dt_1 \int_0^\infty dt_2 \int_0^\infty dt_3 E_{pr}(t-t_3)E^*_{pu}(t')E_{pu}(t'-t_1)\{(R_1 + R_4) \vdots \mathbf{e}_{pr}\mathbf{e}^*_{pu}\mathbf{e}_{pu}\\ \times \exp[i\omega_{pr}t_3 + i\omega_{pu}t_1] + (R_2 + R_3) \vdots \mathbf{e}_{pr}\mathbf{e}_{pu}\mathbf{e}^*_{pu} \exp[i\omega_{pr}t_3 - i\omega_{pu}t_1]\}.\end{aligned} \tag{6.4}$$

In order to take into account the finite pulse-width effect on the pump–probe polarization, the pulse envelope functions are assumed to be a Gaussian form as $E_{pu}(t) = \exp(-w^2t^2/2)$ and $E_{pr}(t) = \exp(-\bar{w}^2t^2/2)$. Hereafter, the pump and probe beams are assumed to be linearly polarized so that $\mathbf{e}_{pu}$ and $\mathbf{e}_{pr}$ are real. Inserting Gaussian pulse envelope functions into Equation 6.4, replacing $R_j(t_3,t_2,t_1)$ with $R_j(t_3,t_2=T,t_1)$, and carrying out multiple integrals, one can find that the pump–probe polarization is given by the sum of two contributions, $\mathbf{P}_{PP}^{SE}(t)$ and $\mathbf{P}_{PP}^{GB}(t)$, that are associated with the stimulated emission (R_1 and R_2) and ground-state bleaching (R_3 and R_4) pathways, respectively, that is,

$$\mathbf{P}_{PP}(t) = \mathbf{P}_{PP}^{SE}(t) + \mathbf{P}_{PP}^{GB}(t) \tag{6.5}$$

where

$$\mathbf{P}_{PP}^{SE}(t) = \frac{-i\pi E_{pr}(t)E_{pu}^2[\boldsymbol{\mu}_{ge}\boldsymbol{\mu}_{eg}\boldsymbol{\mu}_{ge}\boldsymbol{\mu}_{eg}] \vdots \mathbf{e}_{pr}\mathbf{e}_{pu}\mathbf{e}_{pu}}{(\Omega^2+w^2)^{1/2}\left(\Omega^2+\bar{w}^2-\frac{H^2(T)}{\Omega^2+w^2}\right)^{1/2}}\exp(-X^2)$$
$$\times\left\{\exp(-Y^2(T)) + \frac{2i}{\sqrt{\pi}}F(Y(T))\right\} \tag{6.6}$$

$$\mathbf{P}_{PP}^{GB}(\mathrm{k}_s,t) = \frac{-i\pi E_{pr}(t)E_{pu}^2[\boldsymbol{\mu}_{ge}\boldsymbol{\mu}_{eg}\boldsymbol{\mu}_{ge}\boldsymbol{\mu}_{eg}] \vdots \mathbf{e}_{pr}\mathbf{e}_{pu}\mathbf{e}_{pu}}{(\Omega^2+w^2)^{1/2}\left(\Omega^2+\bar{w}^2-\frac{H^2(T)}{\Omega^2+w^2}\right)^{1/2}}\exp(-X^2)$$
$$\times\left\{\exp(-Z^2(T)) + \frac{2i}{\sqrt{\pi}}F(Z(T))\right\}. \tag{6.7}$$

Here, the auxiliary functions in Equations 6.6 and 6.7 are defined as

$$X \equiv \frac{\omega_{pu}-\bar{\omega}_{eg}}{\sqrt{2[\Omega^2+w^2]}}$$

$$Y(T) \equiv \frac{\omega_{pr}-\bar{\omega}_{eg}-2Q(T)-\frac{H(T)}{\Omega^2+w^2}(\omega_{pu}-\bar{\omega}_{eg})}{\sqrt{2\left(\Omega^2+\bar{w}^2-\frac{H^2(T)}{\Omega^2+w^2}\right)}}$$

$$Z(T) \equiv \frac{\omega_{pr}-\bar{\omega}_{eg}-\frac{H(T)}{\Omega^2+w^2}(\omega_{pu}-\bar{\omega}_{eg})}{\sqrt{2\left(\Omega^2+\bar{w}^2-\frac{H^2(T)}{\Omega^2+w^2}\right)}}. \tag{6.8}$$

The Dawson integral, $F(x)$, in Equations 6.6 and 6.7, is defined as[10]

$$F(x) = e^{-x^2}\int_0^x du\, e^{u^2}. \tag{6.9}$$

The two contributions in Equations 6.6 and 6.7 are 2D Gaussian function with respect to the pump and probe field frequencies, ω_{pu} and ω_{pr}. More specifically, each contribution in Equations 6.6 and 6.7, when the imaginary pats are taken into consideration, is given as a product of two Gaussian functions. First of all, $\sqrt{\pi/(\Omega^2 + w^2)} \times \exp(-X^2)$ is a Gaussian function with center at $\omega_{pu} = \bar{\omega}_{eg}$, and its standard deviation is $\sqrt{(\Omega^2 + w^2)}$. The stimulated emission contribution to the pump–probe polarization also depends on another Gaussian function, which is $\sqrt{\pi/(\Omega^2 + \bar{w}^2 - H^2(T)/(\Omega^2 + w^2))} \times \exp(-Y^2(T))$. Note that the width of this Gaussian function changes in time T due to the T-dependent $H(T)$, which was defined in Equation 5.51. Additionally, from the definition of $Y(T)$in Equation 6.8, one can find that the center of the Gaussian function, $\exp(-Y^2(T))$,changes in time T as

$$\omega_{pr} = \bar{\omega}_{eg} + 2Q(T) + \frac{H(T)}{\Omega^2 + w^2}(\omega_{pu} - \bar{\omega}_{eg}). \tag{6.10}$$

Note that the spectral diffusion here was taken into account by $Q(T)$, and that the 2D peak shape is diagonally elongated because of the last term in Equation 6.10. The ground-state bleaching contribution to the pump–probe polarization also contains the similar term determining the line shape along the probe field frequency, which is $\sqrt{\pi/(\Omega^2 + \bar{w}^2 - H^2(T)/(\Omega^2 + w^2))} \exp(-Z^2(T))$ in Equation 6.7. The center of the Gaussian function $\exp(-Z^2(T))$ with respect to ω_{pr} is given as

$$\omega_{pr} = \bar{\omega}_{eg} + \frac{H(T)}{\Omega^2 + w^2}(\omega_{pu} - \bar{\omega}_{eg}). \tag{6.11}$$

Now, following the same line of derivations, one can find that the heterodyne-detected 2D TD and TB spectra are given as

$$S_{TD}(\omega_{pu}, \omega_{pr}; T) = \mathrm{Im}\left[\int_{-\infty}^{\infty} dt\, \mathbf{E}^*_{pr}(t) \cdot \mathbf{P}_{PP}(t;T)\right]$$

$$\propto \frac{-\pi \exp(-X^2)}{(\Omega^2 + w^2)^{1/2}\left(\Omega^2 + \bar{w}^2 - \frac{H^2(T)}{\Omega^2 + w^2}\right)^{1/2}}\{\exp(-Y^2(T)) + \exp(-Z^2(T))\} \tag{6.12}$$

$$S_{TB}(\omega_{pu}, \omega_{pr}; T) = \mathrm{Re}\left[\int_{-\infty}^{\infty} dt\, \mathbf{E}^*_{pr}(t) \cdot \mathbf{P}_{PP}(t;T)\right]$$

$$\propto \frac{\pi \exp(-X^2)}{(\Omega^2 + w^2)^{1/2}\left(\Omega^2 + \bar{w}^2 - \frac{H^2(T)}{\Omega^2 + w^2}\right)^{1/2}}\left\{\frac{2}{\sqrt{\pi}} F(Y(T)) + \frac{2}{\sqrt{\pi}} F(Z(T))\right\}. \tag{6.13}$$

For numerical calculation of these 2D spectra in Equations 6.12 and 6.13, both the spectral density, $\rho(\omega)$, and the solvent reorganization energy, λ, which are required

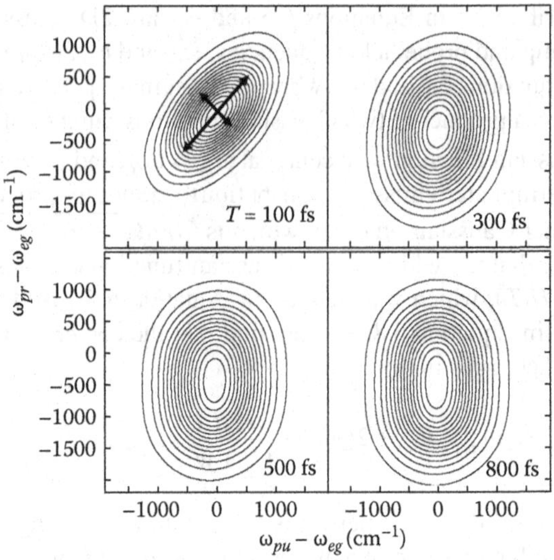

FIGURE 6.1 Two-dimensional transient grating spectra for the model system discussed in Section 5.8. The 2D contour spectra are shown for T = 100, 300, 500, and 800 fs.

to obtain the line-broadening function $g(t)$, should be determined first. Here, we consider the same model 2LS used to numerically simulate the integrated photon echo signal and PEPS in Section 5.8. The spectral density is given in Equation 5.83, and λ is assumed to be 500 cm^{-1} in the present case. For the following numerical simulations, the pump–pulse envelope will be assumed to be identical to that of the probe pulse, and the full-width at half-maximum (FWHM) of each pulse is set to be 50 fs, so that w and $\overline{w}$ are 250 cm^{-1}.

In Figure 6.1, the 2D transient dichroism spectra at T = 100, 300, 500, and 800 fs are plotted. Here, the population relaxation contribution to the signals that can be taken into account by multiplying an exponentially decaying function to the corresponding pump–probe response function has not been included because it does not strongly alter the 2D peak shape except for its widths along the x- and y-axis in the spectrum. The TD spectra at short time T are tilted and elliptical. Particularly, the TD spectrum at τ = 100 fs is diagonally elongated. The degree of slant of the TG and TD contours decreases as the pump–probe delay time T increases. The reason the 2D TD spectra are significantly tilted at short time T is that the memory on the phase space of initially pumped wavepacket is not fully faded out yet within such a short time. That is to say, the solvent inhomogeneity experienced by chromophores is large at short timescale. This memory loss rate is determined by the function, $H(T)$, defined in Equation 5.51, or approximately the solvation correlation function, $S(T)$ (see Equation 5.53).

At sufficiently short time T, the 2D spectrum is diagonally elongated even in the case when there is no static inhomogeneity. From the expression for the TD spectrum in Equation 6.12, one can obtain an approximate result for the FWHM along the diagonal, which is found to be

$$\Delta\omega_{diag}(T) = \left(\frac{8(\ln 2)\{(\Omega^2 + w^2)(\Omega^2 + \overline{w}^2) - H^2(T)\}}{2\Omega^2 + w^2 + \overline{w}^2 - 2H(T)} \right)^{1/2}. \tag{6.14}$$

The FWHM along the antidiagonal is, on the other hand,

$$\Delta\omega_{anti-diag}(T) = \left(\frac{8(\ln 2)\{(\Omega^2 + w^2)(\Omega^2 + \overline{w}^2) - H^2(T)\}}{2\Omega^2 + w^2 + \overline{w}^2 + 2H(T)} \right)^{1/2}. \tag{6.15}$$

Second, the width of the 2D TD spectrum along the ω_{pr} axis at $\omega_{pu} = \omega_{eg}$ increases as the delay time T increases. This is not only because of the $H(T)$-dependent standard deviation of the ω_{pr}-dependent Gaussian function, which is $\sqrt{\Omega^2 + \overline{w}^2 - H^2(T)/(\Omega^2 + w^2)}$, but also because of the spectral diffusion–induced frequency-shift of the 2D peak from the stimulated emission contributions. Due to the spectral diffusion function, $Q(T)$, the center frequency of $\sqrt{\pi/(\Omega^2 + \overline{w}^2 - H^2(T)/(\Omega^2 + w^2))}\exp(-Y^2(T))$ along the ω_{pr} axis at long time T shifts toward the value of $\omega_{eg} - 2\lambda/\hbar$. This can be easily understood by noting that the TD signals at large T are given by a sum of two 2D Gaussian functions centered at ($\omega_{pu} = \omega_{eg}$, $\omega_{pr} = \omega_{eg}$) and ($\omega_{pu} = \omega_{eg}$, $\omega_{pr} = \omega_{eg} - 2\lambda/\hbar$), that is,

$$S_{TD}(T \to \infty) \approx \frac{\pi \exp(-X^2)}{(\Omega^2 + w^2)^{1/2}(\Omega^2 + \overline{w}^2)^{1/2}} \{\exp(-Y^2(\infty)) + \exp(-Z^2(\infty))\}, \tag{6.16}$$

where

$$Y(\infty) \equiv \frac{\omega_{pr} - \omega_{eg} + 2\lambda/\hbar}{\sqrt{2(\Omega^2 + \overline{w}^2)}} \quad \text{and} \quad Z(\infty) \equiv \frac{\omega_{pr} - \omega_{eg}}{\sqrt{2(\Omega^2 + \overline{w}^2)}}. \tag{6.17}$$

As can be seen in the contour plots in Figure 6.1, the center position of the 2D TD spectrum, which is given by two 2D Gaussian functions originating from ground-state bleaching and stimulated emission contributions, changes with respect to the delay time T, and its location is at ($\omega_{pu} = \omega_{eg}$ and $\omega_{pr} = \omega_{eg} + \delta\omega(T)$), where the T-dependent frequency shift $\delta\omega(T)$ is found to be

$$\delta\omega(T) = Q(T) = S(T) - \frac{\lambda}{\hbar}. \tag{6.18}$$

Therefore, the T-dependent $\delta\omega(T)$ obtained from experimentally measured series of 2D TD spectra can directly provide quantitative information on the correlation function, $S(T)$, which is related to the frequency–frequency correlation function (see Equations 5.52 and 5.53).

EXERCISE 6.1

Using the model system discussed below Equation 6.13, numerically calculate the 2D TD spectrum at T = 1000 fs. From the simulated spectrum, estimate $\Delta\omega_{diag}$ and $\Delta\omega_{anti\text{-}diag}$ values and compare them with the results obtained with Equations 6.14 and 6.15.

Next, consider the 2D transient birefringence spectra numerically calculated by using the same model parameters (see Figure 6.2). Each spectrum contains both positive and negative peaks, which is a characteristic dispersive feature. Note that the two peaks at the maximum and the minimum are separated from each other, and that the magnitude of peak separation, $\Delta(T)$, increases as the interpulse delay time T increases. In addition, it is found that the 2D TB contour plot has a nodal line, and its slope is close to 1 at short time T but decreases to zero at long time. The slope of the nodal line will be denoted as $\sigma(T)$. Then, consider the contour line of $S_{TB}(\omega_{pu},\omega_{pr};T)=0$. The slope of the tangential line of this specific contour line in the region between the positive and negative peaks should be $\sigma(T)$. Because the Dawson's integral, $F(x)$, reaches the maximum value at x=0.92,[10] $|F(Y(T))|$ and $|F(Z(T))|$ become maximum when, for $\omega_{pu}=\omega_{eg}$,

$$\frac{\omega_{pr}-\omega_{eg}-2Q(T)}{\sqrt{2\left(\Omega^2-\frac{H^2(T)}{\Omega^2+w^2}+\bar{w}^2\right)}}=0.92 \quad \text{and} \quad \frac{\omega_{pr}-\omega_{eg}}{\sqrt{2\left(\Omega^2-\frac{H^2(T)}{\Omega^2+w^2}+\bar{w}^2\right)}}=0.92. \tag{6.19}$$

Therefore, the location of the midpoint between the positive and negative peaks is at

$$\omega^*_{pu}=\omega_{eg} \quad \text{and} \quad \omega^*_{pr}=0.92\sqrt{2\left(\Omega^2-\frac{H^2(T)}{\Omega^2+w^2}+\bar{w}^2\right)}+\omega_{eg}+Q(T). \tag{6.20}$$

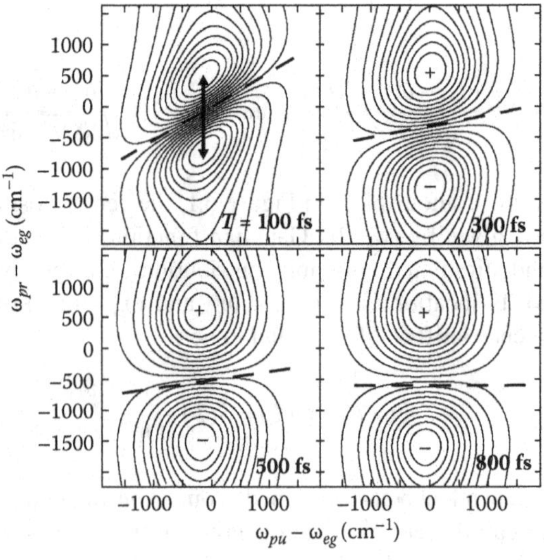

FIGURE 6.2 Two-dimensional transient birefringence spectra of the same model system used in Figure 6.1.

From this, the slope of the nodal line is found to be

$$\sigma(T) = \frac{H(T)}{\Omega^2 + w^2} \cong \left(\frac{2}{\hbar\beta}\right)\frac{S(T)}{\Omega^2 + w^2}. \tag{6.21}$$

This shows that the correlation function $S(T)$ can be experimentally measured from the T-dependent change of the slope of the 2D TB nodal line also.

Up until now, the static inhomogeneity has not been included in the description of 2D pump–probe spectrum of a model 2LS. If the static inhomogeneity is approximately given as a Gaussian with standard deviation Σ, one should simply perform the following replacements in all the equations in this section:

$$\Omega^2 \rightarrow \Omega^2 + \Sigma^2$$

$$H(T) \rightarrow H(T) + \Sigma^2. \tag{6.22}$$

In this case, the 2D TD and TB contours remain to be tilted regardless of the delay time T. For instance, the asymptotic value of the slope, $\sigma(T \rightarrow \infty)$, would approach to a finite value, and it is directly related to the width of the static inhomogeneity as

$$\sigma(T \rightarrow \infty) = \frac{\Sigma^2}{\Omega^2 + \Sigma^2 + w^2}. \tag{6.23}$$

This relationship would be of use in determining the width of static inhomogeneity distribution, Ω. Note that the value Ω^2 is the homogeneous line-broadening factor that can be estimated from the antidiagonal line-width in Equation 6.15 and the pump pulse width w can be experimentally measured. Thus, from the measured $\sigma(T \rightarrow \infty)$ value and Equation 6.23, Ω^2 can be quantitatively estimated.

6.3 TWO-DIMENSIONAL PUMP–PROBE SPECTRUM OF AN ANHARMONIC OSCILLATOR

In the previous section, 2D pump–probe spectroscopy of a 2LS was considered in detail. However, when the chromophore is a vibrational oscillator, not only the first vibrationally excited state but also the second excited (overtone) state are involved in a 2D four-wave-mixing process. If the oscillator is perfectly harmonic, the 2D vibrational response function vanishes. However, for a realistic vibration, the potential energy surface is anharmonic so that the corresponding response function does not vanish and the measured 2D spectrum provides critical information on the vibrational anharmonicity for a single oscillator system.

Here, the three vibrational levels are denoted as $|g\rangle$, $|e\rangle$, and $|f\rangle$, where $|f\rangle$ is the overtone (second excited) state. Due to the presence of the third state, in addition to the four diagrams in Equation 6.3, one should consider two more contributions:

$$\langle\mu \xleftarrow{\underset{e}{\overset{f\ e}{}}} |g\rangle\langle g| \rangle$$

$$\langle\mu \xleftarrow{\underset{e}{\overset{f\ \ e}{}}} |g\rangle\langle g| \rangle. \tag{6.24}$$

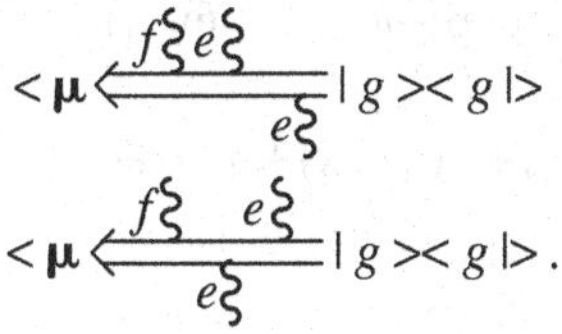

Hereafter, the corresponding response function components associated with the above two diagrams will be denoted as R_5 and R_6, respectively. They involve population ($\rho_{ee}^{(2)}$) evolution during the second time period t_2. Then, the third radiation–matter interaction induces one quantum transition from e to f. Therefore, these two contributions are called the *excited-state absorption* (EA). The expressions for the corresponding third-order response function components can be obtained from Equations 5.26 and 5.29, which are valid for an arbitrary four-level system. In the case of the weakly anharmonic oscillator, the transition dipole matrix element $|\boldsymbol{\mu}_{fe}|$ is related to $|\boldsymbol{\mu}_{eg}|$ as $|\boldsymbol{\mu}_{fe}| \cong \sqrt{2}\,|\boldsymbol{\mu}_{eg}|$. Furthermore, the vibrational chromophore-solvent interaction induces fluctuation of the vibrational force constant so that the fluctuating part of the transition frequency between g and f states is twice as large as that between g and e states, that is,

$$U_{fg}(t) \cong 2U_{eg}(t). \tag{6.25}$$

Therefore, the correlation functions representing correlation amplitudes between fluctuating transition frequencies are related to one another as[1, 11]

$$C_{ee}(t) = \frac{1}{4}C_{ff}(t) = \frac{1}{2}C_{ef}(t) = \frac{1}{2}C_{fe}(t) \tag{6.26}$$

where

$$C_{ff}(t) = \frac{1}{\hbar^2} < U_{fg}(t)U_{fg}(0)\rho_B >_B$$

$$C_{ef}(t) = \frac{1}{\hbar^2} < U_{eg}(t)U_{fg}(0)\rho_B >_B$$

$$C_{fe}(t) = \frac{1}{\hbar^2} < U_{fg}(t)U_{eg}(0)\rho_B >_B . \tag{6.27}$$

Using these relationships, one can obtain the expressions for the two diagrams in Equation 6.24, in terms of the line-broadening function $g(t)$, as

$$R_5(t_3, t_2, t_1) = -[\boldsymbol{\mu}_{ge}\boldsymbol{\mu}_{ef}\boldsymbol{\mu}_{fe}\boldsymbol{\mu}_{eg}]\exp\{-i\bar{\omega}_{fe}t_3 + i\bar{\omega}_{eg}t_1\}$$

$$\times \exp\{-g(t_3) - g^*(t_1) + g(t_2) - g^*(t_1+t_2) - g(t_2+t_3) + g^*(t_1+t_2+t_3)\}$$

$$R_6(t_3, t_2, t_1) = -[\boldsymbol{\mu}_{ge}\boldsymbol{\mu}_{ef}\boldsymbol{\mu}_{fe}\boldsymbol{\mu}_{eg}]\exp\{-i\bar{\omega}_{fe}t_3 - i\bar{\omega}_{eg}t_1\}$$

$$\times \exp\{-g(t_3) - g(t_1) - g^*(t_2) + g(t_1+t_2) + g^*(t_2+t_3) - g(t_1+t_2+t_3)\}. \tag{6.28}$$

By using the short-time approximation again and by considering the well-separated pulse limit, the excited-state absorption contribution to the pump–probe polarization, $\mathbf{P}_{PP}(\mathbf{k}_s,t)$, is found to be

$$\mathbf{P}_{PP}^{EA}(t) = \frac{2i\pi E_{pr}(t)E_{pu}^2[\boldsymbol{\mu}_{ef}\boldsymbol{\mu}_{fe}\boldsymbol{\mu}_{eg}\boldsymbol{\mu}_{ge}]\vdots\mathbf{e}_{pr}\mathbf{e}_{pu}\mathbf{e}_{pu}}{(\Omega^2+w^2)^{1/2}\left(\Omega^2-\frac{H^2(T)}{\Omega^2+w^2}+\overline{w}^2\right)^{1/2}}\exp(-X^2)$$

$$\times\left\{\exp(-W^2(T))+\frac{2i}{\sqrt{\pi}}F(W(T))\right\} \tag{6.29}$$

where

$$W(T) \equiv \frac{\omega_{pr}-\overline{\omega}_{fe}-2Q(T)-\frac{H(T)}{\Omega^2+w^2}(\omega_{pu}-\overline{\omega}_{eg})}{\sqrt{2\left(\Omega^2-\frac{H^2(T)}{\Omega^2+w^2}+\overline{w}^2\right)}}. \tag{6.30}$$

Note that $\mathrm{P}_{PP}^{EA}(t)$ differs from $\mathrm{P}_{PP}^{SE}(t)$ by (1) the factor of 2 originating from the relationship $|\boldsymbol{\mu}_{fe}|^2 = 2|\boldsymbol{\mu}_{eg}|^2$, (2) the sign that the excited-state absorption contributes to the PP signal negatively, and (3) $\omega_{pr}-\overline{\omega}_{eg}\rightarrow\omega_{pr}-\overline{\omega}_{fe}$.

Therefore, for an effectively three-vibrational-level system, the total pump–probe polarization is given by a sum of three contributions:

$$\mathbf{P}_{PP}(t) = \mathbf{P}_{PP}^{SE}(t)+\mathbf{P}_{PP}^{GB}(t)+\mathbf{P}_{PP}^{EA}(t). \tag{6.31}$$

Due to the phase difference $e^{i\pi}$ (= −1) between $P_{PP}^{EA}(t)$ and $P_{PP}^{SE}(t)+P_{PP}^{GB}(t)$, the additional excited-state absorption contribution interferes destructively in the region where the spectral overlap is large. Combining the results in Equations 6.12 and 6.13 with the EA contribution to the 2D pump–probe spectrum, one can find that the 2D TD and TB signals of an anharmonic oscillator are

$$S_{TD}(\omega_{pu},\omega_{pr};T) \propto \frac{\pi\exp(-X^2)}{(\Omega^2+w^2)^{1/2}\left(\Omega^2-\frac{H^2(T)}{\Omega^2+w^2}+\overline{w}^2\right)^{1/2}}$$

$$\times\{2\exp(-W^2(T))-\exp(-Y^2(T))-\exp(-Z^2(T))\} \tag{6.32}$$

$$S_{TB}(\omega_{pu},\omega_{pr};T) \propto \frac{\pi\exp(-X^2)}{(\Omega^2+w^2)^{1/2}\left(\Omega^2-\frac{H^2(T)}{\Omega^2+w^2}+\overline{w}^2\right)^{1/2}}$$

$$\times\left\{\frac{2}{\sqrt{\pi}}F(Y(T))+\frac{2}{\sqrt{\pi}}F(Z(T))-\frac{4}{\sqrt{\pi}}F(W(T))\right\}. \tag{6.33}$$

The 2D TD spectrum consists of three 2D Gaussian functions. The peak positions of the three independent terms are

$$\begin{aligned}
\text{Ground-state bleaching (GB):} &\quad (\omega_{pu} = \bar{\omega}_{eg}, \omega_{pr} = \bar{\omega}_{eg}) \\
\text{Stimulated emission (SE):} &\quad (\omega_{pu} = \bar{\omega}_{eg}, \omega_{pr} = \bar{\omega}_{eg} + 2Q(T)) \\
\text{Excited-state absorption (EA):} &\quad (\omega_{pu} = \bar{\omega}_{eg}, \omega_{pr} = \bar{\omega}_{fe} + 2Q(T)).
\end{aligned}$$

Noting that $\bar{\omega}_{fe} = \bar{\omega}_{eg} - \delta\omega_{anh}$, where $\delta\omega_{anh}$ is the overtone anharmonic frequency shift, one can find that the peak position of the EA contribution is at $(\omega_{pu} = \bar{\omega}_{eg}$, $\omega_{pr} = \bar{\omega}_{eg} - \delta\omega_{anh} + 2Q(T))$.

Perfectly harmonic case. If there is no overtone anharmonicity, that is, perfectly harmonic oscillator, $\bar{\omega}_{fe} = \bar{\omega}_{eg}$ and the relation $|\mu_{fe}| = \sqrt{2}\,|\mu_{eg}|$ is exact, then, the magnitude of the GB+SE term is identical to that of the EA contribution and the pump–probe signal vanishes. However, all real molecular vibrations are intrinsically anharmonic.

Strongly anharmonic case. In the limiting case when the overtone anharmonic frequency shift $\delta\omega_{anh}$ is much larger than the absorption bandwidth and solvent reorganization energy, that is, $\delta\omega_{anh} \gg \Omega$ and $\delta\omega_{anh} \gg \lambda/\hbar$, the TD spectrum will exhibit two peaks with opposite signs and the peak-to-peak frequency difference is simply identical to $\delta\omega_{anh}$.

Weakly anharmonic case. When $\delta\omega_{anh}$ is comparable to the absorption bandwidth, which is approximately Ω (root mean square fluctuation amplitude of vibrational transition frequency), the peak-to-peak frequency difference is a complicated function of $\delta\omega_{anh}$, Ω, and pulse widths. This case is considered below.

First of all, the functional form of the spectral density, $\rho(\omega)$, will be assumed to be the same with Equation 5.83, but the solvent reorganization energy, λ, is assumed to be 10 cm^{-1} in the present case of anharmonic oscillator. Note that the vibrational Stokes shift, which is the solvation energy change upon vibrational excitation, is typically one to two orders of magnitude smaller than that of electronic transition. The IR pump–pulse envelop is assumed to be identical to that of the IR probe pulse, and the FWHM of each pulse is set to be 200 fs so that w and $\bar{w}$ are 63 cm^{-1}. Due to the nonzero vibrational anharmonicity, we assume that the overtone anharmonic frequency shift $\delta\omega_{anh} = \omega_{eg} - \omega_{fe}$ is 30 cm^{-1}. The 2D TD spectra for varying delay time T are plotted in Figure 6.3. At short time (see the contour plot at $T = 100$ fs), the positive and negative contours are diagonally elongated and the nodal line between the two peaks has a finite slope. As T increases, the slope changes and approaches zero, in the case when there is no static inhomogeneity.

For a weakly anharmonic oscillator, the peak-to-peak frequency difference in the present model system is estimated to be about 180 cm^{-1}, which is much larger than the overtone anharmonic frequency shift 30 cm^{-1}. Furthermore, the two peak positions along the ω_{pr}-axis change in time T via the spectral diffusion process described by $Q(T)$. Note that the two contributions from EA and SE+GB, which are $2\exp(-W^2(T))$ and $-\exp(-Y^2(T)) - \exp(-Z^2(T))$, respectively, are Gaussian functions centered at $\omega_{pr} = \bar{\omega}_{eg} - \delta\omega_{anh} + 2Q(T)$ and $\omega_{pr} = \bar{\omega}_{eg} + Q(T)$, respectively. The maximum values of $2\exp(-W^2(T))$ and $\exp(-Y^2(T)) + \exp(-Z^2(T))$ are in this case almost the same. Thus, the slice of the 2D TD spectrum at $\omega_{pu} = \bar{\omega}_{eg}$ can be recast in the form

$$S_{TD}(\omega_{pu} = \bar{\omega}_{eg}, \omega_{pr}; T) \propto \exp\left(-A(T)\{x - x_1(T)\}^2\right) - \exp\left(-A(T)\{x - x_2(T)\}^2\right) \quad (6.34)$$

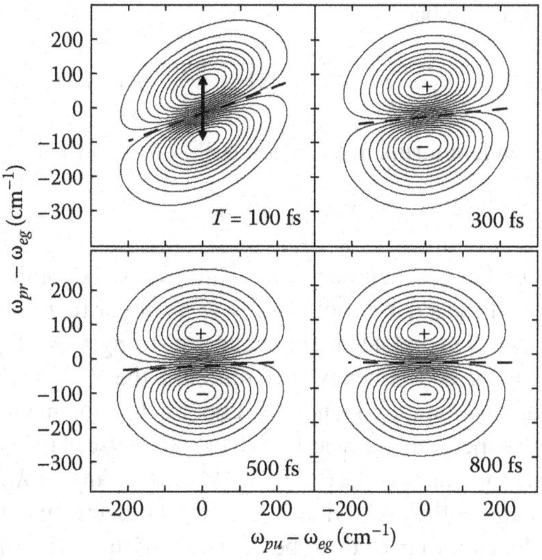

FIGURE 6.3 Two-dimensional transient dichroism spectra of anharmonic oscillator.

where

$$x \equiv \omega_{pr} - \omega_{eg}$$

$$x_1(T) \equiv 2Q(T) - \delta\omega_{anh}$$

$$x_2(T) \equiv Q(T)$$

$$A(T) \equiv \frac{1}{2(\Omega^2 - H^2(T)[\Omega^2 + w^2]^{-1} + \bar{w}^2)}. \tag{6.35}$$

The two (positive and negative) peak positions can be found by solving the following nonlinear equation, obtained from $\partial S_{TD}(\omega_{pu} = \bar{\omega}_{eg}, \omega_{pr}; T)/\partial x = 0$, for x,

$$\frac{x - x_1(T)}{x - x_2(T)} = \exp\left\{-A(T)\left[2(x_1(T) - x_2(T))x - x_1^2(T) + x_2^2(T)\right]\right\}. \tag{6.36}$$

One cannot analytically solve the above nonlinear equation to find two roots. However, in the weakly anharmonic case, it should be noted that, regardless of T, for x in the range from $[x_1(T) + x_2(T)]/2 - \sqrt{\Omega^2 + \bar{w}^2}$ to $[x_1(T) + x_2(T)]/2 + \sqrt{\Omega^2 + \bar{w}^2}$, we have

$$|A(T)[2(x_1(T) - x_2(T))x]| << 1. \tag{6.37}$$

Thus, Equation 6.36 can be recast in the form of a quadratic equation of $(\omega_{pr} - \bar{\omega}_{eg})$. Thus, the magnitude of the peak-to-peak frequency difference, denoted as $\Delta\omega(T)$, is approximately found to be

$$\Delta\omega(T) \cong \sqrt{4(\Omega^2 - H^2(T)[\Omega^2 + w^2]^{-1} + \bar{w}^2) + Q^2(T)}. \tag{6.38}$$

Ignoring the T-dependent terms in Equation 6.38, one can further simplify it as

$$\Delta\omega \cong 2\sqrt{\Omega^2 + \bar{w}^2}. \tag{6.39}$$

which is 180 cm^{-1} in the present model case. Thus, for weakly anharmonic oscillator, it is concluded that, if the square root of $\Omega^2 + \bar{w}^2$ is larger than the sum of $\delta\omega_{anh}$ and $\lambda/\hbar$, or if the two (positive and negative) peaks are strongly overlapped in frequency domain, the peak-to-peak frequency difference in the 2D TD spectrum is determined not by the anharmonic frequency shift but by the root mean square fluctuation amplitude Ω and the spectral bandwidth of the probe pulse. This is indeed the model case studied above, for example, $\sqrt{\Omega^2 + \bar{w}^2} = 90$ cm$^{-1} > \delta\omega_{anh} + \lambda/\hbar = 40$ cm^{-1}.

Secondly, the slope of the nodal line in the 2D TD spectrum is found to be related to the function $S(T)$. Defining $\sigma(\tau)$ to be the slope of the nodal line (see the dashed line in Figure 6.3) at $\omega_{pu} = \bar{\omega}_{eg}$ and $\omega_{pr} = \bar{\omega}_{eg} + [x_1(T) + x_2(T)]/2$, we find

$$\sigma(T) = \frac{H(T)}{\Omega^2 + w^2} \cong \left(\frac{2}{\hbar\beta}\right)\frac{S(T)}{\Omega^2 + w^2}. \tag{6.40}$$

Again, once the slope $\sigma(T)$ is experimentally measured as a function of T, the solvation dynamics function $S(T)$ can be obtained by using the above relationship, Equation 6.40.

Although the time-dependent 2D TB spectrum of an anharmonic oscillator has not been discussed in detail in this chapter, using the formal expression given in Equation 6.33 and performing numerical calculations of the Dawson integrals, one can find spectroscopic signatures of solvation dynamics and vibrational transition frequency-frequency correlation functions from the 2D TB measurements. In addition, similar to the case of 2LS, the static inhomogeneity effects on various pump–probe spectra of anharmonic oscillator can be understood by performing the same replacements in Equation 6.22. Again, the asymptotic value of the inverse slope, $\sigma(T \to \infty)$, will provide quantitative information on the existence and magnitude of static inhomogeneity.

In this chapter, theoretical descriptions of 2D pump–probe spectroscopy of two- and three-level systems, which are good models for an electronic chromophore and an anharmonic oscillator, respectively, were presented. The expressions for the 2D pump–probe signals presented here will be of use in the investigations of pure dephasing, static inhomogeneity, and chromophore-solvent dynamics of two- and three-level systems. However, it should be noted that the 2D pump–probe spectroscopy requires frequency-scanning of the pump field. In contrast, the photon echo spectroscopy with ultrashort pulses is useful for directly obtaining the entire 2D spectrum by scanning the interpulse delay times followed by 2D Fourier transformation. Thus, the photon echo method has been considered to be a convenient 2D vibrational or electronic spectroscopy. This will be discussed in the following chapter.

REFERENCES

1. Kwac, K.; Cho, M., Two-color pump–probe spectroscopies of two- and three-level systems: 2-dimensional line shapes and solvation dynamics. *Journal of Physical Chemistry A* 2003, 107, 5903–5912.
2. Cho, M., Coherent two-dimensional optical spectroscopy. *Chemical Reviews* 2008, 108, 1331–1418.
3. Kwak, K.; Cho, M.; Fleming, G. R.; Agarwal, R.; Prall, B. S., Two-color transient grating spectroscopy of a two-level system. *Bulletin of the Korean Chemical Society* 2003, 24, 1069–1074.
4. Woutersen, S.; Hamm, P., Nonlinear two-dimensional vibrational spectroscopy of peptides. *Journal of Physics-Condensed Matter* 2002, 14, R1035–R1062.
5. Mukamel, S., Femtosecond optical spectroscopy: A direct look at elementary chemical events. *Annual Review of Physical Chemistry* 1990, 41, 647–681.
6. Mukamel, S., *Principles of nonlinear optical spectroscopy*. Oxford University Press: Oxford, 1995.
7. Hamm, P.; Lim, M.; Hochstrasser, R. M., Structure of the amide I band of peptides measured by femtosecond nonlinear infrared spectroscopy. *Journal of Physical Chemistry B* 1998, 102, 6123–6138.
8. DeCamp, M. F.; Tokmakoff, A., Single-shot two-dimensional spectrometer. *Optics Letters* 2006, 31, 113–115.
9. DeCamp, M. F.; DeFlores, L. P.; Jones, K. C.; Tokmakoff, A., Single-shot two-dimensional infrared spectroscopy. *Optics Express* 2007, 15, 233–241.
10. Abramowitz, M.; Stegun, I. A., *Handbook of mathematical functions with formulas, graphs, and mathematical tables*. Dover Publications: New York, 1974.
11. Kwac, K.; Cho, M., Molecular dynamics simulation study of N-methylacetamide in water. II. Two-dimensional infrared pump–probe spectra. *Journal of Chemical Physics* 2003, 119, 2256–2263.

7 Two-Dimensional Photon Echo Spectroscopy

Electronic or vibrational photon echo has been considered to be an optical analog of the NMR spin echo.[1–6] In an optical photon echo experiment typically utilizing three light pulses, a phase-matching geometry based on momentum conservation of the photons is used to detect the echo signal field propagating in the direction that is different from those of incident beams (see Figure 3.3). An early purpose of photon echo investigation was to exploit the correlation between the initial excitation frequency and the final detection (emission or probing) frequency in time and to eliminate the static inhomogeneous line-broadening contribution by measuring the rephasing echo signal.[5, 7, 8] In the limiting case when the line shape is dictated by a large inhomogeneous broadening, the echo signal field will peak at $t = \tau$ due to the rephasing process (see Section 5.6). However, chromophores in solution do not have truly static inhomogeneity due to the ultrafast spectral diffusion and solvation process so that the echo signal field amplitude varies in the detection time t, which is the time after the third pulse in a three-pulse photon echo experiment.

The phase-matched photon echo signal field should then satisfy the following wave vector equality: $\mathbf{k}_s = -\mathbf{k}_1 + \mathbf{k}_2 + \mathbf{k}_3$. The corresponding diagrams have been called the rephasing ones. The "mirror image" echo appears at $\mathbf{k}_s = \mathbf{k}_1 - \mathbf{k}_2 + \mathbf{k}_3$, and the corresponding nonlinear optical transition pathways were called the nonrephasing diagrams. At short time ($<\tau_{sol}$ or $\tau_{decoherence}$), the rephasing echo and the mirror image (nonrephasing) echo signals, with respect to the first coherence period, τ, do not completely overlap,[9] and the time difference between the two peaks was defined as the three-pulse PEPS denoted as $\tau^*(T)$.[7, 10, 11] It turned out that the PEPS as a function of the second delay time T between the second and third pulses in the three-pulse photon echo was shown to be directly related to the transition frequency–frequency correlation function, and its asymptotic value is related to the static inhomogeneity directly reflecting unequal environments around different chromophores.[7, 11] The delay time T was called the waiting or population evolution time in the literatures. Usually, the conventional integrated photon echo signal depends on two time variables τ and T, and the echo field intensity (not amplitude) was detected. Therefore, the integrated photon echo measurement method cannot provide the 2D photon echo spectrum unless notable quantum beats exist.

In a real 2D photon echo measurement, a femtosecond optical (either visible or infrared) pulse whose spectral bandwidth is sufficiently broad enough to simultaneously excite a manifold of excited or delocalized excitonic states can create quantum coherences $\rho_{eg}^{(1)}(\tau)$ between the ground and excited states. The second pulse interacts with the system, and either the ground-state population $\rho_{gg}^{(2)}(\tau, T)$ or excited-state coherence $\rho_{ee'}^{(2)}(\tau, T)$ (for $e \neq e'$) or population $\rho_{ee}^{(2)}(\tau, T)$ is created. Note that the density matrix $\rho^{(2)}(\tau, T)$ is second order with respect to the external electric field *amplitude*. The third field-matter interaction finally generates the third-order perturbation-expanded density matrix elements such as $\rho^{(3)}_{e'g}(\tau, T, t)$, which in turn radiate the echo signal field via a spontaneous emissive interaction with the vaccum field. Detecting the photon echo signal field with respect to τ, *T*, and *t* and Fourier transforming it with respect to τ and *t*, one can obtain the 2D photon echo spectrum $S_{PE}(\omega_t, T, \omega_\tau)$ as a function of the waiting time *T*. One can use different methods to control the pulse-to-pulse delay time, phases between pulses, center frequencies of each pulse, and so forth, but regardless of detailed experimental approaches, the 2D photon echo spectroscopy is essentially to measure the third-order response function with respect to τ, *T*, and *t*. In this regard, it can be considered a 3D spectroscopic method,[12] since one can carry out an additional Fourier transformation of the third-order response function with respect to *T* too. However, for the sake of simplicity in plotting the 3D function and for clear interpretation, the 2D spectrum $S_{PE}(\omega_t, T, \omega_\tau)$ has been reported with respect to the waiting time *T*. In the present chapter, we will mainly consider the 2D photon echo spectroscopy of simple model systems, such as 2LS and anharmonic oscillator. Furthermore, a few simplified 2D peak shape models will be discussed here.

7.1 PHASE AND AMPLITUDE DETECTION OF TWO-DIMENSIONAL PHOTON ECHO SIGNAL FIELDS

There are a number of different ways to detect weak and transient signal electric fields. For instance, one can use a time-gated pulse combined with an upconversion detection technique to measure the temporal amplitude of a weak signal field.[13–16] A variety of heterodyne detection methods have also been developed over the years, but the so-called Fourier transform spectral interferometry (FTSI) has been most extensively used among them.[17–25] Here, the phase-and-amplitude detection of the weak signal field via the FTSI is discussed in detail, not only because it has been widely used in both 2D IR and 2D electronic spectroscopy based on a photon echo scheme, but also because it is a fundamentally important and quite versatile detection scheme used in many other applications.

To fully extract information on nonlinear molecular responses against a train of interrogating pulses, one should be able to characterize the signal field in terms of its phase and amplitude. To achieve such a goal, a heterodyne detection method in frequency domain based on the Mach-Zehnder interferometer (see Figure 7.1) has been widely used because fast response array detector is available. The three-pulse photon echo experimental setup is inside the Echo EXP box in Figure 7.1. Then, the generated signal field E_s is combined with the reference (local oscillator) field E_0. The two fields then interfere with each other, and the total intensity, which is the absolute square of the sum of the two electric fields, is then detected, that is,

$$I(\omega) = |E_0(\omega) + E_s(\omega)|^2 = |E_0(\omega)|^2 + |E_s(\omega)|^2 + 2\,\mathrm{Re}[E_0^*(\omega)E_s(\omega)]. \quad (7.1)$$

Often the second term on the right-hand side of Equation 7.1 is much smaller than the last interference term since the latter is linearly proportional to the reference field amplitude. Using a chopper properly placed in one of the arms of the Mach-Zehnder

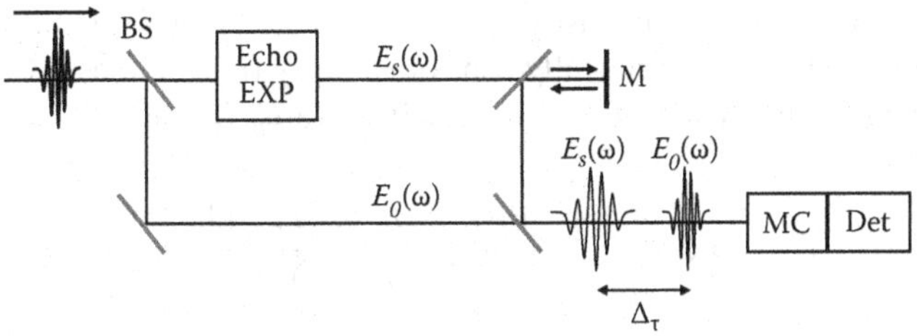

FIGURE 7.1 Fourier transform spectral interferometer for heterodyne-detection of photon echo signal field $E_s(\omega)$. The photon echo experimental setup is inside the Echo EXP box. The generated photon echo signal field is delayed from the reference pulse $E_0(\omega)$ by a finite time Δ_τ. Here, BS is beam splitter; MC, monochromator; M, mirror; Det, multichannel array detector.

interferometer in Figure 7.1 and taking difference intensity, one can selectively measure the heterodyned signal $I_h = 2\,\text{Re}[E_0^*(\omega)E_s(\omega)]$.

When the reference pulse and signal field are temporally overlapped at the detector, the interference term is likely to be very large. However, in order to enhance the spectral resolution and to selectively eliminate the contribution from the reference pulse spectrum to the measured heterodyned signal, the reference pulse is deliberately made to precede the signal by a fixed time delay Δ_τ.[17] The delay time Δ_τ is chosen to be large enough to reduce the temporal overlap between the reference pulse and signal field but small enough to make the interference signal measurably large. In this case, the interference part of the measured signal has an additional phase-factor originating from the finite delay time Δ_τ as

$$I_h(\omega) = 2\,\text{Re}\left[E_0^*(\omega)E_s(\omega)e^{i\omega\Delta_\tau}\right]. \tag{7.2}$$

To obtain the complex spectrum of the signal field, it is necessary to manipulate the heterodyne-detected spectral interferogram as

$$E_s(\omega) = \frac{F\left[\theta(t)F^{-1}\{I_h(\omega)\}\right]e^{-i\omega\Delta_\tau}}{E_0^*(\omega)}, \tag{7.3}$$

where $F[\cdots]$ and $F^{-1}[\cdots]$ are the Fourier and inverse Fourier transforms, respectively. $\theta(t)$ is the heavy-side step function.

EXERCISE 7.1
Derive Equation 7.3 from 7.2.

In a photon echo experiment, the echo field is put into a spectral interferometer to allow its interference with the reference pulse. In this case, the transient profile of the echo signal field as a function of detection time t is not directly measured but indirectly characterized by using this FTSI in frequency domain. Here, the heterodyne-detected signal intensity $I_h(\omega_t, T, \tau)$ corresponds to the echo signal depending on the two experimentally controlled delay times τ and T. Therefore, the 2D photon echo signal field can be extracted from $I_h(\omega_t, T, \tau)$ as

$$E_{echo}(\omega_t, T, \tau) = \frac{F\left[\theta(t)F^{-1}\{I_h(\omega_t, T, \tau)\}\right]e^{-i\omega_t\Delta_\tau}}{E_0^*(\omega_t)}. \quad (7.4)$$

The 2D photon echo spectrum is finally obtained by performing a numerical Fourier transformation with respect to the first coherence delay time, τ, as

$$\tilde{E}_{echo}(\omega_t, T, \omega_\tau) = \int_{-\infty}^{\infty} d\tau \, E_{echo}(\omega_t, T, \tau)\exp(i\omega_\tau \tau). \quad (7.5)$$

This has become the standard procedure for a spectral interferometric heterodyne-detected 2D photon echo experiment. Certainly, one can use a pulse-shaping technology to keep the phase between pulses constant and to control the delay time τ in an automated fashion. Nevertheless, the essential idea is that the double Fourier transformations of the echo signal field $E_{echo}(t, T, \tau)$ with respect to τ and t are required to obtain the 2D photon echo spectrum.

Since thus obtained 2D photon echo spectrum is complex and depends on the phase-matching condition used, there exist different ways to present the 2D photon echo spectra. For the phase-matching scheme with $\mathbf{k}_s = -\mathbf{k}_1 + \mathbf{k}_2 + \mathbf{k}_3$, the real and imaginary parts of $\tilde{E}_{echo}(\omega_t, T, \omega_\tau)$ can be separately measured and have been reported. The absolute magnitude spectrum defined as $|\tilde{E}_{echo}(\omega_t, T, \omega_\tau)|$ was also used in some cases and often discussed in literatures. An absorptive 2D photon echo spectrum obtained as the sum of equally weighted rephasing and nonrephasing photon echo spectra was also considered to be of use. Most of the photon echo spectroscopy experiments were based on a noncollinear four-wave-mixing scheme with a specific phase-matching condition mentioned above, where incident beams propagate slightly differently (see Figure 7.2) in space. Phase-matching method has a clear

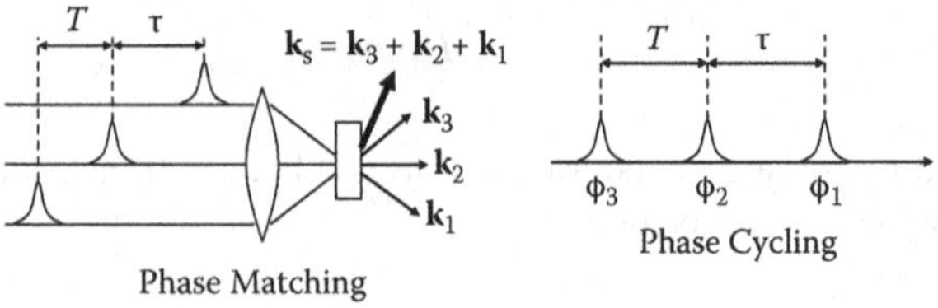

FIGURE 7.2 Phase-matching and phase-cycling beam configurations for photon echo mesurement. In the former case, the three incident beams are noncollinear, and the generated echo signal field radiated in the direction of k_s wavevector is selectively detected by using one of the heterodyne-detection methods. On the other hand, the phase-cycling method uses three collinear pulses, but the relative phase of each pulse is precisely controlled and a proper combination of phase-cycled signals gives the echo signal.

advantage of spatial separation of the desired and undesired signals, as can be seen in Figure 7.2. Note that the signal field propagates in a different direction.

However, the direct optical analog of 2D NMR utilizing the phase-cycling technique was also experimentally demonstrated to be feasible.[26, 27] The phases of the three collinearly propagating pulses are controlled so that the echo polarization becomes a function of the input pulse phases $\phi_1 - \phi_3$ (see Figure 7.2). The echo polarization has a unique phase dependence on the input pulses. Then, the photon echo peaks can be selectively measured by combining sixteen different phase combinations, that is, sixteen-step phase cycling. It should be mentioned that there are certain advantages of phase-cycling technique over phase matching: (1) coherently averaging away the specific interaction mechanism can enhance signal intensity, (2) collinear approach decreases the number of required data points, and (3) phase-matching technique works in extended systems with many chromophores, but the collinear phase-cycling technique is not strongly limited by the size of the sample. For the sake of experimental demonstration, rubidium atomic vapor was chosen, where rubidium atom can be considered a four-level system consisting of the ground state $5S_{1/2}$, two singly excited states $5P_{1/2}$ and $5P_{3/2}$, and one doubly excited state 5D. Despite the success of the optical 2D spectroscopy with employing a phase-cycling technique, it needs to be developed further to allow its application to a variety of 2D electronic and vibrational spectroscopic investigations of complicated molecular systems such as proteins, molecular complexes, and the like.

7.2 TWO-DIMENSIONAL PHOTON ECHO SPECTRUM OF A TWO-LEVEL SYSTEM

In Chapter 5, a theoretical description of the three-pulse photon echo polarization was presented in terms of the third-order electric-dipole response function and its triple convolution with pulsed electric fields. In particular, the rephasing echo measurement is to detect the emitted signal field in the direction of $-\mathbf{k}_1 + \mathbf{k}_2 + \mathbf{k}_3$. Then, only the rephasing diagrams are important due to the resonance conditions, and Section 5.6 showed the temporal envelope of the photon echo polarization:

$$\mathbf{P}_{PE}(t,T,\tau) = \left(\frac{i}{\hbar}\right)^3 \int_0^\infty dt_1 \int_0^\infty dt_2 \int_0^\infty dt_3 \{R_2(t_3,t_2,t_1) + R_3(t_3,t_2,t_1)\} : \mathbf{e}_3\mathbf{e}_2\mathbf{e}_1^* E_3(t-t_3)$$

$$\times E_2(t+T-t_3-t_2)E_1^*(t+\tau+T-t_3-t_2-t_1)\exp\{i\omega t_3 - i\omega t_1\}. \quad (7.6)$$

Here, the two rephasing diagrams representing $R_2(t_3,t_2,t_1)$ and $R_3(t_3,t_2,t_1)$ contributions are, for 2LS,

$$<\mu \xleftarrow[\substack{e\zeta \\ g\zeta \quad e\zeta}]{} |g><g|>$$

$$<\mu \xleftarrow[\substack{e\zeta \\ g\zeta e\zeta}]{} |g><g|>. \quad (7.7)$$

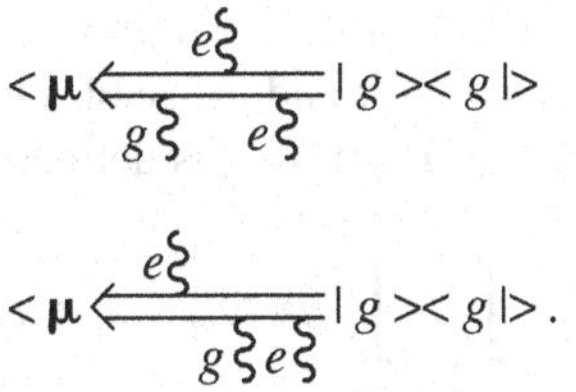

Using the short-time approximate expressions for $R_2(t_3, t_2, t_1)$ and $R_3(t_3, t_2, t_1)$, Equation 7.6 can be rewritten as

$$\mathbf{P}_{PE}(t,T,\tau) = -i\hbar^{-3}[\boldsymbol{\mu}_{ge}\boldsymbol{\mu}_{eg}\boldsymbol{\mu}_{ge}\boldsymbol{\mu}_{eg}]\vdots\mathbf{e}_3\mathbf{e}_2\mathbf{e}_1^*\int_0^\infty dt_1\int_0^\infty dt_2\int_0^\infty dt_3\, M(t_3,t_2,t_1)$$

$$\{\exp(i(\omega-\bar{\omega}_{eg}-2Q(t_2))t_3 - i(\omega-\bar{\omega}_{eg})t_1) + \exp(i(\omega-\bar{\omega}_{eg})t_3$$

$$-i(\omega-\bar{\omega}_{eg})t_1)\}\, E_3(t-t_3)E_2(t+T-t_3-t_2)E_1^*(t+\tau+T-t_3-t_2-t_1), \tag{7.8}$$

where the line-shape function $M(t_3, t_2\ t_1)$ commonly appearing in $R_2(t_3, t_2\ t_1)$ and $R_3(t_3, t_2\ t_1)$ is defined as

$$M(t_3,t_2,t_1) \equiv \exp\left\{-\frac{1}{2}\Omega^2 t_1^2 - \frac{1}{2}\Omega^2 t_3^2 + H(t_2)t_1t_3\right\}. \tag{7.9}$$

If the temporal envelopes of the three pulses are sufficiently short, the above integrations can be approximately performed to find that

$$\mathbf{P}_{PE}(t,T,\tau) \propto -i\hbar^{-3}E_3E_2E_1^*[\boldsymbol{\mu}_{ge}\boldsymbol{\mu}_{eg}\boldsymbol{\mu}_{ge}\boldsymbol{\mu}_{eg}]\vdots\mathbf{e}_3\mathbf{e}_2\mathbf{e}_1^* M(t,T,\tau)$$

$$\times\{\exp(i(\omega-\bar{\omega}_{eg}-2Q(T))t - i(\omega-\bar{\omega}_{eg})\tau)$$

$$+\exp(i(\omega-\bar{\omega}_{eg})t - i(\omega-\bar{\omega}_{eg})\tau)\}. \tag{7.10}$$

Note that the first term inside the curly bracket of Equation 7.10 originates from the stimulated emission pathway involving excited-state population evolution $\rho_{ee}^{(2)}(T,\tau)$ during T, whereas the second does from the ground-state bleaching pathway involving ground-state evolution $\rho_{gg}^{(2)}(T,\tau)$ during T.

From the photon echo polarization in Equation 7.10, the generated echo field amplitude is

$$\mathbf{E}_{PE}(t,T,\tau) \propto i\mathbf{P}_{PE}(t,T,\tau) \propto [\boldsymbol{\mu}_{ge}\boldsymbol{\mu}_{eg}\boldsymbol{\mu}_{ge}\boldsymbol{\mu}_{eg}]\vdots\mathbf{e}_3\mathbf{e}_2\mathbf{e}_1^* M(t,T,\tau)$$

$$\times\{\exp(i(\omega-\bar{\omega}_{eg}-2Q(T))t - i(\omega-\bar{\omega}_{eg})\tau)$$

$$+\exp(i(\omega-\bar{\omega}_{eg})t - i(\omega-\bar{\omega}_{eg})\tau)\}. \tag{7.11}$$

In general, there are three possibilities of 2D Fourier-transforming the above echo field amplitude by choosing a pair of time variables from τ, T, and t. However, the most popular choice has been to take τ and t variables for the transformation, and the 2D Fourier–Laplace transform of $\mathbf{E}_{PE}(t, T, \tau)$ is defined as

$$\tilde{\mathbf{E}}_{PE}(\bar{\omega}_t,T,\bar{\omega}_\tau) = \int_0^\infty dt\int_0^\infty d\tau\, \mathbf{E}_{PE}(t,T,\tau)\exp(i\bar{\omega}_t t + i\bar{\omega}_\tau\tau). \tag{7.12}$$

Inserting Equation 7.11 into 7.12 and carrying out the integrations, one can obtain the 2D spectrum. For the sake of notational simplicity, let us define two frequencies as

$$\omega_\tau \equiv \omega - \bar{\omega}_\tau$$

$$\omega_t \equiv \omega + \bar{\omega}_t. \tag{7.13}$$

Then, we get

$$\tilde{\mathbf{E}}_{PE}(\omega_t, T, \omega_\tau) = \tilde{\mathbf{E}}_{PE}^{SE}(\omega_t, T, \omega_\tau) + \tilde{\mathbf{E}}_{PE}^{GB}(\omega_t, T, \omega_\tau), \tag{7.14}$$

where

$$\tilde{\mathbf{E}}_{PE}^{SE}(\omega_t, T, \omega_\tau) = \frac{\pi[\boldsymbol{\mu}_{ge}\boldsymbol{\mu}_{eg}\boldsymbol{\mu}_{ge}\boldsymbol{\mu}_{eg}]\vdots\mathbf{e}_3\mathbf{e}_2\mathbf{e}_1}{(\Omega^4 - H^2(T))^{1/2}} \exp(-x^2)$$
$$\times\left\{\exp(-y^2(T)) + \frac{2i}{\sqrt{\pi}} F(y(T))\right\} \tag{7.15}$$

$$\tilde{\mathbf{E}}_{PE}^{GB}(\omega_t, T, \omega_\tau) = \frac{\pi[\boldsymbol{\mu}_{ge}\boldsymbol{\mu}_{eg}\boldsymbol{\mu}_{ge}\boldsymbol{\mu}_{eg}]\vdots\mathbf{e}_3\mathbf{e}_2\mathbf{e}_1}{(\Omega^4 - H^2(T))^{1/2}} \exp(-x^2)$$
$$\times\left\{\exp(-z^2(T)) + \frac{2i}{\sqrt{\pi}} F(z(T))\right\}. \tag{7.16}$$

The Dawson integral, $F(x)$, was defined in Equation 6.9, and the auxiliary functions in Equations 7.15 and 7.16 are defined as

$$x \equiv \frac{\omega_\tau - \bar{\omega}_{eg}}{\sqrt{2\Omega^2}}$$

$$y(T) \equiv \frac{\omega_t - \bar{\omega}_{eg} - 2Q(T) - \frac{H(T)}{\Omega^2}(\omega_\tau - \bar{\omega}_{eg})}{\sqrt{2\left(\Omega^2 - \frac{H^2(T)}{\Omega^2}\right)}}$$

$$z(T) \equiv \frac{\omega_t - \bar{\omega}_{eg} - \frac{H(T)}{\Omega^2}(\omega_\tau - \bar{\omega}_{eg})}{\sqrt{2\left(\Omega^2 - \frac{H^2(T)}{\Omega^2}\right)}}. \tag{7.17}$$

The resultant 2D photon echo spectrum in Equation 7.14 is identical to the 2D pump–probe spectrum in Equation 6.7 if the pulse widths w and $\bar{w}$ are assumed to be zero. Therefore, one can carry out the same line-shape analyses of the 2D photon echo spectrum for a 2LS. Before that, it should be mentioned that from Equations 7.15 and 7.16, the 2D line widths at $T = 0$ approaches zero, which is an unrealistic behavior. This is simply caused by the short-time approximation to the third-order response function as well as by the assumption that the pulses are extremely short. Thus, the above approximate results should be of use only when the three pulses are well separated in time and when the pulses are sufficiently shorter than any other nuclear dynamics affecting changes of the response function. If one is interested in the 2D photon echo spectrum at a very short time where the three pulses are significantly overlapped in time, not only the rephasing diagrams but also the other nonrephasing diagrams are to be included in the numerical simulation and in the interpretation of the experimentally measured signal. Then, the more general expression beyond Equation 7.6 should be used. However, in this chapter we will not present any discussion along this line anymore, because not only is such extension conceptually and numerically complicated but also it does not add much to the general picture on how useful the 2D photon echo method is to understanding various interesting chemical and physical processes of molecular complexes.

From Equation 7.16, it is noted that the ground-state bleaching contribution to the real part of the photon echo, $\mathrm{Re}[\tilde{\mathbf{E}}_{PE}(\omega_t,T,\omega_\tau)]$, appears as a 2D Gaussian function with center frequency at $\omega_\tau = \bar{\omega}_{eg}$ and $\omega_t = \bar{\omega}_{eg}$. On the other hand, the stimulated emission contribution to $\mathrm{Re}[\tilde{\mathbf{E}}_{PE}(\omega_t,T,\omega_\tau)]$, which is also a 2D Gaussian function, peaks at $\omega_\tau = \bar{\omega}_{eg}$ and $\omega_t = \bar{\omega}_{eg} + 2Q(T)$. Due to the spectral diffusion process described by $Q(T)$, the center position of the stimulated emission term shifts in time and asymptotically approaches to $\omega_t = \bar{\omega}_{eg} - 2\lambda/\hbar$ as $T \rightarrow \infty$. If the solvent reorganization energy is sufficiently large, the width of the 2D $\mathrm{Re}[\tilde{\mathbf{E}}_{PE}(\omega_t,T,\omega_\tau)]$ spectrum along the ω_t axis will change in time T, and its increasing pattern is determined by $S(T)$.

At a sufficiently short time T, the rephasing 2D photon echo spectrum $\mathrm{Re} \times [\tilde{\mathbf{E}}_{PE}(\omega_t,T,\omega_\tau)]$ is diagonally elongated due to the short-time inhomogeneity of local environments around chromophores, but as T increases the 2D $\mathrm{Re}[\tilde{\mathrm{E}}_{PE}(\omega_t,T,\omega_\tau)]$ spectrum becomes a symmetric round shape.[28–30] From Equations 7.15 and 7.16, the FWHM along the diagonal is found to be

$$\Delta\omega_{diag}(T) = 2\sqrt{\{\Omega^2 + H(T)\}\ln 2}, \tag{7.18}$$

whereas that along the antidiagonal is

$$\Delta\omega_{anti-diag}(T) = 2\sqrt{\{\Omega^2 - H(T)\}\ln 2}. \tag{7.19}$$

Within the short-time approximation to the frequency-frequency correlation function (FFCF), it was shown that the FWHM of the absorption spectrum is $2\sqrt{\ln 2}\,\Omega$ (see Equation 3.51). Therefore, the diagonal FWHM of the 2D photon echo spectrum is always larger than that of the linear absorption spectrum, whereas the antidiagonal FWHM is smaller than $2\sqrt{\ln 2}\,\Omega$. As T increases, the ratio $\Delta\omega_{diag}(T)/\Delta\omega_{anti-diag}(T)$ becomes approximately linearly proportional to H(T) or $S(T)$ as

$$\frac{\Delta\omega_{diag}(T)}{\Delta\omega_{anti-diag}(T)} \cong 1 + \frac{H(T)}{\Omega^2} \cong 1 + \frac{2S(T)}{\hbar\beta\Omega^2}. \tag{7.20}$$

Thus, the ratio of the diagonal FWHM to the antidiagonal FWHM can be used to determine the FFCF or salvation dynamics function $S(T)$ experimentally.

The imaginary part of the photon echo spectrum, $\mathrm{Im}[\tilde{E}_{PE}(\omega_t, T, \omega_\tau)]$, is related to the transient birefringence spectrum discussed in Chapter 6 for the 2D pump–probe spectroscopy. Typical spectral shape of $\mathrm{Im}[\tilde{E}_{PE}(\omega_t, T, \omega_\tau)]$ is similar to those in Figure 6.2. Then, again the slope of the nodal line, denoted as $\sigma(T)$, is T-dependent and given as

$$\sigma(T) = \frac{H(T)}{\Omega^2} \cong \frac{2S(T)}{\hbar\beta\Omega^2}. \tag{7.21}$$

In the case when there is finite static inhomogeneity reflecting inhomogeneously distributed local environments around optical chromophores, the above results should be slightly modified by performing the following replacements:

$$\Omega^2 \to \Omega^2 + \Sigma^2$$
$$H(T) \to H(T) + \Sigma^2, \tag{7.22}$$

where Σ is the standard deviation of the Gaussian function representing the static inhomogeneous line broadening. Then, the real and imaginary parts of the 2D photon echo spectrum remain to be tilted even for a long time T later. For instance, the asymptotic value of the slope, $\sigma(\tau \to \infty)$, would approach to finite value as $\sigma(\tau \to \infty) = \Sigma^2/(\Omega^2 + \Sigma^2)$.

7.3 TWO-DIMENSIONAL NONREPHASING PHOTON ECHO SPECTRUM OF A TWO-LEVEL SYSTEM

A characteristic feature of the rephasing echo spectrum in two dimensions is that it is diagonally elongated at short time. This shows that the excitation frequency, which is the oscillation frequency of the coherence $\rho_{ge}^{(1)}(t_1)$ during t_1 period, positively correlates with the emission frequency, which is the oscillation frequency of the coherence during t_3 period. Now, let us consider the nonrephasing photon echo experiment, where the radiated signal field in the direction of $\mathbf{k}_1 - \mathbf{k}_2 + \mathbf{k}_3$ is measured.

As shown in Section 5.7, the temporal envelope of the nonrephasing photon echo polarization is given as

$$\mathbf{P}_{NR\text{-}PE}(t,T,\tau) = \left(\frac{i}{\hbar}\right)^3 \int_0^\infty dt_1 \int_0^\infty dt_2 \int_0^\infty dt_3 \{R_1(t_3,t_2,t_1) + R_4(t_3,t_2,t_1)\} \vdots \mathbf{e}_3\mathbf{e}_2^*\mathbf{e}_1 E_3(t-t_3)$$
$$\times E_2^*(t+T-t_3-t_2) E_1(t+\tau+T-t_3-t_2-t_1) \exp\{i\omega t_3 + i\omega t_1\}. \tag{7.23}$$

Here, the two diagrams representing $R_1(t_3, t_2, t_1)$ and $R_4(t_3, t_2, t_1)$ contributions to the polarization are

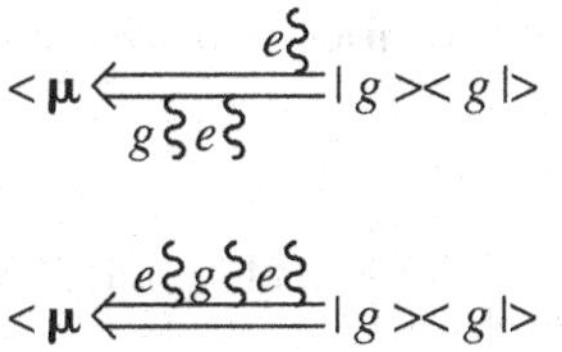

(7.24)

The coherence $\rho_{eg}^{(1)}$ during t_1 time period has the same oscillatory behavior with that during t_3. For the sake of simplicity, let us use the short-time approximate expressions for $R_1(t_3, t_2, t_1)$ and $R_4(t_3, t_2, t_1)$ to rewrite Equation 7.23 as

$$\mathbf{P}_{NR-PE}(t,T,\tau) = -i\hbar^{-3}[\boldsymbol{\mu}_{ge}\boldsymbol{\mu}_{eg}\boldsymbol{\mu}_{ge}\boldsymbol{\mu}_{eg}]\vdots\mathbf{e}_3\mathbf{e}_2^*\mathbf{e}_1\int_0^\infty dt_1\int_0^\infty dt_2\int_0^\infty dt_3\, N(t_3,t_2,t_1)$$

$$\{\exp(i(\omega-\bar{\omega}_{eg}-2Q(t_2))t_3+i(\omega-\bar{\omega}_{eg})t_1)$$

$$+\exp(i(\omega-\bar{\omega}_{eg})t_3+i(\omega-\bar{\omega}_{eg})t_1)\}$$

$$\times E_3(t-t_3)E_2^*(t+T-t_3-t_2)E_1(t+\tau+T-t_3-t_2-t_1), \quad (7.25)$$

where

$$N(t_3,t_2,t_1) \equiv \exp\left\{-\frac{1}{2}\Omega^2t_1^2-\frac{1}{2}\Omega^2t_3^2-H(t_2)t_1t_3\right\}. \quad (7.26)$$

Note that the only difference between the line shape function $N(t_3, t_2, t_1)$ for the nonrephasing photon echo polarization and that for rephasing photon echo polarization, which was denoted as $M(t_3, t_2, t_1)$ in Equation 7.9, is the sign of the term $H(t_2)t_1t_3$ in the exponents. By assuming that the temporal envelopes of the three pulses are sufficiently short, the above integrations in Equation 7.25 can be performed to find

$$\mathbf{P}_{NR-PE}(t,T,\tau) = -i\hbar^{-3}E_3E_2^*E_1[\boldsymbol{\mu}_{ge}\boldsymbol{\mu}_{eg}\boldsymbol{\mu}_{ge}\boldsymbol{\mu}_{eg}]\vdots\mathbf{e}_3\mathbf{e}_2^*\mathbf{e}_1N(t,T,\tau)$$

$$\times\{\exp(i(\omega-\bar{\omega}_{eg}-2Q(T))t+i(\omega-\bar{\omega}_{eg})\tau)$$

$$+\exp(i(\omega-\bar{\omega}_{eg})t+i(\omega-\bar{\omega}_{eg})\tau)\}. \quad (7.27)$$

From the nonrephasing echo polarization, one can show that the signal electric field amplitude is

$$\mathbf{E}_{NR-PE}(t,T,\tau) \propto i\mathbf{P}_{NR-PE}(t,T,\tau) = [\boldsymbol{\mu}_{ge}\boldsymbol{\mu}_{eg}\boldsymbol{\mu}_{ge}\boldsymbol{\mu}_{eg}]\vdots\mathbf{e}_3\mathbf{e}_2^*\mathbf{e}_1N(t,T,\tau)$$

$$\times\{\exp(i(\omega-\bar{\omega}_{eg}-2Q(T))t+i(\omega-\bar{\omega}_{eg})\tau)$$

$$+\exp(i(\omega-\bar{\omega}_{eg})t+i(\omega-\bar{\omega}_{eg})\tau)\}. \quad (7.29)$$

From this, the corresponding 2D Fourier–Laplace transform of $\mathbf{E}_{NR-PE}(t,T,\tau)$, which is defined as

$$\tilde{\mathbf{E}}_{NR-PE}(\bar{\omega}_t,T,\bar{\omega}_\tau) = \int_0^\infty dt\int_0^\infty d\tau\,\mathbf{E}_{NR-PE}(t,T,\tau)\exp(i\bar{\omega}_t t+i\bar{\omega}_\tau\tau),$$

is found to be

$$\tilde{\mathbf{E}}_{NR-PE}(\omega_t, T, \omega_\tau) = \tilde{\mathbf{E}}^{SE}_{NR-PE}(\omega_t, T, \omega_\tau) + \tilde{\mathbf{E}}^{GB}_{NR-PE}(\omega_t, T, \omega_\tau), \tag{7.29}$$

where

$$\tilde{\mathbf{E}}^{SE}_{NR-PE}(\omega_t, T, \omega_\tau) = \frac{\pi[\boldsymbol{\mu}_{ge}\boldsymbol{\mu}_{eg}\boldsymbol{\mu}_{ge}\boldsymbol{\mu}_{eg}]\vdots\mathbf{e}_3\mathbf{e}_2^*\mathbf{e}_1}{(\Omega^4 - H^2(T))^{1/2}}\exp(-x^2)$$
$$\times\left\{\exp\left(-y^2_{NR-PE}(T)\right) + \frac{2i}{\sqrt{\pi}}F(y_{NR-PE}(T))\right\}$$

$$\tilde{\mathbf{E}}^{GB}_{NR-PE}(\omega_t, T, \omega_\tau) = \frac{\pi[\boldsymbol{\mu}_{ge}\boldsymbol{\mu}_{eg}\boldsymbol{\mu}_{ge}\boldsymbol{\mu}_{eg}]\vdots\mathbf{e}_3\mathbf{e}_2^*\mathbf{e}_1}{(\Omega^4 - H^2(T))^{1/2}}\exp(-x^2)$$
$$\times\left\{\exp\left(-z^2_{NR-PE}(T)\right) + \frac{2i}{\sqrt{\pi}}F(z_{NR-PE}(T))\right\}. \tag{7.30}$$

Here, the two frequencies in Equation 7.29 were newly defined as $\omega_\tau \equiv \omega + \bar{\omega}_\tau$ and $\omega_t \equiv \omega + \bar{\omega}_t$. The auxiliary function x was defined in Equation 7.17, and the two other functions $y_{NR-PE}(T)$ and $z_{NR-PE}(T)$ are slightly different from those for the rephasing echo signal, and they are

$$y_{NR-PE}(T) \equiv \frac{\omega_t - \bar{\omega}_{eg} - 2Q(T) + \frac{H(T)}{\Omega^2}(\omega_\tau - \bar{\omega}_{eg})}{\sqrt{2\left(\Omega^2 - \frac{H^2(T)}{\Omega^2}\right)}}$$

$$z_{NR-PE}(T) \equiv \frac{\omega_t - \bar{\omega}_{eg} + \frac{H(T)}{\Omega^2}(\omega_\tau - \bar{\omega}_{eg})}{\sqrt{2\left(\Omega^2 - \frac{H^2(T)}{\Omega^2}\right)}}. \tag{7.31}$$

In order to compare the 2D peak shape of nonrephasing spectrum with that of rephasing photon echo spectrum, the same model 2LS discussed in Section 5.8 and used in the previous chapter is considered. The real and imaginary parts of the rephasing and nonrephasing photon echo spectra are plotted in Figure 7.3. Here, the waiting time T is assumed to be 100 fs. The real and imaginary parts of $\tilde{E}_{PE}(\omega_t, T, \omega_\tau)$, which are in the far right upper and lower panels in Figure 7.3, are diagonally elongated at such a short time. On the other hand, those of the nonrephasing spectrum, $\tilde{E}_{NR-PE}(\omega_t, T, \omega_\tau)$, shown in the middle of the upper and lower panels in Figure 7.3 are antidiagonally elongated. Often, the absorptive 2D spectrum is defined as the sum of the rephasing and nonrephasing photon echo spectra. The real and imaginary parts of the 2D absorptive spectrum ($= \tilde{E}_{PE}(\omega_t, T, \omega_\tau) + \tilde{E}_{NR-PE}(\omega_t, T, \omega_\tau)$) are plotted in Figure 7.3 also. Indeed, regardless of the presence of short-time inhomogeneity, the line shapes are symmetric without any elongations along the diagonal

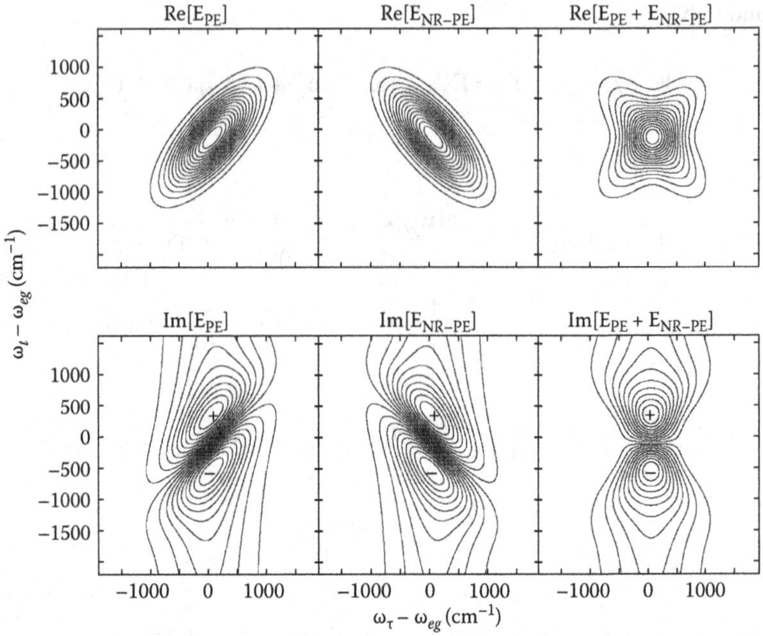

FIGURE 7.3 Real (upper-left two figures) and imaginary (lower-left two figures) parts of the rephasing and nonrephasing echo spetra. The real and imaginary parts of the sum of rephasing and nonrephasing echo spectra are shown in the upper-right and lower-right panels, respetively.

nor antidiagonal directions. From these results, it is possible to draw a conclusion that the information content extracted from the rephasing photon echo spectrum is the same with that from the nonrephasing spectrum within the approximations used in this chapter. Throughout this book, the rephasing photon echo will only be considered and discussed in detail, but in practice the absorptive spectrum, which is given by the sum of the rephasing photon echo and nonrephasing spectra, has been shown to be spectrally narrow and exhibits certain enhancement of frequency resolution. Therefore, one might prefer measuring the purely absorptive 2D spectrum instead of the rephasing photon echo.

7.4 TWO-DIMENSIONAL PHOTON ECHO SPECTRUM OF AN ANHARMONIC OSCILLATOR

When an anharmonic oscillator is under investigation by using the 2D vibrational photon echo method, it was shown that 3LS is a good model for this. In Section 6.3, the 2D pump–probe spectroscopy of an anharmonic oscillator was discussed in detail. In addition to the ground-state bleaching and stimulated emission contributions, the excited state absorption by the first excited state molecules should also be included to fully describe the photon echo phenomenon. In the case of the pump–probe spectroscopy, two different diagrams shown in Equation 6.24 should be included. However, only the first is one of the rephasing diagrams, that is

$$<\mu \xleftarrow[e\xi]{f\xi e\xi} | g><g|>. \tag{7.32}$$

By using the same approximations discussed in Section 6.3, one can find that the photon echo is given as the sum of three terms as

$$\tilde{\mathbf{E}}_{PE}(\omega_t,T,\omega_\tau)=\tilde{\mathbf{E}}_{PE}^{SE}(\omega_t,T,\omega_\tau)+\tilde{\mathbf{E}}_{PE}^{GB}(\omega_t,T,\omega_\tau)+\tilde{\mathbf{E}}_{PE}^{EA}(\omega_t,T,\omega_\tau), \tag{7.33}$$

where the first two terms involving $g \leftrightarrow e$ transitions were already discussed in Equations 7.15 and 7.16. The excited-state absorption contribution to the 2D photon echo spectrum is

$$\begin{aligned}\tilde{\mathbf{E}}_{PE}^{EA}(\omega_t,T,\omega_\tau) &= -\frac{\pi[\boldsymbol{\mu}_{ef}\boldsymbol{\mu}_{fe}\boldsymbol{\mu}_{eg}\boldsymbol{\mu}_{ge}]\vdots\mathbf{e}_3\mathbf{e}_2\mathbf{e}_1^*}{(\Omega^4-H^2(T))^{1/2}}\exp(-x^2)\\ &\times\left\{\exp(-w^2(T))+\frac{2i}{\sqrt{\pi}}F(w(T))\right\}\end{aligned} \tag{7.34}$$

where

$$w(T)\equiv\frac{\omega_t-\bar{\omega}_{fe}-2Q(T)-\frac{H(T)}{\Omega^2}(\omega_\tau-\bar{\omega}_{eg})}{\sqrt{2\left(\Omega^2-\frac{H^2(T)}{\Omega^2}\right)}}. \tag{7.35}$$

Since the ensemble average frequency $\bar{\omega}_{fe}$ is different from $\bar{\omega}_{eg}$ by the overtone anharmonic frequency shift $\delta\omega_{anh}$, as $\bar{\omega}_{fe}=\bar{\omega}_{eg}-\delta\omega_{anh}$, the excited-state absorption term, $\tilde{\mathbf{E}}_{PE}^{EA}(\omega_t,T,\omega_\tau)$, peaks at different position. Furthermore, since the excited-state absorption contribution is negative, there is a nodal line in the region where the SE+GB spectrum overlaps with the EA spectrum.

Now, let us consider the real part of $\tilde{\mathbf{E}}_{PE}(\omega_t,T,\omega_\tau)$ here. When the overtone anharmonicity is very large in comparison with the absorption bandwidth, the 2D spectrum of $\mathrm{Re}[\tilde{\mathbf{E}}_{PE}^{EA}]$ is frequency resolved from that of $\mathrm{Re}[\tilde{\mathbf{E}}_{PE}^{SE}+\tilde{\mathbf{E}}_{PE}^{GB}]$. The peak-to-peak frequency difference in this case would be identical to $\delta\omega_{anh}$. However, for a weakly anharmonic oscillator, where $\delta\omega_{anh}$ is comparable to or smaller than the absorption bandwidth, the frequency difference between the positive and negative peaks along the ω_t-axis is a function of the absorption bandwidth and $\delta\omega_{anh}$. Assuming that $\boldsymbol{\mu}_{fe}=\sqrt{2}\boldsymbol{\mu}_{eg}$ for this weekly anharmonic oscillator, one can find that the slice of the 2D spectrum $(\mathrm{Re}[\tilde{\mathbf{E}}_{PE}(\omega_t,T,\omega_\tau)])$ at $\omega_\tau=\bar{\omega}_{eg}$ can be recast in the form

$$S_{PE}(\omega_t,T,\omega_\tau=\bar{\omega}_{eg})\propto\exp\left(-A(T)\{x-x_1(T)\}^2\right)-\exp\left(-A(T)\{x-x_2(T)\}^2\right) \tag{7.36}$$

where

$$x \equiv \omega_t - \bar{\omega}_{eg}$$

$$x_1(T) \equiv 2Q(T) - \delta\omega_{anh}$$

$$x_2(T) \equiv Q(T)$$

$$A(T) \equiv \frac{1}{2(\Omega^2 - H^2(T)/\Omega^2)}. \qquad (7.37)$$

The two (positive and negative) peak positions can be found by solving the following nonlinear equation for x,

$$\frac{x - x_1(T)}{x - x_2(T)} = \exp\left\{-A(T)\left[2(x_1(T) - x_2(T))x - x_1^2(T) + x_2^2(T)\right]\right\}. \qquad (7.38)$$

In this case, since $|A(T)[2(x_1(T) - x_2(T))x]| << 1$, one can find that the peak-to-peak frequency difference, denoted as $\Delta\omega(T)$, is approximately given as

$$\Delta\omega(T) \cong \sqrt{4(\Omega^2 - H^2(T)/\Omega^2) + Q^2(T)}. \qquad (7.39)$$

As T increases, we have

$$\lim_{T\to\infty} \Delta\omega(T) = \sqrt{4\Omega^2 + (\lambda/\hbar)^2}. \qquad (7.40)$$

The results presented in this section can be used to interpret 2D vibrational spectroscopy of a single anharmonic oscillator.

7.5 SIMPLE TWO-DIMENSIONAL LORENTZIAN PEAK SHAPE

In this and previous chapters, the 2D peak shapes of the pump–probe and photon echo spectra were discussed in detail by using the short-time-approximated third-order response function in Section 5.3. Most of the salient features found in the time-dependent 2D spectral evolutions could be understood and connected to the fluctuating transition FFCF or the corresponding spectral densities. However, as the number of quantum states increases for a coupled multi-chromophore system, the formal expressions for the diagonal and cross-peaks in a given 2D spectrum become quite complicated. Therefore, it will be necessary to simplify the spectral shape of each peak for the sake of notational simplicity. One of the conventional approaches is to invoke Markovian approximation to the FFCFs as discussed in Section 5.2. Then, for a 2LS, the four response function components are simplified as

$$R_1(t_3,t_2,t_1) = \boldsymbol{\mu}_{ge}\boldsymbol{\mu}_{eg}\boldsymbol{\mu}_{ge}\boldsymbol{\mu}_{eg}\exp(-i\bar{\omega}_{eg}t_3 - i\bar{\omega}_{eg}t_1)\exp\{-\gamma_{ee}t_3 - t_2/T_e - \gamma_{ee}t_1\}$$

$$R_2(t_3,t_2,t_1) = \boldsymbol{\mu}_{ge}\boldsymbol{\mu}_{eg}\boldsymbol{\mu}_{ge}\boldsymbol{\mu}_{eg}\exp(-i\bar{\omega}_{eg}t_3 + i\bar{\omega}_{eg}t_1)\exp\{-\gamma_{ee}t_3 - t_2/T_e - \gamma_{ee}t_1\}$$

$$R_3(t_3,t_2,t_1) = \boldsymbol{\mu}_{ge}\boldsymbol{\mu}_{eg}\boldsymbol{\mu}_{ge}\boldsymbol{\mu}_{eg}\exp(-i\bar{\omega}_{eg}t_3 + i\bar{\omega}_{eg}t_1)\exp\{-\gamma_{ee}t_3 - t_2/T_e - \gamma_{ee}t_1\}$$

$$R_4(t_3,t_2,t_1) = \boldsymbol{\mu}_{ge}\boldsymbol{\mu}_{eg}\boldsymbol{\mu}_{ge}\boldsymbol{\mu}_{eg}\exp(-i\bar{\omega}_{eg}t_3 - i\bar{\omega}_{eg}t_1)\exp\{-\gamma_{ee}t_3 - t_2/T_e - \gamma_{ee}t_1\}, \quad (7.41)$$

where γ_{ee} and T_e are the dephasing constant of the *e-g* coherence and the lifetime of the excited state, respectively. Here, it is assumed that the ground-state hole has the same lifetime, which means that the excited-state population can only relax down to the ground state without any intermediate state involved.

Carrying out the 2D Fourier–Laplace transformation of Equation 7.41, one can find that the 2D photon echo spectrum of a 2LS is simply written as

$$\tilde{\mathbf{E}}_{PE}(\omega_t,T,\omega_\tau) = 2[\boldsymbol{\mu}_{ge}\boldsymbol{\mu}_{eg}\boldsymbol{\mu}_{ge}\boldsymbol{\mu}_{eg}]\vdots\mathbf{e}_3\mathbf{e}_2\mathbf{e}_1^* e^{-T/T_e}L(\bar{\omega}_{eg},\gamma_{ee},\bar{\omega}_{eg},\gamma_{ee}), \quad (7.42)$$

where the 2D Lorentzian function $L(y, \gamma_y, x, \gamma_x)$ is defined as

$$L(y,\gamma_y,x,\gamma_x) \equiv \frac{1}{(\omega_t - y + i\gamma_y)(\omega_\tau - x - i\gamma_x)}. \quad (7.43)$$

In Figure 7.4, the real and imaginary parts and the absolute magnitude of the above 2D Lorentzian function are plotted to show their general shapes in 2D frequency domain.

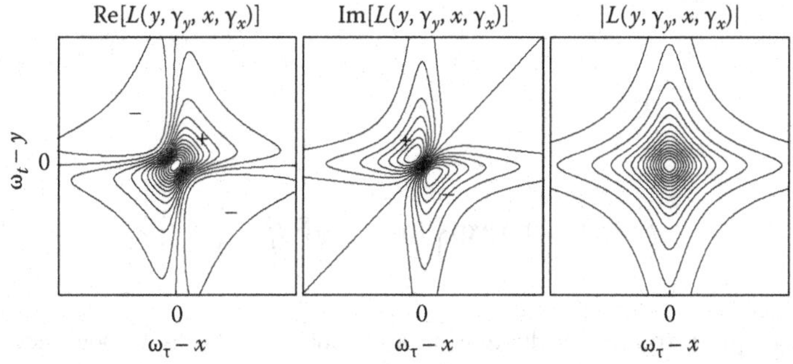

FIGURE 7.4 Typical shapes of the real and imaginary parts and the absolute magntiude of the 2D Lorentzian peak shape function $L(y, \gamma_y, x, \gamma_x)$ defined in Equation 7.43.

For an anharmonic oscillator system, the 2D photon echo spectrum within the 2D Lorentzian shape approximation, is

$$\tilde{\mathbf{E}}_{PE}(\omega_t,T,\omega_\tau)=2[\boldsymbol{\mu}_{ge}\boldsymbol{\mu}_{eg}\boldsymbol{\mu}_{ge}\boldsymbol{\mu}_{eg}]\vdots\mathbf{e}_3\mathbf{e}_2\mathbf{e}_1^*e^{-T/T_e}L(\bar{\omega}_{eg},\gamma_{ee},\bar{\omega}_{eg},\gamma_{ee})$$

$$-[\boldsymbol{\mu}_{ef}\boldsymbol{\mu}_{fe}\boldsymbol{\mu}_{eg}\boldsymbol{\mu}_{ge}]\vdots\mathbf{e}_3\mathbf{e}_2\mathbf{e}_1^*e^{-T/T_e}L(\bar{\omega}_{fe},\gamma_{ff},\bar{\omega}_{eg},\gamma_{ee}). \quad (7.44)$$

7.6 SIMPLE TWO-DIMENSIONAL GAUSSIAN PEAK SHAPE

Quite often the 2D photon echo spectrum appears to be a Gaussian function in 2D frequency domain. Therefore, it will be quite useful to introduce simplified 2D Gaussian peak shape function to approximately describe the shape of 2D photon echo spectrum in many cases. This can be achieved by ignoring the t_2-dependent auxiliary terms in the short-time approximate expressions of the third-order response function components.[30–32] That is to say, the four terms in Equations 5.26 with 5.29 are simplified as

$$R_1(t_3,t_2,t_1)=\sum_{abc}[A_2]_{gc}[A_3]_{cb}[B]_{ba}[A_1]_{ag}\exp\{-i\bar{\omega}_{ab}t_3-i\bar{\omega}_{ac}t_2-i\bar{\omega}_{ag}t_1\}F_1(t_3,t_2,t_1)$$

$$R_2(t_3,t_2,t_1)=\sum_{abc}[A_1]_{gc}[A_3]_{cb}[B]_{ba}[A_2]_{ag}\exp\{-i\bar{\omega}_{ab}t_3-i\bar{\omega}_{ac}t_2-i\bar{\omega}_{gc}t_1\}F_2(t_3,t_2,t_1)$$

$$R_3(t_3,t_2,t_1)=\sum_{abc}[A_1]_{gc}[A_2]_{cb}[B]_{ba}[A_3]_{ag}\exp\{-i\bar{\omega}_{ab}t_3-i\bar{\omega}_{gb}t_2-i\bar{\omega}_{gc}t_1\}F_3(t_3,t_2,t_1)$$

$$R_4(t_3,t_2,t_1)=\sum_{abc}[B]_{gc}[A_3]_{cb}[A_2]_{ba}[A_1]_{ag}\exp\{-i\bar{\omega}_{cg}t_3-i\bar{\omega}_{bg}t_2-i\bar{\omega}_{ag}t_1\}F_4(t_3,t_2,t_1)$$

$$(7.45)$$

where

$$F_j(t_3,t_2,t_1)=\exp\left\{f_j(t_2)-\frac{1}{2}\delta_j^2t_1^2-\frac{1}{2}\Delta_j^2t_3^2\right\}. \quad (7.46)$$

The mean square frequency fluctuation amplitudes of the first coherence during t_1 and of that during t_3 are denoted as δ_j^2 and Δ_j^2, respectively. When the system is on yet another coherence during t_2, the corresponding response function component oscillates in time t_2. This appears as quantum beats in the transient grating, photon echo, or other four-wave-mixing spectroscopy probing the system evolution during the t_2 period. The decay of the quantum beat is in that case determined by $\exp\{f_j(t_2)\}$, which is a decaying function. From the results in Section 5.3, ignoring the contributions from the spectral diffusion $Q_j(t_2)$ and correlation $H_j(t_2)$, we get

$$f_1(t_2) = -g_{cc}^*(t_2) - g_{aa}(t_2) + 2\,\mathrm{Re}[g_{ca}(t_2)]$$

$$f_2(t_2) = f_1(t_2) = -g_{cc}^*(t_2) - g_{aa}(t_2) + 2\,\mathrm{Re}[g_{ca}(t_2)]$$

$$f_3(t_2) = -g_{bb}^*(t_2)$$

$$f_4(t_2) = -g_{bb}(t_2).$$

$$\delta_1^2 = C_{ca}(0)$$

$$\delta_2^2 = C_{ca}(0)$$

$$\delta_3^2 = C_{cc}(0) - C_{cb}(0)$$

$$\delta_4^2 = C_{aa}(0) - C_{ba}(0).$$

$$\Delta_1^2 = C_{bb}(0) - C_{cb}(0) - C_{ba}(0) + C_{ca}(0)$$

$$\Delta_2^2 = C_{bb}(0) + C_{ca}(0) - C_{cb}(0) - C_{ba}(0)$$

$$\Delta_3^2 = C_{aa}(0) - C_{ba}(0)$$

$$\Delta_4^2 = C_{cc}(0) - C_{cb}(0). \tag{7.47}$$

As an example, let us consider the 2D photon echo of a 2LS. Ignoring the spectral diffusion process, one can find that the 2D photon echo spectrum can be recast in a 2D Gaussian form as

$$\tilde{\mathbf{E}}_{PE}(\omega_t, T, \omega_\tau) = 2[\boldsymbol{\mu}_{ge}\boldsymbol{\mu}_{eg}\boldsymbol{\mu}_{ge}\boldsymbol{\mu}_{eg}]\vdots\mathbf{e}_3\mathbf{e}_2\mathbf{e}_1^*\Gamma(\bar{\omega}_{eg}, \Omega^2, \bar{\omega}_{eg}, \Omega^2). \tag{7.48}$$

Here, $\Gamma(y, \sigma_y^2, x, \sigma_x^2)$ is the 2D Fourier–Laplace transform of the 2D Gaussian function in time domain, and it is defined

$$\Gamma\left(y, \sigma_y^2, x, \sigma_x^2\right) = \frac{\pi}{\sigma_y \sigma_x} \exp\left(-\frac{(\omega_\tau - x)^2}{2\sigma_x^2}\right)\left\{\exp\left(-\frac{(\omega_t - y)^2}{2\sigma_y^2}\right) + \frac{2i}{\sqrt{\pi}} F\left(\frac{\omega_t - y}{\sqrt{2}\sigma_y}\right)\right\}. \tag{7.49}$$

The real part of the photon echo spectrum is a single 2D Gaussian function, whereas the imaginary part shows dispersive shape determined by the Dawson's integral.

For an anharmonic oscillator system, the 2D photon echo spectrum contains the excited-state absorption contribution so that we get

$$\tilde{\mathbf{E}}_{PE}(\omega_t, T, \omega_\tau) = 2[\boldsymbol{\mu}_{ge}\boldsymbol{\mu}_{eg}\boldsymbol{\mu}_{ge}\boldsymbol{\mu}_{eg}] \vdots \mathbf{e}_3\mathbf{e}_2\mathbf{e}_1^* \Gamma(\bar{\omega}_{eg}, \Omega^2, \bar{\omega}_{eg}, \Omega^2)$$
$$-[\boldsymbol{\mu}_{ef}\boldsymbol{\mu}_{fe}\boldsymbol{\mu}_{eg}\boldsymbol{\mu}_{ge}] \vdots \mathbf{e}_3\mathbf{e}_2\mathbf{e}_1^* \Gamma(\bar{\omega}_{fe}, \Omega^2, \bar{\omega}_{eg}, \Omega^2). \quad (7.50)$$

The real part of the photon echo spectrum in this case exhibits two frequency-resolved 2D Gaussian peaks. The positive peak originating from the $g \leftrightarrow e$ transitions is determined by the first term in Equation 7.50. The negative peak originating from the excited-state absorption is represented by the second term. Due to the overtone anharmonic frequency shift, we have $\bar{\omega}_{fe} \neq \bar{\omega}_{eg}$, and the two peaks are separated in the ω_t frequency domain.

In this and previous sections, we presented two popular models for the shape of 2D spectrum, that is, 2D Lorentzian or Gaussian forms. However, in reality the real 2D spectrum shows a bit more complicated features. At the absorption maximum, the 2D spectrum is well fitted to a 2D Gaussian function, but the tail parts of the spectrum appear to be Lorentzian. Thus, one can develop a theoretical model that is an extension of the Voigh profile in 1D spectrum. However, we shall not explore any further extension along this line because the general expressions for the nonlinear response function were already presented before in this book and they are quite general enough to cover the Gaussian to Lorentzian limits. Instead, throughout this book, the simplified 2D Gaussian peak shape function $\Gamma(y, \sigma_y^2, x, \sigma_x^2)$ will be used except for the cases when one needs to analyze detailed 2D peak shapes of experimentally measured spectrum, which was found to significantly deviate from a 2D Gaussian form.

REFERENCES

1. Hahn, E. L., Spin echoes. *Physical Review* 1950, 80, 580–594.
2. Ernst, R. R.; Bodenhausen, G.; Wokaun, A., *Nuclear magnetic resonance in one and two dimensions*. Oxford University Press: Oxford, 1987.
3. Warren, W. S.; Zewail, A. H., Optical analogs of NMR phase coherent multiple pulse spectroscopy. *Journal of Chemical Physics* 1981, 75, 5956–5958.
4. Zanni, M. T.; Hochstrasser, R. M., Two-dimensional infrared spectroscopy: A promising new method for the time resolution of structures. *Current Opinion in Structural Biology* 2001, 11, 516–522.
5. Fleming, G. R.; Cho, M., Chromophore-solvent dynamics. *Annual Review of Physical Chemistry* 1996, 47, 109–134.
6. Mukamel, S., *Principles of nonlinear optical spectroscopy*. Oxford University Press: Oxford, 1995.
7. Cho, M.; Yu, J.-Y.; Joo, T.; Nagasawa, Y.; Passino, S. A.; Fleming, G. R., The Integrated photon echo and solvation dynamics. *Journal of Physical Chemsitry* 1996, 100, 11944–11953.
8. de Boeij, W. P.; Pshenichnikov, M. S.; Wiersma, D. A., Ultrafast solvation dynamics explored by femtosecond photon echo spectroscopies. *Annual Review of Physical Chemistry* 1998, 49, 99–123.

9. Weiner, A. M.; Desilvestri, S.; Ippen, E. P., Three-pulse scattering for femtosecond dephasing studies: Theory and experiment. *Journal of the Optical Society of America B-Optical Physics* 1985, 2, 654–662.
10. Joo, T. H.; Jia, Y. W.; Yu, J. Y.; Lang, M. J.; Fleming, G. R., Third-order nonlinear time domain probes of solvation dynamics. *Journal of Chemical Physics* 1996, 104, 6089–6108.
11. de Boeij, W.; Pshenichnikov, M. S.; Wiersma, D. A., On the relation between the echo peak shift and Brownian oscillator correlation function. *Chemical Physics Letters* 1996, 253, 53–60.
12. Cho, M., Nonlinear response functions for the three-dimensional spectroscopies. *Journal of Chemical Physics* 2001, 115, 4424.
13. Vohringer, P.; Arnett, D. C.; Yang, T. S.; Scherer, N. F., Time-gated photon-echo spectroscopy in liquids. *Chemical Physics Letters* 1995, 237, 387–398.
14. Vohringer, P.; Arnett, D. C.; Westervelt, R. A.; Feldstein, M. J.; Scherer, N. F., Optical dephasing on femtosecond time scales: Direct measurement and calculation from solvent spectral densities. *Journal of Chemical Physics* 1995, 102, 4027–4036.
15. deBoeij, W. P.; Pshenichnikov, M. S.; Wiersma, D. A., Mode suppression in the non-Markovian limit by time-gated stimulated photon echo. *Journal of Chemical Physics* 1996, 105, 2953–2960.
16. de Boeij, W. P.; Pshenichnikov, M. S.; Wiersma, D. A., System–bath correlation function probed by conventional and time-gated stimulated photon echo. *Journal of Physical Chemistry* 1996, 100, 11806–11823.
17. Lepetit, L.; Cheriaux, G.; Joffre, M., Linear techniques of phase measurement by femtosecond spectral interferometry for applications in spectroscopy. *Journal of the Optical Society of America B-Optical Physics* 1995, 12, 2467–2474.
18. Lepetit, L.; Joffre, M., Two-dimensional nonlinear optics using Fourier-transform spectral interferometry. *Optics Letters* 1996, 21, 564–566.
19. Likforman, J. P.; Joffre, M.; Thierry-Mieg, V., Measurement of photon echoes by use of femtosecond Fourier-transform spectral interferometry. *Optics Letters* 1997, 22, 1104–1106.
20. Segonds, P.; Canioni, L.; LeBoiteux, S.; Joffre, M.; Bousquet, B.; Li, W.; Sarger, L., Femtosecond interferometry and photon echo: Steady state and transient processes in spectroscopy. *Journal of Luminescence* 1997, 72–4, 849–850.
21. Asplund, M. C.; Zanni, M. T.; Hochstrasser, R. M., Two-dimensional infrared spectroscopy of peptides by phase-controlled femtosecond vibrational photon echoes. *Proceedings of the National Academy of Sciences of the USA* 2000, 97, 8219–8224.
22. Gallagher, S. M.; Albrecht, A. W.; Hybl, T. D.; Landin, B. L.; Rajaram, B.; Jonas, D. M., Heterodyne detection of the complete electric field of femtosecond four-wave mixing signals. *Journal of the Optical Society of America. B, Optical Physics* 1998, 15, 2338–2345.
23. Hybl, J. D.; Albrecht, A. W.; Gallagher Faeder, S. M.; Jonas, D. M., Two-dimensional electronic spectroscopy. *Chemical Physics Letters* 1998, 297, 307–313.
24. Brixner, T.; Stiopkin, I. V.; Fleming, G. R., Tunable two-dimensional femtosecond spectroscopy. *Optics Letters* 2004, 29, 884–886.
25. Brixner, T.; Mancal, T.; Stiopkin, I. V.; Fleming, G. R., Phase-stabilized two-dimensional electronic spectroscopy. *Journal of Chemical Physics* 2004, 121, 4221–4236.
26. Tian, P.; Keusters, D.; Suzaki, Y.; Warren, W. S., Femtosecond phase-coherent two-dimensional spectroscopy. *Science* 2003, 300, 1553–1555.
27. Jonas, D. M., Optical analogs of 2D NMR. *Science* 2003, 300, 1515–1517.

28. Tokmakoff, A., Two-dimensional line shapes derived from coherent third-order nonlinear spectroscopy. *Journal of Physical Chemistry A* 2000, 104, 4247–4255.
29. Cho, M.; Brixner, T.; Stiopkin, I.; Vaswani, H.; Fleming, G. R., Two dimensional electronic spectroscopy of molecular complexes. *Journal of the Chinese Chemical Society* 2006, 53, 15–24.
30. Cho, M., Coherent two-dimensional optical spectroscopy. *Chemical Reviews* 2008, 108, 1331–1418.
31. Kwac, K.; Cho, M., Two-color pump–probe spectroscopies of two- and three-level systems: 2-dimensional line shapes and solvation dynamics. *Journal of Physical Chemistry A* 2003, 107, 5903–5912.
32. Cho, M.; Vaswani, H. M.; Brixner, T.; Stenger, J.; Fleming, G. R., Exciton analysis in 2D electronic spectroscopy. *Journal of Physical Chemistry B* 2005, 109, 10542–10556.

8 Coupled Multi-Chromophore System

The linear spectroscopic signal is fully characterized by the associated linear response function and provides information on optical transition frequencies, transition amplitudes such as dipole strength, light-scattering cross-section, and so forth, as well as chromophore–bath interaction-induced line broadenings. If two different chromophores are spatially close to each other, quantum states of the two chromophores cannot be written as simple product states and become delocalized over the two chromophores due to finite couplings. Such coupling-induced effects, such as mode mixing, excitation transfer processes and so forth are however quite weak so that their signatures and characteristc features in a typical 1D spectrum are often completely hidden under the primary spectroscopy properties.[1] As demonstrated over the last decade, this spectral congestion and masking problem can be partly overcome by using 2D spectroscopic methods.

In Chapters 6 and 7, theoretical descriptions of 2D spectroscopy for 2LS and 3LS were presented and discussed in detail. It was shown that solvation dynamics as well as homogeneous and inhomogeneous line-broadening processes could be studied by analyzing the 2D peak shape of time-dependent pump–probe or photon echo spectra.[2,3] However, the more interesting case would involve those coupled multi-chromophore systems. When N two- or three-level chromophores are spatially close to each other due to intermolecular or covalent bonding interaction, they are electronically coupled to one another.[4] Then, the excited states can be delocalized over a number of chromophores, depending on the relevant coupling strengths, and the corresponding 2D spectrum could exhibit multiple peaks along the diagonal as well as on the off-diagonal region.[1, 5–7] These diagonal peaks and off-diagonal cross-peaks reveal critical information on the inter-chromophore coupling strengths, excitation transfers, coherence-to-coherence transfers, chemical reaction and exchange rates, and so forth.[1]

As an example, consider photosynthetic light-harvesting complexes consisting of tens to hundreds of chlorophylls.[8] The constituent chlorophylls are electronically coupled to one another to form spatially delocalized excitons when they are optically excited. Such delocalizations of excited states could improve light-absorption efficiency over a wide range of frequencies. In addition, high quantum yield and ultrafast energy transfer processes within the complex could occur, and such excitation migration happens between two different excitonic states after its photo-excitation by sunlight photons.[9] The 2D photon echo spectrum as a function of waiting time T thus provides direct information on the exciton state-to-state population transfers as well as coherence transfers.[10, 11]

Another important example of the coupled multi-chromophore system involves the amide I vibrations in polypeptides and proteins.[12, 13] Amide I vibration is relatively localized carbonyl stretching mode in a single peptide bond.[14] However, such amide I oscillators are coupled to one another via electrostatic interactions such as transition dipole-dipole coupling and hydrogen bonds.[14–16] Consequently, amide I normal modes are formed in polypeptides and proteins. Therefore, the amide I vibrational excitations of protein should be treated in terms of delocalized states. The cross-peaks in the 2D IR spectrum thus reveal the electrical and mechanical couplings between two modes. Therefore, it is necessary to develop an appropriate model for such coupled multi-chromophore systems to quantitatively describe a variety of interesting observed 2D spectroscopic features. Among many different theoretical models, the Frenkel Hamiltonian has been considered to be the most useful, conceptually simple, and easy to apply to many seemingly unrelated problems.[4] In this chapter, the delocalized state representation of the excited states for the coupled multi-chromophore system will be presented and discussed.[17] The multi-chromophore system based on the Frenkel Hamiltonian can be considered to be the standard and reference model for future theoretical development on molecular complexes, but it shouldn't be the only one for describing 2D optical spectroscopic results.

The main purpose of the present chapter is to provide a systematic theory on the optical and vibrational properties of coupled multi-chromophore systems. In the following chapters, we will discuss 2D vibrational and electronic spectroscopy of rather simple systems like coupled 2LS dimer and coupled anharmonic oscillators. Thus, those who are not interested in the generalized description of arbitrary multi-chromophore system can skip this chapter. Note that the discussions in the following chapters, from Chapter 9 on, do not heavily rely on detailed knowledge on the multi-chromophore system.

8.1 FRENKEL HAMILTONIAN IN SITE REPRESENTATION

In order to describe a variety of nonlinear optical properties of molecular complexes and aggregates, the Frenkel exciton theory will be discussed in this section. Denoting as $a_m^\dagger$ and a_m the creation and annihilation operators of an electronic excitation at the mth two-level chromophore, the zero-order Hamiltonian can be written as

$$H_0 = \sum_{m=1}^{N} \hbar\omega_m a_m^\dagger a_m + \sum_{m}^{N}\sum_{n\neq m}^{N} \hbar J_{mn} a_m^\dagger a_n + H_B, \tag{8.1}$$

where the excited-state energy of the mth chromophore, the electronic coupling constant between the mth and nth chromophores, and the bath Hamiltonian were denoted as $\hbar\omega_m$, J_{mn}, and H_B, respectively (see Figure 8.1). If each monomeric chromophore is an anharmonic oscillator instead of a two-electronic-level system, the zero-order Hamiltonian should be written as

$$H_0 = \sum_{m=1}^{N} \hbar\omega_m a_m^\dagger a_m + \sum_{m}^{N}\sum_{n\neq m}^{N} \hbar J_{mn} a_m^\dagger a_n - \sum_{m}^{N}\sum_{n}^{N} \hbar\Delta_{mn} a_m^\dagger a_n^\dagger a_m a_n + H_B \tag{8.2}$$

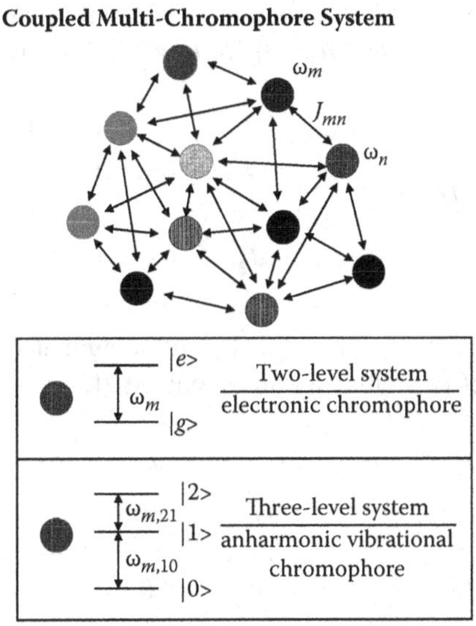

FIGURE 8.1 Schematic representation of coupled multi-chromophore system. The *m*th chromophore excitation frequency (site energy) is denoted as ω_m ($\hbar\,\omega_m$), and the coupling constant between the *m*th and *n*th chromophore transitions is denoted as J_{mn}. Each circle in this schematic figure represents a single chromophore that can be modeled as either a 2LS or a 3LS.

Note that the third term on the right-hand side of Equation 8.2 describes potential anharmonic frequency shifts.

The chromophore–bath interactions and the changes of inter-chromophore distance and orientation induce fluctuations of site energies and coupling constants. Thus, the general system–bath interaction Hamiltonian is written as

$$H_{SB} = \sum_m \sum_n \hbar x_{mn}(\mathbf{q}) a_m^\dagger a_n \tag{8.3}$$

where $x_{mn}(\mathbf{q})$ is an operator of bath coordinates, $\mathbf{q}$, and it is assumed that their average values with respect to the bath Hamiltonian describing thermal equilibrium at temperature T, $\langle x_{mn}(\mathbf{q})\rangle_B$, are zero (note that if $\langle x_{mn}(\mathbf{q})\rangle_B$ values are finite they can be included in the zero-order Hamiltonian). The q-dependence of $x_{mn}(\mathbf{q})$ for $m \neq n$ can vary the strength of the excitation-transfer coupling. The total matter Hamiltonian can therefore be written as

$$H = H_0 + H_{SB} + H_B. \tag{8.4}$$

For any general four-wave-mixing spectroscopy, it is necessary to consider three well-separated manifolds of quantum states: the ground state |0>, N singly excited states, and $N(N \mp 1)/2$ doubly excited states (note that the upper (lower) sign in $N(N \mp 1)/2$ corresponds to the case when the chromophore is modeled as a 2LS

(3LS)). From the zero-order Hamiltonian, the Hamiltonian matrix of the singly excited states with the basis set $\{a_m^+|0>\}$ for $m = 1 \sim N$ is given as

$$\tilde{H}_0^{(1)} = \begin{bmatrix} \varepsilon_1 & J_{12} & \cdots & J_{1N} \\ J_{12} & \varepsilon_2 & \cdots & J_{2N} \\ \vdots & \vdots & \ddots & \vdots \\ J_{1N} & J_{2N} & \cdots & \varepsilon_N \end{bmatrix}, \tag{8.5}$$

where it was assumed that $J_{mn} = J_{nm}$. The Hamiltonian matrix of the doubly excited states with the basis set $\{a_m^+ a_n^+|0>\}$ for an N coupled 2LS is

$$\tilde{H}_0^{(2)} = \begin{bmatrix} \varepsilon_1+\varepsilon_2 & J_{23} & \cdots & J_{2N} & J_{13} & \cdots & 0 \\ J_{23} & \varepsilon_1+\varepsilon_3 & \cdots & J_{3N} & J_{12} & \cdots & 0 \\ \vdots & \vdots & \ddots & \vdots & \vdots & \cdots & \vdots \\ J_{2N} & J_{3N} & \cdots & \varepsilon_1+\varepsilon_N & 0 & \cdots & J_{1(N-1)} \\ J_{13} & J_{12} & \cdots & 0 & \varepsilon_2+\varepsilon_3 & \cdots & 0 \\ \vdots & \vdots & \vdots & \vdots & \vdots & \ddots & \vdots \\ 0 & 0 & \cdots & J_{1(N-1)} & 0 & \cdots & \varepsilon_{N-1}+\varepsilon_N \end{bmatrix}. \tag{8.6}$$

In the case of the N coupled anharmonic oscillator system, the Hamiltonian matrix of the doubly excited states is slightly different from Equation 8.6 due to the presence of overtone states.

8.2 DELOCALIZED EXCITON REPRESENTATION

In order to obtain the eigenvalues and eigenvectors of delocalized singly and doubly excited states, one should perform diagonalizations of the $\tilde{H}_0^{(1)}$- and $\tilde{H}_0^{(2)}$-matrices in Equations 8.5 and 8.6 as

$$U^{-1}\tilde{H}_0^{(1)}U = \hbar\tilde{\Omega} \tag{8.7}$$

$$V^{-1}\tilde{H}_0^{(2)}V = \hbar\tilde{W}, \tag{8.8}$$

where the singly and doubly excited-state eigenvalues are the diagonal matrix elements of $\hbar\tilde{\Omega}$ and $\hbar\tilde{W}$, respectively. The corresponding eigenfunctions are linear combinations of singly and doubly excited-state wavefunctions as

$$|e_j> = \sum_m U_{jm}^{-1}|m> \tag{8.9}$$

$$|f_k> = \sum_{m=1}^{N-1}\sum_{n=m+1}^{N} v_{mn}^{(k)}|m,n>, \tag{8.10}$$

where $|m> = a_m^+|0>$ and $|m,n> = a_m^+ a_n^+|0>$ are the basis states. The eigenvector elements of the jth singly excited state e_j and of the kth doubly excited state f_k are denoted as U_{jm}^{-1} and $v_{mn}^{(k)}$, respectively. The matrix elements of $v^{(k)}$ correspond to the elements of the kth row of the matrix V^{-1}.

The system–bath interaction Hamiltonian matrices $H_{SB}^{(1)}$ and $H_{SB}^{(2)}$ in the site representation are

$$[\tilde{H}_{SB}^{(1)}(\mathbf{q})]_{mn} = \hbar x_{mn}(\mathbf{q}) \tag{8.11}$$

$$\tilde{H}_{SB}^{(2)}(\mathbf{q}) = \hbar \begin{bmatrix} x_{11}+x_{22} & x_{23} & \cdots & x_{2N} & x_{13} & \cdots & 0 \\ J_{23} & x_{11}+x_{33} & \cdots & x_{3N} & x_{12} & \cdots & 0 \\ \vdots & \vdots & \ddots & \vdots & \vdots & \cdots & \vdots \\ x_{2N} & x_{3N} & \cdots & x_{11}+x_{NN} & 0 & \cdots & x_{1(N-1)} \\ x_{13} & x_{12} & \cdots & 0 & x_{22}+x_{33} & \cdots & 0 \\ \vdots & \vdots & \vdots & \vdots & \vdots & \ddots & \vdots \\ 0 & 0 & \cdots & x_{1(N-1)} & 0 & \cdots & x_{(N-1)(N-1)}+x_{NN} \end{bmatrix}. \tag{8.12}$$

In the delocalized state representation, they are to be transformed as

$$\hbar\tilde{\Xi}_{SB}^{(1)}(\mathbf{q}) = U^{-1}\tilde{H}_{SB}^{(1)}(\mathbf{q})U \tag{8.13}$$

$$\hbar\tilde{\Xi}_{SB}^{(2)}(\mathbf{q}) = V^{-1}\tilde{H}_{SB}^{(2)}(\mathbf{q})V. \tag{8.14}$$

The diagonal matrix elements, $[\tilde{\Xi}_{SB}^{(1)}(\mathbf{q})]_{jj}$ and $[\tilde{\Xi}_{SB}^{(2)}(\mathbf{q})]_{kk}$, describe the energy fluctuations induced by the chromophore-bath interactions of the jth singly excited and the kth doubly excited states, respectively. The off-diagonal matrix elements of $\tilde{\Xi}_{SB}^{(1)}(\mathbf{q})$ and $\tilde{\Xi}_{SB}^{(2)}(\mathbf{q})$ are then responsible for excitation transfers within the singly and doubly excited-state manifolds, respectively.

8.3 DELOCALIZED STATE ENERGY AND TRANSITION DIPOLE MATRIX ELEMENT

From the diagonalization of the $\tilde{H}_0^{(1)}$ matrix and the transformed system–bath interaction Hamiltonian $\tilde{\Xi}_{SB}^{(1)}(\mathbf{Q})$, one can find that the energy of the jth singly excited state including the chromophore-bath interaction potential is given as

$$\hbar\Omega_j(\mathbf{q}) = \hbar\tilde{\Omega}_{jj} + \hbar\left[\tilde{\Xi}_{SB}^{(1)}(\mathbf{q})\right]_{jj} = \hbar\tilde{\Omega}_{jj} + \hbar\sum_m\sum_n U_{jm}^{-1} x_{mn}(\mathbf{q}) U_{nj}. \tag{8.15}$$

Usually, the fluctuation amplitudes of the coupling constants, x_{mn} (for $m \neq n$), are smaller than the fluctuation amplitudes of site energies (diagonal elements), that is,

$$< x_{mm}^2 >_B \gg < x_{np}^2 >_B \text{ for all } m, n, \text{ and } p, \text{ and } n \neq p. \tag{8.16}$$

Therefore, making use of the orthogonality of the transformation, one can simplify Equation 8.15 as

$$\hbar\Omega_j(\mathbf{q}) \cong \hbar\tilde{\Omega}_{jj} + \hbar\sum_m U_{mj}^2 x_{mm}(\mathbf{q}). \tag{8.17}$$

Fluctuations of the jth singly excited-state energy are induced by the second term in Equation 8.17, which is determined by the square of eigenvector elements and the interaction between each chromophore and bath degrees of freedom. If site-state $|m\rangle$ does not contribute to exciton state $|j\rangle$, fluctuation in the site energy ε_m does not affect the exciton energy $\hbar\Omega_j$.

Similarly, the kth doubly excited-state energy including the chromophore-bath interaction potential is written as

$$\hbar W_k(\mathbf{q}) = \hbar\tilde{W}_{kk} + \hbar\left[\tilde{\Xi}_{SB}^{(2)}(\mathbf{q})\right]_{kk} = \hbar\tilde{W}_{kk} + \hbar\sum_m\sum_n V_{jm}^{-1}\left[\tilde{H}_{SB}^{(2)}(\mathbf{q})\right]_{mn} V_{nj}$$

$$\cong \hbar\tilde{W}_{kk} + \hbar\sum_{m=1}^{N-1}\sum_{n=m+1}^{N}\left(v_{mn}^{(k)}\right)^2\{x_{mm}(\mathbf{q}) + x_{nn}(\mathbf{q})\}. \tag{8.18}$$

The site energy fluctuation of the mth chromophore, which is described by the $\hbar x_{mm}(\mathbf{q})$ operator, modulates both the singly and doubly excited-state energies. The relative weighting factors are again determined by the associated eigenvector elements $v_{mn}^{(k)}$. From Equations 8.17 and 8.18, one can deduce the fact that the fluctuation of the jth singly excited-state transition frequency is intrinsically correlated with the fluctuations of other singly or doubly excited-state transition frequencies. Because of this instantaneous correlation resulting from the electronic couplings, the 2D photon echo spectrum of coupled multi-chromophore system can exhibit cross-peaks even at very short waiting time T (see Chapter 9 for a more detailed discussion on this point).

Once the eigenvectors of the singly and doubly excited states are determined, the transition dipole matrix elements can be expressed as linear combinations of transition dipoles of constituent chromophores, that is,

$$\boldsymbol{\mu}_{e_j g} \equiv \langle e_j|\boldsymbol{\mu}|g\rangle = \sum_m U_{jm}^{-1}\mathbf{d}_m \tag{8.19}$$

$$\boldsymbol{\mu}_{f_k e_j} = \langle f_k|\boldsymbol{\mu}|e_j\rangle = \sum_{m=1}^{N-1}\sum_{n=m+1}^{N} v_{mn}^{(k)}(U_{jn}^{-1}\mathbf{d}_m + U_{jm}^{-1}\mathbf{d}_n)$$

(coupled two-level systems) (8.20)

$$\boldsymbol{\mu}_{f_k e_j} = \sum_{m=1}^{N}\sum_{n=m}^{N} v_{m,n}^{(k)}\left\{(U_{j,m}^{-1}\mathbf{d}_n + U_{j,n}^{-1}\mathbf{d}_m)(1-\delta_{mn}) + \sqrt{2}U_{j,m}^{-1}\mathbf{d}_m\delta_{mn}\right\}$$

(coupled anharmonic oscillator systems) (8.21)

where $\mathbf{d}_m$ is the transition dipole vector of the mth chromophore, that is, $\mathbf{d}_m \equiv \langle 0 | a_m \boldsymbol{\mu} | 0 \rangle$. The transition dipole matrix elements in Equations 8.19–8.21 can be used to calculate various 2D spectroscopic response functions of coupled multi-chromophore systems.

8.4 TRANSITION FREQUENCY–FREQUENCY CORRELATION FUNCTIONS

For the multilevel system considered here, both the auto- and cross-correlation functions of the singly and doubly excited-state transition frequencies are required to calculate the nonlinear response functions associated with various 2D spectroscopic methods. Using the approximate expressions (Equation 8.17) for the singly excited-state energies, one can obtain the time-correlation between any given pair of singly excited-state transition frequencies as

$$< \delta\Omega_j(t)\delta\Omega_k(0) >_B = \sum_m \sum_n U_{mj}^2 U_{nk}^2 < x_{mm}(t) x_{nn}(0) >_B, \tag{8.22}$$

where $\delta\Omega_j(\mathbf{q}) = \Omega_j(\mathbf{q}) - \tilde{\Omega}_{jj}$ and $\delta\Omega_j(t) = \exp(iH_B t/\hbar)\delta\Omega_j(\mathbf{q})\exp(-iH_B t/\hbar)$. If the transition frequency fluctuation of the mth chromophore is assumed to be statistically uncorrelated with that of the nth chromophore, the following approximation (IBA: Independent Bath Approximation) can be used to greatly simplify the theoretical derivation of the nonlinear response function,[17]

$$< x_{mm}(t) x_{nn}(0) >_B = \delta_{mn} < x_{mm}(t) x_{mm}(0) >_B . \tag{8.23}$$

Then, Equation 8.22 is simplified as

$$< \delta\Omega_j(t)\delta\Omega_k(0) >_B = \sum_m U_{mj}^2 U_{mk}^2 < x_{mm}(t) x_{mm}(0) >_B = \sum_m U_{mj}^2 U_{mk}^2 C_m(t). \tag{8.24}$$

Further assuming that the site energy fluctuation correlation functions $< x_{mm}(t)\, x_{mm}(0) >_B$ are all identical (HBA: Homogeneous Bath Approximation), we have

$$< x_{mm}(t) x_{mm}(0) >_B = C_m(t) = C(t) \quad \text{(for all } m\text{)}. \tag{8.25}$$

The single chromophore transition FFCF $C(t)$ can be expressed in terms of the spectral density as discussed in Chapter 3. Nevertheless, it should be mentioned that the two approximations IBA and HBA given in Equations 8.23 and 8.25 are not always necessary to ultimately calculate the nonlinear response function.

By using these IBA and HBA approximations, Equation 8.24 is further simplified as

$$< \delta\Omega_j(t)\delta\Omega_k(0) >_B = \left(\sum_m U_{mj}^2 U_{mk}^2 \right) C(t). \tag{8.26}$$

Next, the correlation functions between a pair doubly excited-state transition frequencies are found to be

$$<\delta W_j(t)\delta W_k(0)>_B = \sum_{m=1}^{N-1}\sum_{n=m+1}^{N}\sum_{r=1}^{N-1}\sum_{s=r+1}^{N}\left(v_{mn}^{(j)}\right)^2\left(v_{rs}^{(k)}\right)^2\langle\{x_{mm}(t)+x_{nn}(t)\}\{x_{rr}(0)+x_{ss}(0)\}\rangle_B$$

$$\cong\left(\sum_{m=1}^{N-1}\sum_{n=m+1}^{N}\left(v_{mn}^{(j)}\right)^2\{P_m^{(k)}+P_n^{(k)}\}\right)C(t), \tag{8.27}$$

where the second equality was obtained by invoking the two approximations, IBA and HBA, and

$$P_m^{(k)} \equiv \sum_{j=1}^{m-1}\left(v_{jm}^{(k)}\right)^2+\sum_{j=m+1}^{N}\left(v_{mj}^{(k)}\right)^2. \tag{8.28}$$

Finally, the cross-correlation functions between $\delta\Omega_j(t)$ and $\delta W_k(0)$ are also required in calculating the nonlinear response functions. They are

$$<\delta\Omega_j(t)\delta W_k(0)>_B = \sum_{m=1}^{N}\sum_{r=1}^{N-1}\sum_{s=r+1}^{N}U_{mj}^2(v_{rs}^{(k)})^2<x_{mm}(t)\{x_{rr}(0)+x_{ss}(0)\}>_B$$

$$\cong\left(\sum_{m=1}^{N}U_{mj}^2P_m^{(k)}\right)C(t). \tag{8.29}$$

In this section, by invoking the two approximations mentioned above, it was shown that the auto- and cross-correlation functions of fluctuating transition frequencies of singly and doubly excited states can be written in terms of the FFCF of a single chromophore, *C*(*t*). This approach is quite useful for numerical simulations of linear and nonlinear optical spectra of coupled multi-chromophore systems in general, but one can carry out more time-consuming but realistic numerical calculations without relying on these approximations if all the necessary parameters and quantities are sufficiently known.

8.5 EXCHANGE-NARROWING EFFECT ON ABSORPTION SPECTRUM

In Equations 8.26, 8.27, and 8.29, three different time-correlation functions of singly and doubly excited-state frequency fluctuations were obtained. In order to understand the effects of chromophore–chromophore couplings on spectroscopic properties, let us first consider the mean square fluctuation amplitude of the *j*th singly excited-state transition frequency, $<\delta\Omega_j^2>_B$. From Equation 8.26, we find

$$<\delta\Omega_j^2>_B = C(0)\sum_m U_{mj}^4 = \frac{C(0)}{N_j}. \tag{8.30}$$

Note that the inverse participation ratio N_j is usually defined as

$$N_j = \left[\sum_m U_{mj}^4\right]^{-1}. \tag{8.31}$$

The probability that the excitation j is localized at site m is $P_m(j) = U_{mj}^2$. The approximate number of sites participating in the jth exciton is therefore $N_j = 1/< P_m(j) > = 1/\Sigma_m P_m(j)P_m(j) = 1/\Sigma_m U_{mj}^4$. The inverse participation ratio N_j is a measure of how many molecular excited states are involved in a given delocalized singly excited state. The ratio $< \delta\Omega_j^2 >_B / C(0)$ therefore provides direct evidence on the extent of delocalization of the jth excited state of coupled multi-chromophore system. In the limit of the complete localization, $(\Sigma_m U_{mj}^4)^{-1} = 1$ for all j and $< \delta\Omega_j^2 >_B = C(0)$. On the other hand, if the jth delocalized state is fully delocalized over all N chromophores, we have $U_{mj} = 1/\sqrt{N}$, and the ratio $< \delta\Omega_j^2 >_B / C(0)$ becomes $1/N$. In this case, the mean square fluctuation amplitude of the jth delocalized excited state becomes very small (by the factor of $1/N$) in comparison to that of an isolated chromophore.

The absorption spectrum of the N-coupled multi-chromophore system is then given as the sum of N sub-bands associated with optical transitions to N singly excited states, that is,

$$\kappa(\omega) \propto \mathrm{Im}[\chi(\omega)] = \mathrm{Im}\left[\sum_j |\mu_{gj}|^2 \frac{i}{\hbar}\int_0^\infty dt\,\{e^{-i(\varpi_{jg}-\omega)t - g_{jj}(t)} - e^{i(\varpi_{jg}+\omega)t - g_{jj}^*(t)}\}\right]. \tag{8.32}$$

Defining the line-broadening function of a single chromophore as

$$g_0(t) = \int_0^t d\tau_2 \int_0^{\tau_2} d\tau_1\, C(\tau_1), \tag{8.33}$$

one can rewrite the absorption spectrum in Equation 8.32 as

$$\kappa(\omega) \propto \mathrm{Im}\left[\sum_j |\mu_{gj}|^2 \frac{i}{\hbar}\int_0^\infty dt\,\{e^{-i(\varpi_{jg}-\omega)t - g_0(t)/N_j} - e^{i(\varpi_{jg}+\omega)t - g_0^*(t)/N_j}\}\right]. \tag{8.34}$$

Here, it should be noted that

$$\begin{aligned} g_{jj}(t) &= \int_0^t d\tau_2 \int_0^{\tau_2} d\tau_1 < \delta\Omega_j(\tau_1)\delta\Omega_j(0) > \\ &= \frac{1}{N_j}\int_0^t d\tau_2 \int_0^{\tau_2} d\tau_1\, C(\tau_1) \\ &= \frac{1}{N_j} g_0(t). \end{aligned}$$

For the sake of simplicity, consider the Markovian limit, that is, $g_0(t) = \gamma_0 t$ (see Section 3.2), to obtain

$$\kappa(\omega) \propto \frac{1}{\hbar}\mathrm{Im}\left[\sum_j |\mu_{gj}|^2 \left\{ \frac{1}{\bar{\omega}_{jg} - \omega - i\gamma_0/N_j} + \frac{1}{\bar{\omega}_{jg} + \omega + i\gamma_0/N_j} \right\}\right]. \tag{8.35}$$

This result suggests that that the jth sub-band associated with the transition from the ground state to the jth singly excited state is much narrower by the factor N_j than the absorption spectrum of an uncoupled chromophore in the same condensed phase. This phenomenon is the well-known exchange-narrowing effect.[18] Although, in Equation 8.35, only the Markovian limit is considered, the same line-narrowing process occurs for other cases of line-broadenings as well.

8.6 MEASUREMENTS OF AUTO- AND CROSS-FREQUENCY–FREQUENCY CORRELATION FUNCTIONS

In Section 5.8, the three-pulse photon echo peak shift of a 2LS was discussed and shown to be useful in measuring the FFCF $C_R(t)$ or in the classical limit the solvation correlation function. If the singly excited-state energies of an N-coupled multi-chromophore system are discretely distributed so that the frequency resolution of such excited states is achievable, it is possible to use the one-color PEPS technique to measure individual time-correlation functions $C_R(t)$ for each state by properly tuning the incident beam frequency.

When the three pulses used for the PEPS measurement have the same frequency ω and it is close to the jth transition frequency, that is, $\omega = \tilde{\Omega}_{jj}$, the corresponding PEPS signal, from Equation 5.81, is given as[19]

$$\tau^*(T;\omega = \tilde{\Omega}_{jj}) = \frac{\sqrt{N_j C(0)}\,\mathrm{Re}[C_R(T)]}{\sqrt{\pi}\left\{C^2(0) - C_R^2(T)\right\}}. \tag{8.36}$$

It is interesting to note that the PEPS value is linearly proportional to the square root of the inverse participation ratio, that is, $\sqrt{N_j}$. This result shows that a series of one-color PEPS experiments varying the center frequency of the incident pulses can provide critical information on the extent of delocalization of the jth singly excited state of the N-coupled multi-chromophore system.

Although the auto-correlation function of $\delta\Omega_j(t)$ can be experimentally measured by using the one-color PEPS technique, a cross-correlation function such as $<\delta\Omega_j(t)\delta\Omega_k(0)>_B$ for $j \neq k$ requires the two-color PEPS measurement method. Two-color photon echo spectroscopy is carried out by choosing the frequencies of the first two pulses to be different from the third pulse (see Figure 8.2).[20–22] Since the two incident field frequencies ω and ω' can be independently tuned, two different singly excited states are excited by such a two-color rephasing photon echo process. For instance, let us consider the case when the ω-field is resonant with

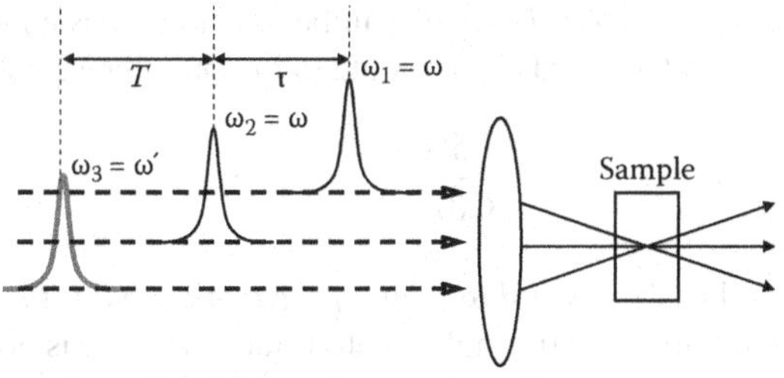

FIGURE 8.2 Experimental beam configuration for general two-color photon echo measurement. The first two pulses have the same center frequency $\omega_1 = \omega_2 = \omega$, whereas the third one has a different frequency $\omega_3 = \omega'$.

the jth transition and the ω'-field is resonant with the kth transition with $j \neq k$. The corresponding rephasing diagram associated with this case is

$$<\mu \overset{e_k\wr}{\underset{g\wr e_j\wr}{\Longleftarrow}} |g><g|>. \tag{8.37}$$

The first coherence created by the interaction of the molecule with the first ω-field is $\rho^{(1)}_{ge_j}$, and its oscillation frequency is given by $\tilde{\Omega}_{jj}$, that is, $\exp(i\tilde{\Omega}_{jj}t_1)$. After the first delay time τ, the second radiation–matter interaction puts the molecular system on the population on either the ground or jth excited state. The third interaction with the ω'-field then creates the coherence $\rho^{(3)}_{e_kg}$, and its oscillation is determined by the $\exp(-i\tilde{\Omega}_{kk}t_3)$. Noting that the one-color PEPS is useful to the measurement of the correlation between the transition frequency of the chromophore during the t_1 period, and that during the t_3 period, one can show that the two-color PEPS described above provides information on the correlation between $\delta\Omega_j(0)$ and $\delta\Omega_k(T)$ when $\omega = \tilde{\Omega}_{jj}$ and $\omega' = \tilde{\Omega}_{kk}$. Therefore, if the transition frequency fluctuation of the jth state does not correlate with that of the kth state due to *zero coupling*, the cross-correlation function $<\delta\Omega_j(t)\delta\Omega_k(0)>_B$ vanishes and the two-color PEPS also vanishes. Unfortunately, the two-color PEPS of the coupled multi-chromophore system is a much more complicated experiment than the one-color PEPS, because of the other contributions from doubly excited-state transitions, excitation transfer processes in the manifold of singly excited states, coherence-to-coherence transfers, and so forth. Consequently, its interpretation requires detailed understanding of the various chemical and physical processes involved.

Nevertheless, it is useful to consider further the magnitude of the cross-correlation function, $<\delta\Omega_j(t)\delta\Omega_k(0)>_B$. The ratio $<\delta\Omega_j\delta\Omega_k>_B/C(0)$ is given by

$$\frac{<\delta\Omega_j\delta\Omega_k>_B}{C(0)} = \sum_m U_{mj}^2 U_{mk}^2. \tag{8.38}$$

Noting that the vector, $\vec{p}_j = (U_{1j}^2, U_{2j}^2, \cdots)$, can be understood as a probability density distribution of the jth delocalized excited state in the site representation, we have

$$\frac{<\delta\Omega_j \delta\Omega_k>_B}{C(0)} = \vec{p}_j \cdot \vec{p}_k \tag{8.39}$$

which can be viewed as the *spatial overlap of the two probability–density distributions*, $\vec{p}_j$ and $\vec{p}_k$, of the jth and kth singly excited states. If there is no coupling among the constituent chromophores, the spatial overlap $\vec{p}_j \cdot \vec{p}_k$ is zero, and consequently the magnitude of $<\delta\Omega_j \delta\Omega_k>_B$ vanishes. This means that if two different delocalized states do not share common molecular (site) excited states, the transition frequency fluctuations of the two delocalized states are uncorrelated and $<\delta\Omega_j \delta\Omega_k>_B$ vanishes. Consequently, an experimental method such as the two-color photon echo measuring $<\delta\Omega_j \delta\Omega_k>_B$ can provide spatial information about a pair of delocalized singly excited states that have different transition frequencies.

We next consider the cross-correlation between the jth singly excited-state frequency fluctuation and the kth doubly excited-state frequency fluctuation, $<\delta\Omega_j(t)\delta W_k(0)>_B$. Its amplitude divided by $C(0)$ is

$$\frac{<\delta\Omega_j \delta W_k>_B}{C(0)} = \sum_{m=1}^{N} U_{mj}^2 P_m^{(k)}. \tag{8.40}$$

In order to understand the physical meaning of the quantity, $\sum_{m=1}^{N} U_{mj}^2 P_m^{(k)}$, let us define the projection operator, $\hat{P}_m = a_m^\dagger a_m$, where $|m>$ denotes the singly excited state of the mth chromophore. Then, one can show that

$$P_m^{(k)} = \langle f_k | \hat{P}_m | f_k \rangle \tag{8.41}$$

where $|f_k\rangle$ is the kth two-exciton state wavefunction, that is,

$$|f_k\rangle = \sum_{m=1}^{N-1} \sum_{n=m+1}^{N} v_{mn}^{(k)} |m,n>. \tag{8.42}$$

Therefore, $P_m^{(k)}$ is the expectation value of $a_m^\dagger a_m$ in the kth doubly excited state, and is considered to be the "amount" of the mth chromophore excitation in the kth doubly excited state. In other words, the elements of the vector $\vec{P}_k \equiv (P_1^{(k)}, P_2^{(k)}, \cdots)$ give the *probability density* of each single-site excitation in the kth doubly excited state. Therefore, Equation 8.40 can be rewritten as

$$\frac{<\delta\Omega_j \delta W_k>_B}{C(0)} = \vec{p}_j \cdot \vec{P}_k, \tag{8.43}$$

which can be interpreted as the spatial overlap between the probability density of the jth singly excited state and the reduced probability density of the kth doubly excited.

Finally, the mean square fluctuation amplitude of the kth doubly excited state is found to be

$$\frac{<\delta W_k^2>_B}{C(0)} = \sum_{m=1}^{N-1}\sum_{n=m+1}^{N}\left(v_{mn}^{(k)}\right)^2\left\{P_m^{(k)} + P_n^{(k)}\right\}. \tag{8.44}$$

This result suggests that $<\delta W_k^2>_B$ is determined by the overlap of the probability density of the kth doubly excited state in the $|m,n>$ basis and the projected (reduced) probability densities.

8.7 EXCITON POPULATION TRANSFER

Later in Chapter 13, we will discuss one of the examples where the population and coherence transfers are critical in understanding the time-dependent changes of 2D spectra of coupled multi-chromophore systems, such as photosynthetic light-harvesting complexes. In this section, a brief discussion on the theory of exciton population transfer rate is therefore presented. Among many different approaches, we will focus on the projection operator technique. Suppose that the molecular Hamiltonian can be divided into two parts as

$$H = H_0 + H' \tag{8.45}$$

where H_0 and H' represent the reference and perturbation Hamiltonians, respectively. For example, if the site representation Hamiltonian in Equation 8.1 is used, the inter-chromophore couplings (the second term in Equation 8.1) and the off-diagonal matrix elements in the system–bath interaction Hamiltonian in Equation 8.3 can be considered as the perturbation Hamiltonian, which are responsible for excitation transitions between two different chromophores. On the other hand, in the delocalized exciton representation, the system–bath interactions in Equations 8.13 and 8.14 are the perturbation Hamiltonians for the singly and doubly excited states.

The time evolution of molecular density matrix is then described by the following quantum Liouville equation:

$$\frac{\partial\rho(t)}{\partial t} = -iL\rho(t) = -i(L_0 + L')\rho(t). \tag{8.46}$$

Now, let us introduce the projection operator:

$$\mathbf{P} = \mathbf{P}_0 + \sum_{\mu}\mathbf{P}_{\mu} \tag{8.47}$$

where the definitions of the individual terms are

$$\mathbf{P}_\mu \rho \equiv |\mu> \rho_{\mu\mu}^{eq} <\mu| Tr_B[\rho_{\mu\mu}]$$

$$\rho_{\mu\mu}^{eq} = \frac{\exp\left[-\beta H_\mu^0\right]}{Z}. \tag{8.48}$$

$\mathbf{P}_0$ is just the projection operator for the electronic ground state. Here, μ can be either a singly or doubly excited-site state or a one or two exciton state, depending on the choice of representation and $H_\mu^0 \equiv <\mu| H_0 |\mu>$. Then, the complementary operator $\mathbf{Q}$, which projects the density matrix onto the manifold of off-diagonal (coherence) density matrix components, is defined as

$$\mathbf{Q} = 1 - \mathbf{P}. \tag{8.49}$$

Using the projection operator method,[23–25] one can obtain the equations describing the time evolutions of diagonal and off-diagonal density operators, which describe population and coherence evolutions, respectively, as

$$\frac{\partial \mathbf{P}\rho(t)}{\partial t} = -i\mathbf{P}L\mathbf{P}\rho(t) - \int_0^t d\tau\, \mathbf{P}L\mathbf{Q}e^{-i(t-\tau)\mathbf{Q}L}\mathbf{Q}L\mathbf{P}\rho(\tau) - i\mathbf{P}Le^{-it\mathbf{Q}L}\mathbf{Q}\rho(0) \tag{8.50}$$

$$\frac{\partial \mathbf{Q}\rho(t)}{\partial t} = -i\mathbf{Q}L\mathbf{Q}\rho(t) - \mathbf{Q}L\int_0^t d\tau e^{-i(t-\tau)\mathbf{P}L}\mathbf{P}L\mathbf{Q}\rho(\tau) - i\mathbf{Q}Le^{-it\mathbf{P}L}\mathbf{P}\rho(0). \tag{8.51}$$

Equation 8.50 describes the population transfer process between eigenstates since it determines time–evolutions of *diagonal* density matrix elements, whereas Equation 8.51 does coherence transfer processes between two different coherences.[26]

Population transfer rate. At time zero, if the system is in thermal equilibrium with the bath, we have $\mathbf{Q}\rho(0) = 0$, and the last term in Equation 8.50 vanishes. Then, up to the second-order terms with respect to H', one finds that Equation 8.50 can be approximately written as

$$\frac{\partial \mathbf{P}\rho(t)}{\partial t} = -\int_0^t d\tau\, \mathbf{P}L'e^{-i(t-\tau)L_0}L'\mathbf{P}\rho(\tau). \tag{8.52}$$

Here, the formulas, $\mathbf{P}^2 = \mathbf{P}$, $L_0\mathbf{P} = \mathbf{P}L_0 = 0$, and $\mathbf{P}L'\mathbf{P} = 0$, were used. This is the starting point for further derivation of a Markovian relaxation equation (quantum master equation) for the projected density matrix elements (populations)

$$\frac{\partial \rho_{\alpha\alpha}(t)}{\partial t} = -\sum_{\beta\neq\alpha} K_{\beta\beta,\alpha\alpha}\rho_{\alpha\alpha}(t) + \sum_{\beta\neq\alpha} K_{\alpha\alpha,\beta\beta}\rho_{\beta\beta}(t). \tag{8.53}$$

The rate constant $K_{\beta\beta,\alpha\alpha}$ in the Markovian limit, which describes population transfer from α to β state, is given as

$$K_{\beta\beta,\alpha\alpha} = 2\,\mathrm{Re}\int_0^\infty d\tau\, Tr_B\left[e^{iH_\alpha^0\tau}H'_{\alpha\beta}e^{-iH_\beta^0\tau}H'_{\beta\alpha}\rho_{\alpha\alpha}^{eq}\right]. \tag{8.54}$$

Depending on the choice of H_0 and H', one can obtain the Förster energy transfer rate, Redfield rate, or generalized Redfield rate.[27] If the site representation is chosen and if the second term in Equation 8.1 is selected as the perturbation Hamiltonian, the resultant rate constant corresponds to the Förster theory. On the other hand, if the reference eigenstates are delocalized excitonic states with neglect of the diagonal Hamiltonian matrix elements in Equation 8.13, then the rate constants obtained with Equation 8.54 correspond to the Redfield expressions for the population transfer processes. However, if the diagonal Hamiltonian matrix elements in Equation 8.13 are also included in the zero-order Hamiltonian H_0, one can obtain the modified Redfield theory expressions for the population transfer-rate constants.[28]

More specifically, in the Förster regime, the rate constant $K_{\beta\beta,\alpha\alpha}$, where α and β represent the excited states of the αth and βth chromophores, is given as

$$K_{\beta\beta,\alpha\alpha} = \frac{|J_{\beta\alpha}|^2}{2\pi}\int_{-\infty}^{\infty} d\omega\, A_\beta(\omega)F_\alpha(\omega), \tag{8.55}$$

where $A_\beta(\omega)$ and $F_\alpha(\omega)$ are the line-shape functions of the absorption and fluorescence of the αth and βth chromophores, respectively. Note that the rate constant in Equation 8.55 is linearly proportional to both the square of the coupling constant and the spectral overlap between $A_\beta(\omega)$ and $F_\alpha(\omega)$.

In the Redfield regime, the population transfer rate from the jth exciton state to the kth exciton state is[29]

$$K_{kk,jj} = 2\,\mathrm{Re}\int_0^{\infty} dt \left\langle \left[U^{-1}H_{SB}^{(1)}(\mathbf{q}(t))U\right]_{jk}\left[U^{-1}H_{SB}^{(1)}(\mathbf{q}(0))U\right]_{kj}\right\rangle \exp\{-i\Delta\Omega_{kj}t\} \tag{8.56}$$

where the frequency difference between the kth and jth singly excited (one-exciton) states is denoted as $\Delta\Omega_{kj}$. Then, Equation 8.56 can be rewritten as, from Equation 8.13,

$$\begin{aligned}
K_{kk,jj} &= 2\,\mathrm{Re}\int_0^{\infty} dt \sum_{m,n}\sum_{m',n'} U_{jm}^{-1}U_{nk}U_{km'}^{-1}U_{n'j}\langle x_{mn}(\mathbf{q}(t))x_{m'n'}(\mathbf{q}(0))\rangle \exp\{-i\Delta\Omega_{kj}t\} \\
&\cong 2\,\mathrm{Re}\int_0^{\infty} dt \sum_{m}\sum_{m'} U_{jm}^{-1}U_{mk}U_{km'}^{-1}U_{m'j}\langle x_{mm}(\mathbf{q}(t))x_{m'm'}(\mathbf{q}(0))\rangle \exp\{-i\Delta\Omega_{kj}t\} \\
&\cong 2\,\mathrm{Re}\int_0^{\infty} dt \sum_{m} U_{mk}^2U_{mj}^2\langle x_{mm}(\mathbf{q}(t))x_{mm}(\mathbf{q}(0))\rangle \exp\{-i\Delta\Omega_{kj}t\} \\
&\cong \left(\sum_m U_{mk}^2U_{mj}^2\right) 2\,\mathrm{Re}\int_0^{\infty} dt\, C(t)\exp\{-i\Delta\Omega_{kj}t\} \\
&= \left(\sum_m U_{mk}^2U_{mj}^2\right) \pi|\Delta\Omega_{kj}|^2 \left\{\coth\left(\frac{\beta\hbar|\Delta\Omega_{kj}|}{2}\right)\pm 1\right\}\rho(|\Delta\Omega_{kj}|).
\end{aligned} \tag{8.57}$$

Here, a series of approximations, Equations 8.16, 8.23, and 8.25, was invoked. Furthermore, we used the expression for $C(t)$ in terms of spectral density (see Equations 3.62 and 3.63). In Equation 8.57, the upper (lower) sign is the case of downhill (uphill) transition, that is, $\Delta\Omega_{kj} < 0$ ($\Delta\Omega_{kj} > 0$). This sign factor ensures detailed balance. Note that the factor $\sum_m U_{mk}^2 U_{mj}^2$, which appeared in Equation 8.57, is the spatial overlap of the probability density distributions of the kth and jth singly excited states. This quantity is spectroscopically measurable, as discussed in Section 8.6, via two-color photon echo measurements in principle.[22] If a given pair of exciton wavefunctions is spatially overlapped with each other, the Redfield excitation transfer rate can be large, as long as the spectral density at frequency $\Delta\Omega_{kj}$ is sizable.[17, 30]

REFERENCES

1. Cho, M., Coherent two-dimensional optical spectroscopy. *Chemical Reviews* 2008, 108, 1331–1418.
2. Kwac, K.; Cho, M., Two-color pump–probe spectroscopies of two- and three-level systems: 2-dimensional line shapes and solvation dynamics. *Journal of Physical Chemistry A* 2003, 107, 5903–5912.
3. Kwac, K.; Cho, M., Molecular dynamics simulation study of N-methylacetamide in water. II. Two-dimensional infrared pump–probe spectra. *Journal of Chemical Physics* 2003, 119, 2256–2263.
4. Zhang, W. M.; Chernyak, V.; Mukamel, S., Multidimensional femtosecond correlation spectroscopies of electronic and vibrational excitons. *Journal of Chemical Physics* 1999, 110, 5011–5028.
5. Cho, M.; Brixner, T.; Stiopkin, I.; Vaswani, H.; Fleming, G. R., Two dimensional electronic spectroscopy of molecular complexes. *Journal of the Chinese Chemical Society* 2006, 53, 15–24.
6. Ge, N. H.; Hochstrasser, R. M., Femtosecond two-dimensional infrared spectroscopy: IR-COSY and THIRSTY. *Phys. Chem. Comm.* 2002, 17–26.
7. Khalil, M.; Demirdoven, N.; Tokmakoff, A., Coherent 2D IR spectroscopy: Molecular structure and dynamics in solution. *Journal of Physical Chemistry A.* 2003, 107, 5258–5279.
8. van Amerongen, H.; Valkunas, L.; van Grondelle, R., *Photosynthetic excitons*. World Scientific: Singapore, 2000.
9. Yang, M.; Damjanovic, A.; Vaswani, H. M.; Fleming, G. R., Energy transfer in photosystem I of cyanobacteria *Synechococcus elongatus*: Model study with structure-based semi-empirical Hamiltonian and experimental spectral density. *Biophysics Journal* 2003, 85, 140–158.
10. Brixner, T.; Stenger, J.; Vaswani, H. M.; Cho, M.; Blankenship, R. E.; Fleming, G. R., Two-dimensional spectroscopy of electronic couplings in photosynthesis. *Nature* 2005, 434, 625–628.
11. Engel, G. S.; Calhoun, T. R.; Read, E. L.; Ahn, T. K.; Mancal, T.; Cheng, Y. C.; Blankenship, R. E.; Fleming, G. R., Evidence for wavelike energy transfer through quantum coherence in photosynthetic systems. *Nature* 2007, 446, 782–786.
12. Zanni, M. T.; Hochstrasser, R. M., Two-dimensional infrared spectroscopy: a promising new method for the time resolution of structures. *Current Opinion in Structural Biology* 2001, 11, 516–522.
13. Hamm, P.; Lim, M. H.; Hochstrasser, R. M., Structure of the amide I band of peptides measured by femtosecond nonlinear infrared spectroscopy. *Journal of Physical Chemistry B* 1998, 102, 6123–6138.

14. Krimm, S.; Bandekar, J., Vibrational spectroscopy and conformation of peptides, polypeptides, and proteins. *Advances in Protein Chemistry* 1986, 38, 181.
15. Cheam, T. C.; Krimm, S., Transition dipole interaction in polypeptides: abinitio calculation of transition dipole parameters. *Chemical Physics Letters* 1984, 107, 613–616.
16. Torii, H., Tasumi, M. Theoretical analyses of the amide I of infrared bands of globular proteins. In *Infrared spectroscopy of biomolecules*. In Mantsch, H. H., Chapman, D. ed.; Wiley-Liss: New York, 1996; p 1.
17. Cho, M.; Vaswani, H. M.; Brixner, T.; Stenger, J.; Fleming, G. R., Exciton analysis in 2D electronic spectroscopy. *Journal of Physical Chemistry B* 2005, 109, 10542–10556.
18. Kobayashi, T., *J-aggregates*. World Scientific: Singapore, 1996.
19. Cho, M.; Yu, J.-Y.; Joo, T.; Nagasawa, Y.; Passino, S. A.; Fleming, G. R., The integrated photon echo and solvation dynamics. *Journal of Physical Chemistry* 1996, 100, 11944–11953.
20. Yang, M.; Fleming, G. R., Two-color three-pulse photon echoes as a probe of electronic coupling in molecular complexes. *Journal of Chemical Physics* 1999, 110, (6), 2983–2990.
21. Prall, B. S.; Parkinson, D. Y.; Fleming, G. R.; Yang, M.; Ishikawa, N., Two-dimensional optical spectroscopy: Two-color photon echoes of electronically coupled phthalocyanine dimers. *Journal of Chemical Physics* 2004, 120, 2537–2540.
22. Cho, M.; Fleming, G. R., The integrated photon echo and solvation dynamics. II. Peak shifts and two-dimensional photon echo of a coupled chromophore system. *Journal of Chemical Physics* 2005, 123, 114506.
23. Zwanzig, R., Memory effects in irreversible thermodynamics. *Physical Review* 1961, 124, 983.
24. Mori, H., Transport collective motion and Brownian motion. *Progress of Theoretical Physics* 1965, 33, 423.
25. Harp, G. D.; Berne, B. J., Time-correlation functions, memory functions, and molecular dynamics. *Physical Review A* 1970, 2, 975.
26. Hyeon-Deuk, K.; Tanimura, Y.; Cho, M., Ultrafast exciton-exciton coherent transfer in molecular aggregates and its application to light-harvesting systems. *Journal of Chemical Physics* 2007, 127, 075101.
27. Yang, M.; Fleming, G. R., Influence of phonons on exciton transfer dynamics: comparison of the Redfield, Forster, and modified Redfield equations. *Chemical Physics* 2002, 275, 355–372.
28. Zhang, W. M.; Meier, T.; Chernyak, V.; Mukamel, S., Exciton migration and three-pulse femtosecond optical spectroscopies of photosynthetic antenna complexes. *Journal of Chemical Physics* 1998, 108, 7763–7774.
29. Ernst, R. R.; Bodenhausen, G.; Wokaun, A., *Nuclear magnetic resonance in one and two dimensions*. Oxford University Press: Oxford, 1987.
30. Kuhn, O.; Sundstrom, V., Energy transfer and relaxation dynamics in light-harvesting antenna complexes of photosynthetic bacteria. *Journal of Physical Chemistry B* 1997, 101, (17), 3432–3440.

9 Two-Dimensional Spectroscopy of Coupled Dimers

Two-dimensional spectroscopy is a useful method for studying coupling-induced phenomena such as band splitting and excitation transfer as well as for determining the molecular structure of complex molecules in solution. For a coupled dimer, the existence of cross-peaks is good evidence of coupling between the two constituent chromophores. As an example, by measuring the cross-peak amplitude in the 2D amide I IR spectrum of dipeptide consisting of two peptide bonds, it becomes possible to determine the solution structure of dipeptide, as the vibrational coupling strength between the two amide I local modes has been shown be strongly dependent on the backbone conformation of the dipeptide.[1–9] Similarly, for coupled electronic chromophores, not only two singly excited states are energetically separated from each other due to coupling but also the downhill and uphill energy transfers between the two excited states occur in time. The latter effects on the diagonal and cross-peak amplitude when a series of time-resolved 2D spectra are measured.[10]

In the previous chapter, a general model Hamiltonian for an N-coupled multi-chromophore system was presented and discussed. However, fundamental aspects of 2D spectroscopy can be understood by considering simple coupled dimer systems, where the constituent chromophores are modeled as either a 2LS or 3LS. A model Hamiltonian for a coupled (2LS) dimer will be discussed in the delocalized exciton representation. Using the approximate third-order response function obtained by using the cumulant expansion method and invoking the short-time approximation discussed in Chapter 5, one can obtain the 2D photon echo spectrum of a coupled dimer. A few model calculation results will be presented to demonstrate how 2D spectroscopy can be of use to study chemical and physical processes of coupled dimer systems.

9.1 MODEL HAMILTONIAN OF A COUPLED TWO-LEVEL SYSTEM DIMER

From the N-coupled multi-chromophore system Hamiltonian in Equation 8.1, we have the zero-order Hamiltonian of a coupled dimer system:

$$H_0 = \varepsilon_1 a_1^\dagger a_1 + \varepsilon_2 a_2^\dagger a_2 + \hbar J (a_1^\dagger a_2 + a_2^\dagger a_1) + H_B, \tag{9.1}$$

where $a_m^\dagger$ and a_m are the creation and annihilation operators of excitation at the mth chromophore. The mth site energy, electronic coupling constant between the mth and nth chromophores, and bath Hamiltonian are denoted as ε_m, J, and H_B, respectively. From the transition dipole coupling theory, which is based on the assumption that a transition dipole of one chromophore couples to that of another chromophore via dipole-dipole interaction, one can estimate the coupling constant J as

$$J = \mathbf{d}_1 \cdot \mathbf{T}_{12} \cdot \mathbf{d}_2 = (\mathbf{d}_1 \cdot \mathbf{d}_2) R_{12}^{-3} - 3(\mathbf{d}_1 \cdot \mathbf{R}_{12})(\mathbf{R}_{12} \cdot \mathbf{d}_2) R_{12}^{-5}, \tag{9.2}$$

where the two local transition dipoles are denoted as d_j and the angle between them will be denoted as ϕ. In Equation 9.2, the vector connecting the two point dipoles is denoted as $\mathbf{R}_{12}$. Although the transition dipole coupling model has been extensively used to estimate the coupling strength, as the inter-chromophore distance decreases, simple dipole-dipole approximation breaks down.[6, 7, 11, 12] Then, the transition charge–transition charge interaction or transition charge density model can become a more accurate description for quantitatively determining the coupling constant J than the above transition dipole coupling model simply based on a dipole-dipole interaction.[12, 13] Furthermore, the site energies effectively depend on the inter-chromophore distance and interaction strength so that an appropriate model that is capable of taking into account these effects should be used to properly apply the coupled dimer model to a real system.

In the case of dimeric molecular systems in condensed phases, chromophore-bath interaction and inter-chromophore distance and orientation fluctuations will induce fluctuations of both site energies and coupling constants. Thus, one of the useful chromophore-bath interaction Hamiltonian models is

$$H_{SB} = \hbar x_1(\mathbf{q}) a_1^\dagger a_1 + \hbar x_2(\mathbf{q}) a_2^\dagger a_2 + \hbar x_c(\mathbf{q})(a_1^\dagger a_2 + a_2^\dagger a_1), \tag{9.3}$$

where $x(\mathbf{q})$'s are operators of bath coordinates, $\mathbf{q}$, and the expectation values calculated over the bath states, $\langle x_m(\mathbf{q})\rangle_B$ for $m = 1$, 2, and c, are assumed to be zero. $x_1(\mathbf{q})$ and $x_2(\mathbf{q})$ describe the site energy fluctuations and $x_c(\mathbf{q})$ accounts for the coupling constant fluctuation.

Now, let us consider a coupled 2LS dimer with finite coupling constant J. The unitary transformation of the singly excited-state Hamiltonian matrix obtained from Equation 9.1 can be performed to find eigenvalues and eigenfunctions of the two singly excited states.[14] They will be denoted as e_1 and e_2, and the doubly excited state will be denoted as f (see Figure 9.1). Often, in the literatures, the singly and doubly excited states have been referred to as one- and two-exciton states, respectively.[15] Throughout this book both terms are used. First of all, the two singly excited states are given as

$$\begin{pmatrix} |e_1> \\ |e_2> \end{pmatrix} = U^{-1} \begin{pmatrix} a_1^\dagger |0> \\ a_2^\dagger |0> \end{pmatrix} = \begin{pmatrix} \cos\theta & \sin\theta \\ -\sin\theta & \cos\theta \end{pmatrix} \begin{pmatrix} a_1^\dagger |0> \\ a_2^\dagger |0> \end{pmatrix}, \tag{9.4}$$

where $|0>$ is the ground ket-state. The unitary transformation matrix U was defined in the above equation. The mixing angle θ varies from 0 to $\pi/2$, and is a function of J, ε_1, and ε_2 as

$$\theta = \frac{1}{2} \arctan\left(\frac{2J}{\varepsilon_1 - \varepsilon_2} \right). \tag{9.5}$$

The two singly excited-state energies, denoted as $\hbar\,\Omega_1$ and $\hbar\,\Omega_2$, are found to be

$$\begin{aligned} \hbar\Omega_1 &= \varepsilon_1 \cos^2\theta + \varepsilon_2 \sin^2\theta + 2J\cos\theta\sin\theta \\ \hbar\Omega_2 &= \varepsilon_1 \sin^2\theta + \varepsilon_2 \cos^2\theta - 2J\cos\theta\sin\theta. \end{aligned} \tag{9.6}$$

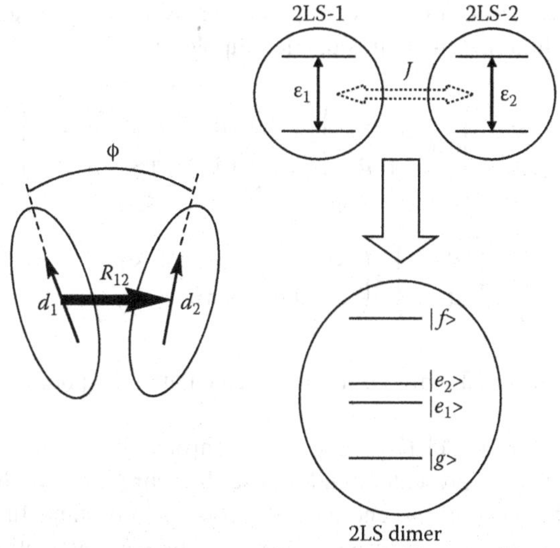

FIGURE 9.1 Coupled two-level system dimer. The coupling constant between two transition dipoles is denoted as J. The transition dipoles of the two chromophores are denoted as d_1 and d_2, and the angle between the two is ϕ. The vector pointing from the center of d_1 dipole to that of d_2 dipole is R_{12}. After diagonalizing the zero-order Hamiltonian, one can obtain the two singly excited-state energies and eigenfunctions (e_1 and e_2) and one doubly excited state f.

The doubly excited-state wavefunction and its energy $\hbar\,\Omega_f$ are

$$| f >= a_1^+ a_2^+ | 0 >$$

$$\hbar\Omega_f = \varepsilon_1 + \varepsilon_2 = \hbar\Omega_1 + \hbar\Omega_2. \tag{9.7}$$

In a real system, the doubly excited-state energy might be different from the sum of two singly excited-state energies, because the two excited-state molecules within the dimer interact with each other to make the doubly excited-state energy change. This is known as the exciton–exciton binding (or repulsion) interaction. Such an effect on the doubly excited-state energy cannot be described by the simplified model Hamiltonian in Equation 9.1. One might have to include $\hbar\Delta a_2^\dagger a_1^\dagger a_2 a_1$ to Equation 9.1 to describe such biexciton binding energy. However, we will ignore such effects in this chapter for the sake of simplicity.

Now, by including the solvation (solvent reorganization) energies, the ensemble-averaged vertical transition energies one- and two-exciton states are written as

$$\hbar\bar{\omega}_{e_1g} = \hbar\Omega_1 + \lambda_1 \cos^2\theta + \lambda_2 \sin^2\theta + 2\lambda_c \cos\theta \sin\theta \tag{9.8}$$

$$\hbar\bar{\omega}_{e_2g} = \hbar\Omega_2 + \lambda_1 \sin^2\theta + \lambda_2 \cos^2\theta - 2\lambda_c \cos\theta \sin\theta \tag{9.9}$$

$$\hbar\bar{\omega}_{fg} = \hbar\Omega_f + \lambda_1 + \lambda_2 = \hbar\bar{\omega}_{e_1g} + \hbar\bar{\omega}_{e_2g}, \tag{9.10}$$

where λ_j, for $j = 1, 2$, or c, are the corresponding solvent reorganization energies.

Next, one can find that the four transition dipoles are given as

$$\begin{pmatrix} \boldsymbol{\mu}_{e_1g} \\ \boldsymbol{\mu}_{e_2g} \end{pmatrix} = U^{-1}\begin{pmatrix} \mathbf{d}_1 \\ \mathbf{d}_2 \end{pmatrix} = \begin{pmatrix} \cos\theta & \sin\theta \\ -\sin\theta & \cos\theta \end{pmatrix}\begin{pmatrix} \mathbf{d}_1 \\ \mathbf{d}_2 \end{pmatrix} \tag{9.11}$$

$$\begin{pmatrix} \boldsymbol{\mu}_{e_1f} \\ \boldsymbol{\mu}_{e_2f} \end{pmatrix} = \begin{pmatrix} \sin\theta & \cos\theta \\ \cos\theta & -\sin\theta \end{pmatrix}\begin{pmatrix} \mathbf{d}_1 \\ \mathbf{d}_2 \end{pmatrix}. \tag{9.12}$$

Equations 9.11 and 9.12 will be used to calculate 2D photon echo transition amplitude.

In Equation 9.3, a model Hamiltonian for chromophore–bath interaction for a coupled 2LS dimer was presented, and it describes chromophore–bath interaction-induced fluctuations of the site energies and coupling constant. In the delocalized exciton representation, the transformed chromophore–bath interaction Hamiltonians for the singly and doubly excited states should be considered. For the singly and doubly excited states, the transformed Hamiltonians are, respectively,

$$\begin{aligned} \tilde{\Xi}_{SB}^{(1)}(\mathbf{q}) &= U^{-1}H_{SB}^{(1)}(\mathbf{q})U \\ &= \begin{pmatrix} x_1\cos^2\theta + x_2\sin^2\theta + 2x_c\cos\theta\sin\theta & -(x_1 - x_2)\cos\theta\sin\theta + x_c\cos 2\theta \\ -(x_1 - x_2)\cos\theta\sin\theta + x_c\cos 2\theta & x_1\sin^2\theta + x_2\cos^2\theta - 2x_c\cos\theta\sin\theta \end{pmatrix} \end{aligned} \tag{9.13}$$

$$\tilde{\Xi}_{SB}^{(2)}(\mathbf{q}) = x_1(\mathbf{q}) + x_2(\mathbf{q}). \tag{9.14}$$

The diagonal matrix element $[\tilde{\Xi}_{SB}^{(1)}(\mathbf{q})]_{jj}$ describes fluctuation of the jth singly excited-state energy, whereas the off-diagonal matrix element $[\tilde{\Xi}_{SB}^{(1)}(\mathbf{q})]_{jk}$ induces an excitation transfer between the two different singly excited states e_j and e_k. Finally, $\tilde{\Xi}_{SB}^{(2)}(\mathbf{q})$ induces fluctuation of the doubly excited-state energy.

9.2 DELOCALIZED EXCITED-STATE ENERGY FLUCTUATIONS AND TIME CORRELATION FUNCTIONS

From the transformed Hamiltonian in Equations 9.13 and 9.14, the fluctuating parts of the transition frequencies are

$$\begin{aligned} \delta\Omega_1(\mathbf{q}) &= (x_1\cos^2\theta + x_2\sin^2\theta + 2x_c\cos\theta\sin\theta)/\hbar \\ \delta\Omega_2(\mathbf{q}) &= (x_1\sin^2\theta + x_2\cos^2\theta - 2x_c\cos\theta\sin\theta)/\hbar \\ \delta W(\mathbf{q}) &= (x_1 + x_2)/\hbar. \end{aligned} \tag{9.15}$$

Now, let us consider various frequency–frequency correlation functions. First, invoking the IBA (independent bath approximation) we have, for m and $n = 1, 2$, or c,

$$< x_m(t)x_n(0) >_B = 0 \quad \text{for} \quad m \neq n. \tag{9.16}$$

This means that the site transition frequency fluctuation of the mth chromophore is statistically uncorrelated with that of the nth chromophore. In other words, the bath degrees of freedom coupled to different chromophore transitions are statistically independent.

For the sake of notational simplicity, we define the quantity κ that is a measure of the delocalization of the excited states as

$$\kappa \equiv \cos\theta \sin\theta. \tag{9.17}$$

As shown in Chapter 7 for a 2LS, the line-broadening of linear absorption spectrum and the line width of the diagonal peak in a given 2D spectrum are determined by the FFCF. For a coupled dimer, the corresponding auto-correlation functions are

$$\begin{aligned} C_{e_1e_1}(t) &= < \delta\Omega_1(t)\delta\Omega_1(0) >_B = C_1(t)\cos^4\theta + C_2(t)\sin^4\theta + 4C_c(t)\kappa^2 \\ C_{e_2e_2}(t) &= < \delta\Omega_2(t)\delta\Omega_2(0) >_B = C_1(t)\sin^4\theta + C_2(t)\cos^4\theta + 4C_c(t)\kappa^2 \\ C_{ff}(t) &= < \delta W(t)\delta W(0) >_B = C_1(t) + C_2(t), \end{aligned} \tag{9.18}$$

where the FFCFs of $x_m(t)$ ($\equiv \exp(iH_B t/\hbar)x_m(\mathbf{q})\exp(-iH_B t/\hbar)$) for $m = 1, 2$, and c are defined as

$$C_m(t) = < x_m(t)x_m(0) >_B. \tag{9.19}$$

Next, let us consider the cross correlation functions:

$$\begin{aligned} C_{e_1e_2}(t) &= C_{e_2e_1}(t) = < \delta\Omega_1(t)\delta\Omega_2(0) >_B = \{C_1(t) + C_2(t) - 4C_c(t)\}\kappa^2 \\ C_{e_1f}(t) &= C_{fe_1}(t) = < \delta\Omega_1(t)\delta W(0) >_B = C_1(t)\cos^2\theta + C_2(t)\sin^2\theta \\ C_{e_2f}(t) &= C_{fe_2}(t) = < \delta\Omega_2(t)\delta W(0) >_B = C_1(t)\sin^2\theta + C_2(t)\cos^2\theta. \end{aligned} \tag{9.20}$$

It is interesting to note that the correlation between the transition frequencies of the delocalized singly excited states e_1 and e_2 (between $\delta\Omega_1(t)$ and $\delta\Omega_2(0)$) is proportional to κ^2 ($= \cos^2\theta \sin^2\theta$). Therefore, if the two chromophores are not coupled to each other, that is, $\theta = 0$ or $\pi/2$, we have $\kappa = 0$ and expect that the cross-correlation function $< \delta\Omega_1(t)\delta\Omega_2(0) >_B$ vanishes. In this zero coupling limit, there will be no cross-peaks, as will be shown below.

9.3 COUPLED TWO-LEVEL SYSTEM DIMER: QUANTUM BEATS AT SHORT TIME

In Section 7.2, the 2D photon echo spectroscopy of a single 2LS was discussed in detail. Now, if two chromophores are coupled to each other to form delocalized singly excited states, the total number of quantum states one needs to consider is four, as can be seen in Figure 9.1. Therefore, in addition to the two diagonal peaks originating from the singly excited states e_1 and e_2, there are also two off-diagonal cross-peaks produced by the inter-chromophore coupling. In this section, the very short-time regime in which excitation transfer between the two singly excited states e_1 and e_2 does not play significant roles will be considered in detail.

Since there are two singly excited states e_1 and e_2 as well as a doubly excited state f, there are a number of different nonlinear optical transition pathways (diagrams) contributing to the 2D photon echo spectrum. For a single 2LS, it was shown that the following two diagrams should be taken into consideration:

$$<\mu \xLeftarrow[g\wr \quad e\wr]{e\wr} |g><g|.$$

$$<\mu \xLeftarrow[g\wr e\wr]{e\wr} |g><g|. \tag{9.21}$$

In addition, due to the presence of doubly excited state f, it is necessary to include the following diagram:

$$<\mu \xLeftarrow[e\wr]{f\wr e\wr} |g><g|. \tag{9.22}$$

Now, for a coupled 2LS dimer, there are twelve diagrams in total, which represent different polarization components. One can classify those twelve diagrams into four groups, depending on the center frequencies of the corresponding peaks in the 2D PE spectrum.

The first group of diagrams, which produces the diagonal peak at $\omega_\tau = \bar{\omega}_{e_1g}$ and $\omega_t = \bar{\omega}_{e_1g}$, consists of the following two diagrams, which will be denoted as D1-SE (diagonal peak 1-stimulated emission) and D1-GB (diagonal peak 1-ground-state bleach):

$$<\mu \xLeftarrow[g\wr \quad e_1\wr]{e_1\wr} |g><g| \quad \propto \exp\{-i\bar{\omega}_{e_1g}t_3 - i\bar{\omega}_{ge_1}t_1\}$$

$$<\mu \xLeftarrow[g\wr e_1\wr]{e_1\wr} |g><g| \quad \propto \exp\{-i\bar{\omega}_{e_1g}t_3 - i\bar{\omega}_{ge_1}t_1\}. \tag{9.23}$$

In the above equations, only the coherence oscillation factor is shown. These two contributions have the same coherence oscillation term $\exp\{-i\bar{\omega}_{e_1g}t_3 - i\bar{\omega}_{ge_1}t_1\}$.

The second group of diagrams (D2-SE and D2-GB) shown below is associated with another diagonal peak at $\omega_\tau = \bar{\omega}_{e_2g}$ and $\omega_t = \bar{\omega}_{e_2g}$:

$$<\mu \xLeftarrow[g\wr \quad e_2\wr]{e_2\wr} |g><g| \quad \propto \exp\{-i\bar{\omega}_{e_2g}t_3 - i\bar{\omega}_{ge_2}t_1\}$$

$$<\mu \xLeftarrow[g\wr e_2\wr]{e_2\wr} |g><g| \quad \propto \exp\{-i\bar{\omega}_{e_2g}t_3 - i\bar{\omega}_{ge_2}t_1\}. \tag{9.24}$$

The third group of diagrams (C12-SE, C12-GB, C12-EA1, and C12-EA2) below is related to the cross-peak at $\omega_\tau = \bar{\omega}_{e_1g}$ and $\omega_t = \bar{\omega}_{e_2g}$:

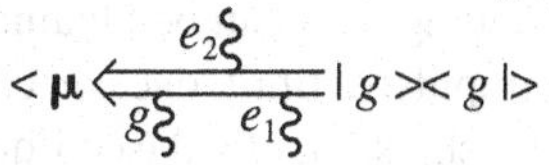
$$\propto \exp\{-i\bar{\omega}_{e_2g}t_3 - i\bar{\omega}_{e_2e_1}t_2 - i\bar{\omega}_{ge_1}t_1\}$$

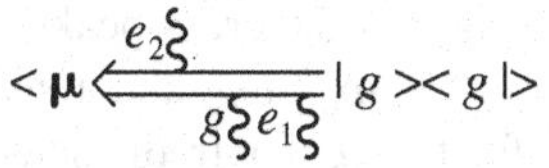
$$\propto \exp\{-i\bar{\omega}_{e_2g}t_3 - i\bar{\omega}_{ge_1}t_1\}$$

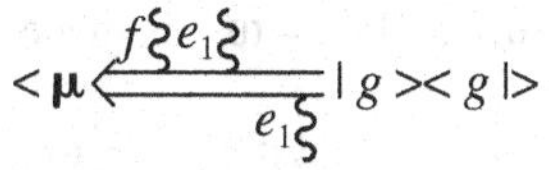
$$\propto \exp\{-i\bar{\omega}_{fe_1}t_3 - i\bar{\omega}_{ge_1}t_1\}$$

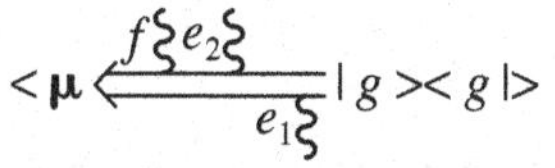
$$\propto \exp\{-i\bar{\omega}_{fe_1}t_3 - i\bar{\omega}_{e_2e_1}t_2 - i\bar{\omega}_{ge_1}t_1\}. \tag{9.25}$$

The first in Equation 9.25 is associated with a quantum beat contribution to the cross-peak amplitude, since it oscillates in time t_2 as $\exp\{-i\bar{\omega}_{e_2e_1}t_2\}$. The fourth term also oscillates in time during t_2 as $\exp\{-i\bar{\omega}_{e_2e_1}t_2\}$. These oscillatory contributions appear as quantum beats in the transient grating or pump–probe signal from the dimer. The same quantum beat can be observed by measuring the oscillatory amplitude of the associated cross-peak. From the coherence oscillation term associated with the second term in Equation 9.25, it is clear that they are associated with the cross-peak at $\omega_\tau = \bar{\omega}_{e_1g}$ and $\omega_t = \bar{\omega}_{e_2g}$. In addition, the third term in Equation 9.25 also contributes to the cross-peak at $\omega_\tau = \bar{\omega}_{e_1g}$ and $\omega_t = \bar{\omega}_{e_2g}$, because the frequency difference between the f and e_1 states is very close to that between the e_2 and g states, that is, $\bar{\omega}_{fe_1} \cong \bar{\omega}_{e_2g}$, when the exciton–exciton binding energy is negligible.

Finally, the remaining four diagrams (C21-SE, C21-GB, C21-EA1, and C21-EA2) producing the cross-peak at $\omega_\tau = \bar{\omega}_{e_2g}$ and $\omega_t = \bar{\omega}_{e_1g}$ are given as

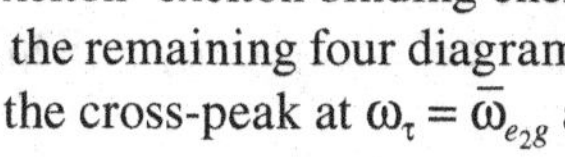
$$\propto \exp\{-i\bar{\omega}_{e_1g}t_3 - i\bar{\omega}_{e_1e_2}t_2 - i\bar{\omega}_{ge_2}t_1\}$$

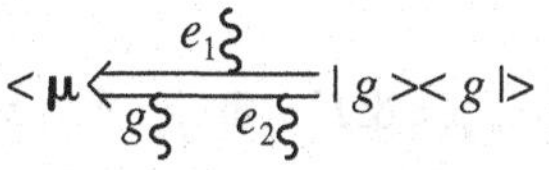
$$\propto \exp\{-i\bar{\omega}_{e_1g}t_3 - i\bar{\omega}_{ge_2}t_1\}$$

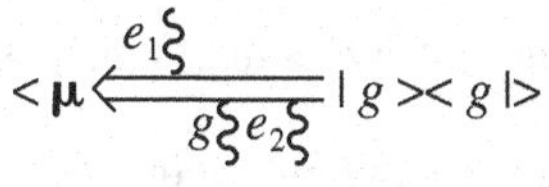
$$\propto \exp\{-i\bar{\omega}_{fe_2}t_3 - i\bar{\omega}_{ge_2}t_1\}$$

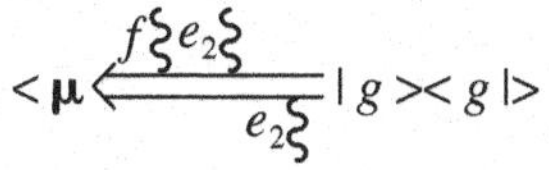
$$\propto \exp\{-i\bar{\omega}_{fe_2}t_3 - i\bar{\omega}_{e_1e_2}t_2 - i\bar{\omega}_{ge_2}t_1\}. \tag{9.26}$$

Again, the first and fourth terms are responsible for quantum beats of the cross-peak at $\omega_\tau = \bar{\omega}_{e_2g}$ and $\omega_t = \bar{\omega}_{e_1g}$. In addition to the second term, the third term also contributes to this cross-peak because $\bar{\omega}_{fe_2} \cong \bar{\omega}_{e_1g}$. Due to the quantum beat contributions originating from the first and fourth terms, the cross-peak amplitude at $\omega_\tau = \bar{\omega}_{e_2g}$ and $\omega_t = \bar{\omega}_{e_1g}$ oscillates in time t_2, and its amplitude decays by the quantum beat dephasing process.

The next step is to obtain the expressions for the two diagonal peaks and the two cross-peaks. The short-time approximations to the nonlinear response function components that directly correspond to the above twelve diagrams can be obtained by using the results presented in Section 5.3. Then, in the impulsive limit, one can carry out the 2D Fourier-Laplace transformation of the photon echo signal field (see Equation 7.12) to obtain the 2D Gaussian shape–approximated diagonal and cross-peaks.

First of all, the two diagonal peaks at $\omega_\tau = \bar{\omega}_{e_1g}$ and $\omega_t = \bar{\omega}_{e_1g}$ and at $\omega_\tau = \bar{\omega}_{e_2g}$ and $\omega_t = \bar{\omega}_{e_2g}$ are identical to Equation 7.48 except for the center frequencies and other auxiliary functions. The diagonal peak at $\omega_\tau = \bar{\omega}_{e_1g}$ and $\omega_t = \bar{\omega}_{e_1g}$ is given as

$$\tilde{\mathbf{E}}_{D1}(\omega_t,T,\omega_\tau) = 2[\boldsymbol{\mu}_{ge_1}\boldsymbol{\mu}_{e_1g}\boldsymbol{\mu}_{ge_1}\boldsymbol{\mu}_{e_1g}]\vdots\mathbf{e}_3\mathbf{e}_2\mathbf{e}_1^*\Gamma\left(\omega_t = \bar{\omega}_{e_1g}, <\delta\Omega_1^2>, \omega_\tau = \bar{\omega}_{e_1g}, <\delta\Omega_1^2>\right) \tag{9.27}$$

where the approximate 2D Gaussian peak shape function (see Equation 7.49) is used. The two contributions in Equation 9.23 are the same in this limiting case so that the factor 2 appears in Equation 9.27. Similarly, the diagonal peak at $\omega_\tau = \bar{\omega}_{e_2g}$ and $\omega_t = \bar{\omega}_{e_2g}$ is

$$\tilde{\mathbf{E}}_{D2}(\omega_t,T,\omega_\tau) = 2[\boldsymbol{\mu}_{ge_2}\boldsymbol{\mu}_{e_2g}\boldsymbol{\mu}_{ge_2}\boldsymbol{\mu}_{e_2g}]\vdots\mathbf{e}_3\mathbf{e}_2\mathbf{e}_1^*\Gamma\left(\omega_t = \bar{\omega}_{e_2g}, <\delta\Omega_2^2>, \omega_\tau = \bar{\omega}_{e_2g}, <\delta\Omega_2^2>\right). \tag{9.28}$$

We next consider the two cross-peaks. Again, using the approximate 2D Gaussian peak shape function theory in Section 7.6, one can find that the cross-peak at $\omega_\tau = \bar{\omega}_{e_1g}$ and $\omega_t = \bar{\omega}_{e_2g}$ is given as

$$\begin{aligned}
\tilde{\mathbf{E}}_{C12}(\omega_t,T,\omega_\tau) = &[\boldsymbol{\mu}_{ge_2}\boldsymbol{\mu}_{e_1g}\boldsymbol{\mu}_{e_2g}\boldsymbol{\mu}_{ge_1}]\vdots\mathbf{e}_3\mathbf{e}_2\mathbf{e}_1^*\Gamma(\bar{\omega}_{e_2g}, <\delta\Omega_1\delta\Omega_2>, \bar{\omega}_{e_1g}, <\delta\Omega_1\delta\Omega_2>) \\
&\times \exp\{-i\bar{\omega}_{e_2e_1}T - f_{12}(T)\} \\
&+[\boldsymbol{\mu}_{ge_2}\boldsymbol{\mu}_{e_2g}\boldsymbol{\mu}_{e_1g}\boldsymbol{\mu}_{ge_1}]\vdots\mathbf{e}_3\mathbf{e}_2\mathbf{e}_1^*\Gamma\left(\bar{\omega}_{e_2g}, <\delta\Omega_2^2>, \bar{\omega}_{e_1g}, <\delta\Omega_1^2>\right) \\
&-[\boldsymbol{\mu}_{e_1f}\boldsymbol{\mu}_{fe_1}\boldsymbol{\mu}_{e_1g}\boldsymbol{\mu}_{ge_1}]\vdots\mathbf{e}_3\mathbf{e}_2\mathbf{e}_1^*\Gamma\left(\bar{\omega}_{fe_1}, <\delta\Omega_2^2>, \bar{\omega}_{e_1g}, <\delta\Omega_1^2>\right) \\
&-[\boldsymbol{\mu}_{e_1f}\boldsymbol{\mu}_{fe_2}\boldsymbol{\mu}_{e_2g}\boldsymbol{\mu}_{ge_1}]\vdots\mathbf{e}_3\mathbf{e}_2\mathbf{e}_1^*\Gamma(\bar{\omega}_{fe_1}, <\delta\Omega_1\delta\Omega_2>, \bar{\omega}_{e_1g}, <\delta\Omega_1\delta\Omega_2>) \\
&\times \exp\{-i\bar{\omega}_{e_2e_1}T - f_{12}(T)\},
\end{aligned} \tag{9.29}$$

where the relaxation of the quantum beat with frequency of $\bar{\omega}_{e_2e_1}$ is determined by $\exp\{-f_{12}(T)\}$. Here, $f_{12}(T)$ is given as

$$f_{12}(T) = g^*_{e_1e_1}(T) + g_{e_2e_2}(T) - 2\,\mathrm{Re}[g_{e_1e_2}(T)]. \tag{9.30}$$

Due to the first and fourth terms oscillating in the waiting time T, the cross-peak amplitude is modulated by these quantum beating contributions. However, it decays very rapidly. Taking the short-time approximation of $f_{12}(T)$ up to the second order with respect to T, one can find that

$$\exp\{-f_{12}(T)\} \cong \exp\left\{-\frac{1}{2}\left(<\delta\Omega_1^2> + <\delta\Omega_2^2> -2<\delta\Omega_1\delta\Omega_2>\right)T^2\right\}. \tag{9.31}$$

This is a Gaussian decay function, and it becomes vanishingly small after the chromophore-bath interaction-induced decoherence time $\tau_{decoherence}(=\sqrt{\hbar^2 \ln 2/\lambda k_B T})$ at room temperature.

By using the same procedure, one can obtain the cross-peak at $\omega_\tau = \bar{\omega}_{e_2 g}$ and $\omega_t = \bar{\omega}_{e_1 g}$,

$$\begin{aligned}\tilde{\mathbf{E}}_{C21}(\omega_t,T,\omega_\tau) = {} & [\boldsymbol{\mu}_{ge_1}\boldsymbol{\mu}_{e_2g}\boldsymbol{\mu}_{e_1g}\boldsymbol{\mu}_{ge_2}]\vdots\mathbf{e}_3\mathbf{e}_2\mathbf{e}_1^*\Gamma(\bar{\omega}_{e_1g},<\delta\Omega_1\delta\Omega_2>,\bar{\omega}_{e_2g},<\delta\Omega_1\delta\Omega_2>)\\ & \times\exp\{-i\bar{\omega}_{e_1e_2}T - f_{12}^*(T)\}\\ & +[\boldsymbol{\mu}_{ge_1}\boldsymbol{\mu}_{e_1g}\boldsymbol{\mu}_{e_2g}\boldsymbol{\mu}_{ge_2}]\vdots\mathbf{e}_3\mathbf{e}_2\mathbf{e}_1^*\Gamma\left(\bar{\omega}_{e_1g},<\delta\Omega_1^2>,\bar{\omega}_{e_2g},<\delta\Omega_2^2>\right)\\ & -[\boldsymbol{\mu}_{e_2f}\boldsymbol{\mu}_{fe_2}\boldsymbol{\mu}_{e_2g}\boldsymbol{\mu}_{ge_2}]\vdots\mathbf{e}_3\mathbf{e}_2\mathbf{e}_1^*\Gamma\left(\bar{\omega}_{fe_2},<\delta\Omega_1^2>,\bar{\omega}_{e_2g},<\delta\Omega_2^2>\right)\\ & -[\boldsymbol{\mu}_{e_2f}\boldsymbol{\mu}_{fe_1}\boldsymbol{\mu}_{e_1g}\boldsymbol{\mu}_{ge_2}]\vdots\mathbf{e}_3\mathbf{e}_2\mathbf{e}_1^*\Gamma(\bar{\omega}_{fe_2},<\delta\Omega_1\delta\Omega_2>,\bar{\omega}_{e_2g},<\delta\Omega_1\delta\Omega_2>)\\ & \times\exp\{-i\bar{\omega}_{e_1e_2}T - f_{12}^*(T)\}.\end{aligned} \tag{9.32}$$

Again, there are two quantum beat contributions, which decay very rapidly. The second and third terms on the right-hand side of Equation 9.32 contribute to the cross-peak even after time T greater than $\tau_{decoherence}$.

From the results in Equations 9.27, 9.28, 9.29, and 9.32, the total 2D photon echo spectrum of a coupled 2LS dimer is given as

$$\tilde{\mathbf{E}}_{PE}(\omega_t,T,\omega_\tau) = \tilde{\mathbf{E}}_{D1}(\omega_t,T,\omega_\tau) + \tilde{\mathbf{E}}_{D2}(\omega_t,T,\omega_\tau) + \tilde{\mathbf{E}}_{C12}(\omega_t,T,\omega_\tau) + \tilde{\mathbf{E}}_{C21}(\omega_t,T,\omega_\tau). \tag{9.33}$$

From the resultant expressions for the two cross-peaks, one can show that they vanish when the coupling constant J is zero. In the zero coupling limit, e_1 and e_2 are completely localized states on the two chromophores separately and the f state is just a product of the two localized excited states. Then, the first term in Equation 9.29 cancels out the fourth term in the equation. Similarly, the second term in Equation 9.29 cancels out the third term. This is why the presence of cross-peaks in an experimentally measured 2D spectrum of a dimer system is critical evidence of a nonzero coupling between the two electric-dipole-allowed transitions of the individual chromophores.

For the sake of simplicity, let us consider the homodimer system with a sufficiently large coupling constant. That is to say, it is assumed that the widths of the diagonal or cross-peaks are smaller than the coupling constant J, that is,

$$J > \sqrt{<\delta\Omega^2>}. \tag{9.34}$$

In this case, the two singly excited states are frequency resolved in both 1D and 2D spectra. A schematic 2D spectrum for this strong coupling case is shown in

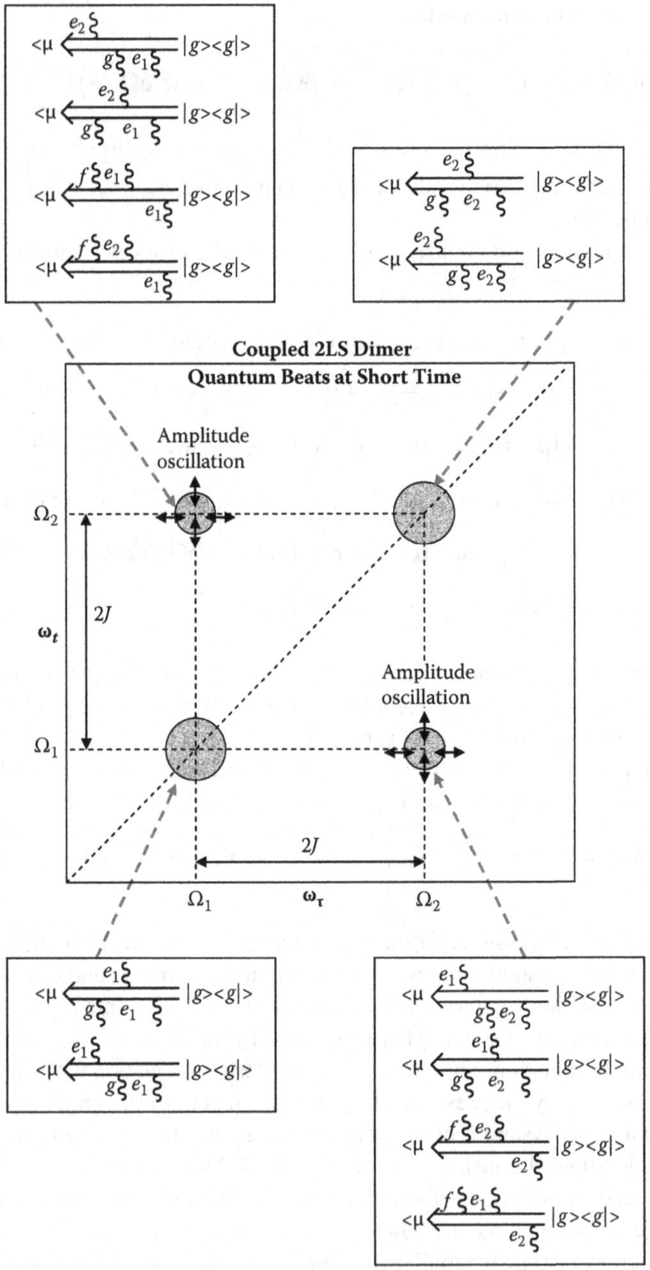

FIGURE 9.2 Quantum beat contributions to the 2D photon echo spectrum of coupled homodimer. The two diagonal peaks are separated by $2J$ in frequency. Each cross-peak is associated with four different diagrams as shown here. The cross-peak amplitudes oscillate in time T at time shorter than the system–bath interaction-induced decoherence time.

Figure 9.2, where only the real part of the 2D spectrum is depicted. The two diagonal peaks are separated by $2J$ in frequency. Two cross-peaks appear, and they oscillate in time T with frequency of $\bar{\omega}_{e_2e_1}$ (= $2J$). The associated diagrams are also shown in the figure. Analyzing the time-dependent changes of cross-peak amplitudes, one can extract information on the decoherence time.

9.4 COUPLED TWO-LEVEL SYSTEM DIMER: INTERMEDIATE TIME REGION

As shown in the previous section, the cross-peak amplitudes oscillate in time T due to the created coherence between e_1 and e_2 states. However, such quantum beats only last for a short time because the corresponding quantum beat relaxation rate given in Equation 9.31 is in general quite fast and similar to the timescale of free-induction decay. Therefore, at waiting times sufficiently longer than the quantum beat relaxation time, that is, $T > \tau_{decoherence} = \sqrt{\hbar^2 \ln 2/\lambda k_B T}$, the diagonal and cross-peaks are given as

$$\tilde{\mathbf{E}}_{D1}(\omega_t, T, \omega_\tau) = 2[\boldsymbol{\mu}_{ge_1}\boldsymbol{\mu}_{e_1g}\boldsymbol{\mu}_{ge_1}\boldsymbol{\mu}_{e_1g}] \vdots \mathbf{e}_3\mathbf{e}_2\mathbf{e}_1^*\Gamma\left(\bar{\omega}_{e_1g}, <\delta\Omega_1^2>, \bar{\omega}_{e_1g}, <\delta\Omega_1^2>\right)$$

$$\tilde{\mathbf{E}}_{D2}(\omega_t, T, \omega_\tau) = 2[\boldsymbol{\mu}_{ge_2}\boldsymbol{\mu}_{e_2g}\boldsymbol{\mu}_{ge_2}\boldsymbol{\mu}_{e_2g}] \vdots \mathbf{e}_3\mathbf{e}_2\mathbf{e}_1^*\Gamma\left(\bar{\omega}_{e_2g}, <\delta\Omega_2^2>, \bar{\omega}_{e_2g}, <\delta\Omega_2^2>\right)$$

$$\tilde{\mathbf{E}}_{C12}(\omega_t, T, \omega_\tau) = [\boldsymbol{\mu}_{ge_2}\boldsymbol{\mu}_{e_2g}\boldsymbol{\mu}_{e_1g}\boldsymbol{\mu}_{ge_1}] \vdots \mathbf{e}_3\mathbf{e}_2\mathbf{e}_1^*\Gamma\left(\bar{\omega}_{e_2g}, <\delta\Omega_2^2>, \bar{\omega}_{e_1g}, <\delta\Omega_1^2>\right)$$
$$-[\boldsymbol{\mu}_{e_1f}\boldsymbol{\mu}_{fe_1}\boldsymbol{\mu}_{e_1g}\boldsymbol{\mu}_{ge_1}] \vdots \mathbf{e}_3\mathbf{e}_2\mathbf{e}_1^*\Gamma\left(\bar{\omega}_{fe_1}, <\delta\Omega_2^2>, \bar{\omega}_{e_1g}, <\delta\Omega_1^2>\right)$$

$$\tilde{\mathbf{E}}_{C21}(\omega_t, T, \omega_\tau) = [\boldsymbol{\mu}_{ge_1}\boldsymbol{\mu}_{e_1g}\boldsymbol{\mu}_{e_2g}\boldsymbol{\mu}_{ge_2}] \vdots \mathbf{e}_3\mathbf{e}_2\mathbf{e}_1^*\Gamma\left(\bar{\omega}_{e_1g}, <\delta\Omega_1^2>, \bar{\omega}_{e_2g}, <\delta\Omega_2^2>\right)$$
$$-[\boldsymbol{\mu}_{e_2f}\boldsymbol{\mu}_{fe_2}\boldsymbol{\mu}_{e_2g}\boldsymbol{\mu}_{ge_2}] \vdots \mathbf{e}_3\mathbf{e}_2\mathbf{e}_1^*\Gamma\left(\bar{\omega}_{fe_2}, <\delta\Omega_1^2>, \bar{\omega}_{e_2g}, <\delta\Omega_2^2>\right). \quad (9.35)$$

Hereafter, let us consider the case when the three incident pulses are linearly polarized along the X-axis in a laboratory-fixed frame and when the X-component of the photon echo field vector is detected. For the sake of simplicity, assume that the two local transition dipoles d_1 and d_2 have the same magnitudes, $d = |\mathbf{d}_1| = |\mathbf{d}_2|$. Then, after performing the rotational average of the relevant fourth-rank tensor (XXXX) element, one can estimate the amplitudes $\{\hat{S}_{jk}^0\}$ of the four peaks at their maxima (or minima):

(1) Diagonal peak at ($\omega_\tau = \bar{\omega}_{e_1g}$, $\omega_t = \bar{\omega}_{e_1g}$)

$$\hat{S}_{11}^0 = \frac{2\pi}{<\delta\Omega_1^2>}\left\{2\left[\boldsymbol{\mu}_{e_1g}^4\right]_{XXXX}\right\} = \frac{2\pi d^4}{<\delta\Omega_1^2>}\{12(1+2\kappa\cos\phi)^2\}. \quad (9.36)$$

(2) Diagonal peak at ($\omega_\tau = \bar{\omega}_{e_2g}$, $\omega_t = \bar{\omega}_{e_2g}$)

$$\hat{S}_{22}^0 = \frac{2\pi}{<\delta\Omega_2^2>}\left\{2\left[\boldsymbol{\mu}_{e_2g}^4\right]_{XXXX}\right\} = \frac{2\pi d^4}{<\delta\Omega_2^2>}\{12(1-2\kappa\cos\phi)^2\}. \quad (9.37)$$

(3) Cross-peak at $(\omega_\tau = \bar{\omega}_{e_1g}, \omega_t = \bar{\omega}_{e_2g})$

$$\hat{S}^0_{12} = \frac{2\pi}{\sqrt{<\delta\Omega_1^2><\delta\Omega_2^2>}}\left\{\left[\mu^2_{e_1g}\mu^2_{e_2g}\right]_{XXXX} - [\mu_{ge_1}\mu_{e_1f}\mu_{fe_1}\mu_{e_1g}]_{XXXX}\right\}$$

$$= -\frac{2\pi d^4}{\sqrt{<\delta\Omega_1^2><\delta\Omega_2^2>}}\{8(2\kappa^2 + 3\kappa\cos\phi + 4\kappa^2\cos^2\phi)\}. \quad (9.38)$$

(4) Cross-peak at $(\omega_\tau = \bar{\omega}_{e_2g}, \omega_t = \bar{\omega}_{e_1g})$

$$\hat{S}^0_{21} = \frac{2\pi}{\sqrt{<\delta\Omega_1^2><\delta\Omega_2^2>}}\left\{\left[\mu^2_{e_2g}\mu^2_{e_1g}\right]_{XXXX} - [\mu_{ge_2}\mu_{e_2f}\mu_{fe_2}\mu_{e_2g}]_{XXXX}\right\}$$

$$= -\frac{2\pi d^4}{\sqrt{<\delta\Omega_1^2><\delta\Omega_2^2>}}\{8(2\kappa^2 - 3\kappa\cos\phi + 4\kappa^2\cos^2\phi)\}. \quad (9.39)$$

Here, κ, defined in Equation 9.17, is a measure of delocalization of excited states. ϕ is the angle between the two local transition dipoles $\mathbf{d}_1$ and $\mathbf{d}_2$ (see Figure 9.1). The highly simplified expressions given in the above can provide a guideline for the interpretation of experimentally measured amplitudes of the diagonal and cross-peaks and can be used to estimate the angle between the two local transition dipole vectors. It is again clear that, in the zero coupling case, the delocalization factor κ is zero and the cross-peak amplitudes $\hat{S}^0_{12}$ and $\hat{S}^0_{21}$ vanish. This is because e_1 and e_2 states are each completely localized on one of the chromophores so that $\mu_{e_1g} = \mathbf{d}_1$ and $\mu_{e_2g} = \mathbf{d}_2$. Then, in this zero-coupling case we have $[\mu^2_{e_1g}\mu^2_{e_2g}]_{XXXX} = [\mu_{ge_1}\mu_{e_1f}\mu_{fe_1}\mu_{e_1g}]_{XXXX}$ and $[\mu^2_{e_2g}\mu^2_{e_1g}]_{XXXX} = [\mu_{ge_2}\mu_{e_2f}\mu_{fe_2}\mu_{e_2g}]_{XXXX}$. Therefore, the two contributions exactly cancel out (destructively interfering with each other at the amplitude-level), and the cross-peaks vanish.

If we further assume that the two chromophores are identical, that is, a homodimer, the delocalization factor κ is 0.5 and the peak amplitudes are simplified as

$$\hat{S}^0_{11} = \frac{24\pi\,|d|^4}{<\delta\Omega_1^2>}(1+\cos\phi)^2$$

$$\hat{S}^0_{22} = \frac{24\pi\,|d|^4}{<\delta\Omega_2^2>}(1-\cos\phi)^2$$

$$\hat{S}^0_{12} = -\frac{8\pi\,|d|^4}{\sqrt{<\delta\Omega_1^2><\delta\Omega_2^2>}}(\cos\phi+1)(2\cos\phi+1)$$

$$\hat{S}^0_{21} = -\frac{8\pi\,|d|^4}{\sqrt{<\delta\Omega_1^2><\delta\Omega_2^2>}}(\cos\phi-1)(2\cos\phi-1). \quad (9.40)$$

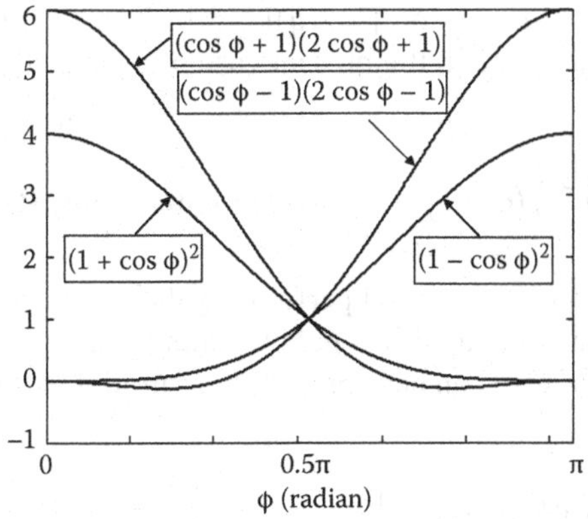

FIGURE 9.3 The ϕ-dependent functions in Equation 9.40.

In Figure 9.3, the ϕ-dependent functions in Equation 9.40 are plotted. When the two local transition dipole vectors are parallel to each other, that is, $\phi = 0$, then $\widehat{S}_{22}^0 = \widehat{S}_{21}^0 = 0$. If the two vectors are antiparallel, then $\widehat{S}_{11}^0 = \widehat{S}_{12}^0 = 0$. If the two local transition dipole vectors are perpendicular to each other, we have $\widehat{S}_{11}^0 = \widehat{S}_{22}^0$ and $\widehat{S}_{12}^0 = \widehat{S}_{21}^0$. Therefore, the relative orientations of the two chromophores can be estimated by analyzing the diagonal and cross-peak amplitudes with the results in Equation 9.40.

9.5 COUPLED TWO-LEVEL SYSTEM DIMER: POPULATION TRANSFER EFFECTS

In this section we will consider the population transfer effects on the 2D PE spectrum of a coupled 2LS dimer system. As can be seen in Equation 9.13, the transformed chromophore–bath interaction Hamiltonian is not completely diagonalized, and the off-diagonal matrix elements of $\tilde{\Xi}_{SB}^{(1)}(\mathbf{q})$ are

$$\left[\tilde{\Xi}_{SB}^{(1)}(\mathbf{q})\right]_{12} = \left[\tilde{\Xi}_{SB}^{(1)}(\mathbf{q})\right]_{21} = (x_2 - x_1)\kappa + x_c \cos 2\theta. \tag{9.41}$$

Therefore, population transfer processes between the two singly excited states occur, and the 2D peak shape thus changes in time T. Treating $[\tilde{\Xi}_{SB}^{(1)}(\mathbf{q})]_{12}$ as the perturbation Hamiltonian and using second-order perturbation theory, that is, Fermi's golden rule,[16] one can obtain an expression for the population transfer rate constant and the relevant quantum Master equation (see Section 8.7).

The second-order population transfer rate constant from the jth excited state to the kth state was shown to be (see Equation 8.56)

$$K_{kj} = 2\,\mathrm{Re}\int_0^\infty dt \; < \left[\tilde{\Xi}_{SB}^{(1)}(\mathbf{q}(t))\right]_{jk} \left[\tilde{\Xi}_{SB}^{(1)}(\mathbf{q}(0))\right]_{kj} >_B \exp\{-i\bar{\omega}_{kj}t\}. \tag{9.42}$$

The time-correlation function of $[\tilde{\Xi}_{SB}^{(1)}(\mathbf{q})]_{12}$, which is required to complete the calculation of Equation 9.42 in the present case of a coupled 2LS dimer, is found to be

$$< \left[\tilde{\Xi}_{SB}^{(1)}(\mathbf{q}(t))\right]_{12} \left[\tilde{\Xi}_{SB}^{(1)}(\mathbf{q}(0))\right]_{21} >_B = \{C_1(t) + C_2(t)\}\kappa^2 + C_c(t)\cos^2 2\theta. \tag{9.43}$$

Inserting Equation 9.43 into 9.42 and performing the integration over time, one can obtain the two (downhill and uphill) population transfer rate constants. Since the real and imaginary parts of $C_j(t)$ can be expressed in terms of the corresponding spectral density, we get

$$K_{12} = \pi |\bar{\omega}_{12}|^2 \left\{\coth\left(\frac{\beta\hbar|\bar{\omega}_{12}|}{2}\right) + 1\right\}\left\{[\rho_1(|\bar{\omega}_{12}|) + \rho_2(|\bar{\omega}_{12}|)]\kappa^2 + \rho_c(|\bar{\omega}_{12}|)\cos^2 2\theta\right\} \tag{9.44}$$

$$K_{21} = \pi |\bar{\omega}_{21}|^2 \left\{\coth\left(\frac{\beta\hbar|\bar{\omega}_{21}|}{2}\right) - 1\right\}\left\{[\rho_1(|\bar{\omega}_{21}|) + \rho_2(|\bar{\omega}_{21}|)]\kappa^2 + \rho_c(|\bar{\omega}_{21}|)\cos^2 2\theta\right\}. \tag{9.45}$$

The resultant expressions for the rate constants obey the detailed balance condition as

$$\frac{K_{21}}{K_{12}} = \frac{\coth\left(\frac{\beta\hbar|\bar{\omega}_{12}|}{2}\right) - 1}{\coth\left(\frac{\beta\hbar|\bar{\omega}_{12}|}{2}\right) + 1} = \exp(-\hbar|\bar{\omega}_{12}|/k_B T). \tag{9.46}$$

For an N-state system, the conditional probability, $G_{kj}(t)$, for the population to be in a specific state $|k>$ at time t, provided that it was at state $|j>$ at $t = 0$ for an arbitrary pair of j and k, can be obtained by solving the following master equation (see Equation 8.53):

$$\dot{G}_{kj}(t) = \sum_{l \neq k} K_{kl} G_{lj}(t) - \left(\sum_{l \neq k} K_{lk}\right) G_{kj}(t). \tag{9.47}$$

This coupled linear differential equation can be solved by using the Laplace transform method. Denoting the Laplace transform of $G_{kj}(t)$ as $\tilde{G}_{kj}(s)$, one can rewrite the above initial value problem as

$$s\underline{\tilde{G}}(s) + \underline{K}\underline{\tilde{G}}(s) = \underline{I} \tag{9.48}$$

where the underlines in the above equation mean that they are the N by N matrices and $\underline{I}$ is the identity matrix. The $[j,k]$th matrix element of $\underline{\tilde{G}}(s)$ is $\tilde{G}_{jk}(s)$. Diagonalizing the rate constant matrix $\underline{K}$ as

$$\underline{V}^{-1}\underline{K}\underline{V} = \underline{\Lambda} = \begin{pmatrix} \lambda_1 & 0 & \cdots & 0 \\ 0 & \lambda_2 & \cdots & 0 \\ \vdots & \vdots & \ddots & \vdots \\ 0 & 0 & \cdots & \lambda_N \end{pmatrix}, \tag{9.49}$$

one can solve Equation 9.47 for the conditional probabilities by taking the inverse Laplace transformation of Equation 9.48 to find

$$\underline{G}(t) = \underline{V} \begin{pmatrix} e^{-\lambda_1 t} & 0 & \cdots & 0 \\ 0 & e^{-\lambda_2 t} & \cdots & 0 \\ \vdots & \vdots & \ddots & \vdots \\ 0 & 0 & \cdots & e^{-\lambda_N t} \end{pmatrix} \underline{V}^{-1}. \tag{9.50}$$

Now, for the two-state system consisting of e_1 and e_2, the rate constant matrix $\underline{K}$ is simply given as

$$\underline{K} = \begin{pmatrix} K_{21} & -K_{12} \\ -K_{21} & K_{12} \end{pmatrix}. \tag{9.51}$$

Two eigenvalues of this rate constant matrix are 0 and $K_{12} + K_{21}$, and the respective eigenvectors are

$$\begin{pmatrix} \dfrac{K_{12}}{\sqrt{K_{21}^2 + K_{12}^2}} \\ \dfrac{K_{21}}{\sqrt{K_{21}^2 + K_{12}^2}} \end{pmatrix} \text{ and } \begin{pmatrix} -\dfrac{1}{\sqrt{2}} \\ \dfrac{1}{\sqrt{2}} \end{pmatrix}. \tag{9.52}$$

From these results, one can find that the survival and conditional probability functions are

$$G_{11}(t) = \frac{K_{12} + K_{21}\exp\{-(K_{21} + K_{12})t\}}{K_{21} + K_{12}}$$

$$G_{22}(t) = \frac{K_{21} + K_{12}\exp\{-(K_{21} + K_{12})t\}}{K_{21} + K_{12}}$$

$$G_{21}(t) = \frac{K_{21}[1 - \exp\{-(K_{21} + K_{12})t\}]}{K_{21} + K_{12}}$$

$$G_{12}(t) = \frac{K_{12}[1 - \exp\{-(K_{21} + K_{12})t\}]}{K_{21} + K_{12}}. \tag{9.53}$$

Here, the diagonal matrix elements of $\underline{G}(t)$ are usually called the survival probability. For instance, $G_{11}(t)$ is the probability of finding the system to be in e_1 state at time t later when the system was in the same state at time zero.

Now, due to population transfer between the two singly excited states during the waiting time T, the diagonal and cross-peak amplitudes would change in time. Since the population transfer process is comparatively slower than the decoherence timescale, $\tau_{decoherence}$, those diagrams involving quantum beating terms will be ignored. Then, among the remaining eight diagrams in Equations 9.23–9.26, only four of them are stimulated emission contributions that involve population evolution on one of the two singly excited states during time T. Therefore, the population transfers during T affect those four cases. As an example, let us consider the following diagram, which is the first one in Equation 9.23:

$<\mu$ 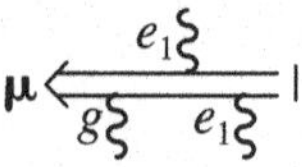

$|g><g|>.$ (9.54)

When there is no population transfer from e_1 to e_2 states within the time delay T, the above diagram contributes to the diagonal peak at $\omega_\tau = \bar{\omega}_{e_1g}$ and $\omega_t = \bar{\omega}_{e_1g}$. However, when the population relaxation time is fast in comparison with the excited-state lifetime, the population on the e_1 state created at $t = t_1$ can end up at the e_2 population or remain at the e_1 population. Such a probability is fully described by the conditional probability matrix $\underline{G}(t)$ discussed above. Therefore, the diagram shown in Equation 9.54 should be rewritten as the sum of two contributions as

$G_{21}(T) <\mu$ 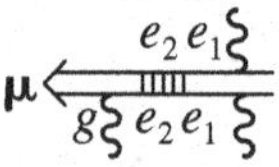

$|g><g|> \quad \propto \exp\{-i\bar{\omega}_{e_2g}t_3 - i\bar{\omega}_{ge_1}t_1\}$ (9.55)

$G_{11}(T) <\mu$ 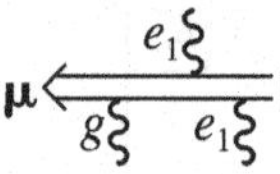

$|g><g|> \quad \propto \exp\{-i\bar{\omega}_{e_1g}t_3 - i\bar{\omega}_{ge_1}t_1\}.$ (9.56)

The first one describes the population transfer from e_1 to e_2 states during T so that the conditional probability $G_{21}(T)$ multiplies the third-order polarization. Furthermore, the coherence oscillation term is given as $\exp\{-i\bar{\omega}_{e_2g}t_3 - i\bar{\omega}_{ge_1}t_1\}$ so that this diagram will contribute to the cross-peak at $\omega_\tau = \bar{\omega}_{e_1g}$ and $\omega_t = \bar{\omega}_{e_2g}$. Consequently, the corresponding cross-peak amplitude will change (increase) due to this additional contribution originating from the population transfer from e_1 to e_2 states. The second diagram in Equation 9.56 is the case where the initially created population on e_1 remains on e_1 even after finite time T. Therefore, the conditional probability (or survival probability) $G_{11}(T)$ multiplies the third-order polarization. This term contributes to the diagonal peak at $\omega_\tau = \bar{\omega}_{e_1g}$ and $\omega_t = \bar{\omega}_{e_1g}$. Overall, the cross-peak amplitude increases, and the corresponding diagonal peak amplitude decreases because of the population transfer.

Taking into consideration the population transfer processes, we find that the diagrams associated with the diagonal and cross-peaks are fully given as

(1) Diagonal peak at $(\omega_\tau = \bar{\omega}_{e_1g},\ \omega_t = \bar{\omega}_{e_1g})$

$$G_{11}(T) < \mu \xleftarrow[g\xi\quad e_1\xi]{e_1\xi} |g><g|>$$

$$< \mu \xleftarrow[g\xi e_1\xi]{e_1\xi} |g><g|>$$

$$G_{21}(T) < \mu \xleftarrow[e_2e_1\xi]{f\xi e_2 e_1\xi} |g><g|> \qquad (9.57)$$

(2) Diagonal peak at $(\omega_\tau = \bar{\omega}_{e_2g},\ \omega_t = \bar{\omega}_{e_2g})$

$$G_{22}(T) < \mu \xleftarrow[g\xi\quad e_2\xi]{e_2\xi} |g><g|>$$

$$< \mu \xleftarrow[g\xi e_2\xi]{e_2\xi} |g><g|>$$

$$G_{12}(T) < \mu \xleftarrow[e_1 e_2\xi]{f\xi e_1 e_2\xi} |g><g|> \qquad (9.58)$$

(3) Cross-peak at $(\omega_\tau = \bar{\omega}_{e_1g},\ \omega_t = \bar{\omega}_{e_2g})$

$$< \mu \xleftarrow[g\xi e_1\xi]{e_2\xi} |g><g|>$$

$$G_{11}(T) < \mu \xleftarrow[e_1\xi]{f\xi e_1\xi} |g><g|>$$

$$G_{21}(T) < \mu \xleftarrow[g\xi e_2 e_1\xi]{e_2 e_1\xi} |g><g|> \qquad (9.59)$$

(4) Cross-peak at $(\omega_\tau = \bar{\omega}_{e_2g},\ \omega_t = \bar{\omega}_{e_1g})$

$$< \mu \xleftarrow[g\xi e_2\xi]{e_1\xi} |g><g|>$$

$$G_{22}(T) < \mu \xleftarrow[e_2\xi]{f\xi e_2\xi} |g><g|>$$

$$G_{12}(T) < \mu \xleftarrow[g\xi e_1 e_2\xi]{e_1 e_2\xi} |g><g|> \qquad (9.60)$$

Then, by using the short-time approximation to the nonlinear response function and 2D Gaussian peak shape function approximation, it is possible to obtain the 2D

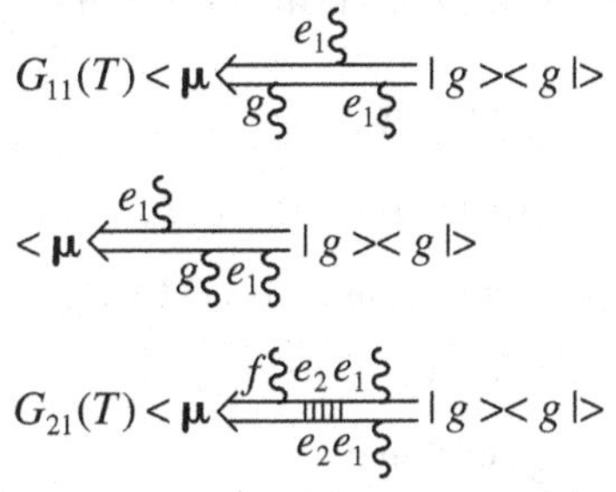

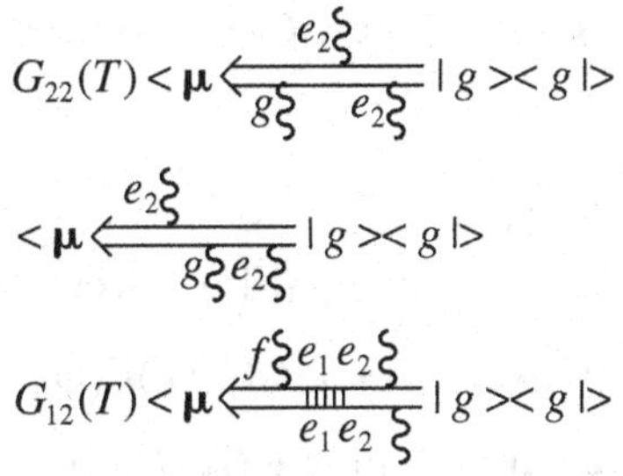

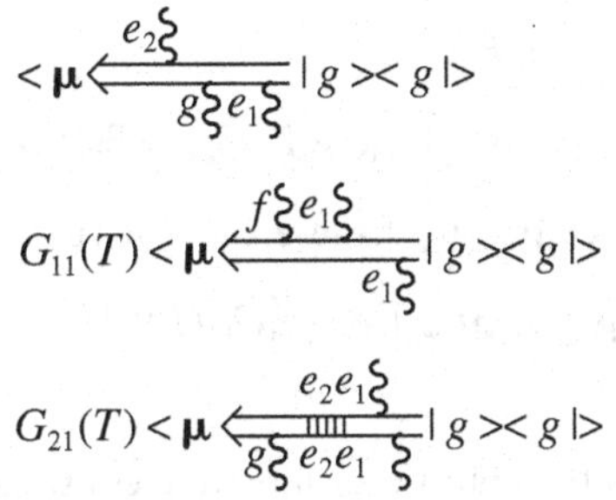

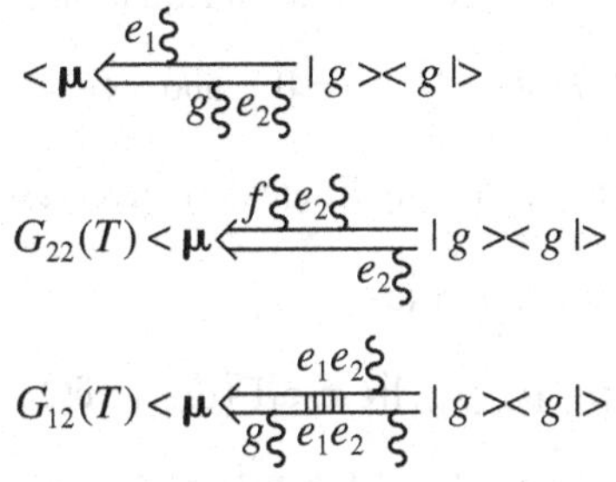

photon echo spectrum of a coupled 2LS dimer undergoing population transfer between two singly excited states. For the diagonal and cross-peaks, we have

(1) Diagonal peak at $(\omega_\tau = \bar{\omega}_{e_1g}, \omega_t = \bar{\omega}_{e_1g})$

$$\tilde{\mathbf{E}}_{D1}(\omega_t,T,\omega_\tau) = [\boldsymbol{\mu}_{ge_1}\boldsymbol{\mu}_{e_1g}\boldsymbol{\mu}_{e_1g}\boldsymbol{\mu}_{ge_1}]\vdots\mathbf{e}_3\mathbf{e}_2\mathbf{e}_1^*\{1+G_{11}(T)\}\Gamma\left(\bar{\omega}_{e_1g},<\delta\Omega_1^2>,\bar{\omega}_{e_1g},<\delta\Omega_1^2>\right)$$
$$-[\boldsymbol{\mu}_{e_2f}\boldsymbol{\mu}_{fe_2}\boldsymbol{\mu}_{e_1g}\boldsymbol{\mu}_{ge_1}]\vdots\mathbf{e}_3\mathbf{e}_2\mathbf{e}_1^*G_{21}(T)\Gamma\left(\bar{\omega}_{fe_2},<\delta\Omega_1^2>,\bar{\omega}_{e_1g},<\delta\Omega_1^2>\right) \tag{9.61}$$

(2) Diagonal peak at $(\omega_\tau = \bar{\omega}_{e_2g}, \omega_t = \bar{\omega}_{e_2g})$

$$\tilde{\mathbf{E}}_{D2}(\omega_t,T,\omega_\tau) = [\boldsymbol{\mu}_{ge_2}\boldsymbol{\mu}_{e_2g}\boldsymbol{\mu}_{e_2g}\boldsymbol{\mu}_{ge_2}]\vdots\mathbf{e}_3\mathbf{e}_2\mathbf{e}_1^*\{1+G_{22}(T)\}\Gamma\left(\bar{\omega}_{e_2g},<\delta\Omega_2^2>,\bar{\omega}_{e_2g},<\delta\Omega_2^2>\right)$$
$$-[\boldsymbol{\mu}_{e_1f}\boldsymbol{\mu}_{fe_1}\boldsymbol{\mu}_{e_2g}\boldsymbol{\mu}_{ge_2}]\vdots\mathbf{e}_3\mathbf{e}_2\mathbf{e}_1^*G_{12}(T)\Gamma\left(\bar{\omega}_{fe_1},<\delta\Omega_2^2>,\bar{\omega}_{e_2g},<\delta\Omega_2^2>\right) \tag{9.62}$$

(3) Cross-peak at $(\omega_\tau = \bar{\omega}_{e_1g}, \omega_t = \bar{\omega}_{e_2g})$

$$\tilde{\mathbf{E}}_{C12}(\omega_t,T,\omega_\tau) = [\boldsymbol{\mu}_{ge_2}\boldsymbol{\mu}_{e_2g}\boldsymbol{\mu}_{e_1g}\boldsymbol{\mu}_{ge_1}]\vdots\mathbf{e}_3\mathbf{e}_2\mathbf{e}_1^*\Gamma\left(\bar{\omega}_{e_2g},<\delta\Omega_2^2>,\bar{\omega}_{e_1g},<\delta\Omega_1^2>\right)$$
$$-[\boldsymbol{\mu}_{e_1f}\boldsymbol{\mu}_{fe_1}\boldsymbol{\mu}_{e_1g}\boldsymbol{\mu}_{ge_1}]\vdots\mathbf{e}_3\mathbf{e}_2\mathbf{e}_1^*G_{11}(T)\Gamma\left(\bar{\omega}_{fe_1},<\delta\Omega_2^2>,\bar{\omega}_{e_1g},<\delta\Omega_1^2>\right)$$
$$+[\boldsymbol{\mu}_{ge_2}\boldsymbol{\mu}_{e_2g}\boldsymbol{\mu}_{e_1g}\boldsymbol{\mu}_{ge_1}]\vdots\mathbf{e}_3\mathbf{e}_2\mathbf{e}_1^*G_{21}(T)\Gamma\left(\bar{\omega}_{e_2g},<\delta\Omega_2^2>,\bar{\omega}_{e_1g},<\delta\Omega_1^2>\right) \tag{9.63}$$

(4) Cross-peak at $(\omega_\tau = \bar{\omega}_{e_2g}, \omega_t = \bar{\omega}_{e_1g})$

$$\tilde{\mathbf{E}}_{C21}(\omega_t,T,\omega_\tau) = [\boldsymbol{\mu}_{ge_1}\boldsymbol{\mu}_{e_1g}\boldsymbol{\mu}_{e_2g}\boldsymbol{\mu}_{ge_2}]\vdots\mathbf{e}_3\mathbf{e}_2\mathbf{e}_1^*\Gamma\left(\bar{\omega}_{e_1g},<\delta\Omega_1^2>,\bar{\omega}_{e_2g},<\delta\Omega_2^2>\right)$$
$$-[\boldsymbol{\mu}_{e_2f}\boldsymbol{\mu}_{fe_2}\boldsymbol{\mu}_{e_2g}\boldsymbol{\mu}_{ge_2}]\vdots\mathbf{e}_3\mathbf{e}_2\mathbf{e}_1^*G_{22}(T)\Gamma\left(\bar{\omega}_{fe_2},<\delta\Omega_1^2>,\bar{\omega}_{e_2g},<\delta\Omega_2^2>\right)$$
$$+[\boldsymbol{\mu}_{ge_1}\boldsymbol{\mu}_{e_1g}\boldsymbol{\mu}_{e_2g}\boldsymbol{\mu}_{ge_2}]\vdots\mathbf{e}_3\mathbf{e}_2\mathbf{e}_1^*G_{12}(T)\Gamma\left(\bar{\omega}_{e_1g},<\delta\Omega_1^2>,\bar{\omega}_{e_2g},<\delta\Omega_2^2>\right). \tag{9.64}$$

In the limiting case when the uphill transition rate constant K_{21} is negligibly small, that is to say, if the energy difference between e_1 and e_2 states is much larger than the thermal energy, the conditional probabilities in Equation 9.53 are simplified as

$$G_{11}(t) \cong 1, \quad G_{22}(t) = \exp(-K_{12}t), \quad G_{21}(t) = 0, \quad \text{and} \quad G_{12}(t) = 1-\exp(-K_{12}t). \tag{9.65}$$

Then, the diagonal and cross-peak amplitudes are given as

(1) Diagonal peak at $(\omega_\tau = \bar{\omega}_{e_1g}, \omega_t = \bar{\omega}_{e_1g})$

$$\tilde{\mathbf{E}}_{D1}(\omega_t,T,\omega_\tau) = 2[\boldsymbol{\mu}_{ge_1}\boldsymbol{\mu}_{e_1g}\boldsymbol{\mu}_{e_1g}\boldsymbol{\mu}_{ge_1}]\vdots\mathbf{e}_3\mathbf{e}_2\mathbf{e}_1^*\Gamma\left(\bar{\omega}_{e_1g},<\delta\Omega_1^2>,\bar{\omega}_{e_1g},<\delta\Omega_1^2>\right)$$
$$-[\boldsymbol{\mu}_{e_2f}\boldsymbol{\mu}_{fe_2}\boldsymbol{\mu}_{e_1g}\boldsymbol{\mu}_{ge_1}]\vdots\mathbf{e}_3\mathbf{e}_2\mathbf{e}_1^*\{1-\exp(-K_{12}t)\}$$
$$\times\Gamma\left(\bar{\omega}_{fe_2},<\delta\Omega_1^2>,\bar{\omega}_{e_1g},<\delta\Omega_1^2>\right) \tag{9.66}$$

(2) Diagonal peak at $(\omega_\tau = \bar{\omega}_{e_2g}, \omega_t = \bar{\omega}_{e_2g})$

$$\tilde{\mathbf{E}}_{D2}(\omega_t, T, \omega_\tau) = [\boldsymbol{\mu}_{ge_2}\boldsymbol{\mu}_{e_2g}\boldsymbol{\mu}_{e_2g}\boldsymbol{\mu}_{ge_2}] \vdots \mathbf{e}_3\mathbf{e}_2\mathbf{e}_1^*\{1+\exp(-K_{12}t)\}$$
$$\times\Gamma\left(\bar{\omega}_{e_2g}, <\delta\Omega_2^2>, \bar{\omega}_{e_2g}, <\delta\Omega_2^2>\right)$$
$$-[\boldsymbol{\mu}_{e_1f}\boldsymbol{\mu}_{fe_1}\boldsymbol{\mu}_{e_2g}\boldsymbol{\mu}_{ge_2}] \vdots \mathbf{e}_3\mathbf{e}_2\mathbf{e}_1^*\{1-\exp(-K_{12}t)\}$$
$$\times\Gamma\left(\bar{\omega}_{fe_1}, <\delta\Omega_2^2>, \bar{\omega}_{e_2g}, <\delta\Omega_2^2>\right) \tag{9.67}$$

(3) Cross-peak at $(\omega_\tau = \bar{\omega}_{e_1g}, \omega_t = \bar{\omega}_{e_2g})$

$$\tilde{\mathbf{E}}_{C12}(\omega_t, T, \omega_\tau) = [\boldsymbol{\mu}_{ge_2}\boldsymbol{\mu}_{e_2g}\boldsymbol{\mu}_{e_1g}\boldsymbol{\mu}_{ge_1}] \vdots \mathbf{e}_3\mathbf{e}_2\mathbf{e}_1^*\Gamma\left(\bar{\omega}_{e_2g}, <\delta\Omega_2^2>, \bar{\omega}_{e_1g}, <\delta\Omega_1^2>\right)$$
$$-[\boldsymbol{\mu}_{e_1f}\boldsymbol{\mu}_{fe_1}\boldsymbol{\mu}_{e_1g}\boldsymbol{\mu}_{ge_1}] \vdots \mathbf{e}_3\mathbf{e}_2\mathbf{e}_1^*\Gamma\left(\bar{\omega}_{fe_1}, <\delta\Omega_2^2>, \bar{\omega}_{e_1g}, <\delta\Omega_1^2>\right) \tag{9.68}$$

(4) Cross-peak at $(\omega_\tau = \bar{\omega}_{e_2g}, \omega_t = \bar{\omega}_{e_1g})$

$$\tilde{\mathbf{E}}_{C21}(\omega_t, T, \omega_\tau) = [\boldsymbol{\mu}_{ge_1}\boldsymbol{\mu}_{e_1g}\boldsymbol{\mu}_{e_2g}\boldsymbol{\mu}_{ge_2}] \vdots \mathbf{e}_3\mathbf{e}_2\mathbf{e}_1^*\Gamma\left(\bar{\omega}_{e_1g}, <\delta\Omega_1^2>, \bar{\omega}_{e_2g}, <\delta\Omega_2^2>\right)$$
$$-[\boldsymbol{\mu}_{e_2f}\boldsymbol{\mu}_{fe_2}\boldsymbol{\mu}_{e_2g}\boldsymbol{\mu}_{ge_2}] \vdots \mathbf{e}_3\mathbf{e}_2\mathbf{e}_1^*\exp(-K_{12}t)$$
$$\times\Gamma\left(\bar{\omega}_{fe_2}, <\delta\Omega_1^2>, \bar{\omega}_{e_2g}, <\delta\Omega_2^2>\right)$$
$$+[\boldsymbol{\mu}_{ge_1}\boldsymbol{\mu}_{e_1g}\boldsymbol{\mu}_{e_2g}\boldsymbol{\mu}_{ge_2}] \vdots \mathbf{e}_3\mathbf{e}_2\mathbf{e}_1^*\{1-\exp(-K_{12}t)\}$$
$$\times\Gamma\left(\bar{\omega}_{e_1g}, <\delta\Omega_1^2>, \bar{\omega}_{e_2g}, <\delta\Omega_2^2>\right). \tag{9.69}$$

These results show that the two diagonal peak amplitudes decrease due to the additional excited-state absorption contributions specified by the second terms in Equations 9.66 and 9.67. The cross-peak at $\omega_\tau = \bar{\omega}_{e_1g}$ and $\omega_t = \bar{\omega}_{e_2g}$ remains the same, whereas that at $\omega_\tau = \bar{\omega}_{e_2g}$ and $\omega_t = \bar{\omega}_{e_1g}$ increases due to the population transition from the upper state e_2 to the lower state e_1. In this limiting case of downhill-only population transfer, the real part of the 2D spectrum is schematically drawn in Figure 9.4. The upper-right diagonal peak amplitude associated with the higher-lying e_2 state decays in time due to population transfer from the e_2 to the e_1 state, whereas the lower-right cross-peak amplitude increases in time T. The two peaks at $\omega_\tau = \bar{\omega}_{e_1g}$ do not change much.

Using the general results presented in this chapter, one can experimentally study quantum beat, coupling, and population transfer processes as well as extract information on the molecular structure of the dimer, such as the relative orientation of the two monomers and the intermolecular interaction strength.

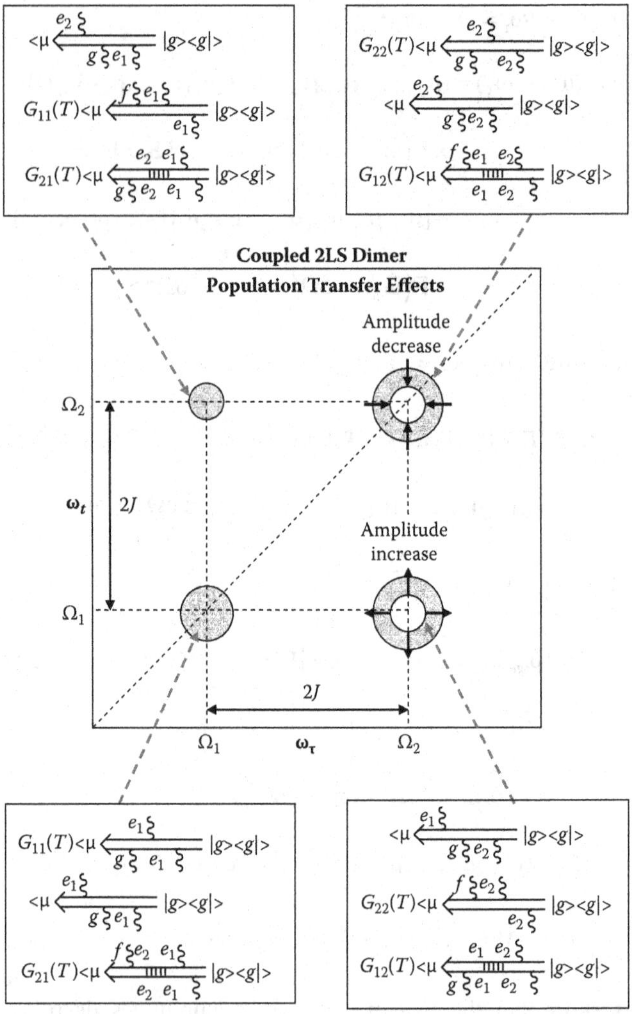

FIGURE 9.4 Population transfer effects on 2D photon echo spectrum of coupled 2LS system. In the limiting case when the uphill population transfer rate is negligibly smaller than the downhill transfer rate, the upper diagonal peak amplitude decreases and the lower-right cross-peak amplitude increases due to population transfer.

9.6 COUPLED ANHARMONIC OSCILLATORS: MODEL HAMILTONIAN

Two-dimensional IR photon echo spectroscopy has been widely used to study *vibrational* couplings between two different amide I local oscillators and eventually to determine peptide conformations and dynamics by examining the 2D peak shape changes with respect to the waiting time T. Unlike the electronic chromophore, the vibrational degrees of freedom should be modeled as a 3LS consisting of the ground,

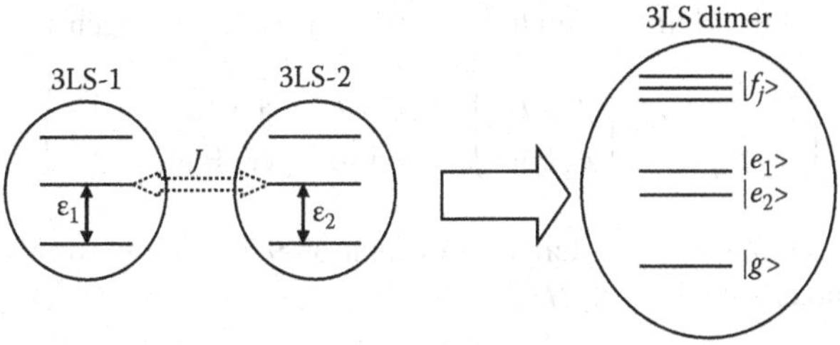

FIGURE 9.5 Coupled anharmonic oscillators. The coupling constant is J. Each anharmonic oscillator is assumed to be a 3LS. Then, the coupled anharmonic oscillators form two singly excited states (e_1 and e_2) and three doubly excited states ($f_1 \sim f_3$).

first excited, and overtone states. When such three-level oscillators are coupled to each other, it is necessary to consider at least six vibrational quantum states (see Figure 9.5). The two singly excited states e_1 and e_2 are delocalized over the two oscillators. The three doubly excited states denoted as f_j in Figure 9.5 are combination and overtone states and are also delocalized over the two oscillators due to nonzero coupling constant J. The model Hamiltonian for this coupled oscillator system is

$$H_0 = \sum_{m=1}^{2} \hbar\omega_m a_m^\dagger a_m + \hbar J\{a_1^\dagger a_2 + a_2^\dagger a_1\} + \hbar\Delta_{11} a_1^\dagger a_1^\dagger a_1 a_1 + \hbar\Delta_{22} a_2^\dagger a_2^\dagger a_2 a_2$$
$$+ 2\hbar\Delta_{12} a_1^\dagger a_2^\dagger a_1 a_2 + H_B. \tag{9.70}$$

Here, $\omega_m (= \varepsilon_m/\hbar)$ is the vibrational frequency of the mth oscillator, and J is the coupling constant. The two overtone anharmonic frequency shifts are denoted as Δ_{mm}, and the combination anharmonic frequency shift as Δ_{12}. The chromophore–bath interaction Hamiltonian is again assumed to be

$$H_{SB} = \hbar x_1(\mathbf{q}) a_1^\dagger a_1 + \hbar x_2(\mathbf{q}) a_2^\dagger a_2 + \hbar x_c(\mathbf{q})\{a_1^\dagger a_2 + a_2^\dagger a_1\}. \tag{9.71}$$

The singly excited states can be described by the following Hamiltonian matrix, when the two basis states are $a_1^\dagger |0>$ and $a_2^\dagger |0>$:

$$\tilde{H}_0^{(1)} = \hbar \begin{bmatrix} \omega_1 & J \\ J & \omega_2 \end{bmatrix}. \tag{9.72}$$

Next, the Hamiltonian matrix of the doubly excited states with the basis set $\{|2,0> = a_1^\dagger a_1^\dagger |0>, |0,2> = a_2^\dagger a_2^\dagger |0>, |1,1> = a_1^\dagger a_2^\dagger |0>\}$ is

$$\tilde{H}_0^{(2)} = \hbar \begin{bmatrix} 2\omega_1 - \Delta_{11} & 0 & \sqrt{2}J \\ 0 & 2\omega_2 - \Delta_{22} & \sqrt{2}J \\ \sqrt{2}J & \sqrt{2}J & \omega_1 + \omega_2 - \Delta_{12} \end{bmatrix}. \tag{9.73}$$

Diagonalization of the Hamiltonian matrix, $\tilde{H}_0^{(1)}$, gives the two eigenstates e_1 and e_2,

$$\begin{pmatrix} |e_1> \\ |e_2> \end{pmatrix} = U^{-1}\begin{pmatrix} a_1^\dagger|0> \\ a_2^\dagger|0> \end{pmatrix} = \begin{pmatrix} \cos\theta & \sin\theta \\ -\sin\theta & \cos\theta \end{pmatrix}\begin{pmatrix} a_1^\dagger|0> \\ a_2^\dagger|0> \end{pmatrix}. \tag{9.74}$$

Here, the mixing angle θ was defined in Equation 9.5. The two singly excited-state energies are the eigenvalues of $\tilde{H}_0^{(1)}$:

$$\begin{aligned} \hbar\Omega_1 &= \varepsilon_1\cos^2\theta + \varepsilon_2\sin^2\theta + 2J\cos\theta\sin\theta \\ \hbar\Omega_2 &= \varepsilon_1\sin^2\theta + \varepsilon_2\cos^2\theta - 2J\cos\theta\sin\theta. \end{aligned} \tag{9.75}$$

Unlike the case of the coupled 2LS dimer, there are three doubly excited states $f_1 - f_3$, which are eigenstates of $\tilde{H}_0^{(2)}$ in Equation (9.73). The elements of the jth eigenstate f_j will be denoted as c_{j1} , c_{j2}, and c_{j3}, that is,

$$\begin{pmatrix} |f_1> \\ |f_2> \\ |f_3> \end{pmatrix} = V^{-1}\begin{pmatrix} |2,0> \\ |0,2> \\ |1,1> \end{pmatrix} = \begin{pmatrix} c_{11} & c_{12} & c_{13} \\ c_{21} & c_{22} & c_{23} \\ c_{31} & c_{32} & c_{33} \end{pmatrix}\begin{pmatrix} |2,0> \\ |0,2> \\ |1,1> \end{pmatrix}. \tag{9.76}$$

The eigenvalues of $\tilde{H}_0^{(2)}$ will be denoted as $\hbar W_j$ $(j = 1 - 3)$.

With the basis sets for the singly and doubly excited states, the system–bath interaction Hamiltonian matrices $H_{SB}^{(1)}$ and $H_{SB}^{(2)}$ are

$$\tilde{H}_{SB}^{(1)}(\mathbf{q}) = \hbar\begin{bmatrix} x_1(\mathbf{q}) & x_c(\mathbf{q}) \\ x_c(\mathbf{q}) & x_2(\mathbf{q}) \end{bmatrix} \tag{9.77}$$

$$\tilde{H}_{SB}^{(2)}(\mathbf{q}) = \hbar\begin{bmatrix} 2x_1(\mathbf{q}) & 0 & \sqrt{2}x_c(\mathbf{q}) \\ 0 & 2x_2(\mathbf{q}) & \sqrt{2}x_c(\mathbf{q}) \\ \sqrt{2}x_c(\mathbf{q}) & \sqrt{2}x_c(\mathbf{q}) & x_1(\mathbf{q}) + x_2(\mathbf{q}) \end{bmatrix}. \tag{9.78}$$

Then, the transformed system–bath interaction Hamiltonian matrixes can be obtained by using the general results in Equations 8.13 and 8.14. The fluctuating parts of the transition frequencies of the e_1 and e_2 states are

$$\begin{aligned} \delta\Omega_1(\mathbf{q}) &= (x_1\cos^2\theta + x_2\sin^2\theta + 2x_c\cos\theta\sin\theta)/\hbar \\ \delta\Omega_2(\mathbf{q}) &= (x_1\sin^2\theta + x_2\cos^2\theta - 2x_c\cos\theta\sin\theta)/\hbar. \end{aligned} \tag{9.79}$$

Those of the three doubly excited states, denoted as $\delta W_j(\mathbf{q})$, can be obtained by considering the diagonal elements of $V^{-1}H_{SB}^{(2)}V$ matrix as

$$\delta W_j(\mathbf{q}) = \left[V^{-1}H_{SB}^{(2)}(\mathbf{q})V\right]_{jj} \tag{9.80}$$

where V-matrix was defined in Equation 9.76.

Also, the transition dipole matrix elements between g and e_1 states and between g and e_2 states and those between one of the two singly excited states e_j (for $j = 1$ and 2) and one of the three doubly excited states f_k ($k = 1 - 3$) can be written as linear combinations of the two local transition dipoles $\mathbf{d}_1$ and $\mathbf{d}_2$ (see Equations 8.19 and (8.21):

$$\begin{pmatrix} \boldsymbol{\mu}_{e_1g} \\ \boldsymbol{\mu}_{e_2g} \end{pmatrix} = U^{-1}\begin{pmatrix} \mathbf{d}_1 \\ \mathbf{d}_2 \end{pmatrix} = \begin{pmatrix} \cos\theta & \sin\theta \\ -\sin\theta & \cos\theta \end{pmatrix}\begin{pmatrix} \mathbf{d}_1 \\ \mathbf{d}_2 \end{pmatrix}$$

$$\boldsymbol{\mu}_{f_1e_1} = (\sqrt{2}c_{11}\cos\theta + c_{13}\sin\theta)\mathbf{d}_1 + (\sqrt{2}c_{12}\sin\theta + c_{13}\cos\theta)\mathbf{d}_2$$

$$\boldsymbol{\mu}_{f_1e_2} = (-\sqrt{2}c_{11}\sin\theta + c_{13}\cos\theta)\mathbf{d}_1 + (\sqrt{2}c_{12}\cos\theta - c_{13}\sin\theta)\mathbf{d}_2$$

$$\boldsymbol{\mu}_{f_2e_1} = (\sqrt{2}c_{21}\cos\theta + c_{23}\sin\theta)\mathbf{d}_1 + (\sqrt{2}c_{22}\sin\theta + c_{23}\cos\theta)\mathbf{d}_2$$

$$\boldsymbol{\mu}_{f_2e_2} = (-\sqrt{2}c_{21}\sin\theta + c_{23}\cos\theta)\mathbf{d}_1 + (\sqrt{2}c_{22}\cos\theta - c_{23}\sin\theta)\mathbf{d}_2$$

$$\boldsymbol{\mu}_{f_3e_1} = (\sqrt{2}c_{31}\cos\theta + c_{33}\sin\theta)\mathbf{d}_1 + (\sqrt{2}c_{32}\sin\theta + c_{33}\cos\theta)\mathbf{d}_2$$

$$\boldsymbol{\mu}_{f_3e_2} = (-\sqrt{2}c_{31}\sin\theta + c_{33}\cos\theta)\mathbf{d}_1 + (\sqrt{2}c_{32}\cos\theta - c_{33}\sin\theta)\mathbf{d}_2. \quad (9.81)$$

Here, the harmonic approximation was used to estimate the transition dipole matrix element between the first excited state and the overtone state of each individual local oscillator, that is, $|\boldsymbol{\mu}_{21}| = \sqrt{2}|\boldsymbol{\mu}_{10}|$.

The transition FFCFs for the present coupled anharmonic oscillator system can be obtained from the results for the general N-coupled anharmonic oscillator system in Chapter 8. Therefore, all the necessary ingredients for calculating the 2D photon echo have been specified by now. In the following section, the short-time approximation to the third-order response function and the 2D Gaussian peak shape approximation will be used to show how many cross-peaks are observable as well as what information can be extracted from the 2D photon echo study of the coupled anharmonic oscillator systems.

9.7 COUPLED ANHARMONIC OSCILLATORS: TWO-DIMENSIONAL PHOTON ECHO SPECTRUM AT SHORT TIME

When two anharmonic oscillators are coupled to each other as discussed above, a number of third-order response function components contribute to the 2D photon echo in addition to those for the coupled 2LS dimer, since there are three doubly excited ($f_1 - f_3$) states that are electric-dipole-allowed from the two singly excited (e_1 and e_2) states. Nevertheless, there appear only two diagonal peaks originating from $g \leftrightarrow e_1$ and $g \leftrightarrow e_2$ transitions, and the corresponding expressions for peak shapes and amplitudes are identical to those of the coupled 2LS dimer.

The third-order polarization associated with the diagonal peak at $\omega_\tau = \bar{\omega}_{e_1g}$ and $\omega_t = \bar{\omega}_{e_1g}$ is given as the sum of stimulated emission and ground-state bleaching diagrams:

$$<\mu \xleftarrow[g\wr \quad e_1\wr]{e_1\wr} |g><g| \quad \text{and} \quad <\mu \xleftarrow[g\wr e_1\wr]{e_1\wr} |g><g|. \tag{9.82}$$

The corresponding 2D photon echo diagonal peak at $\omega_\tau = \bar{\omega}_{e_1g}$ and $\omega_t = \bar{\omega}_{e_1g}$ is given as

$$\tilde{\mathbf{E}}_{D1}(\omega_t, T, \omega_\tau) = 2[\boldsymbol{\mu}_{ge_1}\boldsymbol{\mu}_{e_1g}\boldsymbol{\mu}_{ge_1}\boldsymbol{\mu}_{e_1g}]\vdots\mathbf{e}_3\mathbf{e}_2\mathbf{e}_1\Gamma\left(\bar{\omega}_{e_1g}, <\delta\Omega_1^2>, \bar{\omega}_{e_1g}, <\delta\Omega_1^2>\right). \tag{9.83}$$

The two polarizations producing the diagonal peak at $\omega_\tau = \bar{\omega}_{e_2g}$ and $\omega_t = \bar{\omega}_{e_2g}$ are, similarly,

$$<\mu \xleftarrow[g\wr \quad e_2\wr]{e_2\wr} |g><g| \quad \text{and} \quad <\mu \xleftarrow[g\wr e_2\wr]{e_2\wr} |g><g|. \tag{9.84}$$

The diagonal peak at $\omega_\tau = \bar{\omega}_{e_2g}$ and $\omega_t = \bar{\omega}_{e_2g}$ is then

$$\tilde{\mathbf{E}}_{D2}(\omega_t, T, \omega_\tau) = 2[\boldsymbol{\mu}_{ge_2}\boldsymbol{\mu}_{e_2g}\boldsymbol{\mu}_{ge_2}\boldsymbol{\mu}_{e_2g}]\vdots\mathbf{e}_3\mathbf{e}_2\mathbf{e}_1^*\Gamma\left(\bar{\omega}_{e_2g}, <\delta\Omega_2^2>, \bar{\omega}_{e_2g}, <\delta\Omega_2^2>\right). \tag{9.85}$$

All the other nonlinear optical transition pathways (diagrams) contribute to the off-diagonal peaks in a given 2D photon echo spectrum of coupled anharmonic oscillator system.

In a real experiment utilizing very short pulses, coherence between e_1 and e_2 states can be created and contribute to the photon echo polarization. Despite the fact that there are a number of diagrams contributing to different cross-peaks, one can classify them into two groups. The first group contains diagrams that produce cross-peaks at $\omega_\tau = \bar{\omega}_{e_1g}$, whereas those in the second group produce cross-peaks at $\omega_\tau = \bar{\omega}_{e_2g}$. The diagrams within each group differ from one another by the coherence oscillation frequency during the t_3 period, which determines the center frequency of each cross-peak along the ω_t – axis.

(Group 1) Diagrams producing cross-peaks at $\omega_\tau = \bar{\omega}_{e_1g}$

$$<\mu \xleftarrow[g\wr \quad e_1\wr]{e_2\wr} |g><g| \quad \propto \exp\{-i\bar{\omega}_{e_2g}t_3 - i\bar{\omega}_{e_2e_1}t_2 - i\bar{\omega}_{ge_1}t_1\}$$

$$<\mu \xleftarrow[g\wr e_1\wr]{e_2\wr} |g><g| \quad \propto \exp\{-i\bar{\omega}_{e_2g}t_3 - i\bar{\omega}_{ge_1}t_1\}$$

$$<\mu \xleftarrow[e_1\wr]{f_1\wr e_1\wr} |g><g| \quad \propto \exp\{-i\bar{\omega}_{f_1e_1}t_3 - i\bar{\omega}_{ge_1}t_1\}$$

$$<\mu \xleftarrow[e_1\wr]{f_2\wr e_1\wr} |g><g| \quad \propto \exp\{-i\bar{\omega}_{f_2e_1}t_3 - i\bar{\omega}_{ge_1}t_1\}$$

$$<\mu \overset{f_3 \, e_1}{\underset{e_1}{\Longleftarrow}} |g><g| \quad \propto \exp\{-i\bar{\omega}_{f_3e_1}t_3 - i\bar{\omega}_{ge_1}t_1\}$$

$$<\mu \overset{f_1 \, e_2}{\underset{e_1}{\Longleftarrow}} |g><g| \quad \propto \exp\{-i\bar{\omega}_{f_1e_1}t_3 - i\bar{\omega}_{e_2e_1}t_2 - i\bar{\omega}_{ge_1}t_1\}$$

$$<\mu \overset{f_2 \, e_2}{\underset{e_1}{\Longleftarrow}} |g><g| \quad \propto \exp\{-i\bar{\omega}_{f_2e_1}t_3 - i\bar{\omega}_{e_2e_1}t_2 - i\bar{\omega}_{ge_1}t_1\}$$

$$<\mu \overset{f_3 \, e_2}{\underset{e_1}{\Longleftarrow}} |g><g| \quad \propto \exp\{-i\bar{\omega}_{f_3e_1}t_3 - i\bar{\omega}_{e_2e_1}t_2 - i\bar{\omega}_{ge_1}t_1\} \tag{9.86}$$

(Group 2) Diagrams producing cross-peaks at $\omega_\tau = \bar{\omega}_{e_2g}$

$$<\mu \overset{e_1}{\underset{g \quad e_2}{\Longleftarrow}} |g><g| \quad \propto \exp\{-i\bar{\omega}_{e_1g}t_3 - i\bar{\omega}_{e_1e_2}t_2 - i\bar{\omega}_{ge_2}t_1\}$$

$$<\mu \overset{e_1}{\underset{g \, e_2}{\Longleftarrow}} |g><g| \quad \propto \exp\{-i\bar{\omega}_{e_1g}t_3 - i\bar{\omega}_{ge_2}t_1\}$$

$$<\mu \overset{f_1 \, e_2}{\underset{e_2}{\Longleftarrow}} |g><g| \quad \propto \exp\{-i\bar{\omega}_{f_1e_2}t_3 - i\bar{\omega}_{ge_2}t_1\}$$

$$<\mu \overset{f_2 \, e_2}{\underset{e_2}{\Longleftarrow}} |g><g| \quad \propto \exp\{-i\bar{\omega}_{f_2e_2}t_3 - i\bar{\omega}_{ge_2}t_1\}$$

$$<\mu \overset{f_3 \, e_2}{\underset{e_2}{\Longleftarrow}} |g><g| \quad \propto \exp\{-i\bar{\omega}_{f_3e_2}t_3 - i\bar{\omega}_{ge_2}t_1\}$$

$$<\mu \overset{f_1 \, e_1}{\underset{e_2}{\Longleftarrow}} |g><g| \quad \propto \exp\{-i\bar{\omega}_{f_1e_2}t_3 - i\bar{\omega}_{e_1e_2}t_2 - i\bar{\omega}_{ge_2}t_1\}$$

$$<\mu \overset{f_2 \, e_1}{\underset{e_2}{\Longleftarrow}} |g><g| \quad \propto \exp\{-i\bar{\omega}_{f_2e_2}t_3 - i\bar{\omega}_{e_1e_2}t_2 - i\bar{\omega}_{ge_2}t_1\}$$

$$<\mu \overset{f_3 \, e_1}{\underset{e_2}{\Longleftarrow}} |g><g| \quad \propto \exp\{-i\bar{\omega}_{f_3e_2}t_3 - i\bar{\omega}_{e_1e_2}t_2 - i\bar{\omega}_{ge_2}t_1\} \tag{9.87}$$

It is interesting to note that, within each group, there are four diagrams showing quantum beat patterns or coherence oscillations during t_2 period, when the photon echo signal is measured as a function of the waiting time T (= t_2 in the impulsive limit). From the diagrams in Equations 9.86 and 9.87, one can obtain the corresponding expressions for the 2D photon echo peak shapes. Using the 2D Gaussian peak shape approximation, one can find the expressions for the eight diagrams in Group 1:

$$\tilde{\mathbf{E}}_{G1}(\omega_t,T,\omega_\tau)=[\boldsymbol{\mu}_{ge_2}\boldsymbol{\mu}_{e_1g}\boldsymbol{\mu}_{e_2g}\boldsymbol{\mu}_{ge_1}]\vdots\mathbf{e}_3\mathbf{e}_2\mathbf{e}_1^*\Gamma(\bar{\omega}_{e_2g},<\delta\Omega_1\delta\Omega_2>,\bar{\omega}_{e_1g},<\delta\Omega_1\delta\Omega_2>)$$
$$\times\exp\{-i\bar{\omega}_{e_2e_1}T-f_{12}(T)\}$$
$$+[\boldsymbol{\mu}_{ge_2}\boldsymbol{\mu}_{e_2g}\boldsymbol{\mu}_{e_1g}\boldsymbol{\mu}_{ge_1}]\vdots\mathbf{e}_3\mathbf{e}_2\mathbf{e}_1^*\Gamma\left(\bar{\omega}_{e_2g},<\delta\Omega_2^2>,\bar{\omega}_{e_1g},<\delta\Omega_1^2>\right)$$
$$-[\boldsymbol{\mu}_{e_1f_1}\boldsymbol{\mu}_{f_1e_1}\boldsymbol{\mu}_{e_1g}\boldsymbol{\mu}_{ge_1}]\vdots\mathbf{e}_3\mathbf{e}_2\mathbf{e}_1^*\Gamma(\bar{\omega}_{f_1e_1},<(\delta W_1-\delta\Omega_1)^2>,\bar{\omega}_{e_1g},<\delta\Omega_1^2>)$$
$$-[\boldsymbol{\mu}_{e_1f_2}\boldsymbol{\mu}_{f_2e_1}\boldsymbol{\mu}_{e_1g}\boldsymbol{\mu}_{ge_1}]\vdots\mathbf{e}_3\mathbf{e}_2\mathbf{e}_1^*\Gamma\left(\bar{\omega}_{f_2e_1},<(\delta W_2-\delta\Omega_1)^2>,\bar{\omega}_{e_1g},<\delta\Omega_1^2>\right)$$
$$-[\boldsymbol{\mu}_{e_1f_3}\boldsymbol{\mu}_{f_3e_1}\boldsymbol{\mu}_{e_1g}\boldsymbol{\mu}_{ge_1}]\vdots\mathbf{e}_3\mathbf{e}_2\mathbf{e}_1^*\Gamma\left(\bar{\omega}_{f_3e_1},<(\delta W_3-\delta\Omega_1)^2>,\bar{\omega}_{e_1g},<\delta\Omega_1^2>\right)$$
$$-[\boldsymbol{\mu}_{e_1f_1}\boldsymbol{\mu}_{f_1e_2}\boldsymbol{\mu}_{e_2g}\boldsymbol{\mu}_{ge_1}]\vdots\mathbf{e}_3\mathbf{e}_2\mathbf{e}_1^*\Gamma(\bar{\omega}_{f_1e_1},<(\delta W_1-\delta\Omega_1)(\delta W_1-\delta\Omega_2)>,\bar{\omega}_{e_1g},$$
$$<\delta\Omega_1\delta\Omega_2>)\exp\{-i\bar{\omega}_{e_2e_1}T-f_{12}(T)\}$$
$$-[\boldsymbol{\mu}_{e_1f_2}\boldsymbol{\mu}_{f_2e_2}\boldsymbol{\mu}_{e_2g}\boldsymbol{\mu}_{ge_1}]\vdots\mathbf{e}_3\mathbf{e}_2\mathbf{e}_1^*\Gamma(\bar{\omega}_{f_2e_1},<(\delta W_2-\delta\Omega_1)$$
$$\times(\delta W_2-\delta\Omega_2)>,\bar{\omega}_{e_1g},<\delta\Omega_1\delta\Omega_2>)\exp\{-i\bar{\omega}_{e_2e_1}T-f_{12}(T)\}$$
$$-[\boldsymbol{\mu}_{e_1f_3}\boldsymbol{\mu}_{f_3e_2}\boldsymbol{\mu}_{e_2g}\boldsymbol{\mu}_{ge_1}]\vdots\mathbf{e}_3\mathbf{e}_2\mathbf{e}_1^*\Gamma(\bar{\omega}_{f_3e_1},<(\delta W_3-\delta\Omega_1)$$
$$\times(\delta W_3-\delta\Omega_2)>,\bar{\omega}_{e_1g},<\delta\Omega_1\delta\Omega_2>)\exp\{-i\bar{\omega}_{e_2e_1}T-f_{12}(T)\}. \quad (9.88)$$

The 2D photon echo peaks associated with the second group of diagrams in Equation 9.87 are given as

$$\tilde{\mathbf{E}}_{G2}(\omega_t,T,\omega_\tau)=[\boldsymbol{\mu}_{ge_1}\boldsymbol{\mu}_{e_2g}\boldsymbol{\mu}_{e_1g}\boldsymbol{\mu}_{ge_2}]\vdots\mathbf{e}_3\mathbf{e}_2\mathbf{e}_1^*\Gamma(\bar{\omega}_{e_1g},<\delta\Omega_1\delta\Omega_2>,\bar{\omega}_{e_2g},<\delta\Omega_1\delta\Omega_2>)$$
$$\times\exp\{-i\bar{\omega}_{e_1e_2}T-f_{12}^*(T)\}$$
$$+[\boldsymbol{\mu}_{ge_1}\boldsymbol{\mu}_{e_1g}\boldsymbol{\mu}_{e_2g}\boldsymbol{\mu}_{ge_2}]\vdots\mathbf{e}_3\mathbf{e}_2\mathbf{e}_1^*\Gamma\left(\bar{\omega}_{e_1g},<\delta\Omega_1^2>,\bar{\omega}_{e_2g},<\delta\Omega_2^2>\right)$$
$$-[\boldsymbol{\mu}_{e_2f_1}\boldsymbol{\mu}_{f_1e_2}\boldsymbol{\mu}_{e_2g}\boldsymbol{\mu}_{ge_2}]\vdots\mathbf{e}_3\mathbf{e}_2\mathbf{e}_1^*\Gamma\left(\bar{\omega}_{f_1e_2},<(\delta W_1-\delta\Omega_2)^2>,\bar{\omega}_{e_2g},<\delta\Omega_2^2>\right)$$
$$-[\boldsymbol{\mu}_{e_2f_2}\boldsymbol{\mu}_{f_2e_2}\boldsymbol{\mu}_{e_2g}\boldsymbol{\mu}_{ge_2}]\vdots\mathbf{e}_3\mathbf{e}_2\mathbf{e}_1^*\Gamma\left(\bar{\omega}_{f_2e_2},<(\delta W_2-\delta\Omega_2)^2>,\bar{\omega}_{e_2g},<\delta\Omega_2^2>\right)$$
$$-[\boldsymbol{\mu}_{e_2f_3}\boldsymbol{\mu}_{f_3e_2}\boldsymbol{\mu}_{e_2g}\boldsymbol{\mu}_{ge_2}]\vdots\mathbf{e}_3\mathbf{e}_2\mathbf{e}_1^*\Gamma\left(\bar{\omega}_{f_3e_2},<(\delta W_3-\delta\Omega_2)^2>,\bar{\omega}_{e_2g},<\delta\Omega_2^2>\right)$$
$$-[\boldsymbol{\mu}_{e_2f_1}\boldsymbol{\mu}_{f_1e_1}\boldsymbol{\mu}_{e_1g}\boldsymbol{\mu}_{ge_2}]\vdots\mathbf{e}_3\mathbf{e}_2\mathbf{e}_1^*\Gamma(\bar{\omega}_{f_1e_2},<(\delta W_1-\delta\Omega_1)$$
$$\times(\delta W_1-\delta\Omega_2)>,\bar{\omega}_{e_2g},<\delta\Omega_1\delta\Omega_2>)\times\exp\{-i\bar{\omega}_{e_1e_2}T-f_{12}^*(T)\}$$

$$-[\boldsymbol{\mu}_{e_2f_2}\boldsymbol{\mu}_{f_2e_1}\boldsymbol{\mu}_{e_1g}\boldsymbol{\mu}_{ge_2}]\vdots\mathbf{e}_3\mathbf{e}_2\mathbf{e}_1^*$$

$$\times\Gamma(\bar{\omega}_{f_2e_2},<(\delta W_2-\delta\Omega_1)(\delta W_2-\delta\Omega_2)>,\bar{\omega}_{e_2g},<\delta\Omega_1\delta\Omega_2>)$$

$$\times\exp\{-i\bar{\omega}_{e_1e_2}T-f_{12}^*(T)\}$$

$$-[\boldsymbol{\mu}_{e_2f_3}\boldsymbol{\mu}_{f_3e_1}\boldsymbol{\mu}_{e_1g}\boldsymbol{\mu}_{ge_2}]\vdots\mathbf{e}_3\mathbf{e}_2\mathbf{e}_1^*$$

$$\times\Gamma(\bar{\omega}_{f_3e_2},<(\delta W_3-\delta\Omega_1)(\delta W_3-\delta\Omega_2)>,\bar{\omega}_{e_2g},<\delta\Omega_1\delta\Omega_2>)$$

$$\times\exp\{-i\bar{\omega}_{e_1e_2}T-f_{12}^*(T)\}. \quad (9.89)$$

The above results were obtained by assuming that the population transfer processes between the two singly excited states are negligibly slow. It is interesting to note that one can show that the above results for the two-coupled anharmonic oscillator system reduce to those for the coupled 2LS dimer in the limit that

$$\Delta_{11}\to-\infty$$

$$\Delta_{22}\to-\infty$$

$$\Delta_{12}\to 0. \quad (9.90)$$

In this case, the two eigenvalues, $\hbar W_1$ and $\hbar W_2$, which are the energies of f_1 and f_2 states, approach infinity and become nonresonant with the external fields so that these two states are out of the range of detection. Secondly, $\hbar W_3$ becomes $\varepsilon_1+\varepsilon_2$ and the state f_3 is simply $|1,1>(=a_1^\dagger a_2^\dagger|0>)$. Then, one can show that the results in Equations 9.88 and 9.89 reduce to those in Equation 9.29 and 9.32 for the coupled 2LS dimer.

In this section, the short-time behavior of cross-peak amplitudes for coupled anharmonic oscillator system were theoretically described. In the following sections, we will consider a few simple cases to illustrate the information that can be extracted from the 2D vibrational spectrum of coupled anharmonic oscillator systems.

9.8 COUPLED ANHARMONIC OSCILLATORS: DEGENERATE CASE

When the coupling constant is relatively small in comparison to typical absorption bandwidths, that is, $J\le\sqrt{<\delta\Omega^2>}$, the two diagonal peaks cannot be frequency resolved. Furthermore, if the overtone and combination band anharmonicities are small, that is, $\Delta\le\sqrt{<\delta\Omega^2>}$, the positive peak originating from $g\leftrightarrow e$ transitions spectrally overlaps with the negative peak from excited-state absorption contributions ($e\leftrightarrow f$). Thus, the total 2D spectrum is spectrally congested. In this case, it is quite difficult to interpret the 2D spectrum and to extract structural and dynamical information from peak shape and amplitude changes of the broad peaks. However, when $J > \sqrt{<\delta\Omega^2>}$ and $\Delta > \sqrt{<\delta\Omega^2>}$, the two diagonal and corresponding cross-peaks are frequency resolved in the 2D spectrum, and furthermore, the overtone and combination peaks will appear as cross-peaks at proper positions in the 2D spectrum.

For the sake of simplicity, let us consider a degenerate coupled oscillator system where the two oscillators have the same frequency ω_0. The Hamiltonian matrixes associated with the singly and doubly excited states are then given as

$$\tilde{H}_0^{(1)} = \hbar \begin{bmatrix} \omega_0 & J \\ J & \omega_0 \end{bmatrix}. \tag{9.91}$$

$$\tilde{H}_0^{(2)} = \hbar \begin{bmatrix} 2\omega_0 - \Delta_0 & 0 & \sqrt{2}J \\ 0 & 2\omega_0 - \Delta_0 & \sqrt{2}J \\ \sqrt{2}J & \sqrt{2}J & 2\omega_0 - \Delta_c \end{bmatrix}. \tag{9.92}$$

The overtone anharmonic frequency shift of each local oscillator is Δ_0 and that of the combination state is Δ_c. For this degenerate two-oscillator system, the mixing angle θ is $\pi/4$ so that we get

$$\sin\theta = \cos\theta = 1/\sqrt{2}$$

$$\begin{pmatrix} |e_1> \\ |e_2> \end{pmatrix} = \begin{pmatrix} 1/\sqrt{2} & 1/\sqrt{2} \\ -1/\sqrt{2} & 1/\sqrt{2} \end{pmatrix} \begin{pmatrix} a_1^\dagger |0> \\ a_2^\dagger |0> \end{pmatrix}.$$

$$\Omega_1 = \omega_0 + J$$

$$\Omega_2 = \omega_0 - J. \tag{9.93}$$

From the eigenvector elements of e_1 and e_2 states, one can identify them as symmetric and asymmetric vibrations, respectively. If the two oscillators are C=O stretching modes, the e_1 excited state corresponds to the case when the two C=O stretching vibrations are in phase and symmetric. Depending on the sign and magnitude of J, the symmetric normal mode frequency can be higher or lower than ω_0.

Now, after diagonalizing the $\tilde{H}_0^{(2)}$ Hamiltonian matrix in Equation 9.92, one finds that the three eigenvalues are

$$W_1 = 2\omega_0 - \frac{\Delta_0 + \Delta_c}{2} + \frac{2J}{\sin\xi}$$

$$W_2 = 2\omega_0 - \Delta_0$$

$$W_3 = 2\omega_0 - \frac{\Delta_0 + \Delta_c}{2} - \frac{2J}{\sin\xi}, \tag{9.94}$$

where

$$\xi = \cot^{-1}\left(\frac{\Delta_0 - \Delta_c}{4J}\right). \tag{9.95}$$

Note that ξ defined above is a monotonically decreasing function from $\pi/2$ to zero as $(\Delta_0 - \Delta_c)/4J$ increases from 0 to infinity.

The corresponding eigenvectors are found to be

$$\begin{pmatrix} |f_1> \\ |f_2> \\ |f_3> \end{pmatrix} = V^{-1}\begin{pmatrix} |2,0> \\ |0,2> \\ |1,1> \end{pmatrix} = \begin{pmatrix} \frac{\sin(\xi/2)}{\sqrt{2}} & \frac{\sin(\xi/2)}{\sqrt{2}} & \cos(\xi/2) \\ \frac{1}{\sqrt{2}} & -\frac{1}{\sqrt{2}} & 0 \\ -\frac{\cos(\xi/2)}{\sqrt{2}} & -\frac{\cos(\xi/2)}{\sqrt{2}} & \sin(\xi/2) \end{pmatrix}\begin{pmatrix} |2,0> \\ |0,2> \\ |1,1> \end{pmatrix}. \tag{9.96}$$

From the above eigenvectors of the singly and doubly excited states, the f_1 state can be viewed as the overtone state of the symmetric vibration, whereas the f_3 state is the overtone state of the asymmetric vibration. The f_2 state can be considered the combination state of the symmetric and asymmetric vibrations. The energy of the combination (f_2) state does not depend on the coupling constant, as expected. In Figure 9.6, the relative energy levels of the six vibrational states are shown. Although the two energy levels of singly excited states e_1 and e_2 are just linearly dependent on the coupling constant J, the J-dependencies of the three eigenvalues associated with the doubly excited states $W_1 - W_3$ are not simple. Thus, Figure 9.7 depicts W_j's with respect to J when $\Delta_0 = 30$ cm^{-1} and $\Delta_c = 5$ cm^{-1}.

Now, the corresponding transition dipole matrix elements are found to be

$$\begin{pmatrix} \boldsymbol{\mu}_{e_1g} \\ \boldsymbol{\mu}_{e_2g} \end{pmatrix} = \begin{pmatrix} 1/\sqrt{2} & 1/\sqrt{2} \\ -1/\sqrt{2} & 1/\sqrt{2} \end{pmatrix}\begin{pmatrix} \mathbf{d}_1 \\ \mathbf{d}_2 \end{pmatrix} \tag{9.97}$$

and

$$\boldsymbol{\mu}_{f_1e_1} = \left(\frac{\sin(\xi/2)}{\sqrt{2}} + \frac{\cos(\xi/2)}{\sqrt{2}}\right)(\mathbf{d}_1 + \mathbf{d}_2)$$

$$\boldsymbol{\mu}_{f_1e_2} = -\left(\frac{\sin(\xi/2)}{\sqrt{2}} - \frac{\cos(\xi/2)}{\sqrt{2}}\right)(\mathbf{d}_1 - \mathbf{d}_2)$$

$$\boldsymbol{\mu}_{f_2e_1} = (\mathbf{d}_1 - \mathbf{d}_2)/\sqrt{2}$$

$$\boldsymbol{\mu}_{f_2e_2} = -(\mathbf{d}_1 + \mathbf{d}_2)/\sqrt{2}$$

(Continued)

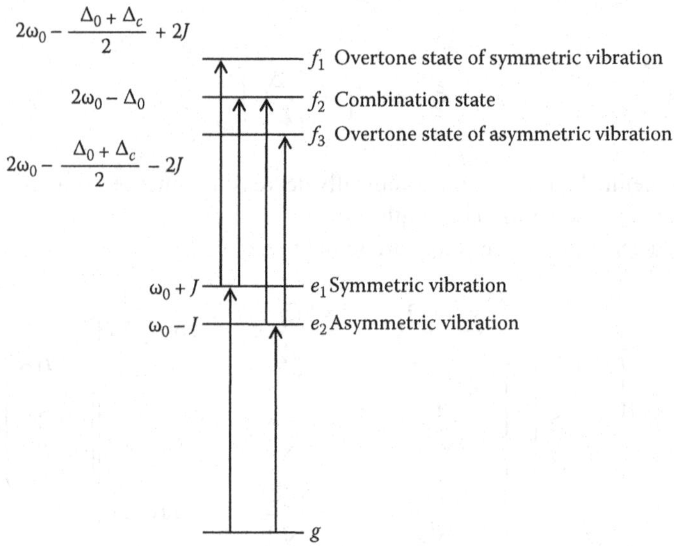

FIGURE 9.6 Energy levels of singly and doubly excited states of coupled anharmonic oscillator system. The two singly excited states are symmetric (e_1) and asymmetric (e_2) vibrations of the two anharmonic oscillators. The three doubly excited states are, on the basis of their eigenvector elements, overtone states of symmetric (f_1) and asymmetric (f_3) vibrations and combination state (f_2). In this figure, the upward arrows show which vibrational transitions are electric dipole-allowed. Vibrational transitions between any two states that are not connected by an arrow are forbidden.

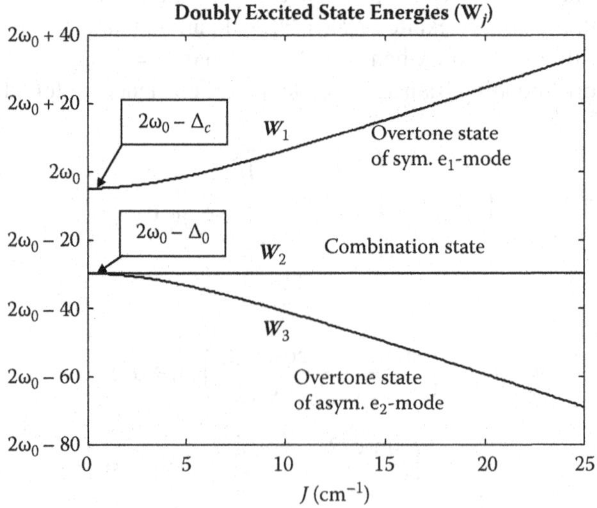

FIGURE 9.7 Eigenvalues of the three doubly excited states, $W1 \sim W3$, versus J (see Equation 9.94). For numerical calculations, the overtone and combination anharmonic frequency shifts are assumed to be 30 and 5 cm^{-1}, respectively.

$$\boldsymbol{\mu}_{f3e_1} = \left(\frac{\sin(\xi/2)}{\sqrt{2}} - \frac{\cos(\xi/2)}{\sqrt{2}} \right)(\mathbf{d}_1 + \mathbf{d}_2)$$

$$\boldsymbol{\mu}_{f3e_2} = \left(\frac{\sin(\xi/2)}{\sqrt{2}} + \frac{\cos(\xi/2)}{\sqrt{2}} \right)(\mathbf{d}_1 - \mathbf{d}_2). \tag{9.98}$$

In this simple case of degenerate coupled anharmonic oscillators, the energies of the singly and doubly excited states, their eigenvectors, and transition dipole matrix elements are fully obtained in terms of the coupling constant and overtone and combination anharmonic frequency shifts. Therefore, it is now possible to calculate the 2D photon echo spectrum by inserting the relevant results into Equations 9.83 and 9.85–9.87. However, still the results are quite complicated, and it appears to be difficult to identify the essential physics behind them. Thus, one may find it useful to consider a few limiting cases.

Hereafter, it is assumed that the absorption bandwidth is smaller than both the coupling constant and anharmonic frequency shifts, that is to say,

$$J > \sqrt{< \delta\Omega^2 >} \quad \text{and} \quad (\Delta_0 + \Delta_c)/2 > \sqrt{< \delta\Omega^2 >}. \tag{9.99}$$

Then, not only the diagonal peaks but also the cross-peaks are frequency resolved, so that the anharmonic frequency shifts and coupling constant can be directly estimated by examining the measured 2D spectrum.

Strong coupling limit $(J > (\Delta_0 + \Delta_c)/2 > \sqrt{< \delta\Omega^2 >})$. First, let us consider the case when the coupling constant is much larger than the average anharmonic frequency shift. Then, the two diagonal peaks originating from $g \leftrightarrow e_1$ and $g \leftrightarrow e_2$ transitions are well separated in frequency, and the splitting is $2J$ (see Equation 9.93). Now, the angle ξ defined in Equation 9.95 approaches $\pi/2$, that is to say,

$$\lim_{(\Delta_0 - \Delta_c)/J \to 0} \xi = \pi/2. \tag{9.100}$$

In this strong coupling limit, the energies of the three doubly excited states are given as

$$W_1 = 2\omega_0 - \frac{\Delta_0 + \Delta_c}{2} + 2J$$

$$W_2 = 2\omega_0 - \Delta_0$$

$$W_3 = 2\omega_0 - \frac{\Delta_0 + \Delta_c}{2} - 2J. \tag{9.101}$$

Furthermore, the six transition dipole matrix elements in Equation 9.98 in a given molecule-fixed frame are simplified as

$$\boldsymbol{\mu}_{f1e_1} = (\mathbf{d}_1 + \mathbf{d}_2)$$

$$\boldsymbol{\mu}_{f1e_2} = 0$$

$$\boldsymbol{\mu}_{f_2e_1} = (\mathbf{d}_1 - \mathbf{d}_2)/\sqrt{2}$$

$$\boldsymbol{\mu}_{f_2e_2} = -(\mathbf{d}_1 + \mathbf{d}_2)/\sqrt{2}$$

$$\boldsymbol{\mu}_{f_3e_1} = 0$$

$$\boldsymbol{\mu}_{f_3e_2} = (\mathbf{d}_1 - \mathbf{d}_2). \tag{9.102}$$

Note that the transition from e_1 to f_3 and from e_2 to f_1 are forbidden (see Figure 9.6, where the upward arrows mean that the vibrational transitions between two states connected by such arrows are electric-dipole-allowed). This selection rule can be understood from the harmonic oscillator picture. Since the f_1 and f_2 states are the overtone state of the symmetric mode and the combination state of the symmetric and asymmetric modes, respectively, the transitions from the e_1 state, which is the first excited state of the symmetric mode, to the two (f_1 and f_2) doubly excited states are harmonically allowed. Similarly, the transitions from the e_2 state, which is the first excited state of the asymmetric mode, to the f_2 and f_3 states are also allowed. All these transitions are one-quantum excitation processes. However, the transition from the symmetric mode excited state e_1 to the asymmetric mode overtone state f_3 should involve one de-excitation of e_1 state to g and a two-quantum excitation of g to f_3, which is a multiquantum process requiring potential anharmonicity in normal mode picture and is harmonically forbidden.

From the general results for the 2D photon echo spectrum of a coupled anharmonic oscillator system presented in the previous section, one finds that, in the strong coupling limit, the 2D spectrum is given by the sum of the following contributions:

$$\tilde{\mathbf{E}}_{D1}(\omega_t, T, \omega_\tau) = 2[\boldsymbol{\mu}_{ge_1}\boldsymbol{\mu}_{e_1g}\boldsymbol{\mu}_{ge_1}\boldsymbol{\mu}_{e_1g}]\vdots\mathbf{e}_3\mathbf{e}_2\mathbf{e}_1^*\Gamma\left(\bar{\omega}_{e_1g}, <\delta\Omega_1^2>, \bar{\omega}_{e_1g}, <\delta\Omega_1^2>\right)$$

$$\tilde{\mathbf{E}}_{D2}(\omega_t, T, \omega_\tau) = 2[\boldsymbol{\mu}_{ge_2}\boldsymbol{\mu}_{e_2g}\boldsymbol{\mu}_{ge_2}\boldsymbol{\mu}_{e_2g}]\vdots\mathbf{e}_3\mathbf{e}_2\mathbf{e}_1^*\Gamma\left(\bar{\omega}_{e_2g}, <\delta\Omega_2^2>, \bar{\omega}_{e_2g}, <\delta\Omega_2^2>\right)$$

$$\begin{aligned}
\tilde{\mathbf{E}}_{G1}(\omega_t, T, \omega_\tau) = {} & [\boldsymbol{\mu}_{ge_2}\boldsymbol{\mu}_{e_1g}\boldsymbol{\mu}_{e_2g}\boldsymbol{\mu}_{ge_1}]\vdots\mathbf{e}_3\mathbf{e}_2\mathbf{e}_1^*\Gamma(\bar{\omega}_{e_2g}, <\delta\Omega_1\delta\Omega_2>, \bar{\omega}_{e_1g}, <\delta\Omega_1\delta\Omega_2>) \\
& \times \exp\{-i\bar{\omega}_{e_2e_1}T - f_{12}(T)\} \\
& + [\boldsymbol{\mu}_{ge_2}\boldsymbol{\mu}_{e_2g}\boldsymbol{\mu}_{e_1g}\boldsymbol{\mu}_{ge_1}]\vdots\mathbf{e}_3\mathbf{e}_2\mathbf{e}_1^*\Gamma\left(\bar{\omega}_{e_2g}, <\delta\Omega_2^2>, \bar{\omega}_{e_1g}, <\delta\Omega_1^2>\right) \\
& - [\boldsymbol{\mu}_{e_1f_1}\boldsymbol{\mu}_{f_1e_1}\boldsymbol{\mu}_{e_1g}\boldsymbol{\mu}_{ge_1}]\vdots\mathbf{e}_3\mathbf{e}_2\mathbf{e}_1^*\Gamma\left(\bar{\omega}_{f_1e_1}, <(\delta W_1 - \delta\Omega_1)^2>, \bar{\omega}_{e_1g}, <\delta\Omega_1^2>\right) \\
& - [\boldsymbol{\mu}_{e_1f_2}\boldsymbol{\mu}_{f_2e_1}\boldsymbol{\mu}_{e_1g}\boldsymbol{\mu}_{ge_1}]\vdots\mathbf{e}_3\mathbf{e}_2\mathbf{e}_1^*\Gamma\left(\bar{\omega}_{f_2e_1}, <(\delta W_2 - \delta\Omega_1)^2>, \bar{\omega}_{e_1g}, <\delta\Omega_1^2>\right) \\
& - [\boldsymbol{\mu}_{e_1f_1}\boldsymbol{\mu}_{f_1e_2}\boldsymbol{\mu}_{e_2g}\boldsymbol{\mu}_{ge_1}]\vdots\mathbf{e}_3\mathbf{e}_2\mathbf{e}_1^* \\
& \times \Gamma(\bar{\omega}_{f_1e_1}, <(\delta W_1 - \delta\Omega_1)(\delta W_1 - \delta\Omega_2)>, \bar{\omega}_{e_1g}, <\delta\Omega_1\delta\Omega_2>) \\
& \times \exp\{-i\bar{\omega}_{e_2e_1}T - f_{12}(T)\}
\end{aligned}$$

$$-[\boldsymbol{\mu}_{e_1f_2}\boldsymbol{\mu}_{f_2e_2}\boldsymbol{\mu}_{e_2g}\boldsymbol{\mu}_{ge_1}]\vdots\mathbf{e}_3\mathbf{e}_2\mathbf{e}_1^*$$
$$\times\Gamma(\bar{\omega}_{f_2e_1},<(\delta W_2-\delta\Omega_1)(\delta W_2-\delta\Omega_2)>,\bar{\omega}_{e_1g},<\delta\Omega_1\delta\Omega_2>)$$
$$\times\exp\{-i\bar{\omega}_{e_2e_1}T-f_{12}(T)\}.$$

$$\tilde{\mathbf{E}}_{G2}(\omega_t,T,\omega_\tau)=[\boldsymbol{\mu}_{ge_1}\boldsymbol{\mu}_{e_2g}\boldsymbol{\mu}_{e_1g}\boldsymbol{\mu}_{ge_2}]\vdots\mathbf{e}_3\mathbf{e}_2\mathbf{e}_1^*\Gamma(\bar{\omega}_{e_1g},<\delta\Omega_1\delta\Omega_2>,\bar{\omega}_{e_2g},<\delta\Omega_1\delta\Omega_2>)$$
$$\times\exp\{-i\bar{\omega}_{e_1e_2}T-f_{12}^*(T)\}$$
$$+[\boldsymbol{\mu}_{ge_1}\boldsymbol{\mu}_{e_1g}\boldsymbol{\mu}_{e_2g}\boldsymbol{\mu}_{ge_2}]\vdots\mathbf{e}_3\mathbf{e}_2\mathbf{e}_1^*\Gamma\left(\bar{\omega}_{e_1g},<\delta\Omega_1^2>,\bar{\omega}_{e_2g},<\delta\Omega_2^2>\right)$$
$$-[\boldsymbol{\mu}_{e_2f_2}\boldsymbol{\mu}_{f_2e_2}\boldsymbol{\mu}_{e_2g}\boldsymbol{\mu}_{ge_2}]\vdots\mathbf{e}_3\mathbf{e}_2\mathbf{e}_1^*\Gamma\left(\bar{\omega}_{f_2e_2},<(\delta W_2-\delta\Omega_2)^2>,\bar{\omega}_{e_2g},<\delta\Omega_2^2>\right)$$
$$-[\boldsymbol{\mu}_{e_2f_3}\boldsymbol{\mu}_{f_3e_2}\boldsymbol{\mu}_{e_2g}\boldsymbol{\mu}_{ge_2}]\vdots\mathbf{e}_3\mathbf{e}_2\mathbf{e}_1^*\Gamma\left(\bar{\omega}_{f_3e_2},<(\delta W_3-\delta\Omega_2)^2>,\bar{\omega}_{e_2g},<\delta\Omega_2^2>\right)$$
$$-[\boldsymbol{\mu}_{e_2f_2}\boldsymbol{\mu}_{f_2e_1}\boldsymbol{\mu}_{e_1g}\boldsymbol{\mu}_{ge_2}]\vdots\mathbf{e}_3\mathbf{e}_2\mathbf{e}_1^*$$
$$\times\Gamma(\bar{\omega}_{f_2e_2},<(\delta W_2-\delta\Omega_1)(\delta W_2-\delta\Omega_2)>,\bar{\omega}_{e_2g},<\delta\Omega_1\delta\Omega_2>)$$
$$\times\exp\{-i\bar{\omega}_{e_1e_2}T-f_{12}^*(T)\}$$
$$-[\boldsymbol{\mu}_{e_2f_3}\boldsymbol{\mu}_{f_3e_1}\boldsymbol{\mu}_{e_1g}\boldsymbol{\mu}_{ge_2}]\vdots\mathbf{e}_3\mathbf{e}_2\mathbf{e}_1^*$$
$$\times\Gamma(\bar{\omega}_{f_3e_2},<(\delta W_3-\delta\Omega_1)(\delta W_3-\delta\Omega_2)>,\bar{\omega}_{e_2g},<\delta\Omega_1\delta\Omega_2>)$$
$$\times\exp\{-i\bar{\omega}_{e_1e_2}T-f_{12}^*(T)\}. \quad (9.103)$$

Figure 9.8 schematically depicts the real part of the 2D PE spectrum of this coupled anharmonic oscillator system in the case when the two local oscillators are degenerate and the coupling constant is much larger than the average anharmonic frequency shift. Eight different peaks appear: two diagonal and six cross-peaks. The two diagonal peaks are positive and the two cross-peaks at $\omega_\tau = \bar{\omega}_{e_1g}$ and $\omega_t = \bar{\omega}_{e_2g}$ and at $\omega_\tau = \bar{\omega}_{e_2g}$ and $\omega_t = \bar{\omega}_{e_1g}$ are also positive. On the other hand, all the other cross-peaks are negative because they all originate from excited-state absorption contributions. Therefore, it is possible to say that the two diagonal (D1 and D2 in Figure 9.8) and two cross- (C12 and C21) peaks all appear as pairs (or couplets) consisting of positive and negative peaks. It is interesting to note that the frequency-splitting magnitudes of the D1 and D2 couplets are identical to each other and that they equal the average anharmonic frequency shift $(\Delta_0 + \Delta_c)/2$. This can be understood from the eigenvalues of the three doubly excited states in Equation 9.101. On the other hand, the frequency-splitting magnitudes of the C12 and C21 cross-peak couplets are determined by the overtone anharmonicity Δ_0. Typically, the overtone anharmonic frequency shift Δ_0 is larger than the combination-state anharmonicity,

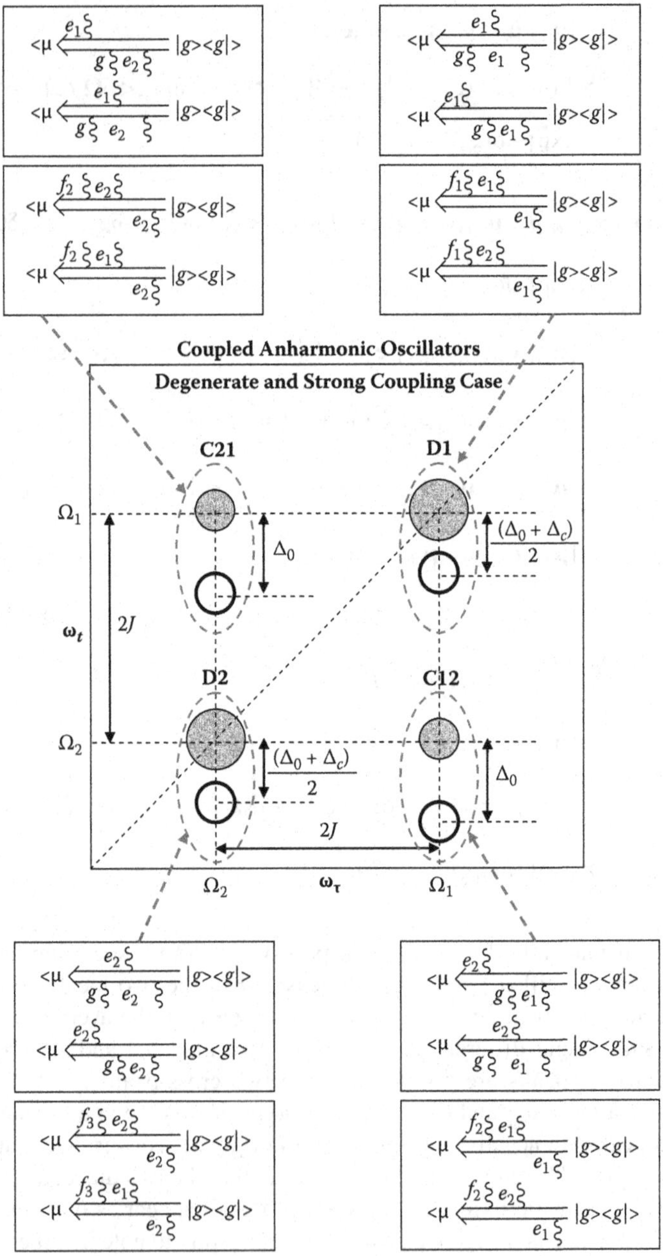

FIGURE 9.8 2D photon echo spectrum of coupled anharmonic oscillator system in the degenerate and strong coupling limit. There appear two diagonal peaks (D1 and D2) and six cross-peaks. The diagrammatic representations of the associated polarizations are also shown.

that is, $\Delta_0 > \Delta_c$, therefore we get

$$\Delta_0 > (\Delta_0 + \Delta_c)/2. \tag{9.104}$$

If the combination anharmonic frequency shift Δ_c is vanishingly small, the frequency splitting of the diagonal peak couplet is just half of that of the cross-peak couplet. These findings show that the experimentally measured frequency-splitting magnitudes of the diagonal and cross-peak couplets can be used to extract information on the overtone and combination anharmonic frequency shifts Δ_0 and Δ_c in the local mode representation.

In a real molecular system, the frequency-splitting magnitudes of the two diagonal peak couplets are in fact different from each other, despite the fact that they are predicted to be the same when the coupled anharmonic oscillator model based on the Frenkel-type Hamiltonian is used. Therefore, there is a certain limitation to the present model, but the present analysis and method should be of use in further developing theoretical models for *N*-coupled anharmonic oscillator systems such as the amide I vibrations of polypeptides and proteins.

Strongly anharmonic case ($(\Delta_0 + \Delta_c)/2 > J > \sqrt{<\delta\Omega^2>}$). When the coupling constant is much smaller than the average anharmonic frequency shift, we get

$$\lim_{(\Delta_0-\Delta_c)/J\to\infty} \xi = 0. \tag{9.105}$$

In this strongly anharmonic case, the asymptotic energies of the three doubly excited states are given as

$$\begin{aligned} W_1 &= 2\omega_0 - \Delta_c \\ W_2 &= W_3 = 2\omega_0 - \Delta_0. \end{aligned} \tag{9.106}$$

The corresponding eigenstates in this limit are simplified as

$$\begin{pmatrix} |f_1> \\ |f_2> \\ |f_3> \end{pmatrix} = V^{-1}\begin{pmatrix} |2,0> \\ |0,2> \\ |1,1> \end{pmatrix} = \frac{1}{\sqrt{2}}\begin{pmatrix} 0 & 0 & \sqrt{2} \\ 1 & -1 & 0 \\ -1 & -1 & 0 \end{pmatrix}\begin{pmatrix} |2,0> \\ |0,2> \\ |1,1> \end{pmatrix}. \tag{9.107}$$

From this expression, one can find that the f_1 state is just the combination state $|1,1>$ in the local mode representation. The f_2 state is the overtone state of the asymmetric mode, whereas the f_3 state is the overtone state of the symmetric mode. The transition dipole matrix elements between *e* and *f* states are found to be

$$\begin{aligned} &\boldsymbol{\mu}_{f1e1} = (\mathbf{d}_1 + \mathbf{d}_2)/\sqrt{2}, \quad \boldsymbol{\mu}_{f1e2} = (\mathbf{d}_1 - \mathbf{d}_2)/\sqrt{2}, \quad \boldsymbol{\mu}_{f2e1} = (\mathbf{d}_1 - \mathbf{d}_2)/\sqrt{2}, \\ &\boldsymbol{\mu}_{f2e2} = -(\mathbf{d}_1 + \mathbf{d}_2)/\sqrt{2}, \quad \boldsymbol{\mu}_{f3e1} = -(\mathbf{d}_1 + \mathbf{d}_2)/\sqrt{2}, \quad \text{and} \quad \boldsymbol{\mu}_{f3e2} = (\mathbf{d}_1 - \mathbf{d}_2)/\sqrt{2}. \end{aligned} \tag{9.108}$$

However, since the coupling constant was assumed to be larger than the absorption bandwidth $\sqrt{<\delta\Omega^2>}$, the diagonal and cross-peaks are still separated in the

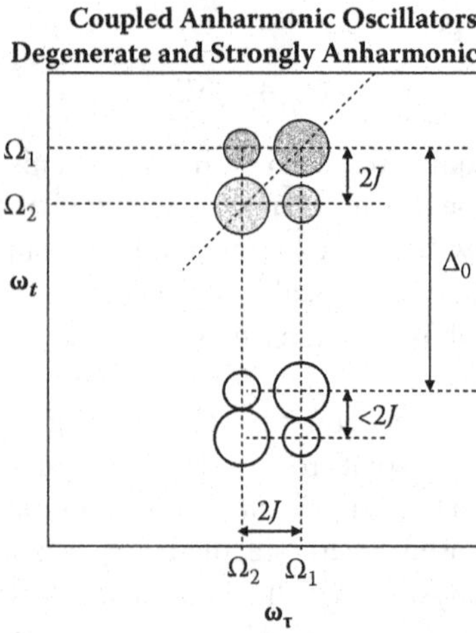

FIGURE 9.9 Two-dimensional photon echo spectrum of coupled anharmonic oscillator system in the degenerate and strongly anharmonic case. Due to the large overtone anharmonic frequency shift, the upper four peaks originating from stimulated emission and ground-state bleaching contributions are separated from the lower four peaks originating from excited-state absorption contributions.

2D frequency domain, and the two doubly excited states (f_2 and f_3) are not degenerate (see Figure 9.7). Nevertheless, all the doubly excited states are accessible from *e* states via electric dipole transitions, and thus every possible transition pathway contributing to the diagonal and cross-peaks should be included. In this particular case, the 2D spectrum is expected to be similar to Figure 9.9, where for the sake of simplicity, the combination anharmonic frequency shift Δ_c is assumed to be negligibly small in comparison to the overtone anharmonic frequency shift Δ_0. The latter assumption is generally acceptable. As shown in Figure 9.9, the upper four peaks including two diagonal and two cross-peaks are positive, and the frequency splitting magnitude is determined by the coupling constant J. The lower four peaks are negative since they involve excited-state absorption processes, and the frequency splitting magnitude along the ω_t-axis is slightly smaller than $2J$ (see the energy difference between f_2 and f_3 states in Figure 9.7). From the experimental measurements of such a strongly anharmonic case, one can estimate the overtone anharmonic frequency shift as well as the coupling constant separately.

9.9 COUPLED ANHARMONIC OSCILLATORS: POPULATION TRANSFER EFFECTS

For a coupled 2LS dimer, it was shown that population transfer between the two singly excited (e_1 and e_2) states affects the diagonal and cross-peak amplitudes in time T. Similarly, one can expect the same behaviors for the coupled anharmonic oscillator system.

The 2D photon echo diagonal peak at $\omega_\tau = \bar{\omega}_{e_1 g}$ and $\omega_t = \bar{\omega}_{e_1 g}$ is produced by the following set of diagrams:

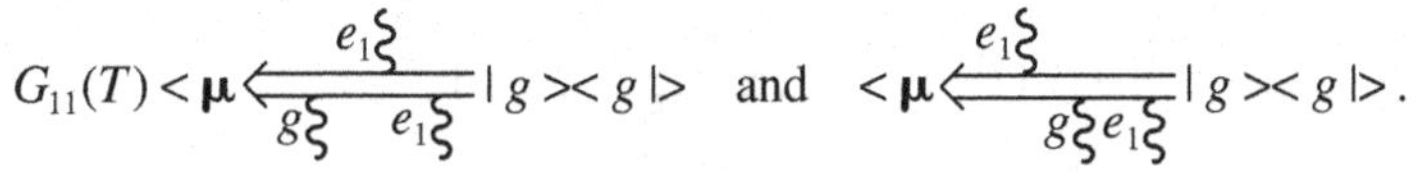

$$G_{11}(T) < \mu \xleftarrow{\substack{e_1 \\ g \quad e_1}} |g><g|> \quad \text{and} \quad <\mu \xleftarrow{\substack{e_1 \\ g \quad e_1}} |g><g|> . \qquad (9.109)$$

The diagonal peak at $\omega_\tau = \bar{\omega}_{e_2 g}$ and $\omega_t = \bar{\omega}_{e_2 g}$ is given by the sum of the following two diagrams:

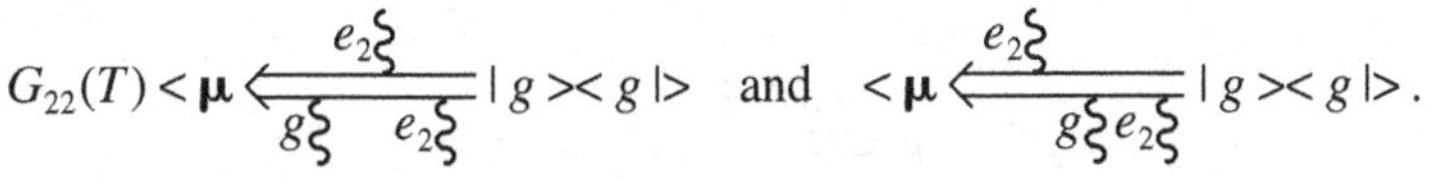

$$G_{22}(T) < \mu \xleftarrow{\substack{e_2 \\ g \quad e_2}} |g><g|> \quad \text{and} \quad <\mu \xleftarrow{\substack{e_2 \\ g \quad e_2}} |g><g|> . \qquad (9.110)$$

The cross-peak at $\omega_\tau = \bar{\omega}_{e_1 g}$ and $\omega_t = \bar{\omega}_{e_2 g}$ is associated with the following polarizations:

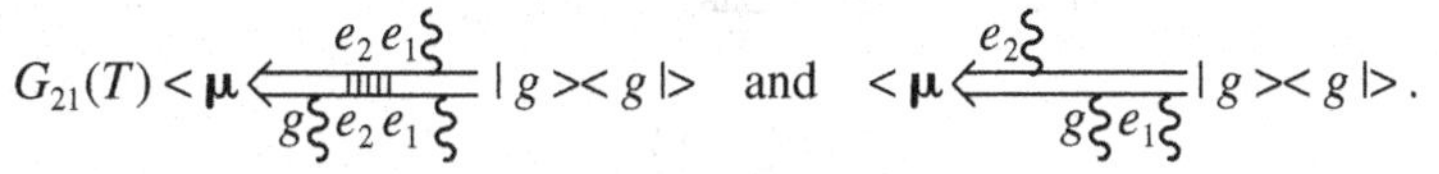

$$G_{21}(T) < \mu \xleftarrow{\substack{e_2 \, e_1 \\ g \quad e_2 e_1}} |g><g|> \quad \text{and} \quad <\mu \xleftarrow{\substack{e_2 \\ g \quad e_1}} |g><g|> . \qquad (9.111)$$

The cross-peak at $\omega_\tau = \bar{\omega}_{e_2 g}$ and $\omega_t = \bar{\omega}_{e_1 g}$ is associated with

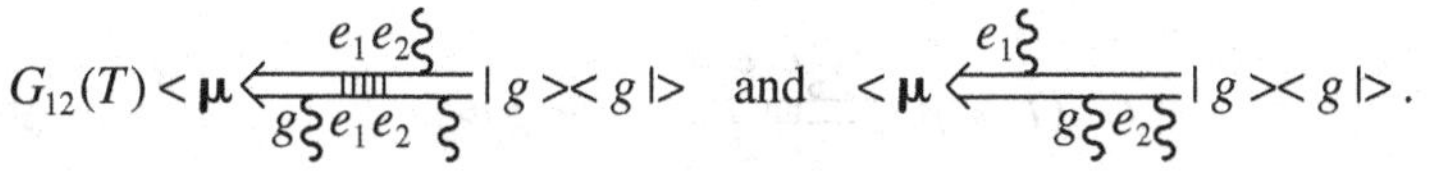

$$G_{12}(T) < \mu \xleftarrow{\substack{e_1 \, e_2 \\ g \quad e_1 e_2}} |g><g|> \quad \text{and} \quad <\mu \xleftarrow{\substack{e_1 \\ g \quad e_2}} |g><g|> . \qquad (9.112)$$

Note that the above contributions are all positive. Furthermore, if the overtone and combination anharmonic frequency shifts are large enough to separate the above $g \leftrightarrow e_j$ diagonal and cross-peaks from other negative cross-peaks involving excited-state absorption, the diagonal peak amplitudes decrease in time due to the time-dependent changes of survival probabilities.

Now, the negative cross-peaks at $\omega_\tau = \bar{\omega}_{e_1 g}$ are associated with the following diagrams:

$$G_{11}(T) < \mu \xleftarrow{\substack{f_1 \, e_1 \\ e_1}} |g><g|>$$

$$G_{11}(T) < \mu \xleftarrow{\substack{f_2 \, e_1 \\ e_1}} |g><g|>$$

$$G_{11}(T) < \mu \xleftarrow{\substack{f_3 \, e_1 \\ e_1}} |g><g|>$$

$$G_{21}(T) < \mu \xleftarrow{\substack{f_1 \, e_2 \, e_1 \\ e_2 \, e_1}} |g><g|>$$

$$G_{21}(T) < \mu \xleftarrow{\substack{f_2 \, e_2 \, e_1 \\ e_2 \, e_1}} |g><g|>$$

$$G_{21}(T) < \mu \xleftarrow{\substack{f_3 \, e_2 \, e_1 \\ e_2 \, e_1}} |g><g|> . \qquad (9.113)$$

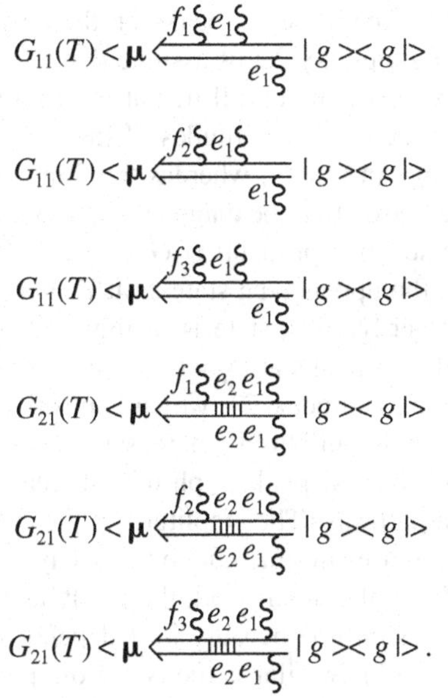

The other negative cross-peaks at $\omega_\tau = \bar{\omega}_{e_2g}$ are associated with the following diagrams:

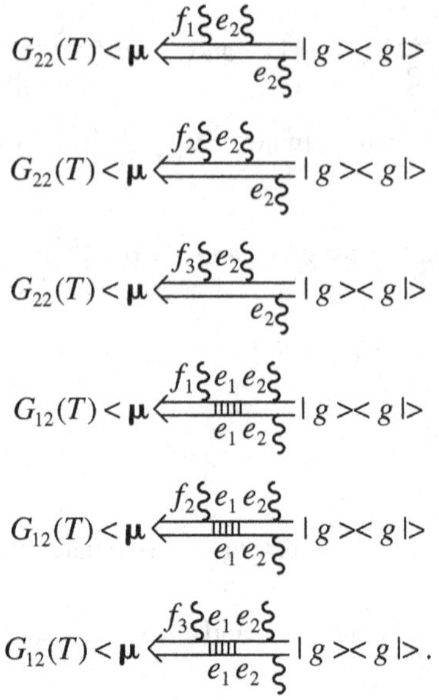

$$G_{22}(T) < \mu \overset{f_1 \} e_2 \}}{\Longleftarrow_{e_2 \}}} |g> <g|>$$

$$G_{22}(T) < \mu \overset{f_2 \} e_2 \}}{\Longleftarrow_{e_2 \}}} |g> <g|>$$

$$G_{22}(T) < \mu \overset{f_3 \} e_2 \}}{\Longleftarrow_{e_2 \}}} |g> <g|>$$

$$G_{12}(T) < \mu \overset{f_1 \} e_1\, e_2 \}}{\Longleftarrow_{e_1\, e_2 \}}} |g> <g|>$$

$$G_{12}(T) < \mu \overset{f_2 \} e_1\, e_2 \}}{\Longleftarrow_{e_1\, e_2 \}}} |g> <g|>$$

$$G_{12}(T) < \mu \overset{f_3 \} e_1\, e_2 \}}{\Longleftarrow_{e_1\, e_2 \}}} |g> <g|>. \qquad (9.114)$$

Due to population transfer processes between the two singly excited states, not only the diagonal peak amplitudes but also the cross-peak amplitudes change in time T, and the entire T-dependency of various peaks is determined by the conditional probability functions in time T.

In order to demonstrate the population transfer effects on the 2D peak shape, let us consider the strong coupling case of degenerate anharmonic oscillators. The transitions from e_1 to f_3 and from e_2 to f_1 are forbidden in this case. Therefore, as can be seen in Figure 9.10, there are six peaks on the line at $\omega_\tau = \bar{\omega}_{e_1g}$ and also at $\omega_\tau = \bar{\omega}_{e_2g}$. For the sake of simplicity, let us assume that the coupling constant is sufficiently large enough to ignore the uphill transition from the low-lying e_2 state to the upper-lying e_1 state. Then, the amplitudes of the diagonal and cross-peaks on the line at $\omega_\tau = \bar{\omega}_{e_1g}$ change in time T, whereas the four peaks at $\omega_\tau = \bar{\omega}_{e_2g}$ remain essentially constant. The reason that the diagonal and cross-peaks at $\omega_\tau = \bar{\omega}_{e_2g}$ do not change much is that the survival probability $G_{22}(T) \cong 1$ and the conditional probability $G_{12}(T)$ of finding the upper-lying state e_1 at T later when the system was on the population on the lower-lying e_2 state is negligibly small in this case. On the other hand, the amplitudes of peaks at $\omega_\tau = \bar{\omega}_{e_1g}$ change drastically. First of all, the amplitude of the upper diagonal peak D1, which is positive, decreases in time, and the main (positive) cross-peak amplitude increases. Furthermore, the other anharmonically frequency-shifted cross-peak amplitudes increase or decrease, depending on the detailed transition pathways. The amplitude of the cross-peak at $\omega_\tau = \bar{\omega}_{e_1g}$ and $\omega_t = \bar{\omega}_{e_1g} - (\Delta_0 + \Delta_c)/2$ decreases in time due to the decay of the survival probability $G_{11}(T)$ with respect to T. On the other hand, the newly appearing peak at $\omega_\tau = \bar{\omega}_{e_1g}$ and $\omega_t = \bar{\omega}_{e_1g} - \Delta_0$ increases in time because its T-dependency is determined by the conditional probability $G_{21}(T)$. Similarly, the two cross-peaks in the bottom of the

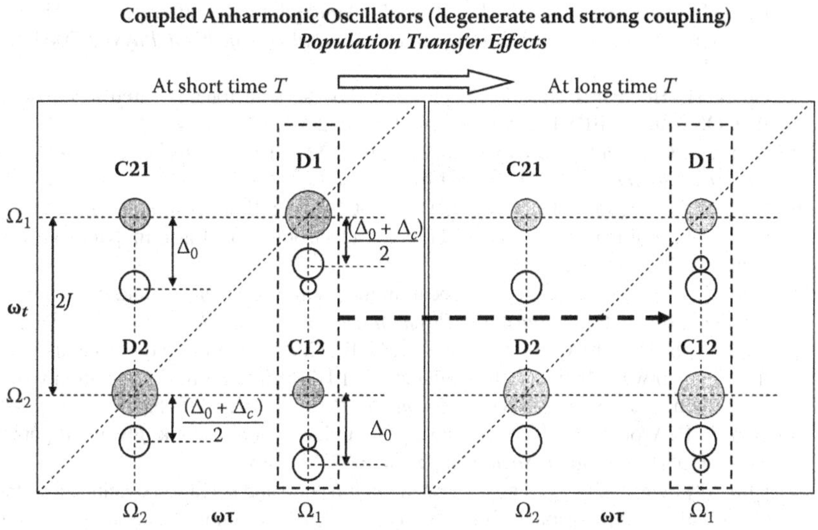

FIGURE 9.10 Population transfer effects on 2D photon echo spectrum of coupled anharmonic oscillator system in the degenerate and strong coupling limit.

dashed box in Figure 9.10 show increasing and decreasing patterns. Using the results presented above, one will be able to analyze the experimental data for an arbitrary coupled anharmonic oscillator system when the population transfer processes are measurably faster than the excited-state lifetimes.

REFERENCES

1. Woutersen, S.; Hamm, P., Structure determination of trialanine in water using polarization sensitive two-dimensional vibrational spectroscopy. *Journal of Physical Chemistry B* 2000, 104, 11316–11320.
2. Woutersen, S.; Hamm, P., Isotope-edited two-dimensional vibrational spectroscopy of trialanine in aqueous solution. *Journal of Chemical Physics* 2001, 114, 2727–2737.
3. Woutersen, S.; Pfister, R.; Hamm, P.; Mu, Y. G.; Kosov, D. S.; Stock, G., Peptide conformational heterogeneity revealed from nonlinear vibrational spectroscopy and molecular dynamics simulations. *Journal of Chemical Physics* 2002, 117, 6833–6840.
4. Torii, H.; Tasumi, M., Ab initio molecular orbital study of the amide I vibrational interactions between the peptide groups in di- and tripeptides and considerations on the conformation of the extended helix. *Journal of Raman Spectroscopy* 1998, 29, 81–86.
5. Kim, Y. S.; Wang, J. P.; Hochstrasser, R. M., Two-dimensional infrared spectroscopy of the alanine dipeptide in aqueous solution. *Journal of Physical Chemistry B* 2005, 109, 7511–7521.
6. Cha, S. Y.; Ham, S. H.; Cho, M., Amide I vibrational modes in glycine dipeptide analog: Ab initio calculation studies. *Journal of Chemical Physics* 2002, 117, 740–750.

7. Ham, S.; Cha, S.; Choi, J.-H.; Cho, M., Amide I modes of tripeptides: Hessian matrix reconstruction and isotope effects. *Journal of Chemical Physics* 2003, 119, 1451–1461.
8. Ge, N. H.; Hochstrasser, R. M., Femtosecond two-dimensional infrared spectroscopy: IR-COSY and THIRSTY. *Phys. Chem. Comm.* 2002, 17–26.
9. Cho, M., Coherent Two-Dimensional Optical Spectroscopy *Bulletin of the Korean Chemical Society* 2006, 27, 1940–1960.
10. Brixner, T.; Stenger, J.; Vaswani, H. M.; Cho, M.; Blankenship, R. E.; Fleming, G. R., Two-dimensional spectroscopy of electronic couplings in photosynthesis. *Nature* 2005, 434, 625–628.
11. Choi, J.-H.; Ham, S.; Cho, M., Local amide I mode frequencies and coupling constants in polypeptides. *Journal of Physical Chemistry B* 2003, 107, 9132–9138.
12. Krueger, B. P.; Scholes, G. D.; Fleming, G. R., Calculation of couplings and energy-transfer pathways between the pigments of LH2 by the ab initio transition density cube method. *Journal of Physical Chemistry B* 1998, 102, 5378–5384.
13. Hamm, P.; Woutersen, S., Coupling of the amide I modes of the glycine dipeptide. *Bulletin of the Chemical Society of Japan* 2002, 75, 985–988.
14. Cho, M.; Fleming, G. R., The integrated photon echo and solvation dynamics. II. Peak shifts and two-dimensional photon echo of a coupled chromophore system. *Journal of Chemical Physics* 2005, 123, 114506.
15. Zhang, W. M.; Chernyak, V.; Mukamel, S., Multidimensional femtosecond correlation spectroscopies of electronic and vibrational excitons. *Journal of Chemical Physics* 1999, 110, 5011–5028.
16. Schatz, G. C., Ratner, M. A., *Quantum mechanics in chemistry*. Prentice-Hall: Englewood Cliffs, 1993.

10 Chemical Exchange and Two-Dimensional Spectroscopy

The 2D spectroscopy of a coupled two-chromophore system was discussed in detail in the previous chapter. Due to the impulsive nature of the incident pulses used for 2D vibrational or electronic spectroscopy, it is possible to create a number of coherences differing from one another by oscillation frequencies, phases, and transition amplitudes and to follow the dynamical evolution of the generated quantum beats at short time. If singly excited-state lifetimes are sufficiently large in comparison to the population transfer timescales, one can measure the population transfer rate constants between the singly excited states by examining cross-peak amplitude changes during time T. However, it should be emphasized that the main cross-peaks originating from $g \leftrightarrow e_1$ and $g \leftrightarrow e_2$ transitions are present even at short time T due to the nonzero coupling between the transition dipoles of the two chromophores.

Similar to the population transfer effects on the 2D spectrum with respect to T, there is another process that affects the amplitudes of the diagonal and cross-peaks in the T-dependent 2D spectra. It is the chemical exchange process including chemical reactions and physical changes of molecules.[1] For instance, the hydrogen-bond formation-dissociation process is a good example for such a chemical exchange.[2–9] Suppose that a molecule M can form a strong hydrogen-bond with a solvent molecule and that M_c denotes the hyrogen-bonded complex and M_f represents the free M in solution. Then, there is a chemical equilibrium between the two forms of solvated M molecule, that is,

$$M_c \rightleftarrows M_f. \tag{10.1}$$

If M_c and M_f have common vibrational oscillators with different frequencies, ω_c and ω_f, these two oscillators can be considered reporters on these two species, M_c and M_f. Here, the two species are not different from each other except for the number of hydrogen-bonded solvent molecules, that is, either 1 or 0. If one carries out a 2D spectroscopic study of this molecular system in its chemical equilibrium, and the equilibrium constant is of order unity, then one can observe time-dependent changes of the diagonal and cross-peak amplitudes. At short time T, there won't be any cross-peaks, because, unlike the coupled dimer system considered in the previous chapter, the two oscillators are not simultaneously present in an individual molecule. Thus, there is no intrinsic coupling between the two oscillators. However, as the waiting time T increases, the cross-peak amplitudes will increase and their time-dependencies are determined by the chemical exchange rates between the two species.

A clear advantage of chemical exchange 2D spectroscopy is that the ultrafast relaxation rates can be measured without relying on an external perturbation such as *T*-jump, pressure-jump, concentration-jump, pH-jump, or and so on to initiate the exchange process. This is because the photo-excitation of one particular species is a kind of tagging process. Then, after the waiting time *T*, the survival probability of the tagged species or the conditional probability of finding other specific species different from the tagged one can be measured by analyzing the corresponding diagonal and cross-peak amplitude changes. In this chapter, chemical exchange effects on the 2D spectrum will be discussed by assuming that the two chemical species are represented by either 2LSs or anharmonic oscillators (effectively 3LS). It also will be shown that, from the peak shape analysis of the 2D spectra with respect to the waiting time *T*, one can extract kinetic information on chemical exchange processes.

10.1 MODEL SYSTEM

There could be a number of cases when the 2D spectroscopy can provide critical information on the kinetic networks and exchange rates among spectroscopically inequivalent species in condensed phases. In the Introduction, hydrogen-bonding dynamics was mentioned as an example. Other examples include chemical reactions, van der Waals complexation, conformational changes of complex molecules such as proteins and nucleic acids, protein–protein complexation, protein–ligand binding, protein-DNA or -RNA binding, and so on. In this chapter, a two-species model will be considered in detail, in which two distinctively different species are in chemical or physical equilibrium, that is,

$$A \underset{k_b}{\overset{k_f}{\rightleftarrows}} B. \tag{10.2}$$

The forward and backward rate constants are denoted as k_f and k_b, respectively. The excited states of these two species will be denoted as A^* and B^*. Suppose that these two excited states can also form a thermal equilibrium state, provided that the lifetimes of these two excited states denoted as T_A and T_B, are sufficiently larger than the chemical exchange times ($1/k_f^*$ and $1/k_b^*$). Then the chemical or physical equilibrium of A^* and B^* is given as

$$A^* \underset{k_b^*}{\overset{k_f^*}{\rightleftarrows}} B^*. \tag{10.3}$$

Note that the exchange rate constants k_f^* and k_b^* could be different from k_f and k_b, because the electronic structures of the excited states are, in general, different from those of the ground states, which in turn make the solute-solvent interactions of the excited states different from those of the ground states.[5, 7] In addition, the

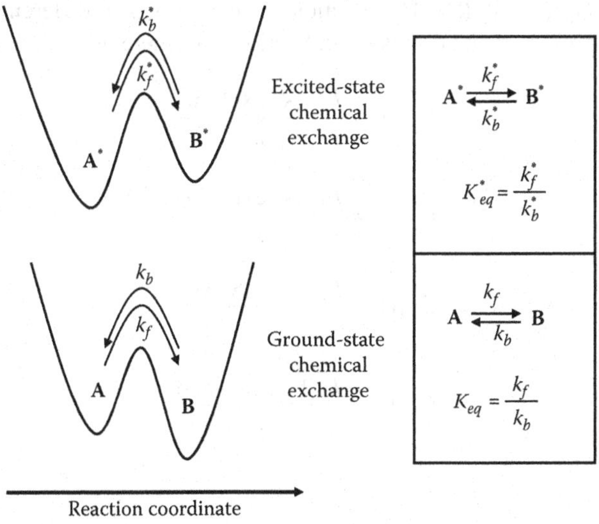

FIGURE 10.1 Reaction potential energy surfaces along the relevant reaction coordinate.

excited-state potential energy surface along the reaction coordinate is likely to be different from the ground-state potential energy surface. In Figure 10.1, a schematic picture of the ground and excited-state potential energy surfaces is shown. Although the chemical exchange processes depicted in this figure are assumed to be barrier-crossing problems, the following results and discussions are quite general as long as a given exchange process involves just two species. In the case of chemical reaction, the two species A and B represent the reactant and the product, respectively. If the process of interest is conformational change of biomolecule such as protein folding and unfolding, and if it is a two-state process, the two species are the native and unfolded proteins. If the chemical exchange of interest is protein-ligand binding such as enzyme-substrate complex formation, the two species may correspond to the free substrate (or enzyme) and the enzyme-substrate complex, respectively.

For the sake of simplicity, the chemical exchange process on the ground state is assumed to be determined by the following master equation:

$$\frac{d}{dt}\begin{pmatrix} G_{AA}(t) & G_{AB}(t) \\ G_{BA}(t) & G_{BB}(t) \end{pmatrix} = \begin{pmatrix} -k_f & k_b \\ k_f & -k_b \end{pmatrix}\begin{pmatrix} G_{AA}(t) & G_{AB}(t) \\ G_{BA}(t) & G_{BB}(t) \end{pmatrix}, \tag{10.4}$$

where $G_{AA}(t)$ ($G_{BB}(t)$) is the survival probability of the A (B) species. The conditional probability of finding B (A) species at t later when it was A (B) initially at time 0 is denoted as $G_{BA}(t)$ $(G_{AB}(t))$. The solutions of these coupled differential equations were already presented and discussed in Section 9.5, where we obtained

$$G_{AA}(t) = \frac{k_b + k_f \exp(-kt)}{k}$$

$$G_{BB}(t) = \frac{k_f + k_b \exp(-kt)}{k}$$

$$G_{BA}(t) = \frac{k_f\{1 - \exp(-kt)\}}{k}$$

$$G_{AB}(t) = \frac{k_b\{1 - \exp(-kt)\}}{k} \tag{10.5}$$

with

$$k = k_f + k_b. \tag{10.6}$$

The conditional and survival probabilities, denoted as $G_{jk}^*(t)$, for the chemical exchange process on their excited states are similarly given except that $k_f \to k_f^*$, $k_b \to k_b^*$, and $k \to k^*$. In the following section, the 2D spectroscopy of chemical exchange dynamics for this two-species model will be discussed.

10.2 CHEMICAL EXCHANGE DIAGRAMS: TWO-LEVEL SYSTEM

In this section, let us consider a 2LS chromophore. If the chemical exchange processes are slow in comparison to the experimental timescale and the excited-state lifetime, the two chemical species that are present in an equilibrium distribution contribute to the 2D spectrum separately. In this slow reaction limit, the 2D photon echo polarization consists of the following four contributions:

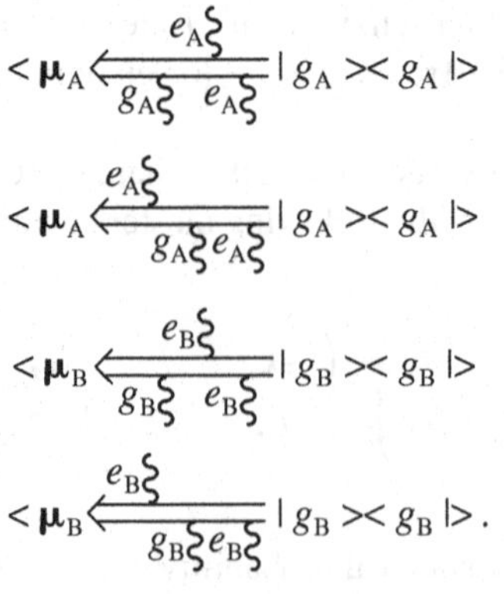

$$< \mu_A \xleftarrow[g_A \; e_A]{e_A} | g_A >< g_A | >$$

$$< \mu_A \xleftarrow[g_A e_A]{e_A} | g_A >< g_A | >$$

$$< \mu_B \xleftarrow[g_B \; e_B]{e_B} | g_B >< g_B | >$$

$$< \mu_B \xleftarrow[g_B e_B]{e_B} | g_B >< g_B | >. \tag{10.7}$$

The first diagram is the stimulated emission contribution from A, whereas the second is the ground-state bleaching contribution from A. Similarly, the third and fourth ones correspond to those from B. Now, since the transition frequencies $\bar{\omega}_{e_A g_A}$ and $\bar{\omega}_{e_B g_B}$ of the two species A and B are assumed to be different from each other, the 2D photon echo spectrum consists of two diagonal peaks at $\omega_\tau = \bar{\omega}_{e_A g_A}$ and $\omega_t = \bar{\omega}_{e_A g_A}$ and at $\omega_\tau = \bar{\omega}_{e_B g_B}$ and $\omega_t = \bar{\omega}_{e_B g_B}$, that is,

$$\tilde{\mathbf{E}}_{PE}(\omega_t, T, \omega_\tau) = 2X_A[\boldsymbol{\mu}_{ge}^A \boldsymbol{\mu}_{eg}^A \boldsymbol{\mu}_{ge}^A \boldsymbol{\mu}_{eg}^A]: \mathbf{e}_3 \mathbf{e}_2 \mathbf{e}_1^* \Gamma\left(\bar{\omega}_{e_A g_A}, \Omega_A^2, \bar{\omega}_{e_A g_A}, \Omega_A^2\right)$$

$$+ 2X_B[\boldsymbol{\mu}_{ge}^B \boldsymbol{\mu}_{eg}^B \boldsymbol{\mu}_{ge}^B \boldsymbol{\mu}_{eg}^B]: \mathbf{e}_3 \mathbf{e}_2 \mathbf{e}_1^* \Gamma\left(\bar{\omega}_{e_B g_B}, \Omega_B^2, \bar{\omega}_{e_B g_B}, \Omega_B^2\right). \tag{10.8}$$

Here, the mean square fluctuation amplitudes of the difference potentials (fluctuating parts of transition frequencies) of A and B species are denoted as Ω_A^2 and Ω_B^2, respectively. The transition dipole matrix element $\boldsymbol{\mu}_{eg}^A$, for example, is defined as $\boldsymbol{\mu}_{eg}^A \equiv <e_A | \boldsymbol{\mu}_A | g_A >$. In Equation 10.8, the mole fractions of A and B species are denoted as X_A and X_B, respectively. Since the relative numbers of A and B species at time zero are determined by the corresponding mole fractions (or concentrations), the two diagonal peak amplitudes are linearly proportional to X_j (for j = A or B).

Next, let us consider the more interesting case when the chemical exchange rates are sufficiently fast to significantly change the 2D spectral peak shape. Typically, the 2D spectrum is obtained by carrying out double Fourier transformations of the echo signal with respect to τ and t. Note that the signal is determined by the electronic coherence present in the system during these two periods so that the required experimental scanning times for τ and t are often very short. Therefore, chemical exchange processes during τ and t can be ignored, but during the waiting time T the electronic population undergoes chemical exchange electronic between the two species. Consequently, we need to take into account more diagrams for the total 2D photon echo polarization. Since not only the ground-state species but also the excited-state species undergo chemical exchanges, both the stimulated emission and ground-state bleaching terms in Equation 10.7 should be divided into two parts that contain either a survival probability or a conditional probability function. Now, the four diagrams in Equation 10.7 should be replaced with the following four diagrams:

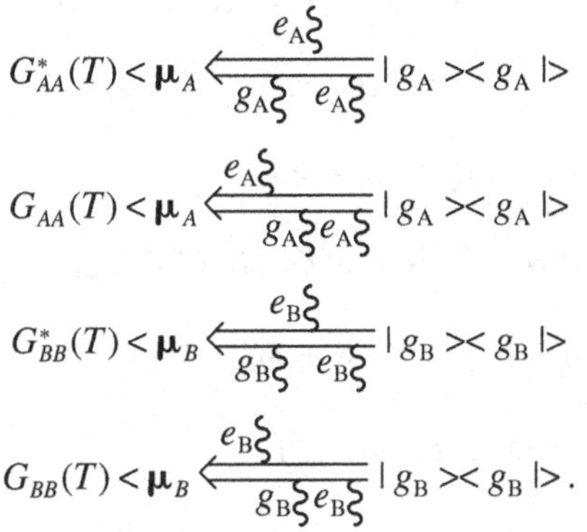

$$G_{AA}^*(T) < \boldsymbol{\mu}_A \xleftarrow[\;g_A\; \;e_A\;]{e_A} |\, g_A > < g_A \,|>$$

$$G_{AA}(T) < \boldsymbol{\mu}_A \xleftarrow[\;g_A\; e_A\;]{e_A} |\, g_A > < g_A \,|>$$

$$G_{BB}^*(T) < \boldsymbol{\mu}_B \xleftarrow[\;g_B\; \;e_B\;]{e_B} |\, g_B > < g_B \,|>$$

$$G_{BB}(T) < \boldsymbol{\mu}_B \xleftarrow[\;g_B\, e_B\;]{e_B} |\, g_B > < g_B \,|>. \tag{10.9}$$

The upper two polarizations in Equation 10.9 contribute to the diagonal peak at $\omega_\tau = \bar{\omega}_{e_A g_A}$ and $\omega_t = \bar{\omega}_{e_A g_A}$, whereas the lower two are associated with the diagonal peak at $\omega_\tau = \bar{\omega}_{e_Bg_B}$ and $\omega_t = \bar{\omega}_{e_Bg_B}$. Since the survival probability functions decay in time T, the diagonal peak amplitudes decrease.

Next, let us consider the diagrams involving chemical exchange from one species to the other during the waiting time T,

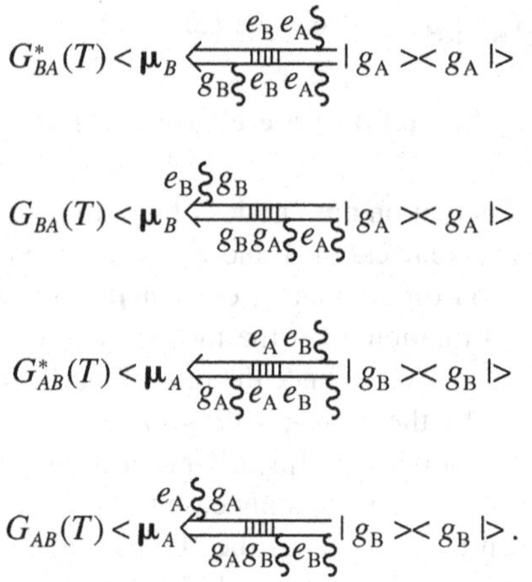

$$G^*_{BA}(T) < \mu_B \overset{e_B \, e_A}{\underset{g_B \, e_B \, e_A}{\Longleftarrow}} | g_A > < g_A |>$$

$$G_{BA}(T) < \mu_B \overset{e_B \, g_B}{\underset{g_B g_A \, e_A}{\Longleftarrow}} | g_A > < g_A |>$$

$$G^*_{AB}(T) < \mu_A \overset{e_A \, e_B}{\underset{g_A \, e_A \, e_B}{\Longleftarrow}} | g_B > < g_B |>$$

$$G_{AB}(T) < \mu_A \overset{e_A \, g_A}{\underset{g_A g_B \, e_B}{\Longleftarrow}} | g_B > < g_B |>. \tag{10.10}$$

These four diagrams show that the coherence during t_1 period in each diagram is different from that during t_3 period, which suggests that they will contribute to cross-peaks. The T-dependent increasing patterns of cross-peak amplitudes are thus determined by the conditional probability functions.

From the generalized diagrams in Equations 10.9 and 10.10, one can show that the diagonal and cross-peaks can be written in terms of the 2D Gaussian peak shape function as,

(1)   Diagonal peak at $(\omega_\tau = \bar{\omega}_{e_Ag_A}, \omega_t = \bar{\omega}_{e_Ag_A})$

$$\tilde{E}_{D1}(\omega_t, T, \omega_\tau) = \left[\mu^A_{ge} \mu^A_{eg} \mu^A_{ge} \mu^A_{eg} \right] : e_3 e_2 e^*_1 X_A \{G^*_{AA}(T) + G_{AA}(T)\}$$

$$\times \Gamma\left(\omega_t = \bar{\omega}_{e_Ag_A}, \Omega^2_A, \omega_\tau = \bar{\omega}_{e_Ag_A}, \Omega^2_A\right) \tag{10.11}$$

(2)   Diagonal peak at $(\omega_\tau = \bar{\omega}_{e_Bg_B}, \omega_t = \bar{\omega}_{e_Bg_B})$

$$\tilde{E}_{D2}(\omega_t, T, \omega_\tau) = \left[\mu^B_{ge} \mu^B_{eg} \mu^B_{ge} \mu^B_{eg} \right] : e_3 e_2 e^*_1 X_B \{G^*_{BB}(T) + G_{BB}(T)\}$$

$$\times \Gamma\left(\omega_t = \bar{\omega}_{e_Bg_B}, \Omega^2_B, \omega_\tau = \bar{\omega}_{e_Bg_B}, \Omega^2_B\right) \tag{10.12}$$

(3)   Cross-peak at $(\omega_\tau = \bar{\omega}_{e_Ag_A}, \omega_t = \bar{\omega}_{e_Bg_B})$

$$\tilde{E}_{AB}(\omega_t, T, \omega_\tau) = \left[\mu^B_{ge} \mu^B_{eg} \mu^A_{ge} \mu^A_{eg} \right] : e_3 e_2 e^*_1 X_A \{G^*_{BA}(T) + G_{BA}(T)\}$$

$$\times \Gamma\left(\omega_t = \bar{\omega}_{e_Bg_B}, \Omega^2_B, \omega_\tau = \bar{\omega}_{e_Ag_A}, \Omega^2_A\right) \tag{10.13}$$

(4) Cross-peak at $(\omega_\tau=\bar{\omega}_{e_Bg_B},\omega_t=\bar{\omega}_{e_Ag_A})$

$$\tilde{\mathbf{E}}_{BA}(\omega_t,T,\omega_\tau)=\left[\boldsymbol{\mu}^A_{ge}\boldsymbol{\mu}^A_{eg}\boldsymbol{\mu}^B_{ge}\boldsymbol{\mu}^B_{eg}\right]\vdots\mathbf{e}_3\mathbf{e}_2\mathbf{e}_1^*X_B\{G^*_{AB}(T)+G_{AB}(T)\}$$
$$\times\Gamma\left(\omega_t=\bar{\omega}_{e_Ag_A},\Omega_A^2,\omega_\tau=\bar{\omega}_{e_Bg_B},\Omega_B^2\right). \quad (10.14)$$

From these results, one finds that no cross-peaks appears at time $T = 0$, since $G_{BA}(0)=G_{AB}(0)=0$ and $G^*_{BA}(0)=G^*_{AB}(0)=0$. In Figure 10.2, a schematic 2D spectrum of the present two-species chemical exchange system is drawn. The T-dependency of the upper (high-energy) diagonal peak amplitude is determined by the average survival probability function $\{G_{BB}(T)+G^*_{BB}(T)\}/2$, which describes the average of $B\to B$ and $B^*\to B^*$ processes. The upper-left cross-peak amplitude

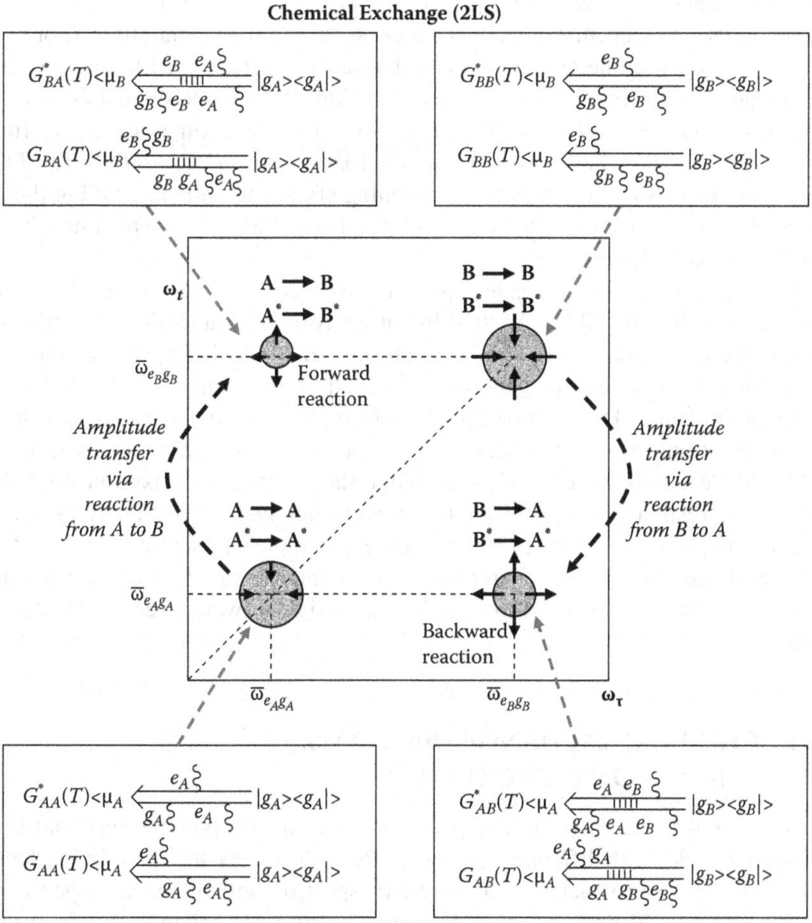

FIGURE 10.2 2D spectrum of two-species chemical exchange system. Each species is modeled as a 2LS.

is determined by the average conditional probability function, $\{G_{BA}(T)+G^*_{BA}(T)\}/2$, which decribes the forward reaction processes, that is, $A \rightarrow B$ and $A^* \rightarrow B^*$. Similarly, one can understand the T-dependencies of the lower (low-energy) diagonal and lower-right cross-peak amplitudes. Thus, measurements of both diagonal and cross-peaks can provide direct information on the forward and backward rate constants, when it is assumed that the rate constants on the ground state are close to those on the excited state.

Before this section is closed, it should be mentioned that the lifetime-broadening effects as well as rotational relaxation contributions should be properly included if necessary. As shown in Section 7.5, the lifetime-broadening effects can be taken into account by multiplying the appropriate exponentially decaying function to the corresponding third-order response function. The lifetime-broadening function for the first two diagrams in Equation 10.7 is simply given by $\exp(-t/2T_{e_A} - T/T_{e_A} - \tau/2T_{e_A})$, where T_{e_A} is the lifetime of the e_A state. The corresponding lifetime-broadening function for the last two diagrams in Equation 10.7 is $\exp(-t/2T_{e_B} - T/T_{e_B} - \tau/2T_{e_B})$. If the system undergoes a chemical exchange process during the waiting time T, one can take the average lifetime of the two excited states to construct the lifetime-broadening function. For the first two diagrams in Equation 10.9, it is approximately given by $\exp(-t/2T_{e_B} - (T^{-1}_{e_A} + T^{-1}_{e_B})T/2 - \tau/2T_{e_A})$. The corresponding lifetime-broadening function for the last two diagrams in Equation 10.9 is $\exp(-t/2T_{e_A} - (T^{-1}_{e_A} + T^{-1}_{e_B})T/2 - \tau/2T_{e_B})$. By including these lifetime-broadening effects properly and taking the 2D Fourier-Laplace transform of the third-order response function, one obtains the lifetime-broadened 2D spectrum.

In addition to lifetime broadening, it is also necessary to consider the rotational relaxation contributions to third-order response functions. Usually, the relevant experimental timescales are determined by dephasing times and lifetimes. Such timescales are generally quite short in comparison to molecular reorientation times. However, if the size of target molecule is sufficiently small and the rotational relaxation timescale is comparable to the above experimental timescales, it is necessary to consider the rotational relaxation contributions to the response funtion. Usually, most target systems are fairly large, for example, peptides, proteins, light-harvesting complexes, semiconductors, and so forth. Therefore, the rotational relaxation contributions won't be considered in detail in this chaper, even though it is a straightforward exercise to include them.

10.3 CHEMICAL EXCHANGE DIAGRAMS: ANHARMONIC OSCILLATOR

When the two characteristic chromophores representing the two species A and B are vibrational modes with different frequencies for each species, the chemical exchange processes can be investigated by using 2D IR spectroscopy. If the exchange time is very slow, the 2D IR photon echo polarization of this equilibrium system is just the sum of polarizations associated with the two species. For the A species, one needs to consider the following three polarizations:

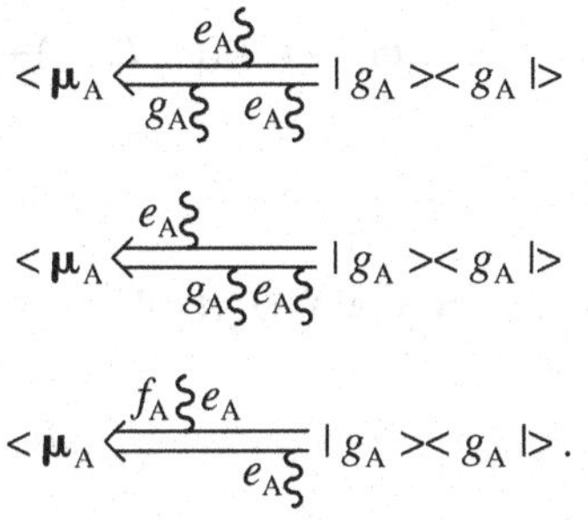

$$< \mu_A \xleftarrow[g_A \zeta \ e_A \zeta]{e_A \zeta} | g_A >< g_A |>$$

$$< \mu_A \xleftarrow[g_A \zeta e_A \zeta]{e_A \zeta} | g_A >< g_A |>$$

$$< \mu_A \xleftarrow[e_A \zeta]{f_A \zeta e_A} | g_A >< g_A |> . \tag{10.15}$$

Note that the third term in the above is the excited-state absorption diagram, which contributes negatively to the 2D photon echo spectrum. Similarly, there are three diagrams for the B species. If the vibrational ground or excited-state molecules undergo chemical exchange processes, the above diagrams should be replaced with those including the survival probability functions. Also, due to the forward and backward reactions, there are new pathways (diagrams) that also contribute to the 2D spectrum.

In addition to the eight diagrams in Equations 10.9 and 10.10 for a chemically exchanging 2LS considered in the previous section, one needs to consider the excited-state absorption contributions whose diagrams are given by

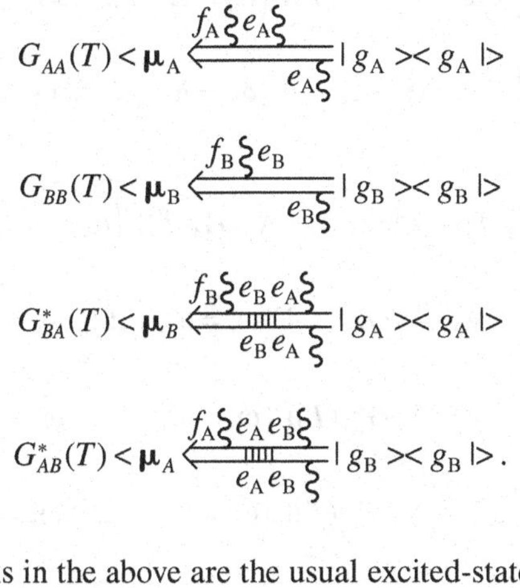

$$G_{AA}(T) < \mu_A \xleftarrow[e_A \zeta]{f_A \zeta e_A \zeta} | g_A >< g_A |>$$

$$G_{BB}(T) < \mu_B \xleftarrow[e_B \zeta]{f_B \zeta e_B} | g_B >< g_B |>$$

$$G_{BA}^*(T) < \mu_B \xleftarrow[e_B e_A \zeta]{f_B \zeta e_B e_A \zeta} | g_A >< g_A |>$$

$$G_{AB}^*(T) < \mu_A \xleftarrow[e_A e_B \zeta]{f_A \zeta e_A e_B \zeta} | g_B >< g_B |> . \tag{10.16}$$

The first two diagrams in the above are the usual excited-state absorption contributions, but their amplitudes are now determined by the corresponding survival probability functions. The latter two diagrams describe the transitions from A to B and from B to A, respectively. Due to these two terms, there will appear two new cross-peaks that are negative.

By combining these four more diagrams in Equation 10.16 with the eight digrams in Equations 10.9 and 10.10 discussed in the previous section, the total 2D spectrum is given by the sum of stimulated emission, ground-state bleaching, and excited-state absorption contributions as

$$\tilde{\mathbf{E}}(\omega_t, T, \omega_\tau) = \tilde{\mathbf{E}}_{SE}(\omega_t, T, \omega_\tau) + \tilde{\mathbf{E}}_{GB}(\omega_t, T, \omega_\tau) + \tilde{\mathbf{E}}_{EA}(\omega_t, T, \omega_\tau), \tag{10.17}$$

where

$$\begin{aligned}
\tilde{\mathbf{E}}_{SE}(\omega_t, T, \omega_\tau) = {} & \left[\boldsymbol{\mu}^A_{ge}\boldsymbol{\mu}^A_{eg}\boldsymbol{\mu}^A_{ge}\boldsymbol{\mu}^A_{eg}\right] \vdots\, \mathbf{e}_3\mathbf{e}_2\mathbf{e}_1^* X_A G^*_{AA}(T)\Gamma\left(\omega_t = \bar{\omega}_{e_Ag_A}, \Omega_A^2, \omega_\tau = \bar{\omega}_{e_Ag_A}, \Omega_A^2\right) \\
& + \left[\boldsymbol{\mu}^B_{ge}\boldsymbol{\mu}^B_{eg}\boldsymbol{\mu}^B_{ge}\boldsymbol{\mu}^B_{eg}\right] \vdots\, \mathbf{e}_3\mathbf{e}_2\mathbf{e}_1^* X_B G^*_{BB}(T)\Gamma\left(\omega_t = \bar{\omega}_{e_Bg_B}, \Omega_B^2, \omega_\tau = \bar{\omega}_{e_Bg_B}, \Omega_B^2\right) \\
& + \left[\boldsymbol{\mu}^B_{ge}\boldsymbol{\mu}^B_{eg}\boldsymbol{\mu}^A_{ge}\boldsymbol{\mu}^A_{eg}\right] \vdots\, \mathbf{e}_3\mathbf{e}_2\mathbf{e}_1^* X_A G^*_{BA}(T)\Gamma\left(\omega_t = \bar{\omega}_{e_Bg_B}, \Omega_B^2, \omega_\tau = \bar{\omega}_{e_Ag_A}, \Omega_A^2\right) \\
& + \left[\boldsymbol{\mu}^A_{ge}\boldsymbol{\mu}^A_{eg}\boldsymbol{\mu}^B_{ge}\boldsymbol{\mu}^B_{eg}\right] \vdots\, \mathbf{e}_3\mathbf{e}_2\mathbf{e}_1^* X_B G^*_{AB}(T)\Gamma\left(\omega_t = \bar{\omega}_{e_Ag_A}, \Omega_A^2, \omega_\tau = \bar{\omega}_{e_Bg_B}, \Omega_B^2\right)
\end{aligned} \tag{10.18}$$

$$\begin{aligned}
\tilde{\mathbf{E}}_{GB}(\omega_t, T, \omega_\tau) = {} & \left[\boldsymbol{\mu}^A_{ge}\boldsymbol{\mu}^A_{eg}\boldsymbol{\mu}^A_{ge}\boldsymbol{\mu}^A_{eg}\right] \vdots\, \mathbf{e}_3\mathbf{e}_2\mathbf{e}_1^* X_A G_{AA}(T)\Gamma\left(\omega_t = \bar{\omega}_{e_Ag_A}, \Omega_A^2, \omega_\tau = \bar{\omega}_{e_Ag_A}, \Omega_A^2\right) \\
& + \left[\boldsymbol{\mu}^B_{ge}\boldsymbol{\mu}^B_{eg}\boldsymbol{\mu}^B_{ge}\boldsymbol{\mu}^B_{eg}\right] \vdots\, \mathbf{e}_3\mathbf{e}_2\mathbf{e}_1^* X_B G_{BB}(T)\Gamma(\omega_t = \bar{\omega}_{e_Bg_B}, \Omega_B^2, \omega_\tau = \bar{\omega}_{e_Bg_B}, \Omega_B^2) \\
& + \left[\boldsymbol{\mu}^B_{ge}\boldsymbol{\mu}^B_{eg}\boldsymbol{\mu}^A_{ge}\boldsymbol{\mu}^A_{eg}\right] \vdots\, \mathbf{e}_3\mathbf{e}_2\mathbf{e}_1^* X_A G_{BA}(T)\Gamma\left(\omega_t = \bar{\omega}_{e_Bg_B}, \Omega_B^2, \omega_\tau = \bar{\omega}_{e_Ag_A}, \Omega_A^2\right) \\
& + \left[\boldsymbol{\mu}^A_{ge}\boldsymbol{\mu}^A_{eg}\boldsymbol{\mu}^B_{ge}\boldsymbol{\mu}^B_{eg}\right] \vdots\, \mathbf{e}_3\mathbf{e}_2\mathbf{e}_1^* X_B G_{AB}(T)\Gamma\left(\omega_t = \bar{\omega}_{e_Ag_A}, \Omega_A^2, \omega_\tau = \bar{\omega}_{e_Bg_B}, \Omega_B^2\right)
\end{aligned} \tag{10.19}$$

$$\begin{aligned}
\tilde{\mathbf{E}}_{EA}(\omega_t, T, \omega_\tau) = {} & -\left[\boldsymbol{\mu}^A_{ef}\boldsymbol{\mu}^A_{fe}\boldsymbol{\mu}^A_{eg}\boldsymbol{\mu}^A_{ge}\right] \vdots\, \mathbf{e}_3\mathbf{e}_2\mathbf{e}_1^* X_A G^*_{AA}(T)\Gamma\left(\omega_t = \bar{\omega}_{f_Ae_A}, \Omega_A^2, \omega_\tau = \bar{\omega}_{e_Ag_A}, \Omega_A^2\right) \\
& - \left[\boldsymbol{\mu}^B_{ef}\boldsymbol{\mu}^B_{fe}\boldsymbol{\mu}^B_{eg}\boldsymbol{\mu}^B_{ge}\right] \vdots\, \mathbf{e}_3\mathbf{e}_2\mathbf{e}_1^* X_B G^*_{BB}(T)\Gamma\left(\omega_t = \bar{\omega}_{f_Be_B}, \Omega_B^2, \omega_\tau = \bar{\omega}_{e_Bg_B}, \Omega_B^2\right) \\
& - \left[\boldsymbol{\mu}^B_{ef}\boldsymbol{\mu}^B_{fe}\boldsymbol{\mu}^A_{eg}\boldsymbol{\mu}^A_{ge}\right] \vdots\, \mathbf{e}_3\mathbf{e}_2\mathbf{e}_1^* X_A G^*_{BA}(T)\Gamma\left(\omega_t = \bar{\omega}_{f_Be_B}, \Omega_B^2, \omega_\tau = \bar{\omega}_{e_Ag_A}, \Omega_A^2\right) \\
& - \left[\boldsymbol{\mu}^A_{ef}\boldsymbol{\mu}^A_{fe}\boldsymbol{\mu}^B_{eg}\boldsymbol{\mu}^B_{ge}\right] \vdots\, \mathbf{e}_3\mathbf{e}_2\mathbf{e}_1^* X_B G^*_{AB}(T)\Gamma\left(\omega_t = \bar{\omega}_{f_Ae_A}, \Omega_A^2, \omega_\tau = \bar{\omega}_{e_Bg_B}, \Omega_B^2\right).
\end{aligned} \tag{10.20}$$

The 2D peak shape of the measured spectrum strongly depends on the magnitudes of the overtone anharmonicities of the two species. Let us denote the overtone anharmonic frequency shifts of the two species as $\delta\omega^A_{anh}$ and $\delta\omega^B_{anh}$, that is,

$$\begin{aligned}
\delta\omega^A_{anh} &= \bar{\omega}_{e_Ag_A} - \bar{\omega}_{f_Ae_A} \\
\delta\omega^B_{anh} &= \bar{\omega}_{e_Bg_B} - \bar{\omega}_{f_Be_B}.
\end{aligned} \tag{10.21}$$

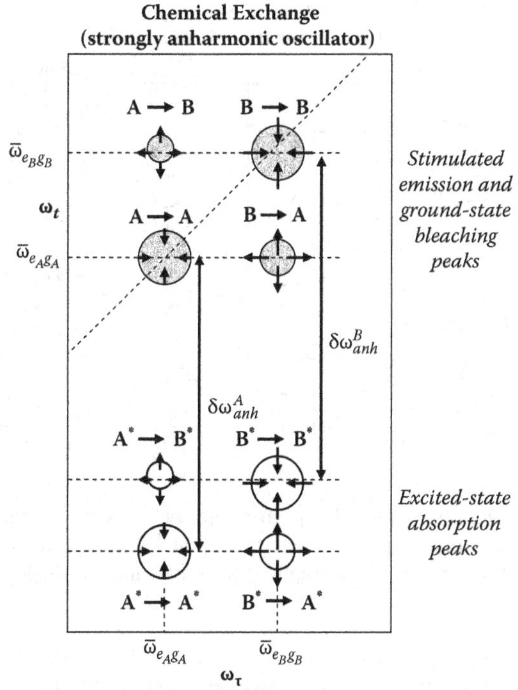

FIGURE 10.3 2D spectrum of two-species chemical exchange system. The two species are anharmonic oscillators with large overtone anharmonic frequency shifts.

In the limiting case that the difference between the fundamental transition frequencies of the oscillators of the species A and B is smaller than the overtone anharmonic frequency shifts, that is,

$$|\bar{\omega}_{e_Bg_B} - \bar{\omega}_{e_Ag_A}| < \delta\omega_{anh}^A \quad \text{and} \quad |\bar{\omega}_{e_Bg_B} - \bar{\omega}_{e_Ag_A}| < \delta\omega_{anh}^B \tag{10.22}$$

the excited-state absorption peaks in the real part of a given 2D spectrum are well-separated from the positive peaks from the stimulated emission and ground-state bleaching peaks.[7] In this large anharmonicity case, the 2D spectrum appears as in Figure 10.3. It should be noted that the time-dependencies of the negative peak amplitudes shown in the bottom part of Figure 10.3 are determined by the chemical exchange processes on the vibrationally excited states, that is, $e_A \leftrightarrow e_B$. The positive diagonal and cross-peaks originating from the stimulated emission and ground-state bleaching contributions, which appear in the upper part of the 2D spectrum in Figure 10.3, are functions of the waiting time T, and their amplitude changes depend on the exchange processes on both the ground and excited states. Therefore, by selectively analyzing the time-dependent changes of the excited-state absorption peak amplitudes with respect to the waiting time T, it is possible to estimate the rates of the chemical exchange processes on the vibrationally excited state only.

If the overtone anharmonic frequency shifts are relatively small in comparison with the magnitude of frequency difference ($|\bar{\omega}_{e_Bg_B} - \bar{\omega}_{e_Ag_A}|$) associated with the

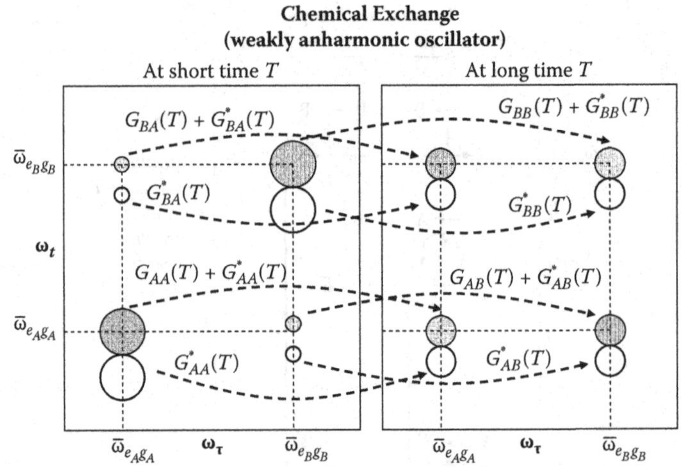

FIGURE 10.4 Chemical exchange 2D spectroscopy of weakly anharmonic oscillator. At short time, there are two main couplets along the diagonal line. As T increases, due to chemical exchange processes, the cross-peak amplitudes increase and the diagonal peak amplitudes decrease in time T.

chemical exchange, the diagonal and cross-peaks show up as a couplet with both positive and negative peaks (see Figure 6.3). When such a single anharmonic oscillator acts as a reporter of the chemical exchange process of interest, only two couplets along the diagonal line should appear at short time. However, as T increases, new cross-peak couplets will appear and their amplitudes grow in time T. In Figure 10.4, schematic 2D spectra for this case are shown. Despite the fact that each peak amplitude is mainly determined by the corresponding transition strength (dipole product), the survival and conditional probabilities do contribute to the peak amplitude changes in time T. As T increases, (a) the diagonal peak amplitudes decrease because of the decaying survival probability functions and (b) the cross-peak amplitudes increase due to the increasing conditional probability functions.

Now, similarly to the case of chemical exchanging 2LS, one can approximately describe and include the lifetime-broadening contributions for the excited-state absorption terms. For the four diagrams in Equation 10.16, the lifetime-broadening functions that should multiply to the corresponding time-domain nonlinear response functions are given as, respectively,

$$\exp(-t/2T_{f_A} - T/T_{e_A} - \tau/2T_{e_A})$$

$$\exp(-t/2T_{f_B} - T/T_{e_B} - \tau/2T_{e_B})$$

$$\exp(-t/2T_{f_B} - \left(T_{e_A}^{-1} + T_{e_B}^{-1}\right)T/2 - \tau/2T_{e_A})$$

$$\exp(-t/2T_{f_A} - (T_{e_A}^{-1} + T_{e_B}^{-1})T/2 - \tau/2T_{e_B}). \quad (10.23)$$

Here, the lifetimes of the overtone states f_A and f_B are denoted as T_{f_A} and T_{f_B}, respectively. If these lifetime broadening effects are significantly large, the corresponding 2D peak shape function should be properly modified by including these contributions.

EXERCISE 10.1

Chemical exchange 2D spectroscopy of two-species model was theoretically discussed. Consider the following three-species chemical exchange process.

$$A \underset{k_{-1}}{\overset{k_1}{\rightleftharpoons}} B \underset{k_{-2}}{\overset{k_2}{\rightleftharpoons}} C$$

Suppose that the reporter chromophores representing these species are the same anharmonic oscillator with different frequencies. (1) What are the diagrams associated with the three diagonal peaks? (2) Obtain the corresponding expressions for these diagonal peaks. (3) What are the diagrams and expressions associated with cross-peaks? (4) Can the chemical exchange 2D spectroscopy be used to distinguish the above chemical equilibrium system from the following case?

$$A \underset{k_{-1}}{\overset{k_1}{\rightleftharpoons}} B$$
$$k_3 \Big\backslash\!\!\Big\backslash k_{-3} \quad k_{-2} \Big/\!\!\Big/ k_2$$
$$C$$

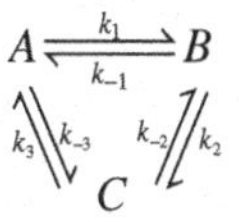

REFERENCES

1. Cho, M., Coherent two-dimensional optical spectroscopy. *Chemical Reviews* 2008, 108, 1331–1418.
2. Woutersen, S.; Mu, Y.; Stock, G.; Hamm, P., Hydrogen-bond lifetime measured by time-resolved 2D-IR spectroscopy: N-methylacetamide in methanol. *Chemical Physics* 2001, 266, 137–147.
3. Kwac, K.; Lee, H.; Cho, M. H., Non-Gaussian statistics of amide I mode frequency fluctuation of N-methylacetamide in methanol solution: Linear and nonlinear vibrational spectra. *Journal of Chemical Physics* 2004, 120, (3), 1477–1490.
4. Kwac, K.; Cho, M. H., Hydrogen bonding dynamics and two-dimensional vibrational spectroscopy: N-methylacetamide in liquid methanol. *Journal of Raman Spectroscopy.* 2005, 36, 326–336.
5. Kim, Y. S.; Hochstrasser, R. M., Chemical exchange 2D IR of hydrogen-bond making and breaking. *Proceedings of the National Academy of Sciences of the USA* 2005, 102, 11185–11190.
6. DeCamp, M. F.; DeFlores, L.; McCracken, J. M.; Tokmakoff, A.; Kwac, K.; Cho, M., Amide I vibrational dynamics of N-methylacetamide in polar solvents: The role of electrostatic interactions. *Journal of Physical Chemistry B* 2005, 109, 11016–11026.
7. Zheng, J. R.; Kwak, K.; Asbury, J.; Chen, X.; Piletic, I. R.; Fayer, M. D., Ultrafast dynamics of solute-solvent complexation observed at thermal equilibrium in real time. *Science* 2005, 309, 1338–1343.
8. Kwac, K.; Lee, C.; Jung, Y.; Han, J.; Kwak, K.; Zheng, J. R.; Fayer, M. D.; Cho, M., Phenol-benzene complexation dynamics: Quantum chemistry calculation, molecular dynamics simulations, and two dimensional IR spectroscopy. *Journal of Chemical Physics* 2006, 125, 244508.
9. Sanda, F.; Mukamel, S., Stochastic simulation of chemical exchange in two dimensional infrared spectroscopy. *Journal of Chemical Physics* 2006, 125, 014507.

11 Polarization-Controlled Two-Dimensional Spectroscopy

Fundamental aspects of 2D photon echo-type spectroscopy have been discussed in detail, such as the effects from chromophore–bath interactions, electronic couplings between chromophores, excitation transfer process, coherence quantum beats, and chemical exchange processes on the frequency distributions, shapes, and amplitudes of diagonal and cross-peaks. When a given pair of singly excited states are energetically close to each other so that the frequency resolution is not perfect, the cross-peaks cannot be easily identified due to the spectral congestion problems. Then, it is not always straightforward to quantitatively estimate the cross-peak amplitudes to extract information on structure and dynamics of coupled multi-chromophore systems. In this regard, the polarization-controlled measurement has been considered to be a useful technique for selectively eliminating the diagonal peaks from the 2D spectrum.[1-4] Sometimes, one can measure the anisotropy of cross-peak to determine the relative angle between two different transition dipoles, which can provide information on the 3D structure of target molecules such as peptides in solution.

In this chapter, we will focus on the photon echo spectroscopy and present results on how the measured diagonal and cross-peak amplitudes depend on the polarization directions of incident beams used to carry out the echo experiment. Since most of the applications of 2D spectroscopy focused on optical samples with chromophores dissolved in solution, the rotational average of the corresponding third-order response function or the relevant echo polarization over randomly oriented molecules in solution is critical. In Chapter 3, a theoretical description of the corresponding rotational average of *n*th-rank tensor was presented and discussed in detail. For model systems such as coupled 2LS dimer and coupled anharmonic oscillators, a few specific cases of experimental beam configurations will be considered in this chapter.

11.1 PARALLEL POLARIZATION *ZZZZ*-ECHO: TWO-LEVEL SYSTEM

One of the critical steps in a theoretical description of 2D photon echo is to carry out a proper rotational average of the fourth-rank tensorial response function. The solution sample with chromophores having random orientations will only be considered in this chapter, but it will be a straightforward exercise to apply the 2D spectroscopic technique to samples with broken centrosymmetry such as molecules adsorbed on the surface or at interface. Nevertheless, because the 2D optical spectroscopy is found to be useful for studying complex molecules in solution, it is important to pay more attention to the rotational averaging calculation for those having a centrosymmetry property.

In Section 3.3, it was shown that the rotationally averaged fourth-rank tensor $\mathbf{T}^{(4)}$ in a laboratory-fixed frame is connected to $\mathbf{t}^{(4)}$ in a molecule-fixed frame as[5]

$$T^{(4)}_{l_1l_2l_3l_4} = I^{(4)}_{l_1l_2l_3l_4;m_1m_2m_3m_4} t^{(4)}_{m_1m_2m_3m_4}, \tag{11.1}$$

where

$$I^{(4)}_{l_1l_2l_3l_4;m_1m_2m_3m_4} = \frac{1}{30}(\delta_{l_1l_2}\delta_{l_3l_4} \quad \delta_{l_1l_3}\delta_{l_2l_4} \quad \delta_{l_1l_4}\delta_{l_2l_3})\begin{pmatrix} 4 & -1 & -1 \\ -1 & 4 & -1 \\ -1 & -1 & 4 \end{pmatrix}\begin{pmatrix} \delta_{m_1m_2}\delta_{m_3m_4} \\ \delta_{m_1m_3}\delta_{m_2m_4} \\ \delta_{m_1m_4}\delta_{m_2m_3} \end{pmatrix}. \tag{11.2}$$

This is a general expression for any arbitrary cases of $l_1 \sim l_4$, which are one of the three Cartesian coordinates in the laboratory-fixed frame.

In Chapter 7, the 2D photon echo spectrum of 2LS was discussed in detail, where the diagonally elongated peak shape and its T-dependency were fully described by using an analytic but approximate expression for the 2D spectrum. However, for the sake of simplicity and to focus on the rotationally averaged transition strength, let us invoke the 2D Gaussian peak shape approximation (see Section 7.6) to the spectrum in this chapter. The 2D spectrum of 2LS was found to be

$$\tilde{\mathbf{E}}_{PE}(\omega_t, T, \omega_\tau) = 2[\boldsymbol{\mu}_{ge}\boldsymbol{\mu}_{eg}\boldsymbol{\mu}_{ge}\boldsymbol{\mu}_{eg}]\vdots\mathbf{e}_3\mathbf{e}_2\mathbf{e}_1^*\Gamma\left(\bar{\omega}_{eg}, \Omega^2, \bar{\omega}_{eg}, \Omega^2\right). \tag{11.3}$$

Note that the amplitude of the complex 2D photon echo spectrum is determined by the transition strength factor, $[\boldsymbol{\mu}_{ge}\boldsymbol{\mu}_{eg}\boldsymbol{\mu}_{ge}\boldsymbol{\mu}_{eg}]\vdots\mathbf{e}_3\mathbf{e}_2\mathbf{e}_1^*$, which is still a vector. Now, let us consider the case when the three incident beams have polarization directions that are parallel to the laboratory Z-axis and also the Z-component of the echo field vector is detected. Then, we have $\mathbf{e}_3 = \mathbf{e}_2 = \mathbf{e}_1 = \hat{Z}$ and need to consider the rotationally averaged fourth-rank tensor element, $[\boldsymbol{\mu}_{ge}\boldsymbol{\mu}_{eg}\boldsymbol{\mu}_{ge}\boldsymbol{\mu}_{eg}]_{ZZZZ}$. Using the relationship in Equation 11.1, we get

$$[\boldsymbol{\mu}_{ge}\boldsymbol{\mu}_{eg}\boldsymbol{\mu}_{ge}\boldsymbol{\mu}_{eg}]_{ZZZZ} = \frac{1}{15}\sum_{m_1,m_2,m_3,m_4=x,y,z}(\delta_{m_1m_2}\delta_{m_3m_4} + \delta_{m_1m_3}\delta_{m_2m_4} + \delta_{m_1m_4}\delta_{m_2m_3}) \times\left[\boldsymbol{\mu}^M_{ge}\boldsymbol{\mu}^M_{eg}\boldsymbol{\mu}^M_{ge}\boldsymbol{\mu}^M_{eg}\right]_{m_1m_2m_3m_4}. \tag{11.4}$$

The transition dipole matrix element $\boldsymbol{\mu}^M_{ge}$ in Equation 11.4 is that in a molecule-fixed frame. For real wavefunctions, we have $\boldsymbol{\mu}^M_{ge} = \boldsymbol{\mu}^M_{eg}$ and it is real. Since the choice of the molecule-fixed frame is arbitrary, it is assumed that the direction of $\boldsymbol{\mu}^M_{ge}$ vector is parallel to the z-axis of the molecule-fixed frame, that is,

$$\boldsymbol{\mu}^M_{ge} = \boldsymbol{\mu}^M_{eg} = \left|\boldsymbol{\mu}^M_{ge}\right|\hat{z}. \tag{11.5}$$

Then, one can find that $[\boldsymbol{\mu}_{ge}\boldsymbol{\mu}_{eg}\boldsymbol{\mu}_{ge}\boldsymbol{\mu}_{eg}]_{ZZZZ}$ in Equation 11.4 is given as

$$[\boldsymbol{\mu}_{ge}\boldsymbol{\mu}_{eg}\boldsymbol{\mu}_{ge}\boldsymbol{\mu}_{eg}]_{ZZZZ} = \frac{1}{5}\left|\boldsymbol{\mu}_{ge}^{M}\right|^{4}. \tag{11.6}$$

Noting that the dipole strength determining the absorption spectrum of the $g \leftrightarrow e$ transition is defined as the square of the transition dipole matrix element $|\boldsymbol{\mu}_{ge}^{M}|^2$, one can find that the *ZZZZ*-echo signal in this case is proportional to the square of the dipole strength. From Equation 11.3 with 11.6, the *ZZZZ*-echo spectrum of a 2LS is

$$\tilde{E}_{PE}^{\|}(\omega_t, T, \omega_\tau) = \frac{2}{5}\left|\boldsymbol{\mu}_{ge}^{M}\right|^{4}\Gamma\left(\bar{\omega}_{eg}, \Omega^2, \bar{\omega}_{eg}, \Omega^2\right). \tag{11.7}$$

The more interesting case is the coupled 2LS dimer, which exhibits a variety of interesting features originating from coupling and delocalized natures of excited states. At short time *T*, one can observe quantum beat contributions to the *T*-dependent 2D spectra. Also, it is possible to observe characteristic changes of the diagonal and cross-peak amplitudes induced by excitation transfers between the two singly excited states. For the sake of simplicity, let us consider the intermediate time region where the population transfer rates are sufficiently slow but the quantum beats are fully relaxed and disappeared.

In this case, as shown in Section 9.4, the 2D photon echo spectrum consists of two diagonal and two cross-peaks as

$$\tilde{\mathbf{E}}_{PE}(\omega_t, T, \omega_\tau) = \tilde{\mathbf{E}}_{D1}(\omega_t, T, \omega_\tau) + \tilde{\mathbf{E}}_{D2}(\omega_t, T, \omega_\tau) + \tilde{\mathbf{E}}_{C12}(\omega_t, T, \omega_\tau) + \tilde{\mathbf{E}}_{C21}(\omega_t, T, \omega_\tau), \tag{11.8}$$

where

$$\tilde{\mathbf{E}}_{D1}(\omega_t, T, \omega_\tau) = 2[\boldsymbol{\mu}_{ge_1}\boldsymbol{\mu}_{e_1g}\boldsymbol{\mu}_{ge_1}\boldsymbol{\mu}_{e_1g}] \vdots \mathbf{e}_3\mathbf{e}_2\mathbf{e}_1^*\Gamma\left(\bar{\omega}_{e_1g}, <\delta\Omega_1^2>, \bar{\omega}_{e_1g}, <\delta\Omega_1^2>\right)$$

$$\tilde{\mathbf{E}}_{D2}(\omega_t, T, \omega_\tau) = 2[\boldsymbol{\mu}_{ge_2}\boldsymbol{\mu}_{e_2g}\boldsymbol{\mu}_{ge_2}\boldsymbol{\mu}_{e_2g}] \vdots \mathbf{e}_3\mathbf{e}_2\mathbf{e}_1^*\Gamma\left(\bar{\omega}_{e_2g}, <\delta\Omega_2^2>, \bar{\omega}_{e_2g}, <\delta\Omega_2^2>\right)$$

$$\begin{aligned}\tilde{\mathbf{E}}_{C12}(\omega_t, T, \omega_\tau) = {} & [\boldsymbol{\mu}_{ge_2}\boldsymbol{\mu}_{e_2g}\boldsymbol{\mu}_{e_1g}\boldsymbol{\mu}_{ge_1}] \vdots \mathbf{e}_3\mathbf{e}_2\mathbf{e}_1^*\Gamma\left(\bar{\omega}_{e_2g}, <\delta\Omega_2^2>, \bar{\omega}_{e_1g}, <\delta\Omega_1^2>\right) \\ & -[\boldsymbol{\mu}_{e_1f}\boldsymbol{\mu}_{fe_1}\boldsymbol{\mu}_{e_1g}\boldsymbol{\mu}_{ge_1}] \vdots \mathbf{e}_3\mathbf{e}_2\mathbf{e}_1^*\Gamma\left(\bar{\omega}_{fe_1}, <\delta\Omega_2^2>, \bar{\omega}_{e_1g}, <\delta\Omega_1^2>\right)\end{aligned}$$

$$\begin{aligned}\tilde{\mathbf{E}}_{C21}(\omega_t, T, \omega_\tau) = {} & [\boldsymbol{\mu}_{ge_1}\boldsymbol{\mu}_{e_1g}\boldsymbol{\mu}_{e_2g}\boldsymbol{\mu}_{ge_2}] \vdots \mathbf{e}_3\mathbf{e}_2\mathbf{e}_1^*\Gamma\left(\bar{\omega}_{e_1g}, <\delta\Omega_1^2>, \bar{\omega}_{e_2g}, <\delta\Omega_2^2>\right) \\ & -[\boldsymbol{\mu}_{e_2f}\boldsymbol{\mu}_{fe_2}\boldsymbol{\mu}_{e_2g}\boldsymbol{\mu}_{ge_2}] \vdots \mathbf{e}_3\mathbf{e}_2\mathbf{e}_1^*\Gamma\left(\bar{\omega}_{fe_2}, <\delta\Omega_1^2>, \bar{\omega}_{e_2g}, <\delta\Omega_2^2>\right).\end{aligned} \tag{11.9}$$

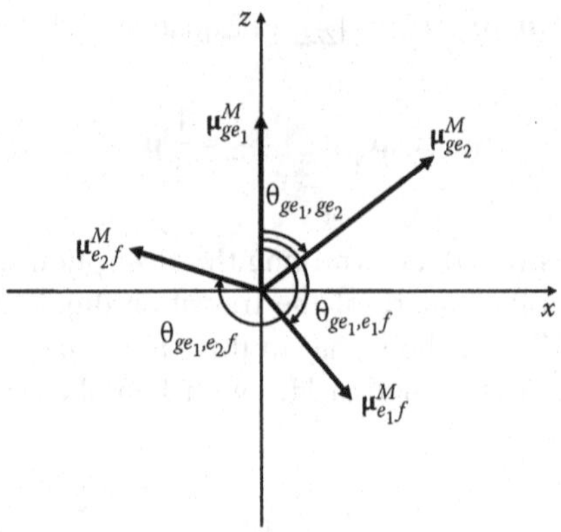

FIGURE 11.1 Transitions dipole vectors of coupled 2LS dimer. They are all on the same plane in a molecule-fixed frame. Angles between two different transition dipole vectors are defined here.

Again, it is assumed that the direction of the transition dipole vector, $\boldsymbol{\mu}^M_{ge_1}$, which determines the amplitude of the $g \leftrightarrow e_1$ transition, is chosen to be parallel to the z-axis in a molecule-fixed frame. Without loss of generality, $\boldsymbol{\mu}^M_{ge_2}$ is assumed to be on the x-z plane in the same molecule-fixed frame by properly choosing the x-axis. Furthermore, one can show that the transition dipole vectors $\boldsymbol{\mu}^M_{e_1f}$ and $\boldsymbol{\mu}^M_{e_2f}$ are on the same x-z molecular plane (see Equation 9.12 and Figure 11.1). Consequently, we have

$$\boldsymbol{\mu}^M_{ge_1} = \left|\boldsymbol{\mu}^M_{ge_1}\right|\hat{z}$$

$$\boldsymbol{\mu}^M_{ge_2} = \left|\boldsymbol{\mu}^M_{ge_2}\right|(\hat{z}\cos\theta_{ge_1,ge_2} + \hat{x}\sin\theta_{ge_1,ge_2})$$

$$\boldsymbol{\mu}^M_{e_1f} = \left|\boldsymbol{\mu}^M_{e_1f}\right|(\hat{z}\cos\theta_{ge_1,e_1f} + \hat{x}\sin\theta_{ge_1,e_1f})$$

$$\boldsymbol{\mu}^M_{e_2f} = \left|\boldsymbol{\mu}^M_{e_2f}\right|(\hat{z}\cos\theta_{ge_1,e_2f} + \hat{x}\sin\theta_{ge_1,e_2f})$$

$$\boldsymbol{\mu}^M_{ge_1}\cdot\boldsymbol{\mu}^M_{ge_2} = \left|\boldsymbol{\mu}^M_{ge_1}\right|\left|\boldsymbol{\mu}^M_{ge_2}\right|\cos\theta_{ge_1,ge_2}.$$

$$\boldsymbol{\mu}^M_{ge_1}\cdot\boldsymbol{\mu}^M_{e_1f} = \left|\boldsymbol{\mu}^M_{ge_1}\right|\left|\boldsymbol{\mu}^M_{e_1f}\right|\cos\theta_{ge_1,e_1f}$$

$$\boldsymbol{\mu}^M_{ge_1}\cdot\boldsymbol{\mu}^M_{e_2f} = \left|\boldsymbol{\mu}^M_{ge_1}\right|\left|\boldsymbol{\mu}^M_{e_2f}\right|\cos\theta_{ge_1,e_2f}. \tag{11.10}$$

Here, the angles $\theta_{m,n}$ of the three transition dipole vectors $\boldsymbol{\mu}^M_{ge_2}$, $\boldsymbol{\mu}^M_{e_1f}$, and $\boldsymbol{\mu}^M_{e_2f}$ with respect to the direction of $\boldsymbol{\mu}^M_{ge_1}$ vector were defined above. Then, the rotationally averaged transition strengths in Equation 11.9 are found to be

$$[\boldsymbol{\mu}_{ge_1}\boldsymbol{\mu}_{e_1g}\boldsymbol{\mu}_{ge_1}\boldsymbol{\mu}_{e_1g}]_{ZZZZ} = \frac{1}{5}\left|\boldsymbol{\mu}^M_{ge_1}\right|^4$$

$$[\boldsymbol{\mu}_{ge_2}\boldsymbol{\mu}_{e_2g}\boldsymbol{\mu}_{ge_2}\boldsymbol{\mu}_{e_2g}]_{ZZZZ} = \frac{1}{5}\left|\boldsymbol{\mu}^M_{ge_2}\right|^4$$

$$[\boldsymbol{\mu}_{ge_2}\boldsymbol{\mu}_{e_2g}\boldsymbol{\mu}_{e_1g}\boldsymbol{\mu}_{ge_1}]_{ZZZZ} = \frac{1}{15}\left|\boldsymbol{\mu}^M_{ge_1}\right|^2\left|\boldsymbol{\mu}^M_{ge_2}\right|^2\left(2\cos^2\theta_{ge_1,ge_2}+1\right).$$

$$[\boldsymbol{\mu}_{e_1f}\boldsymbol{\mu}_{fe_1}\boldsymbol{\mu}_{e_1g}\boldsymbol{\mu}_{ge_1}]_{ZZZZ} = \frac{1}{15}\left|\boldsymbol{\mu}^M_{e_1f}\right|^2\left|\boldsymbol{\mu}^M_{ge_1}\right|^2\left(2\cos^2\theta_{ge_1,e_1f}+1\right)$$

$$[\boldsymbol{\mu}_{e_2f}\boldsymbol{\mu}_{fe_2}\boldsymbol{\mu}_{e_2g}\boldsymbol{\mu}_{ge_2}]_{ZZZZ} = \frac{1}{15}\left|\boldsymbol{\mu}^M_{e_2f}\right|^2\left|\boldsymbol{\mu}^M_{ge_2}\right|^2\left(2\cos^2\{\theta_{ge_1,e_2f}-\theta_{ge_1,ge_2}\}+1\right). \quad (11.11)$$

The resultant *ZZZZ*-spectrum of coupled 2LS dimer is then given as

$$\tilde{E}^{\|}_{D1}(\omega_t,T,\omega_\tau) = \frac{2}{5}\left|\boldsymbol{\mu}^M_{ge_1}\right|^4 \Gamma\left(\bar{\omega}_{e_1g},<\delta\Omega_1^2>,\bar{\omega}_{e_1g},<\delta\Omega_1^2>\right)$$

$$\tilde{E}^{\|}_{D2}(\omega_t,T,\omega_\tau) = \frac{2}{5}\left|\boldsymbol{\mu}^M_{ge_2}\right|^4 \Gamma\left(\bar{\omega}_{e_2g},<\delta\Omega_2^2>,\bar{\omega}_{e_2g},<\delta\Omega_2^2>\right)$$

$$\begin{aligned}\tilde{E}^{\|}_{C12}(\omega_t,T,\omega_\tau) &= \frac{1}{15}\left|\boldsymbol{\mu}^M_{ge_1}\right|^2\left|\boldsymbol{\mu}^M_{ge_2}\right|^2\left(2\cos^2\theta_{ge_1,ge_2}+1\right)\Gamma\left(\bar{\omega}_{e_2g},<\delta\Omega_2^2>,\bar{\omega}_{e_1g},<\delta\Omega_1^2>\right)\\ &-\frac{1}{15}\left|\boldsymbol{\mu}^M_{e_1f}\right|^2\left|\boldsymbol{\mu}^M_{ge_1}\right|^2\left(2\cos^2\theta_{ge_1,e_1f}+1\right)\Gamma\left(\bar{\omega}_{fe_1},<\delta\Omega_2^2>,\bar{\omega}_{e_1g},<\delta\Omega_1^2>\right)\end{aligned}$$

$$\begin{aligned}\tilde{E}^{\|}_{C21}(\omega_t,T,\omega_\tau) &= \frac{1}{15}\left|\boldsymbol{\mu}^M_{ge_1}\right|^2\left|\boldsymbol{\mu}^M_{ge_2}\right|^2\left(2\cos^2\theta_{ge_1,ge_2}+1\right)\Gamma\left(\bar{\omega}_{e_1g},<\delta\Omega_1^2>,\bar{\omega}_{e_2g},<\delta\Omega_2^2>\right)\\ &-\frac{1}{15}\left|\boldsymbol{\mu}^M_{e_2f}\right|^2\left|\boldsymbol{\mu}^M_{ge_2}\right|^2\left(2\cos^2\{\theta_{ge_1,e_2f}-\theta_{ge_1,ge_2}\}+1\right)\Gamma\left(\bar{\omega}_{fe_2},<\delta\Omega_1^2>,\bar{\omega}_{e_2g},<\delta\Omega_2^2>\right).\end{aligned} \quad (11.12)$$

It should be noted that not only the absolute magnitudes of the transition dipoles but also the angles between any two different transition dipole vectors can be written as functions of the mixing angle θ, transition dipoles of the two individual chromophores $\mathbf{d}_1$ and $\mathbf{d}_2$, and the angle between $\mathbf{d}_1$ and $\mathbf{d}_2$ vectors. Here, one should not confuse the mixing angle θ with the angles $\theta_{m,n}$ between two different transition dipole vectors in Equations 11.11 and 11.12. The mixing angle is a function of the coupling constant *J*. Since the coupling constant *J* depends on the relative distance between the two chromophores as well as the relative orientation of the two local transition dipole vectors, the experimentally determined *J* value can provide information on the structure of the 2LS dimer.

It is interesting to note that the amplitudes of C12 and C21 cross-peaks (see Equation 11.12) are mainly determined by the interference between the GB+SE contribution and EA contribution. If the two chromophores are uncoupled, that is, $J = 0$, the coupling-induced mixing angle $\theta = 0$. Then, from Equations 9.11 and 9.12, for $J = 0$, we get

$$\boldsymbol{\mu}_{e_1g} = \mathbf{d}_1, \quad \boldsymbol{\mu}_{e_2g} = \mathbf{d}_2, \quad \boldsymbol{\mu}_{e_1f} = \mathbf{d}_2, \quad \text{and} \quad \boldsymbol{\mu}_{e_2f} = \mathbf{d}_1. \tag{11.13}$$

In this zero-coupling limit, we have $\theta_{ge_1,ge_2} = \phi, \theta_{ge_1,e_1f} = \phi$, and $\theta_{ge_1,e_2f} = 0$, where the angle between the two local transition dipoles $\mathbf{d}_1$ and $\mathbf{d}_2$ was denoted as ϕ. Inserting these results into the expressions for $\tilde{E}_{C12}(\omega_t, T, \omega_\tau)$ and $\tilde{E}_{C21}(\omega_t, T, \omega_\tau)$, one can show that the two cross-peaks vanish, as expected. This indicates that the nonzero cross-peaks are a direct signature of coupling between the transitions of the two 2LS chromophores.

11.2 PERPENDICULAR POLARIZATION *ZYYZ*-ECHO: TWO-LEVEL SYSTEM

The *ZZZZ*-measurement is based on the experimental configuration where the three incident beam polarization directions as well as the detected echo polarization direction are all parallel to the laboratory *Z*-axis. This is often called the parallel polarization photon echo. However, one can control the incident beam polarization directions to carry out the perpendicular polarization photon echo measurement. In this case, the first pulsed beam polarization direction and the detected echo polarization direction are the same and they are paralled to the laboratory *Z*-axis, whereas the second and third beam polarization directions are orthogonal to the first one and assumed to be parallel to the *Y*-axis. Here, it was assumed that the beam propagation directions are all along the *X*-axis.

For a single 2LS chromophore, the *ZYYZ*-echo spectrum requires the rotational average of $[\boldsymbol{\mu}_{ge}\boldsymbol{\mu}_{eg}\boldsymbol{\mu}_{ge}\boldsymbol{\mu}_{eg}]_{ZYYZ}$, and using the relationship in Equation 11.1 one can connect it to the transition strength in a molecule-fixed frame as

$$[\boldsymbol{\mu}_{ge}\boldsymbol{\mu}_{eg}\boldsymbol{\mu}_{ge}\boldsymbol{\mu}_{eg}]_{ZYYZ} = \frac{1}{30} \sum_{m_1,m_2,m_3,m_4=x,y,z} (-\delta_{m_1m_2}\delta_{m_3m_4} - \delta_{m_1m_3}\delta_{m_2m_4} + 4\delta_{m_1m_4}\delta_{m_2m_3}) \times \left[\boldsymbol{\mu}_{ge}^M \boldsymbol{\mu}_{eg}^M \boldsymbol{\mu}_{ge}^M \boldsymbol{\mu}_{eg}^M\right]_{m_1m_2m_3m_4}. \tag{11.14}$$

Again, let us assume that the direction of the $\boldsymbol{\mu}_{ge}^M$ vector is parallel to the molecular z-axis as $\boldsymbol{\mu}_{ge}^M = \boldsymbol{\mu}_{eg}^M = |\boldsymbol{\mu}_{ge}^M|\,\hat{z}$. Then, we get

$$[\boldsymbol{\mu}_{ge}\boldsymbol{\mu}_{eg}\boldsymbol{\mu}_{ge}\boldsymbol{\mu}_{eg}]_{ZYYZ} = \frac{1}{15}\left|\boldsymbol{\mu}_{ge}^M\right|^4. \tag{11.15}$$

The *ZYYZ*-echo spectrum of a 2LS is

$$\tilde{E}_{PE}^{\perp}(\omega_t, T, \omega_\tau) = \frac{2}{15}\left|\boldsymbol{\mu}_{ge}^M\right|^4 \Gamma\left(\bar{\omega}_{eg}, \Omega^2, \bar{\omega}_{eg}, \Omega^2\right). \tag{11.16}$$

This result shows that the *ZYYZ*-echo spectrum is just one-third of the *ZZZZ*-echo spectrum in magnitude, but the shape of the 2D spectrum remains unchanged by the alteration of the beam polarization directions.

Next, let us consider the coupled 2LS dimer in the intermediate time region. The rotationally averaged transition strengths that are needed in the calculations of *ZYYZ*-echo spectrum are

$$[\boldsymbol{\mu}_{ge_1}\boldsymbol{\mu}_{e_1g}\boldsymbol{\mu}_{ge_1}\boldsymbol{\mu}_{e_1g}]_{ZYYZ} = \frac{1}{15}\left|\boldsymbol{\mu}^M_{ge_1}\right|^4$$

$$[\boldsymbol{\mu}_{ge_2}\boldsymbol{\mu}_{e_2g}\boldsymbol{\mu}_{ge_2}\boldsymbol{\mu}_{e_2g}]_{ZYYZ} = \frac{1}{15}\left|\boldsymbol{\mu}^M_{ge_2}\right|^4$$

$$[\boldsymbol{\mu}_{ge_2}\boldsymbol{\mu}_{e_2g}\boldsymbol{\mu}_{e_1g}\boldsymbol{\mu}_{ge_1}]_{ZYYZ} = \frac{1}{30}\left|\boldsymbol{\mu}^M_{ge_1}\right|^2\left|\boldsymbol{\mu}^M_{ge_2}\right|^2\left(3\cos^2\theta_{ge_1,ge_2}-1\right).$$

$$[\boldsymbol{\mu}_{e_1f}\boldsymbol{\mu}_{fe_1}\boldsymbol{\mu}_{e_1g}\boldsymbol{\mu}_{ge_1}]_{ZYYZ} = \frac{1}{30}\left|\boldsymbol{\mu}^M_{e_1f}\right|^2\left|\boldsymbol{\mu}^M_{ge_1}\right|^2\left(3\cos^2\theta_{ge_1,e_1f}-1\right)$$

$$[\boldsymbol{\mu}_{e_2f}\boldsymbol{\mu}_{fe_2}\boldsymbol{\mu}_{e_2g}\boldsymbol{\mu}_{ge_2}]_{ZYYZ} = \frac{1}{30}\left|\boldsymbol{\mu}^M_{e_2f}\right|^2\left|\boldsymbol{\mu}^M_{ge_2}\right|^2\left(3\cos^2\{\theta_{ge_1,e_2f}-\theta_{ge_1,ge_2}\}-1\right). \quad (11.17)$$

Using these results, we find that the perpendicular polarization *ZYYZ*-spectrum of the coupled 2LS dimer is given as

$$\tilde{E}^{\perp}_{D1}(\omega_t,T,\omega_\tau) = \frac{2}{15}\left|\boldsymbol{\mu}^M_{ge_1}\right|^4\Gamma\left(\bar{\omega}_{e_1g},<\delta\Omega_1^2>,\bar{\omega}_{e_1g},<\delta\Omega_1^2>\right)$$

$$\tilde{E}^{\perp}_{D2}(\omega_t,T,\omega_\tau) = \frac{2}{15}\left|\boldsymbol{\mu}^M_{ge_2}\right|^4\Gamma\left(\bar{\omega}_{e_2g},<\delta\Omega_2^2>,\bar{\omega}_{e_2g},<\delta\Omega_2^2>\right)$$

$$\begin{aligned}\tilde{E}^{\perp}_{C12}(\omega_t,T,\omega_\tau) &= \frac{1}{30}\left|\boldsymbol{\mu}^M_{ge_1}\right|^2\left|\boldsymbol{\mu}^M_{ge_2}\right|^2\left(3\cos^2\theta_{ge_1,ge_2}-1\right)\Gamma\left(\bar{\omega}_{e_2g},<\delta\Omega_2^2>,\bar{\omega}_{e_1g},<\delta\Omega_1^2>\right)\\ &-\frac{1}{30}\left|\boldsymbol{\mu}^M_{e_1f}\right|^2\left|\boldsymbol{\mu}^M_{ge_1}\right|^2\left(3\cos^2\theta_{ge_1,e_1f}-1\right)\Gamma\left(\bar{\omega}_{fe_1},<\delta\Omega_2^2>,\bar{\omega}_{e_1g},<\delta\Omega_1^2>\right)\end{aligned}$$

$$\begin{aligned}\tilde{E}^{\perp}_{C21}(\omega_t,T,\omega_\tau) &= \frac{1}{30}\left|\boldsymbol{\mu}^M_{ge_1}\right|^2\left|\boldsymbol{\mu}^M_{ge_2}\right|^2\left(3\cos^2\theta_{ge_1,ge_2}-1\right)\Gamma\left(\bar{\omega}_{e_1g},<\delta\Omega_1^2>,\bar{\omega}_{e_2g},<\delta\Omega_2^2>\right)\\ &-\frac{1}{30}\left|\boldsymbol{\mu}^M_{e_2f}\right|^2\left|\boldsymbol{\mu}^M_{ge_2}\right|^2\left(3\cos^2\{\theta_{ge_1,e_2f}-\theta_{ge_1,ge_2}\}-1\right)\Gamma\left(\bar{\omega}_{fe_2},<\delta\Omega_1^2>,\bar{\omega}_{e_2g},<\delta\Omega_2^2>\right).\end{aligned} \quad (11.18)$$

It is noted that the two diagonal (D1 and D2) peaks in the *ZZZZ*-spectrum are identical to those in the *ZYYZ*-spectrum except for the constant factor 3 between them. However, the cross-peak amplitudes of the present perpendicular polarization echo spectrum are different from those of the parallel polarization echo spectrum.

11.3 DIFFERENCE TWO-DIMENSIONAL PHOTON ECHO SPECTRUM: COUPLED TWO-LEVEL SYSTEM DIMER

Noting that the diagonal peak amplitudes in parallel polarization echo spectrum are just three times larger than those of perpendicular polarization echo spectrum, one can find it useful to consider the difference between parallel polarization echo spectrum and three times the perpendicular polarization echo spectrum.[1, 2, 6] Let us define the different 2D echo spectrum as

$$\Delta\tilde{E}_{PE}(\omega_t,T,\omega_\tau) = 3\tilde{E}^{\perp}_{PE}(\omega_t,T,\omega_\tau) - \tilde{E}^{\parallel}_{PE}(\omega_t,T,\omega_\tau). \tag{11.19}$$

From Equations 11.12 and 11.18, we get

$$\begin{aligned}\Delta\tilde{E}_{PE}(\omega_t,T,\omega_\tau) &= 3\tilde{E}^{\perp}_{C12}(\omega_t,T,\omega_\tau) - \tilde{E}^{\parallel}_{C12}(\omega_t,T,\omega_\tau) + 3\tilde{E}^{\perp}_{C21}(\omega_t,T,\omega_\tau) \\ &\quad - \tilde{E}^{\parallel}_{C21}(\omega_t,T,\omega_\tau) \\ &= -\frac{1}{6}\left|\boldsymbol{\mu}^M_{ge_1}\right|^2\left|\boldsymbol{\mu}^M_{ge_2}\right|^2 \sin^2\theta_{ge_1,ge_2}\Gamma\left(\bar{\omega}_{e_2g},<\delta\Omega_2^2>,\bar{\omega}_{e_1g},<\delta\Omega_1^2>\right) \\ &\quad + \frac{1}{6}\left|\boldsymbol{\mu}^M_{e_1f}\right|^2\left|\boldsymbol{\mu}^M_{ge_1}\right|^2 \sin^2\theta_{ge_1,e_1f}\Gamma\left(\bar{\omega}_{fe_1},<\delta\Omega_2^2>,\bar{\omega}_{e_1g},<\delta\Omega_1^2>\right) \\ &\quad - \frac{1}{6}\left|\boldsymbol{\mu}^M_{ge_1}\right|^2\left|\boldsymbol{\mu}^M_{ge_2}\right|^2 \sin^2\theta_{ge_1,ge_2}\Gamma\left(\bar{\omega}_{e_1g},<\delta\Omega_1^2>,\bar{\omega}_{e_2g},<\delta\Omega_2^2>\right) \\ &\quad + \frac{1}{6}\left|\boldsymbol{\mu}^M_{e_2f}\right|^2\left|\boldsymbol{\mu}^M_{ge_2}\right|^2 \sin^2\{\theta_{ge_1,e_2f} - \theta_{ge_1,ge_2}\}\Gamma\left(\bar{\omega}_{fe_2},<\delta\Omega_1^2>,\bar{\omega}_{e_2g},<\delta\Omega_2^2>\right).\end{aligned} \tag{11.20}$$

It should be noted that the diagonal peaks disappear in this difference spectrum and that only the cross-peaks survive. Furthermore, the cross-peak amplitudes in the difference 2D spectrum are determined by $\sin^2\theta_{m,n}$, where $\theta_{m,n}$ is the angle between the two transition dipole vectors, and again it shouldn't be confused with the mixing angle θ. As the angle $\theta_{m,n}$ approaches 90°, the corresponding cross-peak amplitude increases.

Now, consider a simple homodimer. In this case, the two local transition dipoles $\mathbf{d}_1$ and $\mathbf{d}_2$ have the same magnitudes, that is, $d = |\mathbf{d}_1| = |\mathbf{d}_2|$, but the directions of the two vectors can be different from each other by ϕ (see Section 10.4). Due to the degeneracy of the two site energies, the mixing angle θ is $\pi/4$ and the delocalization factor κ (=$\cos\theta \sin\theta$) is 0.5. In this case, from Equation 11.20, we find that

$$\begin{aligned}\boldsymbol{\mu}_{e_1g} &= \boldsymbol{\mu}_{e_1f} = 2^{-1/2}(\mathbf{d}_1 + \mathbf{d}_2) \\ \boldsymbol{\mu}_{e_2g} &= 2^{-1/2}(-\mathbf{d}_1 + \mathbf{d}_2) \\ \boldsymbol{\mu}_{e_2f} &= 2^{-1/2}(\mathbf{d}_1 - \mathbf{d}_2).\end{aligned} \tag{11.21}$$

The parallel and perpendicular polarization 2D spectra are then highly simplified. The parallel polarization photon echo peaks are given as

$$\tilde{E}^{\parallel}_{D1}(\omega_t,T,\omega_\tau)=\frac{2}{5}d^4(1+\cos\phi)^2\Gamma\left(\bar{\omega}_{e_1g},<\delta\Omega_1^2>,\bar{\omega}_{e_1g},<\delta\Omega_1^2>\right)$$

$$\tilde{E}^{\parallel}_{D2}(\omega_t,T,\omega_\tau)=\frac{2}{5}d^4(1-\cos\phi)^2\Gamma\left(\bar{\omega}_{e_2g},<\delta\Omega_2^2>,\bar{\omega}_{e_2g},<\delta\Omega_2^2>\right)$$

$$\tilde{E}^{\parallel}_{C12}(\omega_t,T,\omega_\tau)=-\frac{2}{15}d^4(1+\cos\phi)(1+2\cos\phi)\Gamma\left(\bar{\omega}_{e_2g},<\delta\Omega_2^2>,\bar{\omega}_{e_1g},<\delta\Omega_1^2>\right)$$

$$\tilde{E}^{\parallel}_{C21}(\omega_t,T,\omega_\tau)=-\frac{2}{15}d^4(1-\cos\phi)(1-2\cos\phi)\Gamma\left(\bar{\omega}_{e_1g},<\delta\Omega_1^2>,\bar{\omega}_{e_2g},<\delta\Omega_2^2>\right). \tag{11.22}$$

We assumed that the exciton-exciton binding energy is negligibly small so that $\bar{\omega}_{fe_1}=\bar{\omega}_{e_2g}$ and $\bar{\omega}_{fe_2}=\bar{\omega}_{e_1g}$. Note that the above results are identical to Equation 9.40, where only the peak amplitudes were considered. Next, the perpendicular polarization photon echo peaks are

$$\tilde{E}^{\perp}_{D1}(\omega_t,T,\omega_\tau)=\frac{2}{15}d^4(1+\cos\phi)^2\Gamma\left(\bar{\omega}_{e_1g},<\delta\Omega_1^2>,\bar{\omega}_{e_1g},<\delta\Omega_1^2>\right)$$

$$\tilde{E}^{\perp}_{D2}(\omega_t,T,\omega_\tau)=\frac{2}{15}d^4(1-\cos\phi)^2\Gamma\left(\bar{\omega}_{e_2g},<\delta\Omega_2^2>,\bar{\omega}_{e_2g},<\delta\Omega_2^2>\right)$$

$$\tilde{E}^{\perp}_{C12}(\omega_t,T,\omega_\tau)=-\frac{1}{30}d^4(1+\cos\phi)(3+\cos\phi)\Gamma\left(\bar{\omega}_{e_2g},<\delta\Omega_2^2>,\bar{\omega}_{e_1g},<\delta\Omega_1^2>\right)$$

$$\tilde{E}^{\perp}_{C21}(\omega_t,T,\omega_\tau)=-\frac{1}{30}d^4(1-\cos\phi)(3-\cos\phi)\Gamma\left(\bar{\omega}_{e_1g},<\delta\Omega_1^2>,\bar{\omega}_{e_2g},<\delta\Omega_2^2>\right). \tag{11.23}$$

From these results, it will be possible to determine the angle between the transition dipoles of two chromophores, which can in turn be used to determine the relative orientation of the two chromophores once the direction of the transition dipole vector of each molecule is known in a molecule-fixed frame.

11.4 PARALLEL POLARIZATION *ZZZZ*-ECHO: ANHARMONIC OSCILLATORS

Except that a single anharmonic oscillator should be effectively treated as a 3LS consisting of *g*, *e*, and *f* states, the polarization dependencies of the 2D IR spectra of coupled anharmonic oscillators are quite similar to those of a coupled 2LS dimer.

The 2D photon echo spectrum of an anharmonic oscillator, within the 2D Gaussian approximation to the spectral peak shape, was shown to be

$$\tilde{\mathbf{E}}_{PE}(\omega_t,T,\omega_\tau)=2[\boldsymbol{\mu}_{ge}\boldsymbol{\mu}_{eg}\boldsymbol{\mu}_{ge}\boldsymbol{\mu}_{eg}]\vdots\mathbf{e}_3\mathbf{e}_2\mathbf{e}_1^*\Gamma\left(\bar{\omega}_{eg},\Omega^2,\bar{\omega}_{eg},\Omega^2\right)$$
$$-[\boldsymbol{\mu}_{ef}\boldsymbol{\mu}_{fe}\boldsymbol{\mu}_{eg}\boldsymbol{\mu}_{ge}]\vdots\mathbf{e}_3\mathbf{e}_2\mathbf{e}_1^*\Gamma\left(\bar{\omega}_{fe},\Omega^2,\bar{\omega}_{eg},\Omega^2\right). \quad (11.24)$$

By following the same procedure, the parallel polarization *ZZZZ*-echo spectrum of an anharmonic oscillator is obtained as

$$\tilde{E}_{PE}^{\parallel}(\omega_t,T,\omega_\tau)=\frac{2}{5}\left|\boldsymbol{\mu}_{ge}^M\right|^4\Gamma\left(\bar{\omega}_{eg},\Omega^2,\bar{\omega}_{eg},\Omega^2\right)-\frac{1}{15}\left|\boldsymbol{\mu}_{ge}^M\right|^2\left|\boldsymbol{\mu}_{ef}^M\right|^2\left(2\cos^2\theta_{ge,ef}+1\right)$$
$$\times\Gamma\left(\bar{\omega}_{fe},\Omega^2,\bar{\omega}_{eg},\Omega^2\right), \quad (11.25)$$

where the angle $\theta_{ge,ef}$ is defined as

$$\cos\theta_{ge,ef}=\frac{\boldsymbol{\mu}_{fe}\cdot\boldsymbol{\mu}_{eg}}{|\boldsymbol{\mu}_{fe}||\boldsymbol{\mu}_{eg}|}. \quad (11.26)$$

Within the harmonic approximation, the dipole matrix element associated with the transition from the first vibrationally excited state to the overtone state is $\boldsymbol{\mu}_{ef}^M=\sqrt{2}\boldsymbol{\mu}_{ge}^M$. Then, the *ZZZZ*-echo spectrum for a weakly anharmonic oscillator is simplified as

$$\tilde{E}_{PE}^{\parallel}(\omega_t,T,\omega_\tau)=\frac{2}{5}\left|\boldsymbol{\mu}_{ge}^M\right|^4\left\{\Gamma\left(\bar{\omega}_{eg},\Omega^2,\bar{\omega}_{eg},\Omega^2\right)-\Gamma\left(\bar{\omega}_{eg}-\delta\omega_{anh},\Omega^2,\bar{\omega}_{eg},\Omega^2\right)\right\}. \quad (11.27)$$

The overtone state lifetime is usually shorter than that of the first excited state, so that the negative peak associated with the excited-state absorption is broader along the ω_t-axis than that of the positive peak. Unless there are other modes acting like energy acceptors from the first excited state, the two peak amplitudes decay in time T as $\exp(-T/T_e)$. This means that the shape, not the amplitude, of 2D spectrum does not change in time. Any deviation from this will be a signature of intramolecular energy transfer from the first excited state to other accepting modes such as bath degrees of freedom or other anharmonically coupled intramolecular vibrational modes.

Next, let us consider the coupled anharmonic oscillators. Again, the intermediate time region is considered for the sake of simplicity. This means that, in Equations 9.88 and 9.89, the quantum beat terms that decay as $\exp(-f_{12}(T))$ are ignored in the following discussion. First of all, the two diagonal peaks are

$$\tilde{E}_{D1}^{\parallel}(\omega_t,T,\omega_\tau)=\frac{2}{5}\left|\boldsymbol{\mu}_{ge_1}^M\right|^4\Gamma\left(\bar{\omega}_{e_1g},<\delta\Omega_1^2>,\bar{\omega}_{e_1g},<\delta\Omega_1^2>\right)$$

$$\tilde{E}_{D2}^{\parallel}(\omega_t,T,\omega_\tau)=\frac{2}{5}\left|\boldsymbol{\mu}_{ge_2}^M\right|^4\Gamma\left(\bar{\omega}_{e_2g},<\delta\Omega_2^2>,\bar{\omega}_{e_2g},<\delta\Omega_2^2>\right). \quad (11.28)$$

The cross-peaks appearing at $\omega_\tau = \bar{\omega}_{e_1g}$, which were collected in the Group 1 in Section 9.7, are

$$\tilde{E}^{\parallel}_{G1}(\omega_t,T,\omega_\tau) = \frac{1}{15}\left|\mu^M_{ge_1}\right|^2\left|\mu^M_{ge_2}\right|^2\left(2\cos^2\theta_{ge_1,ge_2}+1\right)\Gamma\left(\bar{\omega}_{e_2g},<\delta\Omega_2^2>,\bar{\omega}_{e_1g},<\delta\Omega_1^2>\right)$$

$$-\frac{1}{15}\left|\mu^M_{ge_1}\right|^2\left|\mu^M_{e_1f_1}\right|^2\left(2\cos^2\theta_{ge_1,e_1f_1}+1\right)\Gamma\left(\bar{\omega}_{f_1e_1},<(\delta W_1-\delta\Omega_1)^2>,\bar{\omega}_{e_1g},<\delta\Omega_1^2>\right)$$

$$-\frac{1}{15}\left|\mu^M_{ge_1}\right|^2\left|\mu^M_{e_1f_2}\right|^2\left(2\cos^2\theta_{ge_1,e_1f_2}+1\right)\Gamma\left(\bar{\omega}_{f_2e_1},<(\delta W_2-\delta\Omega_1)^2>,\bar{\omega}_{e_1g},<\delta\Omega_1^2>\right)$$

$$-\frac{1}{15}\left|\mu^M_{ge_1}\right|^2\left|\mu^M_{e_1f_3}\right|^2\left(2\cos^2\theta_{ge_1,e_1f_3}+1\right)\Gamma\left(\bar{\omega}_{f_3e_1},<(\delta W_3-\delta\Omega_1)^2>,\bar{\omega}_{e_1g},<\delta\Omega_1^2>\right). \tag{11.29}$$

The Group 2 cross-peaks at $\omega_\tau = \bar{\omega}_{e_2g}$ are

$$\tilde{E}^{\parallel}_{G2}(\omega_t,T,\omega_\tau) = \frac{1}{15}\left|\mu^M_{ge_1}\right|^2\left|\mu^M_{ge_2}\right|^2\left(2\cos^2\theta_{ge_1,ge_2}+1\right)\Gamma\left(\bar{\omega}_{e_1g},<\delta\Omega_1^2>,\bar{\omega}_{e_2g},<\delta\Omega_2^2>\right)$$

$$-\frac{1}{15}\left|\mu^M_{ge_2}\right|^2\left|\mu^M_{e_2f_1}\right|^2\left(2\cos^2\theta_{ge_2,e_2f_1}+1\right)\Gamma\left(\bar{\omega}_{f_1e_2},<(\delta W_1-\delta\Omega_2)^2>,\bar{\omega}_{e_2g},<\delta\Omega_2^2>\right)$$

$$-\frac{1}{15}\left|\mu^M_{ge_2}\right|^2\left|\mu^M_{e_2f_2}\right|^2\left(2\cos^2\theta_{ge_2,e_2f_2}+1\right)\Gamma\left(\bar{\omega}_{f_2e_2},<(\delta W_2-\delta\Omega_2)^2>,\bar{\omega}_{e_2g},<\delta\Omega_2^2>\right)$$

$$-\frac{1}{15}\left|\mu^M_{ge_2}\right|^2\left|\mu^M_{e_2f_3}\right|^2\left(2\cos^2\theta_{ge_2,e_2f_3}+1\right)\Gamma\left(\bar{\omega}_{f_3e_2},<(\delta W_3-\delta\Omega_2)^2>,\bar{\omega}_{e_2g},<\delta\Omega_2^2>\right). \tag{11.30}$$

Depending on (a) the energies of the three doubly excited states f_1 - f_3, (b) the relative angles of the corresponding transition dipole vectors, and (c) their magnitudes, the *ZZZZ*-echo spectrum of coupled anharmonic oscillators change significantly.

11.5 PERPENDICULAR POLARIZATION *ZYYZ*-ECHO: ANHARMONIC OSCILLATORS

It is now a straightforward exercise to obtain the perpendicular polarization *ZYYZ*-echo spectrum of an anharmonic oscillator, and we get

$$\tilde{E}^{\perp}_{PE}(\omega_t,T,\omega_\tau) = \frac{2}{15}\left|\mu^M_{ge}\right|^4\Gamma\left(\bar{\omega}_{eg},\Omega^2,\bar{\omega}_{eg},\Omega^2\right) - \frac{1}{30}\left|\mu^M_{ge}\right|^2\left|\mu^M_{ef}\right|^2\left(3\cos^2\theta_{ge,ef}-1\right)$$

$$\times\Gamma\left(\bar{\omega}_{fe},\Omega^2,\bar{\omega}_{eg},\Omega^2\right). \tag{11.31}$$

Within the harmonic approximation, we have $\boldsymbol{\mu}_{ef}^{M} = \sqrt{2}\boldsymbol{\mu}_{ge}^{M}$ and find that Equation 11.31 is simplified as

$$\tilde{E}_{PE}^{\perp}(\omega_t, T, \omega_\tau) = \frac{2}{15}\left|\boldsymbol{\mu}_{ge}^{M}\right|^4 \left\{\Gamma\left(\bar{\omega}_{eg}, \Omega^2, \bar{\omega}_{eg}, \Omega^2\right) - \Gamma\left(\bar{\omega}_{eg} - \delta\omega_{anh}, \Omega^2, \bar{\omega}_{eg}, \Omega^2\right)\right\}. \tag{11.32}$$

Note that the total *ZYYZ*-spectrum is just one-third of the *ZZZZ*-spectrum in this limiting case, which is similar to the case of the 2LS chromophore.

For the coupled anharmonic oscillators, in the intermediate time region the two diagonal peaks in the *ZYYZ*-echo spectrum are

$$\tilde{E}_{D1}^{\perp}(\omega_t, T, \omega_\tau) = \frac{2}{15}\left|\boldsymbol{\mu}_{ge_1}^{M}\right|^4 \Gamma\left(\bar{\omega}_{e_1g}, <\delta\Omega_1^2>, \bar{\omega}_{e_1g}, <\delta\Omega_1^2>\right)$$

$$\tilde{E}_{D2}^{\perp}(\omega_t, T, \omega_\tau) = \frac{2}{15}\left|\boldsymbol{\mu}_{ge_2}^{M}\right|^4 \Gamma\left(\bar{\omega}_{e_2g}, <\delta\Omega_2^2>, \bar{\omega}_{e_2g}, <\delta\Omega_2^2>\right). \tag{11.33}$$

The cross-peaks at $\omega_\tau = \bar{\omega}_{e_1g}$ are

$$\begin{aligned}\tilde{E}_{G1}^{\perp}(\omega_t, T, \omega_\tau) = &\frac{1}{30}\left|\boldsymbol{\mu}_{ge_1}^{M}\right|^2\left|\boldsymbol{\mu}_{ge_2}^{M}\right|^2\left(3\cos^2\theta_{ge_1,ge_2} - 1\right)\Gamma\left(\bar{\omega}_{e_2g}, <\delta\Omega_2^2>, \bar{\omega}_{e_1g}, <\delta\Omega_1^2>\right)\\
&-\frac{1}{30}\left|\boldsymbol{\mu}_{ge_1}^{M}\right|^2\left|\boldsymbol{\mu}_{e_1f_1}^{M}\right|^2\left(3\cos^2\theta_{ge_1,e_1f_1} - 1\right)\Gamma\left(\bar{\omega}_{f_1e_1}, <(\delta W_1 - \delta\Omega_1)^2>, \bar{\omega}_{e_1g}, <\delta\Omega_1^2>\right)\\
&-\frac{1}{30}\left|\boldsymbol{\mu}_{ge_1}^{M}\right|^2\left|\boldsymbol{\mu}_{e_1f_2}^{M}\right|^2\left(3\cos^2\theta_{ge_1,e_1f_2} - 1\right)\Gamma\left(\bar{\omega}_{f_2e_1}, <(\delta W_2 - \delta\Omega_1)^2>, \bar{\omega}_{e_1g}, <\delta\Omega_1^2>\right)\\
&-\frac{1}{30}\left|\boldsymbol{\mu}_{ge_1}^{M}\right|^2\left|\boldsymbol{\mu}_{e_1f_3}^{M}\right|^2\left(3\cos^2\theta_{ge_1,e_1f_3} - 1\right)\Gamma\left(\bar{\omega}_{f_3e_1}, <(\delta W_3 - \delta\Omega_1)^2>, \bar{\omega}_{e_1g}, <\delta\Omega_1^2>\right).\end{aligned} \tag{11.34}$$

The Group 2 cross-peaks at $\omega_\tau = \bar{\omega}_{e_2g}$ are

$$\begin{aligned}\tilde{E}_{G2}^{\perp}(\omega_t, T, \omega_\tau) = &\frac{1}{30}\left|\boldsymbol{\mu}_{ge_1}^{M}\right|^2\left|\boldsymbol{\mu}_{ge_2}^{M}\right|^2\left(3\cos^2\theta_{ge_1,ge_2} - 1\right)\Gamma\left(\bar{\omega}_{e_1g}, <\delta\Omega_1^2>, \bar{\omega}_{e_2g}, <\delta\Omega_2^2>\right)\\
&-\frac{1}{30}\left|\boldsymbol{\mu}_{ge_2}^{M}\right|^2\left|\boldsymbol{\mu}_{e_2f_1}^{M}\right|^2\left(3\cos^2\theta_{ge_2,e_2f_1} - 1\right)\Gamma\left(\bar{\omega}_{f_1e_2}, <(\delta W_1 - \delta\Omega_2)^2>, \bar{\omega}_{e_2g}, <\delta\Omega_2^2>\right)\\
&-\frac{1}{30}\left|\boldsymbol{\mu}_{ge_2}^{M}\right|^2\left|\boldsymbol{\mu}_{e_2f_2}^{M}\right|^2\left(3\cos^2\theta_{ge_2,e_2f_2} - 1\right)\Gamma\left(\bar{\omega}_{f_2e_2}, <(\delta W_2 - \delta\Omega_2)^2>, \bar{\omega}_{e_2g}, <\delta\Omega_2^2>\right)\\
&-\frac{1}{30}\left|\boldsymbol{\mu}_{ge_2}^{M}\right|^2\left|\boldsymbol{\mu}_{e_2f_3}^{M}\right|^2\left(3\cos^2\theta_{ge_2,e_2f_3} - 1\right)\Gamma\left(\bar{\omega}_{f_3e_2}, <(\delta W_3 - \delta\Omega_2)^2>, \bar{\omega}_{e_2g}, <\delta\Omega_2^2>\right).\end{aligned} \tag{11.35}$$

Similar to the *ZZZZ*-echo spectrum, the *ZYYZ*-echo spectrum also critically depends on the energies of the three doubly excited states $f_1 - f_3$, the relative angles of the corresponding transition dipole vectors, and their magnitudes.

11.6 DIFFERENCE TWO-DIMENSIONAL ECHO SPECTRUM: COUPLED ANHARMONIC OSCILLATORS

From the results on the parallel and perpendicular polarization measurements for coupled anharmonic oscillators, one can eliminate the two major diagonal peaks by taking the difference spectrum $\Delta\tilde{E}_{PE}(\omega_t, T, \omega_\tau)$ defined in Equation 11.19, and it is

$$\begin{aligned}
\Delta\tilde{E}_{PE}(\omega_t,T,\omega_\tau) = &-\frac{1}{6}\left|\boldsymbol{\mu}_{ge_1}^{M}\right|^2\left|\boldsymbol{\mu}_{ge_2}^{M}\right|^2 \sin^2\theta_{ge_1,ge_2}\Gamma\left(\bar{\omega}_{e_2g},<\delta\Omega_2^2>,\bar{\omega}_{e_1g},<\delta\Omega_1^2>\right)\\
&+\frac{1}{6}\left|\boldsymbol{\mu}_{ge_1}^{M}\right|^2\left|\boldsymbol{\mu}_{e_1f_1}^{M}\right|^2 \sin^2\theta_{ge_1,e_1f_1}\Gamma\left(\bar{\omega}_{f_1e_1},<(\delta W_1-\delta\Omega_1)^2>,\bar{\omega}_{e_1g},<\delta\Omega_1^2>\right)\\
&+\frac{1}{6}\left|\boldsymbol{\mu}_{ge_1}^{M}\right|^2\left|\boldsymbol{\mu}_{e_1f_2}^{M}\right|^2 \sin^2\theta_{ge_1,e_1f_2}\Gamma\left(\bar{\omega}_{f_2e_1},<(\delta W_2-\delta\Omega_1)^2>,\bar{\omega}_{e_1g},<\delta\Omega_1^2>\right)\\
&+\frac{1}{6}\left|\boldsymbol{\mu}_{ge_1}^{M}\right|^2\left|\boldsymbol{\mu}_{e_1f_3}^{M}\right|^2 \sin^2\theta_{ge_1,e_1f_3}\Gamma\left(\bar{\omega}_{f_3e_1},<(\delta W_3-\delta\Omega_1)^2>,\bar{\omega}_{e_1g},<\delta\Omega_1^2>\right)\\
&-\frac{1}{6}\left|\boldsymbol{\mu}_{ge_1}^{M}\right|^2\left|\boldsymbol{\mu}_{ge_2}^{M}\right|^2 \sin^2\theta_{ge_1,ge_2}\Gamma\left(\bar{\omega}_{e_1g},<\delta\Omega_1^2>,\bar{\omega}_{e_2g},<\delta\Omega_2^2>\right)\\
&+\frac{1}{6}\left|\boldsymbol{\mu}_{ge_2}^{M}\right|^2\left|\boldsymbol{\mu}_{e_2f_1}^{M}\right|^2 \sin^2\theta_{ge_2,e_2f_1}\Gamma\left(\bar{\omega}_{f_1e_2},<(\delta W_1-\delta\Omega_2)^2>,\bar{\omega}_{e_2g},<\delta\Omega_2^2>\right)\\
&+\frac{1}{6}\left|\boldsymbol{\mu}_{ge_2}^{M}\right|^2\left|\boldsymbol{\mu}_{e_2f_2}^{M}\right|^2 \sin^2\theta_{ge_2,e_2f_2}\Gamma\left(\bar{\omega}_{f_2e_2},<(\delta W_2-\delta\Omega_2)^2>,\bar{\omega}_{e_2g},<\delta\Omega_2^2>\right)\\
&+\frac{1}{6}\left|\boldsymbol{\mu}_{ge_2}^{M}\right|^2\left|\boldsymbol{\mu}_{e_2f_3}^{M}\right|^2 \sin^2\theta_{ge_2,e_2f_3}\Gamma\left(\bar{\omega}_{f_3e_2},<(\delta W_3-\delta\Omega_2)^2>,\bar{\omega}_{e_2g},<\delta\Omega_2^2>\right).
\end{aligned} \quad (11.36)$$

In order to show how the difference spectrum of the present coupled anharmonic oscillators are different from that of the coupled 2LS dimer, let us consider the *degenerate* case when the two constituent oscillators have the same frequency. The general results for this degenerate case were already presented and discussed in Section 9.8. Now, taking the rotational averages of all the contributing response function components, one can obtain the expressions for the difference spectrum $\Delta\tilde{E}_{PE}(\omega_t, T, \omega_\tau)$ in this limiting case.

Degenerate coupled anharmonic oscillators with strong coupling. As shown in Section 9.8, the transitions from e_2 to f_1 state and from e_1 to f_3 state are forbidden in this case. Furthermore, the relative angles $\theta_{m,n}$ are 0, $\pi/2$, or π, depending on a pair of two transition dipoles. Using the results in Section 9.8 for degenerate coupled anharmonic oscillators with a large coupling constant, one can find that the difference 2D photon echo spectrum is highly simplified as

$$\Delta\tilde{E}_{PE}(\omega_t,T,\omega_\tau) = -\frac{d^4\sin^2\phi}{6}\Big\{\Gamma\left(\bar{\omega}_{e_2g},<\delta\Omega_2^2>,\bar{\omega}_{e_1g},<\delta\Omega_1^2>\right)$$

$$-\Gamma\left(\bar{\omega}_{f_2e_1},<(\delta W_2-\delta\Omega_1)^2>,\bar{\omega}_{e_1g},<\delta\Omega_1^2>\right)+\Gamma\left(\bar{\omega}_{e_1g},<\delta\Omega_1^2>,\bar{\omega}_{e_2g},<\delta\Omega_2^2>\right)$$

$$-\Gamma\left(\bar{\omega}_{f_2e_2},<(\delta W_2-\delta\Omega_2)^2>,\bar{\omega}_{e_2g},<\delta\Omega_2^2>\right)\Big\}. \quad (11.37)$$

Interestingly, there are only four cross-peaks, and they all have the same transition strength. Nevertheless, in reality the peak amplitudes could be slightly different from one another since the dephasing constants associated with each term in Equation 11.37 can be different. As shown in Figure 11.2, not only the two diagonal peaks but also the other two cross-peaks that form couplets with the main diagonal peaks D1 and D2 disappear in the difference 2D spectrum (compare Figure 9.8 with Figure 11.2). Also, it should be mentioned that all the peak amplitudes in this spectrum are linearly proportional to $\sin^2\phi$, where ϕ is the angle between the transition dipole vectors of the two *local* oscillators. This ϕ-dependency of $\Delta\tilde{E}_{PE}(\omega_t,T,\omega_\tau)$ would be an interesting property for determining the relative orientation of two

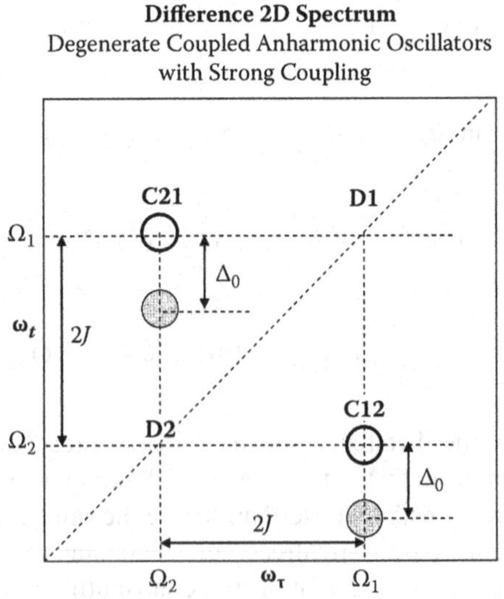

FIGURE 11.2 Difference 2D vibrational spectrum of degenerate coupled anharmonic oscillators. In comparison with Figure 9.8, the two diagonal peak couplets disappear in this difference 2D spectrum.

vibrational chromophores, as long as their transition dipole vectors in a molecule-fixed frame are known.

In the other limiting case when the anharmonic frequency shifts are sufficiently larger than the coupling-induced frequency-splitting magnitude between the two singly excited states, that is, $\Delta_0 > 2J$, there are two groups of peaks originating from SE+GB and EA, as can be seen in Figure 9.9. In that case, there would be four cross-peaks in its difference 2D spectrum, and it will only show cross-peaks in the upper and lower blocks in Figure 9.9.

11.7 GENERALIZED POLARIZATION-CONTROLLED TWO-DIMENSIONAL SPECTROSCOPY

In the previous sections, we have specifically considered two cases, that is, parallel and perpendicular polarization configurations that have been extensively used to selectively eliminate the diagonal peaks to ultimately enhance the frequency resolution of the 2D measurement technique. However, since there are virtually an infinite number of possibilities to control the beam polarization directions and relative propagation directions, it will be of interest to consider the more general situation. Assuming that the three beams propagate almost collinearly, even though, in reality, the angles between the beam propagation directions should not be zero to achieve the phasing-matching detection, there are four polarization directions that can be experimentally controlled. Without loss of generality, we shall assume that the Z-component of the emitted echo field vector is selectively detected and that the three incident beam polarization directions are controllable with respect to the Z-direction.

In this case, the directions of linearly polarized beams are in general written as

$$\mathbf{e}_1 = \hat{Y}\sin\varphi_1 + \hat{Z}\cos\varphi_1$$

$$\mathbf{e}_2 = \hat{Y}\sin\varphi_2 + \hat{Z}\cos\varphi_2$$

$$\mathbf{e}_3 = \hat{Y}\sin\varphi_3 + \hat{Z}\cos\varphi_3$$

$$\mathbf{e}_s = \hat{Z}. \tag{11.38}$$

Here, $\mathbf{e}_s$ is the unit vector of the emitted echo signal field polarization direction. There are three anlges φ_j that can be arbitrarily controlled.

Now, we are interested in finding beam configurations that can selectively remove the main diagonal peaks. As shown in this chapter, regardless of the number of chromophores that are coupled to one another, the diagonal peaks always originate from two-state $g \leftrightarrow e_j$ contributions only. Consequently, one should only consider the rotational average of the tensor element such as $[\boldsymbol{\mu}_{ge}\boldsymbol{\mu}_{eg}\boldsymbol{\mu}_{ge}\boldsymbol{\mu}_{eg}] \otimes \mathbf{e}_s\mathbf{e}_3\mathbf{e}_2\mathbf{e}_1$. Again, it is assumed that the direction of the transition dipole vector $\boldsymbol{\mu}_{ge}^M$ is chosen to be parallel to the molecular z-axis, that is, $\boldsymbol{\mu}_{ge}^{M} = |\boldsymbol{\mu}_{ge}^{M}|\,\hat{z}$. Then, the rotationally averaged tensor element $[\boldsymbol{\mu}_{ge}\boldsymbol{\mu}_{eg}\boldsymbol{\mu}_{ge}\boldsymbol{\mu}_{eg}] \otimes \mathbf{e}_s\mathbf{e}_3\mathbf{e}_2\mathbf{e}_1$ is found to be

$$[\boldsymbol{\mu}_{ge}\boldsymbol{\mu}_{eg}\boldsymbol{\mu}_{ge}\boldsymbol{\mu}_{eg}] \otimes \mathbf{e}_s\mathbf{e}_3\mathbf{e}_2\mathbf{e}_1 = \frac{1}{15}\left|\boldsymbol{\mu}_{ge}^{M}\right|^4 \{3\cos\varphi_1\cos\varphi_2\cos\varphi_3 + \sin\varphi_1\sin\varphi_2\cos\varphi_3$$

$$+\sin\varphi_1\cos\varphi_2\sin\varphi_3 + \cos\varphi_1\sin\varphi_2\sin\varphi_3\}$$

$$= \frac{1}{15}\left|\boldsymbol{\mu}_{ge}^{M}\right|^4 \{\cos(\varphi_1-\varphi_2)\cos\varphi_3 + \cos(\varphi_1-\varphi_3)\cos\varphi_2 + \cos(\varphi_2-\varphi_3)\cos\varphi_1\}. \tag{11.39}$$

Finding a proper set of beam polarization direction angles $(\varphi_1 - \varphi_3)$ that makes the above rotationally averaged transition strength vanish is to solve the following equation:

$$\cos(\varphi_1-\varphi_2)\cos\varphi_3 + \cos(\varphi_1-\varphi_3)\cos\varphi_2 + \cos(\varphi_2-\varphi_3)\cos\varphi_1 = 0. \tag{11.40}$$

We have only one equation, but there are three unknowns. Thus, there are an infinite number of solutions satisfying the above equality. For instance, $\varphi_1 = \varphi_2 = 0$ and $\varphi_3 = \pi/2$, which is the case when $\mathbf{e}_1 = \mathbf{e}_2 = \mathbf{e}_s = \hat{Z}$ and $\mathbf{e}_3 = \hat{Y}$. However, in this particular case, not only the rotationally averaged transition strengths of diagonal peaks but also those of cross-peaks vanish within the electric dipole approximation. This can be easily shown by examining the property of $I^{(4)}_{l_1l_2l_3l_4:m_1m_2m_3m_4}$ in Equation 11.2. More specifically, one should avoid the case when three out of the four polarization directions, that is, $\mathbf{e}_1$, $\mathbf{e}_2$, $\mathbf{e}_3$, and $\mathbf{e}_s$, are parallel to one another as well as when the remaining one is perpendicular to the others, e.g., $\mathbf{e}_1 \parallel \mathbf{e}_2 \parallel \mathbf{e}_3 \perp \mathbf{e}_s$. Bearing this aspect in mind, let us consider two simple cases, which can be of use in practice.

Case 1

$\mathbf{e}_j \parallel \mathbf{e}_s$ (for $j = 1 \sim 3$). In order to reduce the number of possibilities or the number of experimentally controlled variables φ_1, φ_2, and φ_3, let us consider the case when one of the three incident beam polarization directions is parallel to the polarization direction of the radiated echo field vector,

$$\mathbf{e}_j = \mathbf{e}_s = \hat{Z} \text{ for any arbitrary } j\ (=1 \sim 3), \tag{11.41}$$

so that $\varphi_j = 0$. Then, Equation 11.40 is simplified as

$$3\cos\varphi_k\cos\varphi_l + \sin\varphi_k\sin\varphi_l = 0, \tag{11.42}$$

where $k \neq j$, $l \neq j$, and $k \neq l$. From Equation 11.42, it is noted that the two controllable angles φ_k and φ_l are related to each other as

$$\varphi_l = \tan^{-1}(-3\cot\varphi_k) \quad \text{or} \quad \varphi_k = \tan^{-1}(-3\cot\varphi_l). \tag{11.43}$$

In Figure 11.3, φ_l is plotted with respect to φ_k. Although one can choose any values for φ_k and φ_l angles as long as they satisfy Equation 11.43 to make the

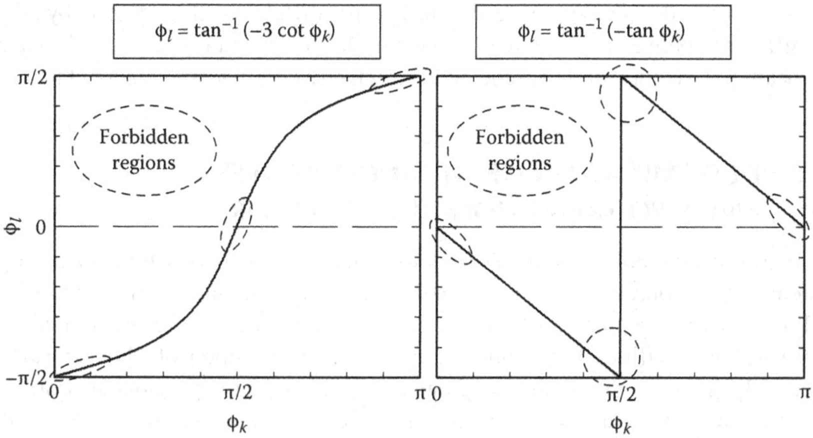

FIGURE 11.3 Plots of Equations 11.43 and 11.45.

diagonal peaks disappear, a pair of angles φ_k and φ_l that are in the forbidden regions should be avoided because those regions are either $\varphi_k = 0$ (or π) or $\varphi_l = 0$. In these cases, as mentioned above, not only do the diagonal peaks vanish, but also the entire 2D echo signal becomes vanishingly small due to the properties of rotational averages within the electric dipole approximation. As an example, if $\varphi_k = \pi/3$ (60°) and $\varphi_l = -\pi/3$ (-60°), the diagonal peaks vanish automatically, but the cross-peaks do not. For instance if $j = 1$, this is the case when the polarization direction angles for the beams 1, 2, 3, and echo field are given as 0°, 60°, −60°, and 0°, respectively.[7]

Case 2

$\mathbf{e}_j \perp \mathbf{e}_s$ (for $j = 1 \sim 3$). Now, let us consider the other limiting case when one ($\mathbf{e}_j$) of the three incident beam polarization directions is controlled to be perpendicular to the emitted echo field polarization direction. In such a case, Equation 11.40 is reduced to

$$\sin\varphi_k \cos\varphi_l + \cos\varphi_k \sin\varphi_l = 0, \tag{11.44}$$

where again $k \neq j$, $l \neq j$, and $k \neq l$. The two controllable angles φ_k and φ_l are then related to each other as

$$\varphi_l = \tan^{-1}(-\tan\varphi_k) \quad \text{or} \quad \varphi_k = \tan^{-1}(-\tan\varphi_l). \tag{11.45}$$

This is simply identical to the following equation:

$$\varphi_l = -\varphi_k \text{ (when } 0 < \varphi_k < \pi/2) \text{ or } \varphi_l = \pi - \varphi_k \text{ (when } \pi/2 < \varphi_k < \pi). \tag{11.46}$$

In Figure 11.3 (right panel), Equation 11.45 is plotted. A pair of angles φ_k and φ_l in the "forbidden regions" should not be chosen, because the entire 2D echo signal, which is rotationally averaged over the randomly oriented molecules in solution, becomes vanishingly small. Now, one of the possible choices is the case when the polarization direction angles for the beams 1, 2, 3, and echo field are given as 90°, 45°, −45°, and 0°, respectively.[7]

As shown in this section, instead of measuring difference 2D spectrum by taking the difference between perpendicular and parallel polarization echo spectra, one can use beam polarization control scheme to selectively eliminate the diagonal peaks.

11.8 DETERMINATION OF THE ANGLE BETWEEN ANY TWO TRANSITION DIPOLE VECTORS

Up until now, the polarization-controlled 2D echo spectroscopy for several model systems was theoretically discussed in detail. Since the polarization directions are additional variables that can be experimentally controlled, there are a number of interesting possibilities for enhancing the spectral resolution of 2D spectrum by selectively enhancing or suppressing particular peaks. In the previous section, only the case when one can selectively eliminate the diagonal peaks was considered in detail. However, one can explore a wide range of possible applications with the generalized polarization-controlled technique. In general, as will be shown below, one can directly and simultaneously measure the angles between two transition dipole vectors by measuring a series of 2D spectra for varying polarization direction angles.

Three relative angles of beam polarizations directions with respect to that of the generated echo field vector are still too many in real experiments, so we will consider one particular case that is likely to be practically useful. First of all, let us assume that the first beam polarization direction is parallel to the emitted echo field polarization direction, that is, $\mathbf{e}_1 \parallel \mathbf{e}_s$. Now, there are two independently controllable variables φ_2 and φ_3. Then, the 2D echo spectrum becomes dependent on these two angles as

$$\tilde{E}_{PE} = \tilde{E}_{PE}(\omega_t, T, \omega_\tau; \varphi_2, \varphi_3). \tag{11.47}$$

For a fixed waiting time T, one can obtain 2D spectra for varying φ_2 and φ_3. Then, as shown in the previous section, when $\varphi_l = \tan^{-1}(-3\cot\varphi_k)$, for example, $\varphi_2 = -\varphi_3 = \pi/3$, the diagonal peaks will disappear. If there are certain cross-peaks that also vanish for this particular beam configuration, one can conclude that the corresponding two transition dipoles are either parallel or antiparallel to each other. However, this is just one limiting case. More generally, one can use the polarization-controlled 2D spectroscopy to extract information on the relative angles between any given pair of transition dipole vectors.

Let us consider the cross-peak at $\omega_\tau = \bar{\omega}_m$ and $\omega_t = \bar{\omega}_n$, where m and n ($\neq m$) represent two different transitions, e.g., $\bar{\omega}_m = \bar{\omega}_{e_1g}$ and $\bar{\omega}_n = \bar{\omega}_{e_2g}$. The corresponding cross-peak is, within the 2D Gaussian peak shape approximation, given as

$$\tilde{\mathbf{E}}_{cross}(\omega_t, T, \omega_\tau) = [\boldsymbol{\mu}_n\boldsymbol{\mu}_n\boldsymbol{\mu}_m\boldsymbol{\mu}_m]\vdots\mathbf{e}_3\mathbf{e}_2\mathbf{e}_1^*\Gamma\left(\bar{\omega}_n, <\delta\Omega_n^2>, \bar{\omega}_m, <\delta\Omega_m^2>\right). \tag{11.48}$$

Here, the amplitude of this cross-peak is determined by the rotationally averaged transition strength $[\boldsymbol{\mu}_n\boldsymbol{\mu}_n\boldsymbol{\mu}_m\boldsymbol{\mu}_m]\vdots\mathbf{e}_3\mathbf{e}_2\mathbf{e}_1^*$. Note that this value depends on the two angles φ_2 and φ_3. Without loss of generality, one can choose the molecular z-axis to be parallel to the direction of $\boldsymbol{\mu}_m^M$ in a molecule-fixed frame, that is, $\boldsymbol{\mu}_m^M = |\boldsymbol{\mu}_m^M|\,\hat{z}$.

If the relative angle of $\boldsymbol{\mu}_n^M$ with respect to the z-axis is $\theta_{n,m}$, one can always write the $\boldsymbol{\mu}_n^M$ vector as

$$\boldsymbol{\mu}_n^M = |\boldsymbol{\mu}_n^M|(\hat{z}\cos\theta_{n,m} + \hat{x}\sin\theta_{n,m}). \tag{11.49}$$

Then, using Equation 11.2, one can find that the rotationally averaged transition strength is given as

$$[\boldsymbol{\mu}_n\boldsymbol{\mu}_n\boldsymbol{\mu}_m\boldsymbol{\mu}_m]_{0,\varphi_3,\varphi_2,0} = \frac{1}{30}|\boldsymbol{\mu}_n^M|^2|\boldsymbol{\mu}_m^M|^2\left\{\cos\varphi_2\cos\varphi_3\left(4\cos^2\theta_{n,m}+2\right)\right.$$

$$\left. + \sin\varphi_2\sin\varphi_3\left(3\cos^2\theta_{n,m}-1\right)\right\}, \tag{11.50}$$

where the subscript "$0,\varphi_3,\varphi_2,0$" means that, by reading it from right to left, the polarization direction angles of the first, second, third, and echo fields are 0, φ_2, φ_3, and 0 degrees from the laboratory *Z*-axis.

Now, let us consider a series of experiments measuring this cross-peak amplitude for varying φ_2 and φ_3. There should be angles φ_2^* and φ_3^* where the rotationally averaged transition strength of the cross-peak vanishes, that is,

$$\cos\varphi_2\cos\varphi_3\left(4\cos^2\theta_{n,m}+2\right)+\sin\varphi_2\sin\varphi_3\left(3\cos^2\theta_{n,m}-1\right)=0 \tag{11.51}$$

or equivalently

$$\cos^2\theta_{n,m} = \frac{\tan\varphi_2^*\tan\varphi_3^* - 2}{4+3\tan\varphi_2^*\tan\varphi_3^*}. \tag{11.52}$$

To make the experiment easier, one can set the φ_2 value to be $\pi/4$ as a constraint, and in this case the cross-peak amplitude is determined by

$$[\boldsymbol{\mu}_n\boldsymbol{\mu}_n\boldsymbol{\mu}_m\boldsymbol{\mu}_m]_{0,\varphi_3,\frac{\pi}{4},0} = \frac{1}{30\sqrt{2}}|\boldsymbol{\mu}_n^M|^2|\boldsymbol{\mu}_m^M|^2\left\{\cos\varphi_3\left(4\cos^2\theta_{n,m}+2\right)+\sin\varphi_3(3\cos^2\theta_{n,m}-1)\right\}. \tag{11.53}$$

For varying φ_3, one can find the angle φ_3^* that makes $[\boldsymbol{\mu}_n\boldsymbol{\mu}_n\boldsymbol{\mu}_m\boldsymbol{\mu}_m]_{0,\varphi_3^*,\frac{\pi}{4},0}$ zero. For this particular angle φ_3^*, we have

$$\cos^2\theta_{n,m} = \frac{\tan\varphi_3^* - 2}{4+3\tan\varphi_3^*}. \tag{11.54}$$

In Figure 11.4, the right-hand side of Equation 11.54 is plotted. Thus, once φ_3^* is determined, it is possible to use Equation 11.54 to determine the important angle $\theta_{n,m}$. Unfortunately, however, it is not possible to distinguish whether $\theta_{n,m}$ is in the range from 0 to $\pi/2$ or in the range from $\pi/2$ to π, because the measured value is $\cos^2\theta_{n,m}$ not $\cos\theta_{n,m}$. In addition, one should be cautious about the

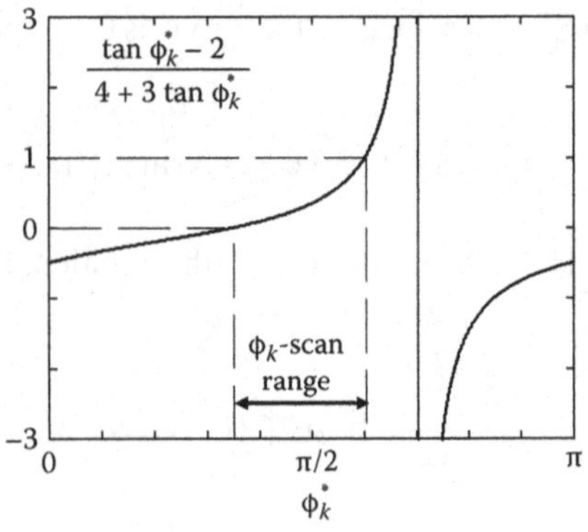

FIGURE 11.4 Plot of the right-hand side of Equation 11.54.

φ_3-scan. Since $\cos^2 \theta_{n,m}$ varies from 0 to 1, φ_3 value should be in the following range in radians:

$$\tan^{-1}(2) < \varphi_3 < \pi + \tan^{-1}(-3) \quad \text{or} \quad \pi + \tan^{-1}(2) < \varphi_3 < 2\pi + \tan^{-1}(-3) \qquad (11.55)$$

or equivalently, in degrees,

$$63.4° < \varphi_3 < 108.4° \quad \text{or} \quad -116.6° < \varphi_3 < -71.6°. \qquad (11.56)$$

The beam polarization directions for this particular φ_3-scan experiment are shown in Figure 11.5, where three polarization directions, $\mathbf{e}_1$, $\mathbf{e}_2$, and $\mathbf{e}_s$, are fixed but only the third beam polarization direction represented by $\mathbf{e}_3$ is varied.

This section showed that polarization-controlled 2D spectroscopy can be a useful technique for selectively measuring cross-peaks by taking the difference

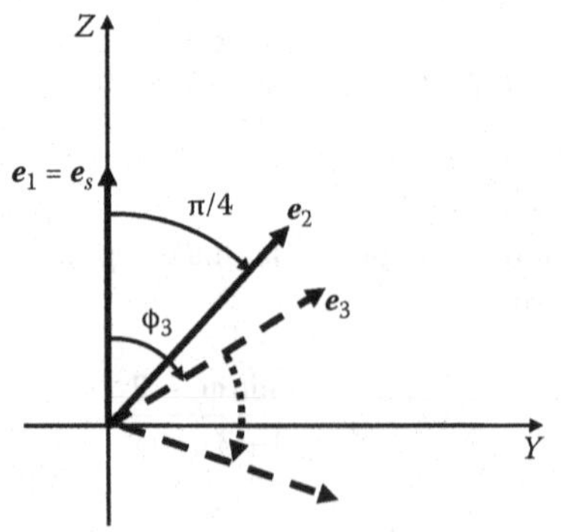

FIGURE 11.5 φ_3-scan experiment. The first beam polarization direction is parallel to the echo field vector. Now, the second beam polarization direction is rotated by $\pi/4$ from the Z-axis in a laboratory-fixed frame. The third beam polarization direction is then scanned from 63.4 to 108.4 degrees, and 2D spectra are measured.

2D spectrum. If a particular cross-peak associated with two different transitions vanishes in the difference 2D spectrum, the corresponding transition dipole vectors should be parallel or antiparallel to each other. The more general scheme is to measure a series of 2D spectra for varying the polarization direction angles. For a given cross-peak, if it vanishes at a specific polarization direction angle, the experimentally measured angle can be connected to the angle between the two transition dipole vectors. This is a remarkable result because the macroscopically controlled beam polarization directions are related to the angles between microscopic (molecular) transition dipoles, even though the molecules have completely random orientations in solution. Once all the angles $\theta_{n,m}$ for all m and n are determined, they can be an extremely useful set of constraints for the determination of 3D structure of complex molecules.

REFERENCES

1. Hochstrasser, R. M., Two-dimensional IR-spectroscopy: Polarization anisotropy effects. *Chemical Physics* 2001, 266, 273–284.
2. Woutersen, S.; Hamm, P., Structure determination of trialanine in water using polarization sensitive two-dimensional vibrational spectroscopy. *Journal of Physical Chemistry B* 2000, 104, 11316–11320.
3. Zanni, M. T.; Ge, N. H.; Kim, Y. S.; Hochstrasser, R. M., Two-dimensional IR spectroscopy can be designed to eliminate the diagonal peaks and expose only the crosspeaks needed for structure determination. *Proceedings of the National Academy of Sciences of the USA* 2001, 98, 11265–11270.
4. Hahn, S.; Kim, S.-S.; Lee, C.; Cho, M., Characteristic two-dimensional IR spectroscopic features of antiparallel and parallel β-sheet polypeptides: Simulation studies. *Journal of Chemical Physics* 2005, 123, 084905.
5. Craig, D. P.; Thirunamachandran, T., *Molecular quantum electrodynamics: An introduction to radiation molecule interactions*. Dover Publications, Inc.: New York, 1998.
6. Ge, N. H.; Hochstrasser, R. M., Femtosecond two-dimensional infrared spectroscopy: IR-COSY and THIRSTY. *Phys. Chem. Comm.* 2002, 17–26.
7. Zanni, M. T.; Ge, N.-H.; Kim, Y. S.; Hochstrasser, R. M., Two-dimensional IR spectroscopy can be designed to eliminate the diagonal peaks and expose only the crosspeaks needed for structure determination. *Proceedings of the National Academy of Sciences of the USA* 2001, 98, 11265–11270.

12 Applications of Two-Dimensional Vibrational Spectroscopy

The 2D vibrational spectroscopic technique based on four-wave-mixing schemes has certain advantages in comparison with conventional 1D vibrational spectroscopy such as IR absorption, Raman scattering, vibrational circular dichroism, and the like.[1–5] Due to the doubly vibrationally resonant condition, IR fields different in frequency can be simultaneously resonant with two different vibrational degrees of freedom, and consequently, cross-peaks in a two-dimensionally displayed spectrum arise from their couplings that are usually difficult to be measured by using 1D method (compare the magnitudes of primary and secondary spectroscopic properties mentioned in Chapter 1). In addition, the two oscillators have to be anharmonic to avoid complete destructive interferences among different nonlinear optical transition pathways. Note that the nonlinear response function of perfectly harmonic oscillators vanishes.

An early attempt to obtain 2D IR spectrum was based on 2D IR pump–probe and dynamic hole-burning techniques, where the pump frequency scanning was required to fully construct the 2D spectrum with respect to the pump and probe frequencies.[1] The 2D IR pump–probe spectra of apamin and scyllatoxin are shown in Figure 12.1, where the *x*- and *y*-axis are the pump and probe frequencies in centimeters^{-1}. Instead of the pump frequency scanning to obtain a series of 1D spectra used to construct a full 2D spectrum, one can scan the first delay time τ in an infrared photon echo experiment to obtain the 2D IR PE spectra of peptides. A number of 2D IR experiments have been performed to study amide I vibrations of polypeptides, since the amide I band shape and center frequency have been known to be highly sensitive to protein secondary structures.[6–8] In addition, it is comparatively easy to introduce isotope-labeled amino acid residue to polypeptides and proteins. Two-dimensional IR spectroscopic investigations of those isotope-labeled amide I modes can provide information on local structure and dynamics around the isotope-labeled peptide. In this chapter, only those representative experimental results and theoretical interpretations are presented. Particularly, the 2D IR photon echo spectroscopic studies of single oscillator systems, coupled two-oscillator systems, coupled multi-oscillator systems, protein folding-unfolding dynamics, and chemical exchange dynamics will be discussed to show how useful the 2D vibrational spectroscopic technique is in studying ultrafast solvent-solute dynamics, protein structure determination, structural changes of proteins, and hydrogen-bonding dynamics.

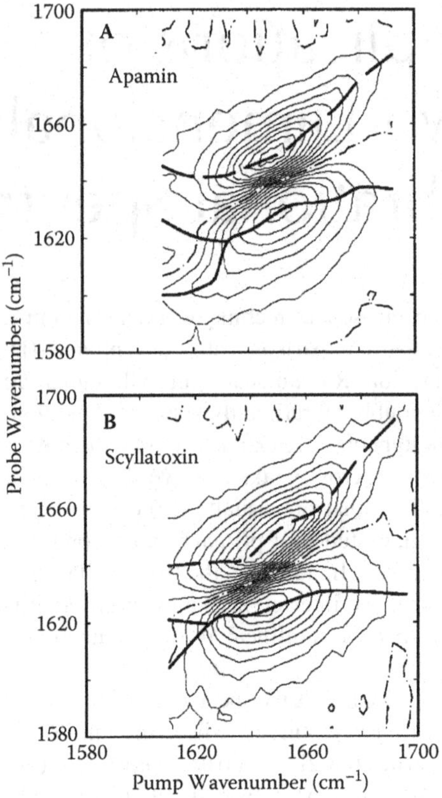

FIGURE 12.1 2D IR pump–probe spectra of apamin and scyllatoxin. A series of dynamic hole-burning experiments were performed to construct these 2D spectra. (From Hamm, P., Lim, M. H., and Hochstrasser, R. M., *Journal of Physical Chemistry B*, 102, 6123, 1998. With permission.)

12.1 SINGLE ANHARMONIC OSCILLATOR SYSTEMS

Despite that the 2D vibrational spectroscopic technique is particularly useful in studying molecular complexes and coupled multi-chromophore systems, its application to single oscillator systems had to be performed first to obtain vital information on the solvent–chromophore (oscillator) interaction dynamics in condensed phases. Two representative examples, which are the amide I vibration of *N*-methylacetamide (NMA) and the O-D (or O-H) stretching mode of HOD in H_2O (HOD in D_2O) will be discussed in this section. NMA is an excellent model system for understanding vibrational dynamics of peptides in solution.[9] In order to understand hydrogen-bonding dynamics and network formation of water, the model systems, HOD in D_2O or HOD in H_2O, have also been extensively studied. The amide I vibrations in NMA or OH (OD) stretch of HOD in D_2O (H_2O) are essentially uncoupled to all the other intramolecular vibrational degrees of freedom or to solvent modes so that they could be treated as a single anharmonic oscillator.

N-methylacetamide. NMA containing a single peptide bond is a prototype model for peptide. By considering it a unit peptide, polypeptide can be described as a collection of such units with certain configurations representing its backbone structure.[10–14] For the NMA in solutions, 2D pump–probe and photon echo experiments were carried out to investigate the peptide-water interaction dynamics.[15–17] The hydrogen bonding interactions between NMA and surrounding protic solvent molecules induce an amide I mode frequency red-shift, where the amide I vibration is mainly C=O stretch + N-H in-plane bend. Since the carbonyl oxygen atom can form one or two hydrogen bonds with surrounding water molecules, the amide I vibrational frequency is sensitive to the number and orientation of hydrogen-bonded water molecules around the carbonyl oxygen atom.[18–20] To quantitatively describe the hydrogen bonding effect on the amide I mode frequency shift, denoted as $\delta\tilde{\nu}_I$, an approximate linear relationship between $\delta\tilde{\nu}_I$ and the hydrogen-bond distance $r(O\cdots H)$ in Å, that is, $\delta\tilde{\nu}_I = -\alpha_{Hyd}\{2.6 - r(O\cdots H)\}$, was used before.[21] Here, the slope α_{Hyd} was assumed to be 30 cm^{-1}/Å. Although this simple relationship between $\delta\tilde{\nu}_I$ and $r(O\cdots H)$ was found to be of use to some extent, its validity is limited only in short-distance range around the optimum hydrogen-bond distance, which is here assumed to be 2.6 Å.[1, 22] Consequently, it was necessary to develop a model that can incorporate the effects from (1) hydrogen-bonding interaction between the N-H group of a given peptide and water oxygen atom, (2) dependency of such a relationship on solvent, and (3) different orientations of hydrogen-bonded solvent molecules.

To elucidate the hydrogen bonding effects on the amide I frequency, *ab initio* calculation studies on the amide I mode frequency shift ($\delta\tilde{\nu}_I$) for a number of NMA-$(D_2O)_n$ ($n = 1 - 5$) clusters were carried out to establish the relationship between $\delta\tilde{\nu}_I$ and electrostatic potentials at six different sites (O, C, N, H, CH_3(C), and CH_3(N)) of the NMA molecule.[23, 24] Here, the electrostatic potential at a given site is created by the distributed partial charges of the surrounding solvent molecules, that is,

$$\tilde{\nu}_I = \tilde{\nu}_I^0 + \delta\tilde{\nu}_I = \tilde{\nu}_I^0 + \sum_{a=1}^{6} l_a \phi_a \tag{12.1}$$

where ϕ_a is the electrostatic potential at the ath site of the NMA. The expansion coefficients, l_a, in the above equation were obtained by carrying out multivariate least square regression analysis with Equation 12.1, for clusters consisting of an NMA and varying number of solvent molecules. The electrostatic potential, ϕ_a, at the site a is

$$\phi_a = \frac{1}{4\pi\varepsilon_0}\sum_m \sum_j \frac{C_{j(m)}^{solvent}}{r_{aj(m)}}, \tag{12.2}$$

where $C_{j(m)}^{solvent}$ denotes the partial charge of the jth site of the mth solvent molecule and $r_{aj(m)}$ is the distance between the NMA site a and the jth site of the mth solvent molecule. The above model in Equations 12.1 and 12.2 is called the electrostatic potential model for solvatochromic frequency shift. The distributed sites on the solute collectively act like an antennae sensing local electrostatic potential distribution, which is highly anisotropic and spatially nonuniform around a solute.

Instead of electrostatic potential calculations at each site, one can employ the vibrational Stark theory to simulate the amide I frequency shift and fluctuation.[20] For the NMA in solution, the amide I frequency is in this case assumed to be linearly dependent on the electric field components as

$$\tilde{\nu}_I = \tilde{\nu}_I^0 + \sum_{i\alpha} c_{i\alpha} E_{i\alpha} \tag{12.3}$$

where $\alpha = \{x, y, z\}$, $E_{i\alpha}$ is the αth component of the electric field vector on the ith atom, i corresponds to either the C, O, N, or D in the deuterated NMA, and $c_{i\alpha}$'s are the expansion coefficients. The electric field vector at the ith atom is calculated as

$$\mathbf{E}_i = \frac{1}{4\pi\varepsilon_0} \sum_{j=1}^{N\times M} \frac{C_j}{r_{ij}^2} \hat{\mathbf{r}}_{ij} \tag{12.4}$$

where j runs over all the charged sites of the surrounding solvent molecules, $\hat{\mathbf{r}}_{ij}$ is a unit vector pointing from the jth solvent atomic site to the ith solute atom, N is the number of solvent molecules, M is the number of charged sites in a single solvent molecule, and r_{ij} denotes the distance between the two sites. If the entire solute-solvent interaction causing frequency shift is dipolar in nature, only one point dipole is required. However, the above model in Equation 12.3 means that the solute-solvent interactions are between properly weighted point dipoles at those distributed sites and solvent polarization. This model is in fact based on the assumption that the solute-solvent interaction is described as the sum of interactions between dipoles distributed on the solute and the solvent electric fields at the centers of the solute's point dipoles. This method utilizing the electric field vector calculation was also found to be quantitatively acceptable in reproducing the amide I band of NMA and the OH stretch band of water.[20]

For the NMA-water solution, by using the above relationship in Equation 12.1 and by carrying out classical MD simulations of the NMA-water solution, it was possible to estimate the amide I mode frequency shift from that of an isolated NMA molecule. Note that the MD simulation trajectories can provide instantaneous solvent configurations around a solute. From them, one can obtain the electrostatic potentials at each site as a function of time, which in turn were used to obtain the amide I frequency trajectory, $\tilde{\nu}_I(t)$. The estimated amide I mode frequency shift, defined as $\langle \delta\tilde{\nu}_I \rangle = \langle \tilde{\nu}_I(t) \rangle - \tilde{\nu}_I^0$, was found to be in good agreement with the experimental value, indicating that the electrostatic interaction between the NMA and solvent water molecules is the principal contribution to the amide I frequency shift and fluctuation.[19] Then, the amide I vibrational dephasing can be investigated by calculating the frequency-frequency correlation function (FFCF) $\langle \delta\tilde{\nu}_I(t)\delta\tilde{\nu}_I(0) \rangle$. The spectral density $\rho(\omega)$ of the coupled bath modes was obtained from the cosine transformation, that is,

$$\rho(\omega) = 2\tanh(\hbar\omega/2k_BT) \int_0^\infty dt \cos(\omega t)\left\{\langle \delta\tilde{\nu}_I(t)\delta\tilde{\nu}_I(0)\rangle / \langle \delta\tilde{\nu}_I^2 \rangle\right\}. \tag{12.5}$$

The resultant $\rho(\omega)$ showed that the librational (hindered rotational) motions of the water molecules directly hydrogen-bonded to the NMA play a critical role in modulating the amide I frequency in time. Once the amide I FFCF $C(t)$ is obtained, the corresponding IR absorption spectrum can be calculated by using Equations 3.97 and 3.38.

In order to study the hydrogen-bonding dynamics of a given peptide in water, 2D IR pump–probe experiment for NMA/D_2O solution was performed. In this chapter, we instead discuss the 2D IR photon echo studies on NMA in D_2O, $CDCl_3$ and DMSO-d_6 solutions for the sake of direct comparisons with theoretical descriptions discussed in Chapter 7.[17] In the top panel of Figure 12.2, four snapshot 2D IR PE spectra at the waiting times of 0, 400, 1000, and 2000 fs are shown. The upper-lying positive peak originates from the $g \leftrightarrow e$ transitions, that is to say, it is the summation of stimulated emission and ground-state bleaching contributions, where the corresponding polarizations are given as, respectively,

$$< \mu \xleftarrow[g\wr \quad e\wr]{e\wr} | g >< g | >$$

$$< \mu \xleftarrow[g\wr e\wr]{e\wr} | g >< g | > . \tag{12.6}$$

The negative peak appearing in the lower frequency region is from the excited-state absorption contribution whose polarization is given as

$$< \mu \xleftarrow[e\wr]{f\wr e\wr} | g >< g | > . \tag{12.7}$$

The frequency separation between the positive and negative peaks is due to the finite overtone anharmonic frequency shift $\delta\omega_{anh}$, which was estimated to be about 16 cm^{-1}. However, since the absorption bandwidth is comparable or even larger than the anharmonic frequency shift, the peak-to-peak frequency difference denoted as $\Delta\omega(T)$ in Chapter 7 is not simply identical to the overtone anharmonic frequency shift, $\delta\omega_{anh}$. In this case of weakly anharmonic limit, Equation 7.39 can be used to approximately estimate the peak-to-peak frequency difference for this case of NMA in D_2O solution. From Figure 12.2, one can estimate $\Delta\omega(T = 2\,\text{ps})$ to be about 25 cm^{-1}. From Equation 7.40 with ignoring the solvent reorganization energy, 2Ω, where Ω is the root mean square of fluctuating amide I frequency, is about 25 cm^{-1}. This is consistent with the absorption bandwidth.

For all three NMA solutions, the 2D IR PE spectra have nodal lines separating the upper positive and lower negative peaks. The slope of the nodal line at $\omega_\tau = \bar{\omega}_{eg}$ varies from 1 to 0 as the waiting time T increases from 0 to a few picoseconds (ps). For a single anharmonic oscillator system, it was shown that this slope is in fact directly related to the FFCF as[25]

$$\sigma(T) = \langle \delta\omega(T)\delta\omega(0) \rangle / \langle \delta\omega^2 \rangle. \tag{12.8}$$

In the case of the NMA/water solution, the slope of the nodal line, $\sigma(T)$, approaches zero in about 2 ps, whereas that of the NMA/DMSO-d_6 solution decreases

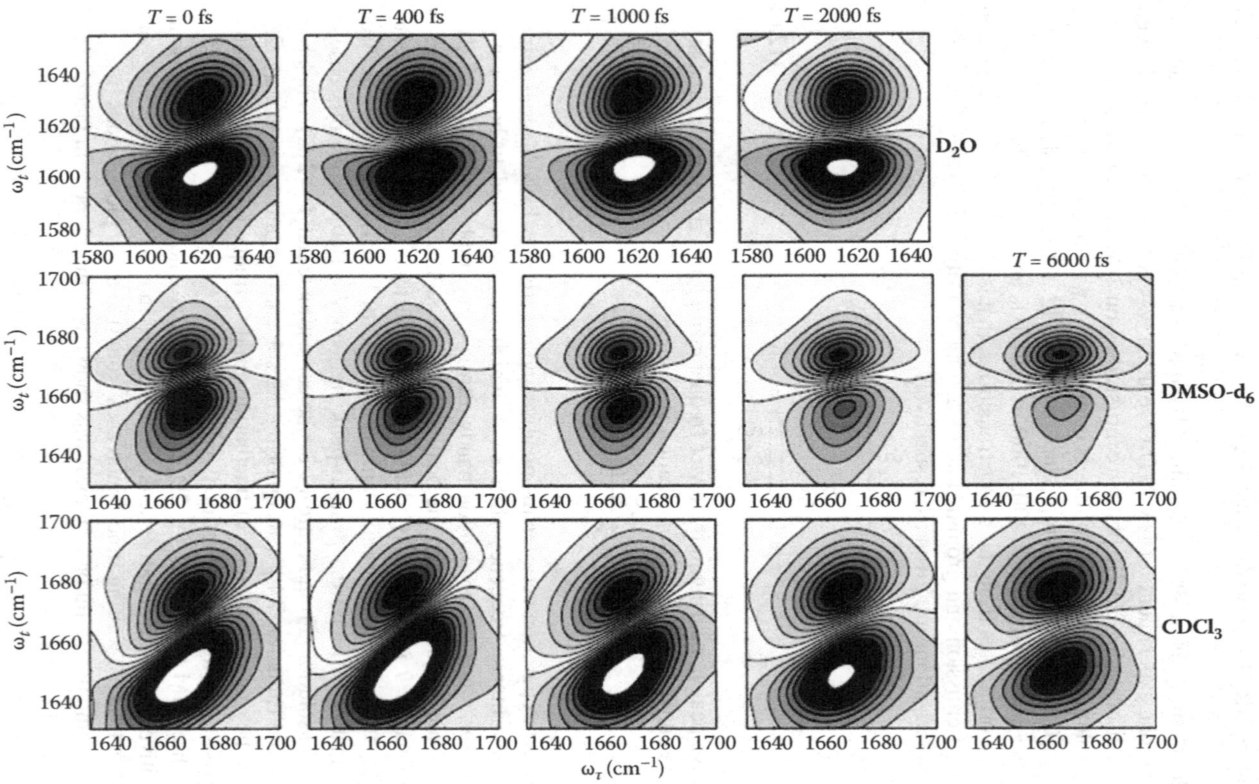

FIGURE 12.2 2D IR photon echo spectra of NMA (*N*-methylacetamide) in D_2O, DMSO-d_6, and $CDCl_3$ solutions. (From DeCamp, M. F., et al., *Journal of Physical Chemistry B*, 109, 11016, 2005. With permission.)

comparatively slowly and is finite even at $T = 6$ ps. An interesting observation for the NMA/$CDCl_3$ solution is that the nodal line at $T = 6$ ps appears to be curvilinear. More specifically, the slope of the nodal line in the lower frequency region decays slower than that in the higher frequency region. This was explained by the presence of improper hydrogen-bonding interaction between the NMA C=O group and the deuterium atoms of $CDCl_3$. From the classical MD simulation, it was found that the NMA molecule can form a single improper hydrogen-bond with a solvent $CDCl_3$ molecule.[17] Therefore, there are two solvation species, either free NMA or NMA with a single hydrogen-bonded $CDCl_3$. Due to this inhomogeneity, the 2D IR PE spectra of NMA/$CDCl_3$ solution appear to be significantly diagonally elongated and asymmetric. This shows the existence of such an improper hydrogen bond and provides a hint on its dynamic timescale.

HOD/H_2O and HOD/D_2O. The dynamics of water is highly important, and it has crucial effects on diverse areas of science. It has been known that a number of water properties are largely related to strong hydrogen bonds that each water molecule can form with its neighbors. Thus, formed hydrogen bond networks are evolving in time, and its time and length scales are critically dependent on the hydrogen bond forming and breaking dynamics.[26] Such hydrogen-bonding dynamics of liquids has been extensively studied by using femtosecond IR spectroscopic methods such as transient absorption experiments and femtosecond IR photon echo studies.[27–47] Here, the 2D IR photon echo studies are primarily discussed and the vibrational chromophore of interest is the O-D stretch of HOD in H_2O.

The 2D IR correlation spectra of the OD stretch of HOD in H_2O with respect to waiting time T show typical positive-negative couplet.[41] At short time $T = 0.1$, the 2D spectrum is diagonally elongated as expected, which indicates inhomogeneous distribution of the OD stretch frequencies. As the waiting time T increases from 0.1 to 1.6 ps, the widths of the peaks increase and the slope $\sigma(T)$ of the nodal line separating the positive peak from the lower negative peak decreases from about 1 to zero.[41] Much like the case of the NMA in heavy water, the inhomogeneity of the hydroxyl stretch frequency distribution persists for a couple of picoseconds, which evidently corresponds to the lifetime of the local hydrogen-bond network around an OD vibrational chromophore.

In order to quantitatively describe the time-dependent change of the 2D IR correlation spectrum, theoretical studies utilizing an MD simulation method were carried out, and the resultant simulated spectra were compared with the experiment.[41] To calculate the instantaneous OD stretch frequencies from the MD trajectory, the vibrational Stark theory, where the electric field component E, which is the projected electric field onto the OD bond, is assumed to be linearly proportional to the frequency shift induced by the electrostatic interaction of the OD group with surrounding solvent molecules, that is,[48]

$$\omega_{OD}(t) = \omega_{OD}^0 + \alpha E(t), \tag{12.9}$$

where ω_{OD}^0 is the OD frequency of an isolated HOD molecule and E is calculated as

$$E = \frac{1}{4\pi\varepsilon_0}\hat{\mathbf{r}}_{OD}\cdot\sum_{j=1}^{3N}\frac{C_j}{r_{jD}^2}\hat{\mathbf{r}}_{jD}. \tag{12.10}$$

The proportionality constant α is known as the vibrational Stark tuning rate. Here, $\hat{\mathbf{r}}_{OD}$ is a unit vector pointing from O to D in the direction of the OD bond; the summation in Equation 12.10 is over all charged sites of solvent water molecules; and $\hat{\mathbf{r}}_{jD}$ is the unit vector pointing from the solvent site j to the D atom of the HOD molecule.

From the *ab initio* calculations of HOD-$(H_2O)_n$ clusters sampled from classical MD trajectories, the expansion coefficient α in Equation 12.9 was obtained and estimated to be -10792 cm^{-1}/au. Because those solvent water molecules around an HOD solute continually change its relative distances and orientations in time, the site-site distances r_{jD} and the projection angles determining the factor of $\hat{\mathbf{r}}_{OD} \cdot \hat{\mathbf{r}}_{jD}$ fluctuate in time. These essentially modulate the electric field component $E(t)$ in Equation 12.9, and the OD stretch frequency fluctuates. From the OD stretch frequency trajectory, the FFCF $< \delta\omega_{OD}(t)\delta\omega_{OD}(0) >$, where $\delta\omega_{OD}(t) = \omega_{OD}(t) - \bar{\omega}_{OD}$, is calculated and used to numerically simulate the corresponding linear and nonlinear vibrational spectra. The FFCF obtained from the MD simulations with employing the above connection formula in Equation 12.9, which was based on the vibrational Stark theory, was found to be in excellent agreement with experimentally retrieved FFCF of which decaying pattern is multimodal with a wide range of different timescales. The fast component (~32 fs) in the correlation function appears to be related to the fluctuations of the hydrogen-bond length coordinate. On the other hand, the slow (~2 ps) component is likely due to hydrogen bond making and breaking dynamics, which is consistent with MD simulations showing that the hydrogen bond lifetime is about 2 ps.

Later, a heterodyne-detected 2D IR photon echo experiment on HOD/D_2O solution was carried out, and the OH stretch frequency fluctuation and ultrafast hydrogen-bond dynamics were investigated.[42, 44–46] One of the issues for understanding hydrogen bond networks in water was the roles of nonhydrogen-bonded configurations and dangling hydrogen bonds.[42] The proposition was that the nonhydrogen-bonded configuration should be considered a transition state in an event of thermally activated hydrogen bond breaking and subsequent new hydrogen bond forming with a different partner. From the ultrafast IR photon echo and MD simulation studies, it was shown that virtually all water molecules in the nonhydrogen-bonded configurations return to a hydrogen bonding partner in 200 fs, strongly indicating that hydrogen bonds in water are broken only fleetingly.[42] Again, the slope of nodal line in the experimentally measured 2D photon echo spectrum decays in time T and its decaying pattern was found to be in agreement with the OH stretch mode FFCF experimentally measured from the photon echo peak shift. The MD simulations suggested that the nonhydrogen-bonded configuration is just a transitory state and that most likely librations on the 50 fs timescale are mainly responsible for making the nonhydrogen-bonded configurations proceed to a new hydrogen bond or return back to the original hydrogen bond. This picture is in contrast to that treating various hydrogen-bonded species such as nonhydrogen-bonded molecules, dangling waters, and hydrogen-bonded molecules with different coordination numbers as chemically distinct states.

12.2 COUPLED TWO-OSCILLATOR SYSTEMS

Solution structures of small oligopeptides have been paid lots of attention, but it was found to be quite difficult to determine their structures in solution. Small peptides containing two peptide bonds have thus been extensively studied by using the 2D IR technique. The amide I band of a dipeptide can be described in terms of two delocalized normal modes, since the two amide I local oscillators are coupled to each other via through-space and through-bond interactions.[13, 49–51] The coupling constant J is then strongly dependent on the relative distance and angle between the two transition dipoles located at the two peptide bonds. For such a coupled-anharmonic-oscillator system, detailed theoretical descriptions of model Hamiltonian and vibrational properties were presented and discussed in Section 9.6.

Two important factors determining the extent of delocalization of vibrationally excited states are (1) two local mode frequencies, ω_1 and ω_2, and (2) coupling constant J. For an isolated dipeptide, the entire map of J with respect to the two dihedral angles ϕ and ψ, which determine the backbone conformation of the dipeptide, was reported.[13, 50, 52] For a glycine dipeptide (Ac-Gly-NHMe), the coupling constants $J(\phi, \psi)$ were calculated and are shown in Figure 12.3. Once the coupling constant J is measured experimentally by analyzing the 2D IR spectrum of a given dipeptide, the map in Figure 12.3 can be of use to obtain information on possible dipeptide conformations.

Acetylproline. As a simple model dipeptide system, acetylated proline amide (Ac-Pro-ND_2) in D_2O solution has been studied by using the 2D IR photon echo

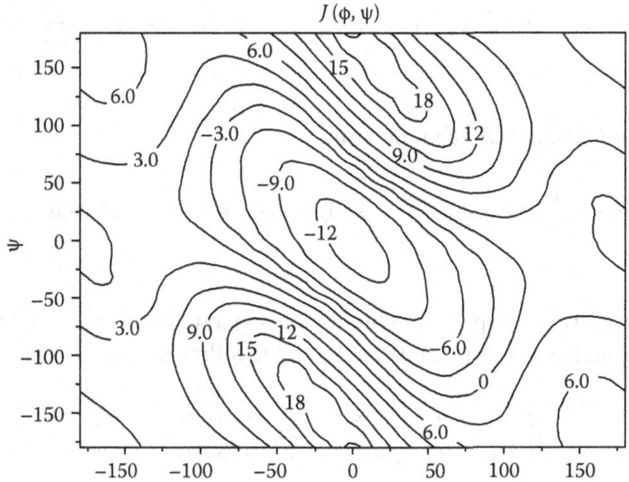

FIGURE 12.3 Amide I vibrational coupling constant J of glycine dipeptide analog for varying dihedral angles ϕ and ψ.

method.[53–56] Due to the five-membered pyrrolidine ring strain, the amide I local-mode frequency of the acetyl-end peptide is about 30 cm^{-1} red-shifted from that of the amide-end peptide.[57] Therefore, the amide I IR band appears as a doublet with two amide I IR sub-bands separated from each other by about 30 cm^{-1}. Interestingly, its backbone conformation changes for varying solvents. For instance, the acetylproline adopts a C_{7eq} conformation when it is dissolved in nonpolar aprotic solvent, because it is stabilized by an intramolecular hydrogen-bonding interaction.[58] On the other hand, if the acetylproline is dissolved in water or other protic solvents, the water molecules actively participate in the intermolecular H-bonding interactions with the two peptide groups so that its backbone conformation changes and becomes close to the so-called polyproline II structure. Therefore, the 2D IR spectrum of the acetylproline in $CDCl_3$ differs from that in D_2O. Now, the extent of mode mixing depends on the conformation-dependent coupling constant J. Note that the cross-peak amplitudes and shapes are determined by the coupling.

In Section 11.4, it was shown that the parallel-polarization *ZZZZ*-echo spectrum for coupled anharmonic oscillators consists of two diagonal peaks, four off-diagonal peaks at $\omega_\tau = \bar{\omega}_{e_1g}$, another four off-diagonal peaks at $\omega_\tau = \bar{\omega}_{e_2g}$. Similarly, the perpendicular-polarization *ZYYZ*-echo spectrum would show those peaks with different amplitudes. If the overtone and combination anharmonic frequency shifts are sufficiently large to make all the off-diagonal peaks frequency-resolvable, one can directly compare one cross-peak in the *ZZZZ*-echo spectrum with that in the *ZYYZ*-echo spectrum to determine the angle between the two transition dipole vectors of normal modes. From Equations 11.29 and 11.30, the cross-peak at $\omega_\tau = \bar{\omega}_{e_1g}$ and $\omega_t = \bar{\omega}_{e_2g}$ in the *ZZZZ*-echo spectrum is given as

$$\tilde{E}^{\parallel}(\omega_t,\omega_\tau) = \frac{1}{15}\left|\boldsymbol{\mu}^M_{ge_1}\right|^2\left|\boldsymbol{\mu}^M_{ge_2}\right|^2\left(2\cos^2\theta_{ge_1,ge_2}+1\right)\Gamma\left(\bar{\omega}_{e_2g},<\delta\Omega_2^2>,\bar{\omega}_{e_1g},<\delta\Omega_1^2>\right), \tag{12.10}$$

whereas that in the *ZYYZ*-echo spectrum is

$$\tilde{E}^{\perp}(\omega_t,\omega_\tau) = \frac{1}{30}\left|\boldsymbol{\mu}^M_{ge_1}\right|^2\left|\boldsymbol{\mu}^M_{ge_2}\right|^2\left(3\cos^2\theta_{ge_1,ge_2}-1\right)\Gamma\left(\bar{\omega}_{e_2g},<\delta\Omega_2^2>,\bar{\omega}_{e_1g},<\delta\Omega_1^2>\right). \tag{12.11}$$

Thus, if these two cross-peak amplitudes are separately measured and their ratio is estimated from them, it is possible to obtain the following simple relation,

$$\frac{\tilde{E}^{\parallel}(\omega_t=\bar{\omega}_{e_2g},\omega_\tau=\bar{\omega}_{e_1g})}{\tilde{E}^{\perp}(\omega_t=\bar{\omega}_{e_2g},\omega_\tau=\bar{\omega}_{e_1g})} = \frac{4\cos^2\theta_{ge_1,ge_2}+2}{3\cos^2\theta_{ge_1,ge_2}-1}. \tag{12.12}$$

From this relationship between the cross-peak amplitude ratio and the angle θ_{ge_1,ge_2} between the two transition dipole vectors, one can estimate θ_{ge_1,ge_2} value in principle, which provides critical information on the dipeptide backbone conformation. This procedure was used to determine the solution structure of acetylpronine with a limited success. Often, it is difficult to use the above strategy using Equation 12.12

to determine θ_{ge_1,ge_2}, because the cross-peaks in the 2D amide I spectrum are not well separated in freqency domain due to spectral congestion. Thus, crude estimations of the cross-peak amplitudes from the spectrally congested 2D spectrum could potentially lead to an erroneous conclusion on the dipeptide conformation. Nevertheless, as shown in Chapter 11, there are alternative ways to determine θ_{ge_1,ge_2} values, and they should be of use in the future.

Alanine dipeptide. There are two different alanine dipeptide systems that contain two peptide bonds each. The first is the trialanine (Ala-Ala-Ala) with free amine and carboxyl groups at the two terminals,[15, 59, 60] and the second is Ac-Ala-NHMe that is an alanine capped by an acetyl group at the amino terminal and by an N-methyl amino group at the carboxyl terminal.[61, 62] Due to the two charged groups in the trialanine at neutral pH, it is believed that the intrinsic peptide backbone conformation is affected by the intramolecular electrostatic interactions. On the other hand, Ac-Ala-NHMe is not.

In order to determine the solution structure of trialanine, the 2D IR pump–probe experiments on the trialanine and its two isotopomers (Ala*-Ala-Ala and Ala-Ala*-Ala) in combination with classical MD simulation studies were carried out.[59, 60] Here, the asterisk in Ala*-Ala-Ala for example means that the amino acid with * has a ^{13}C-isotope labeled carbonyl group. From the measured anisotropy values of these three trialanines, it was possible to estimate the angle ϕ_{12} ($\cong 106°$) between the two amide I transition dipole vectors. Also, from the least-square fit to the experimentally measured 2D IR pump–probe spectrum, the coupling constant J between the two amide I local modes was obtained to be 6 cm^{-1}. Then, by using the maps of the coupling constant in Figure 12.3 as well as of the angle between the two transition dipoles with respect to ϕ and ψ angles, it was shown that the secondary structure of trialanine does not change upon isotope substitution and that the average ϕ and ψ angles are about −60 and 140 degrees. Later, carrying out MD simulation studies with GROMOS96 force field and SPC water, the relative populations of P_{II} and right-handed α-helical (α_R) conformations were found to be about 80 and 20 percent, respectively.[15]

The alanine dipeptide analog (Ac-Ala-NHMe) and its isotopomers were also investigated in detail by using the 2D IR photon echo method. The two amide I modes were found to be fairly localized due to relatively small coupling constant of ~1.5 cm^{-1}. The polarization-controlled experiments discussed in Chapter 11 were carried out, and the results suggested that the allowed angle θ_{ge_1,ge_2} is either 52° or 128°. This indicates that the most probable conformation is polyproline II with Ramachandran angles, $\phi = -70°$ and $\psi = 120°$.[61, 62]

Dicarbonyl metal complex. Dicarbonylacetylacetonato rhodium complex (RDC), which is a square-planar compound with two equivalent CO groups and a bidentate acac ($OC(CH_3)CHC(CH_3)O$) ligand coordinated to the rhodium metal center, has been found to be an excellent model for coupled oscillator system. The CO stretching vibrations in this organometallic compound have very large dipole strengths so that the photon echo signals are comparatively large, which rendered detailed investigations with various nonlinear vibrational spectroscopic techniques.[7] Furthermore, due to the strong coupling between the two CO stretching vibrations, symmetric and asymmetric CO stretching normal modes are formed and the frequency difference was found to be about 70 cm^{-1}, which indicates that the magnitude of coupling constant J is 35 cm^{-1}. In Section 9.8, a detailed theoretical description of this kind of coupled anharmonic oscillators in the degenerate case was presented and discussed. Particularly, the RDC system corresponds to the strong coupling limit, because $J > (\Delta_0 + \Delta_c)/2 > \sqrt{<\delta\Omega^2>}$.

In such a case of strongly coupled degenerate anharmonic oscillators, the energies of the three doubly excited states were found to be

$$W_1 = 2\omega_0 - \frac{\Delta_0 + \Delta_c}{2} + 2J$$

$$W_2 = 2\omega_0 - \Delta_0$$

$$W_3 = 2\omega_0 - \frac{\Delta_0 + \Delta_c}{2} - 2J. \tag{12.13}$$

For this case, one can expect that the experimentally measured 2D spectrum should be similar to Figure 9.8. For the RDC molecule in hexane, the 2D IR (rephasing, nonrephasing, and purely absorptive) spectra were measured, and they are shown in Figure 12.4.[7] One can immediately find that the schematic spectrum in Figure 9.8 is indeed quite similar to the absorptive 2D IR spectrum, which results from the addition of equally weighted rephasing and nonrephasing spectra, in Figure 12.4(c).

From the experimentally measured spectra in Figure 12.4, the anharmonic frequency shifts of the overtone states were found to be 11 and 14 cm^{-1} for the symmetric and asymmetric CO stretch normal modes, respectively. The combination band is red-shifted by 26 cm^{-1} with respect to the sum of the fundamental frequencies, due

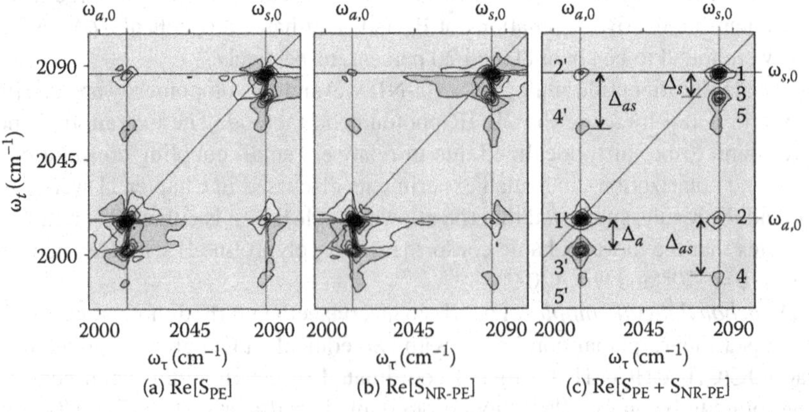

FIGURE 12.4 Real parts of 2D IR spectra of RDC (dicarbonylacetylaceto Rhodium) complex. The rephasing (S_{PE}), nonrephasing ($S_{NR\text{-}PE}$), and absorptive (rephasing + nonrephasing) photon echo spectra are shown in (a), (b), and (c), respectively. In (c), the four peaks 1, 1', 2, and 2' are positive, and all the other cross-peaks are negative in magnitude. (From Khalil, M., Demirdoven, N., and Tokmakoff, A., *Journal of Physical Chemistry A*, 2003, 107, 5258. With permission.)

to the coupling between the carbonyls. The line widths of the two CO stretch bands are about 2.6 cm^{-1}, which is significantly smaller than the anharmonic frequency shifts, that is, $(\Delta_0 + \Delta_c)/2 > \sqrt{<\delta\Omega^2>}$. The two diagonal peaks, denoted as 1' and 1, in the absorptive 2D IR spectrum in Figure 12.4(c) correspond to the asymmetric and symmetric fundamental peaks, respectively, and they can be described by the following expressions:

$$\tilde{\mathbf{E}}_{D1}(\omega_t, T, \omega_\tau) = 2[\boldsymbol{\mu}_{ge_1}\boldsymbol{\mu}_{e_1g}\boldsymbol{\mu}_{ge_1}\boldsymbol{\mu}_{e_1g}]\vdots\mathbf{e}_3\mathbf{e}_2\mathbf{e}_1^*\Gamma\left(\bar{\omega}_{e_1g}, <\delta\Omega_1^2>, \bar{\omega}_{e_1g}, <\delta\Omega_1^2>\right)$$

$$\tilde{\mathbf{E}}_{D2}(\omega_t, T, \omega_\tau) = 2[\boldsymbol{\mu}_{ge_2}\boldsymbol{\mu}_{e_2g}\boldsymbol{\mu}_{ge_2}\boldsymbol{\mu}_{e_2g}]\vdots\mathbf{e}_3\mathbf{e}_2\mathbf{e}_1^*\Gamma\left(\bar{\omega}_{e_2g}, <\delta\Omega_2^2>, \bar{\omega}_{e_2g}, <\delta\Omega_2^2>\right), \quad (12.14)$$

where e_1 and e_2 states are the vibrational excited states of the symmetric and asymmetric CO stretch normal modes, respectively. The negative peaks 3 and 3' in the off-diagonal region are excited-state absorptions from the symmetric and asymmetric mode excited states, e_1 and e_2, to their overtone states, respectively. They are associated with the following terms, respectively,

$$-[\boldsymbol{\mu}_{e_1f_1}\boldsymbol{\mu}_{f_1e_1}\boldsymbol{\mu}_{e_1g}\boldsymbol{\mu}_{ge_1}]\vdots\mathbf{e}_3\mathbf{e}_2\mathbf{e}_1^*\Gamma\left(\bar{\omega}_{f_1e_1}, <(\delta W_1 - \delta\Omega_1)^2>, \bar{\omega}_{e_1g}, <\delta\Omega_1^2>\right)$$

$$-[\boldsymbol{\mu}_{e_2f_3}\boldsymbol{\mu}_{f_3e_2}\boldsymbol{\mu}_{e_2g}\boldsymbol{\mu}_{ge_2}]\vdots\mathbf{e}_3\mathbf{e}_2\mathbf{e}_1^*\Gamma\left(\bar{\omega}_{f_3e_2}, <(\delta W_3 - \delta\Omega_2)^2>, \bar{\omega}_{e_2g}, <\delta\Omega_2^2>\right). \quad (12.15)$$

Due to the overtone frequency shifts, Δ_s and Δ_a, these two peaks appear in the off-diagonal region. The other two cross-peaks 2 and 2' are produced by coupling, and they are associated with the following expressions, respectively,

$$[\boldsymbol{\mu}_{ge_2}\boldsymbol{\mu}_{e_2g}\boldsymbol{\mu}_{e_1g}\boldsymbol{\mu}_{ge_1}]\vdots\mathbf{e}_3\mathbf{e}_2\mathbf{e}_1^*\Gamma\left(\bar{\omega}_{e_2g}, <\delta\Omega_2^2>, \bar{\omega}_{e_1g}, <\delta\Omega_1^2>\right)$$

$$[\boldsymbol{\mu}_{ge_1}\boldsymbol{\mu}_{e_1g}\boldsymbol{\mu}_{e_2g}\boldsymbol{\mu}_{ge_2}]\vdots\mathbf{e}_3\mathbf{e}_2\mathbf{e}_1^*\Gamma(\bar{\omega}_{e_1g}, <\delta\Omega_1^2>, \bar{\omega}_{e_2g}, <\delta\Omega_2^2>). \quad (12.16)$$

Again, due to the anharmonicity of the combination band, Δ_{as}, the conjugate cross-peaks 4 and 4' can be found in the 2D IR spectrum, and their contributions are described as, respectively,

$$-[\boldsymbol{\mu}_{e_1f_2}\boldsymbol{\mu}_{f_2e_1}\boldsymbol{\mu}_{e_1g}\boldsymbol{\mu}_{ge_1}]\vdots\mathbf{e}_3\mathbf{e}_2\mathbf{e}_1^*\Gamma\left(\bar{\omega}_{f_2e_1}, <(\delta W_2 - \delta\Omega_1)^2>, \bar{\omega}_{e_1g}, <\delta\Omega_1^2>\right) \text{ and}$$

$$-[\boldsymbol{\mu}_{e_2f_2}\boldsymbol{\mu}_{f_2e_2}\boldsymbol{\mu}_{e_2g}\boldsymbol{\mu}_{ge_2}]\vdots\mathbf{e}_3\mathbf{e}_2\mathbf{e}_1^*\Gamma\left(\bar{\omega}_{f_2e_2}, <(\delta W_2 - \delta\Omega_2)^2>, \bar{\omega}_{e_2g}, <\delta\Omega_2^2>\right). \quad (12.17)$$

Later, signatures of vibrational coherence transfer processes were investigated by using the time(T)-resolved 2D IR spectroscopy.[63] From the measured absolute value 2D IR rephasing spectra as a function of waiting time T, a few interesting peak amplitude changes were observed. The coherence transfer between the two fundamental vibrations can affect the amplitude of all the peaks. Time evolution of the symmetric and asymmetric superposition state (off-diagonal density matrix) appears as modulated cross- and diagonal-peak amplitudes in the rephasing and nonrephasing spectra, respectively, where the modulation frequency corresponds to the frequency splitting between the two fundamental modes, ~70 cm^{-1}. Population transfers between the two excited states lead to the growth of relaxation-induced cross-peaks. Finally, the slow population relaxation to the ground state induces simultaneous decays of all resonance peaks, and the timescale was estimated to be about 60 ps. Most of the salient features of 2D vibrational spectroscopy of a coupled oscillator system have thus been studied for this simple model system, RDC.

12.3 POLYPEPTIDE SECONDARY STRUCTURES

Proteins in nature contain varying extents of secondary structure polypeptide segments. Therefore, small polypeptide that adopts a specific secondary structure has been considered to be a valuable model system for studying vital factors influencing protein stability and folding. In order to establish the secondary structure–2D vibrational spectrum relationship, steady-state 2D IR spectroscopic studies of secondary structure proteins have been performed. In order to enhance frequency resolution and to study site-specific local backbone conformation in a given chain of polypeptide, isotope-labeling techniques have been extensively used, where $^{12}C{=}O$ in a given peptide bond is replaced with either $^{13}C{=}O$ or $^{13}C{=}^{18}O$. In this section, 2D vibrational spectroscopic investigations of the amide I vibrations of four representative model polypeptides, α-helix, β-sheet, β-hairpin, and 3_{10}-helix, will be briefly discussed.

Right-handed α-helix. Two-dimensional IR pump–probe spectroscopic study of amide I band of *Fs* helix in D_2O was carried out.[64] The *Fs* peptide is an alanine-based 21-residue system with three arginine residues, and it has been known to have a high propensity to form a right-handed α-helix. Its amide I absorption spectrum appears to be a broad and featureless single band with peak maximum at 1637 cm^{-1} at 4°C. Due to the overtone anharmonic frequency shift of amide I oscillators, the 2D IR pump–probe spectrum exhibits positive and negative peaks. Despite that there are some differences in the parallel- and perpendicular-polarization 2D IR pump–probe spectra, the 2D peak shape is featureless.[65] Nevertheless, it was possible to show that there is sizable inhomogeneity associated with conformational disorder. The time-resolved 2D measurements indicated that the conformational fluctuation is in a picosecond timescale. To gain more information on the underlying dynamics of the α-helix in water, MD simulations with employing the electrostatic potential calculation model discussed in Section 12.1 were carried out and conformational fluctuations, frequency-frequency correlations, and delocalization extents of amide I vibrational excited states were studied.[65] If the polypeptide forms a stable and structurally uniform α-helix, the average amide I local mode frequencies for all the peptide bonds are approximately constant.[65, 66] However, each individual amide I local mode frequency (ω_j) fluctuates in time due to the hydrogen-bonding and electrostatic interactions with surrounding water molecules. Despite that the coupling constants (J_{mn}) also fluctuate due to thermally driven conformational fluctuations, their fluctuation amplitudes, that is, standard deviations, are comparatively small, suggesting that the off-diagonal Hamiltonian matrix element (coupling constant) fluctuations and off-diagonal disorders can be ignored in this case of the amide I vibrations of polypeptides. Furthermore, the cross-correlations between any two amide I local mode frequencies ($<\delta\omega_m(t)\delta\omega_n(0)>$ for $m \neq n$) were also found to be negligible so that the independent bath approximation in Equation 8.23 was confirmed to be acceptable in that case.

To extract structural information from the measured 2D spectrum, the 2D IR technique was applied to site-specifically isotope-labeled α-helical polypeptides. Since the amide I vibrational frequency of ^{13}C=O-labeled peptide is red-shifted by about 30 to 40 cm^{-1} from that of normal amide I frequency, such an isotope-labeled amide I peak is separated from the main (unlabeled) amide I band. In order to separate the isotope-peak even farther from the main band, $^{13}C{=}^{18}O$ labeled amino acid was also used and incorporated into a chain of polypeptide or protein. In that case, the amide I frequency shift is as large as 65 cm^{-1}. Since the precise isotope-peak frequency and line shape are known to be sensitive to the local structure around the isotope-labeled residue, Fourier-Transform Infrared (FT-IR) study itself could provide useful information. However, a far more detailed picture was obtained from the 2D IR photon echo studies for a series of doubly isotope-labeled alanine-rich α-helices, Ac-$(A)_4K(A)_4K(A)_4K(A)_4K(A)_4$Y-$NH_2$.[67] Particularly, the 2D spectra of [0,11], [12,13], [11,13], and [11,14], where the notation for these compounds: [alanine residue with $^{13}C{=}^{16}O$, alanine residue with $^{13}C{=}^{18}O$], were measured. The two isotope-labeled peaks that are frequency resolved from each other as well as from the unlabeled amide I band were identified in the 2D IR spectra. The cross-peak between the $^{13}C{=}^{16}O$ and $^{13}C{=}^{18}O$ stretching modes showed that their amplitudes decrease in the following order: [12,13] > [11,14] > [11,13]. The off-diagonal anharmonicity values for [12,13], [11,14], and [11,13] were also estimated to be 0.9, 3.2, and 4.5 cm^{-1}, respectively. The observed trend in the cross-peak amplitudes is in agreement with the trend of coupling constants, that is, $|J_{n,n+1}|$ (6.5 cm^{-1}) > $|J_{n,n+3}|$ (−4.4 cm^{-1}) > $|J_{n,n+2}|$ (-3.4 cm^{-1}).[66] To shed light on the site-specific conformational inhomogeneity, a series of singly $^{13}C{=}^{18}O$-labeled 25-residue α-helical polypeptides was also studied by using the 2D IR spectroscopic method.[68] The labeling site is at residue numbers 11 to 14 in the middle of the helix. Elongation of the diagonal isotope-labeled peak was observed, indicating that there is sizable inhomogeneous contribution. Furthermore, amide I frequencies at the residues 11 and 14 have large inhomogeneous distributions in comparison to those at 12 and 13. This indicates modifications of the intra-helical hydrogen-bond network by the nearby lysine residues, which have positively charged side chains and are spatially close to the residues 11 and 14.

Antiparallel and parallel β-sheet polypeptides. Another well-known and widely studied protein second structure is extended β-sheet conformation, where multiple interstrand hydrogen-bonding interactions stabilize the β-sheet. Due to these strong H-bonds, the coupling constants between two amide I local modes of H-bonded peptides are fairly large, whereas those between two neighboring amide I modes in a given strand are comparatively small.[69–72] In addition, it was found that there are non-negligibly large coupling constants between peptides in neighboring strands. Thus, the amide I normal modes are delocalized over many strands along the chain of H-bonds. Furthermore, the corresponding frequencies of such delocalized amide I normal modes are dependent on the number of strands constituting the β-sheet and become red-shifted as the number of strands increases and reaches to a certain asymptotic value.[69]

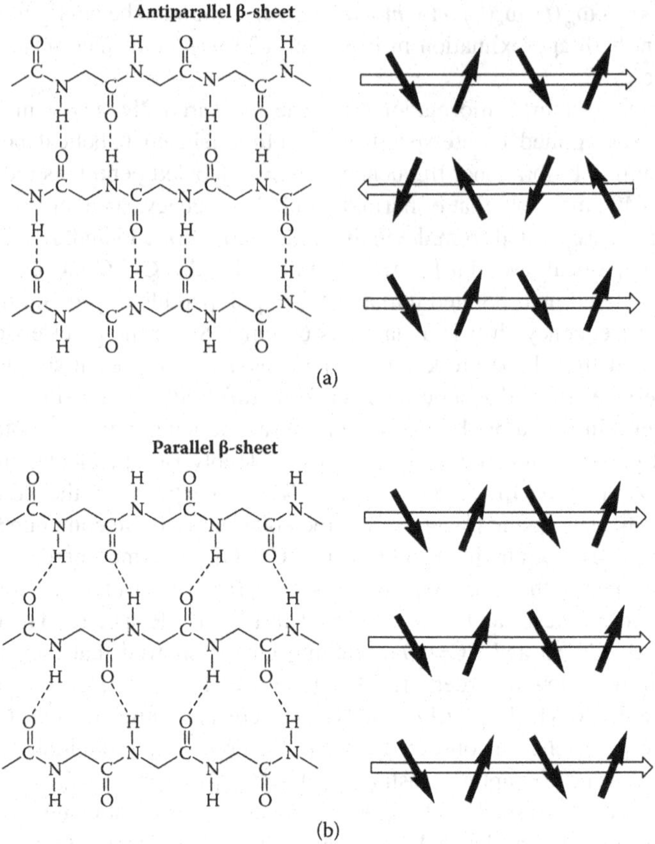

FIGURE 12.5 Antiparallel (a) and parallel (b) β-sheet structures. The corresponding amide I vibrational transition dipole vectors are also shown in this figure. In the case of the antiparallel β-sheet, the amide I local mode transition dipole vectors are aligned in a *zig-zag* fashion along the vertical H-bond chain, whereas those in the parallel β-sheet are all parallel to one another.

An ideal antiparallel β-sheet structure is shown in Figure 12.5. Also, the orientations of the transition dipole vectors (thick arrows) of amide *I local* modes are shown on the right-hand side of this figure. Note that individual amide I transition dipole vector is not parallel to the C=O bond but slightly tilted by 10 to 20 degrees from the C=O bond axis. Figure 12.5 also depicts the molecular structure of parallel β-sheet and the orientations of the corresponding transition dipole vectors of amide I local modes. Except for differences in small tilted orientations, the two β-sheet structures are quite similar in terms of primary spectroscopic properties (see Chapter 1 for a detailed discussion on the hierarchy of spectroscopic properties) such as the most strongly IR-active mode frequency and its dipole strength.[71] Consequently, the amide I IR spectra of these two β-sheet structures have been found to be very similar, but that of antiparallel β-sheet exhibits not only a strong amide I peak at ~1620 cm^{-1}

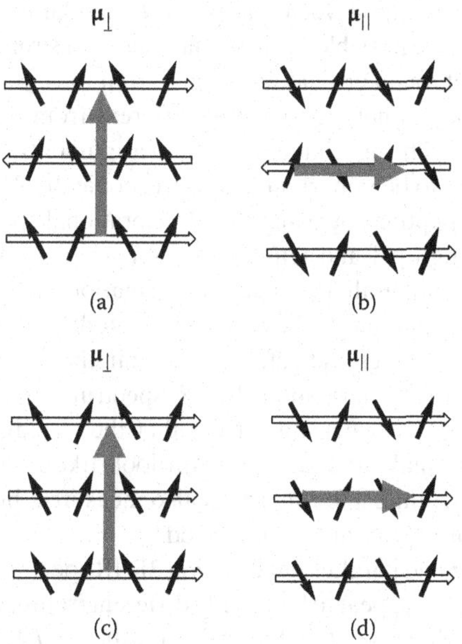

FIGURE 12.6 Transition dipole vectors (long gray arrows) of the two major amide I normal modes in antiparallel and parallel β-sheet polypeptides.

but also a weak peak at ~1680 cm^{-1}, which was considered to be a characteristic feature of antiparallel β-sheet polypeptide. These two amide I vibrations of antiparallel β-sheet polypeptide were denoted as $\omega_\perp$- and $\omega_{||}$-modes, respectively, since the corresponding normal mode transition dipole vectors $\boldsymbol{\mu}_\perp$ and $\boldsymbol{\mu}_{||}$ in an antiparallel β-sheet are perpendicular and parallel to the directions of the constituent strands, respectively. Note that the transition dipole of amide I *normal* mode is a linear combination of the transition dipoles of amide I *local* modes.

The $\boldsymbol{\mu}_\perp$ ($\boldsymbol{\mu}_{||}$) of the antiparallel β-sheet, which is shown as a large gray arrow in Figure 12.6a(b), is produced by the sum of properly weighted amide I local mode transition dipoles (short black arrows in the same figure). Here, the weighting factors are the eigenvector elements of $\omega_\perp$- and $\omega_{||}$-modes. In the case of the antiparallel β-sheet, the frequency of $\omega_\perp$-mode is lower than that of $\omega_{||}$-mode, that is, $\omega_{||} - \omega_\perp =$ ~50 cm^{-1}, and $|\boldsymbol{\mu}_\perp|$ is larger than $|\boldsymbol{\mu}_{||}|$ due to the tilting angle of 10–20 degrees mentioned above. In a real antiparallel β-sheet, however, in addition to these two major amide I normal modes, there are other amide I normal modes whose transition dipoles do not vanish, which in turn complicates the amide I IR spectrum. Nevertheless, it was found that the characteristic $\omega_\perp$- and $\omega_{||}$-modes are important and dominant in determining the line and peak shapes of the linear and 2D IR spectra. Considering only these two representative modes whose frequency difference is sizable, one can easily understand the general features observed in the 2D IR photon echo spectra of antiparallel β-sheet as will be discussed below.

Next, let us consider the amide I vibrations of parallel β-sheet polypeptides. Similar to the antiparallel β-sheet polypeptide, a strongly IR-active $\omega_\perp$-mode is present, and its transition dipole vector $\mu_{\perp}$ is perpendicular to the constituent strands (Figure 12.6c). It was also possible to show that there is a strongly IR-active $\omega_{\parallel}$-mode in this parallel β-sheet, but a critical difference from the antiparallel β-sheet is that the $\omega_{\parallel}$-mode frequency is not significantly different from the $\omega_{\perp}$-mode frequency for the parallel β-sheet. This is related to detailed alignments of amide I vibrations in this sheet and turns out to be important in spectroscopically distinguishing these two different β-sheet polypeptides by using the 2D vibrational spectroscopic method.

Poly-L-Lysine at high pH and temperature greater than 30°C has been known to form an extended antiparallel β-sheet conformation, and it was chosen for 2D IR spectroscopic investigation.[73] The $\omega_{\perp}$- and $\omega_{\parallel}$-mode frequencies were found to be 1611 and 1680 cm^{-1}, which indicates that the number of strands is significantly larger than 5. Its parallel-polarization 2D IR spectrum $\tilde{E}^{\parallel}_{PE}(\omega_t,\omega_\tau)$ was measured and exhibits a Z-shape 2D spectrum.[70] Note that the two diagonal peaks and two additional cross-peaks make the 2D spectrum look like Z. The perpendicular-polarization 2D IR spectrum, $\tilde{E}^{\perp}_{PE}(\omega_t,\omega_\tau)$, was also measured, but its 2D peak shape is quite similar to that of $\tilde{E}^{\parallel}_{PE}(\omega_t,\omega_\tau)$, as expected.

Although the linear and parallel-polarization 2D IR spectra of antiparallel and parallel β-sheet polypeptides appear to be slightly different from each other, the difference 2D IR spectroscopy, which is defined as $\Delta\tilde{E}_{PE}(\omega_t,\omega_\tau) = 3\tilde{E}^{\perp}_{PE}(\omega_t,\omega_\tau) - \tilde{E}^{\parallel}_{PE}(\omega_t,\omega_\tau)$, can provide incisive information for distinguishing the two. In Figure 12.7, the difference 2D IR spectra of model antiparallel and parallel β-sheets are plotted. Since the difference 2D IR spectroscopy is useful for selectively eliminating the diagonal peaks, all the spectral features in Figure 12.7 originate from cross-peaks. The cross-peaks in $\Delta\tilde{E}_{PE}(\omega_t,\omega_\tau)$ of antiparallel β-sheet are significantly larger than those of the cross-peaks near the diagonal line. On the other hand, the cross-peaks in $\Delta\tilde{E}_{PE}(\omega_t,\omega_\tau)$ of the model parallel β-sheet are much weaker than the cross-peak appearing near the diagonal line. The seemingly different $\Delta\tilde{E}_{PE}(\omega_t,\omega_\tau)$'s for the two β-sheets can be easily understood by using the results discussion presented in

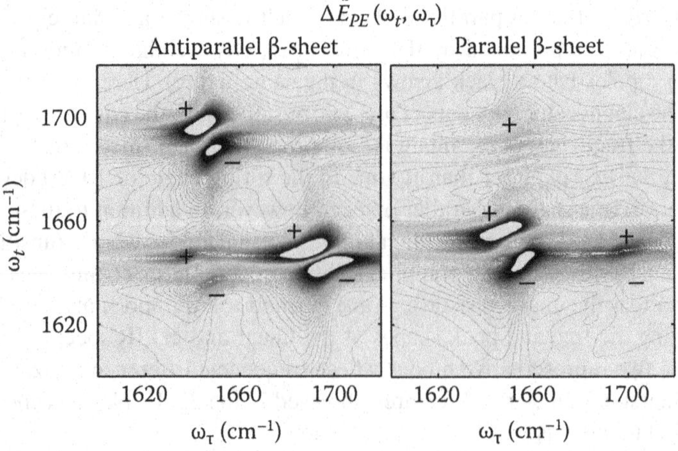

FIGURE 12.7 Difference 2D IR spectra of antiparallel and parallel β-sheet polypeptides.

Section 11.6. It was shown that the cross-peak amplitudes are determined by the corresponding two dipole strengths and the factor $\sin^2\theta_{ge_1,ge_2}$, where θ_{ge_1,ge_2} is the angle between the transition dipole vectors of the two modes.[71] That is to say, the cross-peak amplitude is approximately described as

$$\Delta\tilde{E}_{PE}(\omega_t=\omega_{\|},\omega_\tau=\omega_{\perp})=\Delta\tilde{E}_{PE}(\omega_t=\omega_{\perp},\omega_\tau=\omega_{\|})\propto|\mu_{\perp}|^2|\mu_{\|}|^2\sin^2\theta_{\perp,\|}. \quad (12.18)$$

In the case of the antiparallel β-sheet, the frequency-splitting amplitude between the $\omega_{\perp}$- and $\omega_{\|}$-modes is very large and $\sin^2\theta_{\perp,\|}\approx 1$. Therefore, there should be cross-peaks that are located far from the diagonal line even in the difference 2D IR spectrum. In contrast, the frequency splitting amplitude between the $\omega_{\perp}$- and $\omega_{\|}$-modes for the parallel β-sheet is small so that the corresponding cross-peaks appear very close to the diagonal line in the difference 2D IR spectrum. This explains why the cross-peak amplitudes in the difference 2D IR spectrum of the parallel β-sheet is comparatively weak. This simple example demonstrates that the 2D spectroscopic method, which has an additional capability of measuring the angle θ_{ge_1,ge_2} between two different vibrational transition dipole vectors, can be of critical use in spectroscopically distinguishing two different secondary structure proteins, even though it is not always easy to do so with linear spectroscopic techniques.

β-hairpin. β-hairpin secondary structure motif is critical for 3D structure formation of protein. Furthermore, spectroscopic studies of its thermodynamic stability and conformational fluctuation dynamics have been considered to be important and helpful in understanding protein folding and unfolding dynamics and mechanisms.[72, 74–80] In order to understand the effects of interstrand hydrogen-bonding interactions and couplings on the vibrationally excited amide I states of β-hairpins, quantum chemistry calculation and equilibrium MD simulation studies were carried out. It was shown that the 2D IR spectrum of β-hairpin is largely determined by the amide I normal modes that are delocalized on the peptides in the two antiparallel strands. Tryptophan zipper 2 (Trpzip2: SWTWENGKWTWK), which is a 12-residue peptide with a type I′ turn using the ENGK sequence, was studied by using the 2D IR method.[76] In particular, a series of 2D IR spectra were recorded for varying temperature to study the thermal denaturation process. From the temperature-dependent amide I IR spectra, its melting temperature was estimated to be about 60°C.[81] The amide I IR band of Trpzip2 is peaked at 1636 cm^{-1} and has a shoulder band at ~1676 cm^{-1}, and they can be assigned to the $\omega_{\perp}$- and $\omega_{\|}$-modes, similar to the case of antiparallel β-sheet with just two strands. From the three representative 2D IR spectra at temperatures 25, 63, and 82°C, it was found that the Z-shape pattern in the 2D IR spectrum persists throughout that temperature range. This indicates that the interstrand hydrogen bonding interactions in Trpzip2 remain, even at a high temperature of 82°C.

Later, to further study site-specific denaturation and residue-sensitive local solvation dynamics and structural changes, a 2D IR spectroscopic investigation of site-specifically isotope-labeled Trpzip2 peptides was carried out. The ^{13}C-isotope-labeled peptide was introduced in the terminal (Trp2) or turn (Gly7) region of the hairpin, and these two isotopomers were denoted as L2 and L7, respectively, whereas the unlabeled β-hairpin as UL.[77] Although the isotope peak in the L2 amide I IR spectrum appears as a shoulder band at ~1600 cm^{-1}, that in the L7 IR spectrum is frequency resolved from the main band and appears at ~1590 cm^{-1}. From the amide I IR spectra, it was possible to deduce the fact that the two peptides (Trp2 and Gly7) in the Trpzip2 have different dephasing environments or solvation structures. The observation that the lineshape of UL is quite similar to that of L7 in the frequency range from 1620 to 1700 cm^{-1} suggests that the amide I IR spectrum of β-hairpin is largely determined by the amide I normal modes delocalized on peptide groups in the two strands, and not by those on the turn region. Thus, the isotope-labeling at Trp2 significantly reduces the extent of delocalization of amide I normal modes. The 2D IR spectra of L2 and L7 showed cross-peaks between ^{13}C-labeled and unlabeled modes, which indicate couplings between the amide I local mode of labeled peptide and those of nearby unlabeled ones. Furthermore, the slope of nodal lines, $\sigma(T)$, separating the $v = 0 \leftrightarrow v = 1$ (stimulated emission and ground-state bleaching contributions) and $v = 1 \leftrightarrow v = 2$ (excited-state absorption) transitions were experimentally measured. It turned out that the amide I frequency of Trp2, a terminal residue, has larger inhomogeneity than that of Gly7, a turn-region residue. This is consistent with the picture that the terminal region of β-hairpin is structurally flexible in comparison to the turn region, which has been known as the end-fraying phenomenon.

3_{10}-helix. There have been some attentions on the 3_{10}-helix as one of the secondary structural motifs. With hydrogen bonds between the C=O oxygen of the *j*th amino acid and the N-H hydrogen atom of the (*j*+3)th amino acid, 3_{10}-helix has been known to play important roles in protein structures and functions.[82–87] A transmembrane channel-forming antibiotic contains a large portion of 3_{10}-helical conformation and also the 3_{10}-helical conformation was considered to be an intermediate structure in folding or melting of α-helix.[86, 88, 89] Although a number of spectroscopic investigations exist that identify 3_{10}-helix formation of synthetic model oligopeptides in nonaqueous solutions, a lack of sufficient time resolution of the previous techniques such as electronic and vibrational CD and 2D NMR prohibited discriminating α-helix and 3_{10}-helix at an early stage of the helix formation process. In this regard, the 2D IR spectroscopy was considered to be a useful tool for extracting unambiguous information on transient 3_{10}-helix formation.[90, 91] For three model octapeptides, that is, Z-[L-(αMe)Val]$_8$-O*t*Bu, Z-(Aib)$_8$-O*t*Bu, and Z-(Aib)$_5$-L-Leu-(Aib)$_2$-O*t*Bu, (Z, benzyloxycarbonyl; (αMe)Val, C$^{\alpha}$-methyl valine; Aib, α-aminoisobutyric acid; O*t*Bu, *tert*-butoxy) in organic solvents, 2D IR experiments were performed. Although the amide I IR spectra of these model octapeptides appear as a broad featureless singlet, the [π/4, −π/4, π/2, 0] 2D IR spectrum of 3_{10}-helix (three octapeptides in $CDCl_3$) shows a doublet peak above and below the diagonal line. The readers may find it useful to see Section 11.7 for this polarization-controlled experimental geometry. Particularly, the 2D IR amide I cross-peak pattern was found to be highly sensitive to the difference between 3_{10}- and α-helical structures because these two conformations have quite different vibrational coupling constants.[13] When the octapeptide Z-[L-(αMe)Val]$_8$-O*t*Bu is dissolved in 1,1,1,3,3,3-hexafluoro-2-propanol, the 2D IR spectrum changes in timescale of days. The cross-peak pattern-changes in time and sensitively reflect the 3_{10}-to-α-helix conformational transition process. These experiments demonstrate that the 2D IR spectroscopic technique can be used to study transient structural changes in the helix-coil or coil-helix conformational transition.

12.4 GLOBULAR PROTEINS AND MEMBRANE-BOUND PROTEINS

By focusing on the amide I vibrations in proteins, 2D IR experiments for concanavalin A, ribonuclease A, lysozyme, and myoglobin were performed.[70] A notable difference among the four proteins is the relative fraction of β-sheet structure. The first three proteins contain 46, 32, and 6 percent antiparallel β-sheet and 0, 18, and 31 percent α-helix. Among them, only the concanavalin A has two almost-flat six-stranded antiparallel β-sheets so that its 2D IR correlation spectrum is qualitatively similar to that of poly-L-Lysine, which has been known to form extended antiparallel β-sheet structure. As the extent of β-sheets decreases from concanavalin A to lysozyme, the characteristic Z-form 2D peak shape disappears with concomitant frequency blue-shift of the main peak from 1635 to 1650 cm^{-1}. Furthermore, the 2D peak shape becomes more symmetric in frequency domain as the β-sheet content decreases. The frequency splitting between the $\omega_{\perp}$-mode frequency and the $\omega_{\parallel}$-mode frequency is related to the extent of delocalization of the two characteristic amide I normal modes of β-sheet or to the number of strands involved in the formation of the antiparallel β-sheet. This was confirmed by comparing the 2D spectra of concanavalin A and ribonuclease A. Such experimental results show that the 2D IR spectra of amide I bands of proteins offer a sensitive measure of underlying β-sheet content and detailed structural variables.

Although 2D NMR spectroscopy and X-ray crystallography have proven to be extremely useful to determine protein structures in an atomic resolution, they cannot be easily used to study membrane-bound proteins. In this regard, the 2D IR spectroscopic method should be an alternative tool that is capable of providing structural and dynamic information on the membrane-bound proteins. For CD3ζ peptide segment from residue 31 to 51, where the CD3ζ(31–51) peptide is the transmembrane domain of the *T*-cell receptor, 2D IR spectroscopic studies were carried out.[92–94] Particularly, eleven different isotopomers of CD3ζ, where each peptide at different sites was labeled with $^{13}C{=}^{18}O$, were considered for linear IR and 2D IR studies. The CD3ζ peptide is known to form a tetrameric bundle in the membrane, and the helices are kinked at residue 39-Leu.[95, 96] Therefore, such site-specifically isotope-labeled CD3ζ isotopomers are interesting systems for detailed understanding of site-dependent inhomogeneity of amide I frequencies and vibrational dynamics along the transmembrane peptide backbone. Using the 2D IR spectroscopic techniques with notably enhanced frequency resolution, it was possible to measure the amide I bandwidths and frequencies of the isotope-labeled peaks for those isotopomers.[92] Average frequency is highest in the middle and lowest at the two ends, even though the distribution of amide I local mode frequency along the helix is not symmetric. The experimental 2D IR diagonal line width for the amide I band of inner residues is 25 percent narrower than that of the residue near the water-membrane interfaces. This is consistent with the expectation that the vibrational dynamics of residues in the middle is likely to be different from those near the membrane surface, due to the water solvation dynamics and conformational inhomogeneity of peptide backbone segments near the interfaces. Nevertheless, these two variables, line width and frequency of isotope-labeled peak, do not monotonically change as the distance of the isotope-labeled residue from the surface increases. Note that an isotope labeling does not induce any peptide structure change, unlike electron spin resonance labels or fluorophores introduced in the middle of protein sequence. Thus, the vibrational dynamics of individual amide I modes were successfully probed with 2D IR spectroscopy combined with the isotope-labeling technique.

Another interesting 2D IR experiment was performed for 27-residue human erythrocyte protein Glycophorin A (GpA: KKITLIIFG$_{79}$VMAGVIGTILLISWG$_{94}$IKK), which is a transmembrane helix dimer.[97] Specifically labeling $^{13}C=^{16}O$ or $^{13}C=^{18}O$ to G$_{79}$ and G$_{94}$ in a given GpA sequence, one could generate various combinations of isotope-labeled GpA dimers, that is, homodimers and heterodimers. The isotope-labeled amide I band of the homodimer system with $^{13}C=^{18}O$-labeled at Gly$_{79}$ was found to be asymmetric and consists of two underlying bands with a frequency difference of 8.6 cm^{-1}. This is direct and clear evidence of coupling between the two amide I modes localized on the two Gly$_{79}$ peptides. The cross-peaks between the $^{13}C=^{18}O$-labeled G$_{79}$ in one of the two monomers and the $^{13}C=^{16}O$-labeled G$_{79}$ in the other were observed, whereas there appears no cross-peaks between $^{13}C=^{16}O$-labeled G$_{94}$ in one monomer and $^{13}C=^{18}O$-labeled G$_{79}$ in the other. These observations indicate coupling and spatial proximity between G$_{79}$ peptide groups in the two monomers. In addition, from the polarization-controlled experiments, the angle θ between the transition dipoles of the $^{13}C=^{18}O$-labeled G$_{79}$ amide I local mode in one monomer and that of the $^{13}C=^{16}O$-labeled G$_{79}$ in the other was estimated to be 110°. This could be translated into the helix crossing angle, and it is 45°, which is consistent with NMR results for the same helix dimer.

12.5 NUCLEIC ACIDS

A collection of IR spectra of nucleic acids in solution was presented in a review article, where linear vibrational spectroscopy was shown to be a powerful tool for investigating structural fluctuations and transitions, hydrogen bonding interactions, and global structures of nucleic acid bases, base pairs, and various nucleic acids.[98] Effects of hydrogen bond-induced base pairing, base stacking, coordination of metal ions, and solvation on nucleic acid structure were studied by examining marker band frequency shifts in the IR spectra. In order to understand the natures of delocalized normal modes and vibrational properties of base pairs and DNA oligomers, a series of theoretical investigations were performed.[99–102]

In addition to the linear vibrational spectroscopic investigations, heterodyne-detected 2D IR photon echo technique was used to elucidate the strengths of vibrational couplings and the nature of delocalized normal modes in DNA double helix in heavy water, particularly for a dG$_5$C$_5$ duplex.[103, 104] In addition to four diagonal peaks in the frequency range from 1580 to 1720 cm^{-1}, a number of cross-peaks were observed in the measured parallel-polarization echo spectrum. Among the strongly IR-active modes in that frequency range, guanine and cytosine C=O stretching vibrations mainly contribute to the 2D IR spectrum. From the fits to the linear and 2D IR spectra, the interstrand coupling between the guanine and cytosine C=O stretching modes was estimated to be −7.4 cm^{-1}. Also, the intrastrand couplings between cytosine C=O stretching modes and between guanine C=O stretching modes are 2.3 and 9.7 cm^{-1}, and interstrand coupling between guanine C=O stretching mode at the *j*th base pair and cytosine C=O stretching mode at the (j+1)th base pair is –5.0 cm^{-1}. Anharmonicities of guanine and cytosine C=O stretching modes were found to be 14 and 9 cm^{-1}, respectively.

To elucidate the nature of vibrationally delocalized modes in various DNA double helices, extensive quantum chemistry calculation studies of nucleic acid bases, base pairs, and base pair stacks in H_2O and D_2O were performed.[99–102] Once basis modes and coupling constants are identified and calculated for each base, it becomes possible to quantitatively describe vibrationally delocalized excited states by using the LCBM-Exciton (Linear Combination of Basis Modes-Exciton) theory for coupled multi-anharmonic-oscillator systems discussed in Chapter 8.

Although a few limited experimental studies have been reported, in principle one can apply the 2D IR technique to study polymorphic natures of DNA double helices. DNA structure has been known to depend on a number of different factors such as base composition, water content, pH, counter ions, and so forth. Three representative antiparallel double-stranded helical geometries of DNA are the right-handed A- and B-forms and the left-handed Z-form, and their structures are different from one another by interlayer distance, twist angle between two neighboring base pairs, and other geometric parameters. Motivated by the success of simulating 1D and 2D IR spectrum of the B-form DNA, extensive quantum chemistry calculations to obtain coupling constants, basis mode frequencies, and the associated transition dipoles for A- and Z-form DNA double helices were performed to numerically simulate the corresponding 2D IR spectra of $X(GC)_n$ and $X(AT)_n$ (for X=A, B, or Z). Here, the number of constituent base pairs is denoted as n. Detailed aspects characterizing these three different DNA conformations were discussed and would be of use in further elucidating the natures of delocalized vibrationally excited states in such complicated molecular systems as well as in studying conformational transitions between different polymorphic DNA structures in the time domain.

12.6 HYDROGEN-BONDING DYNAMICS AND CHEMICAL EXCHANGE

Solvents play a critical role in chemistry and biology by actively participating in solvation and energy dissipation and alter thermodynamic and kinetic properties of reactions significantly.[105] Among many different solute-solvent interactions, hydrogen bonding is one of the most crucial ones.[106] Thus, the timescales of H-bond forming and breaking processes are keenly related to thermal equilibrium and dynamics of reactive systems in solvents capable of forming H-bonds.[26] The lifetime of a given H-bond depends on its strength, and typically it is about picoseconds at room temperature. Due to this ultrafast nature of H-bond making and breaking processes, only those femtosecond nonlinear optical spectroscopies can offer a means of probing rapid dynamics and chemical evolutions along H-bond reaction coordinates. This is a good example of chemical exchange processes in condensed phases so that the 2D IR spectroscopy can be a useful tool to directly probe dynamic aspects of hydrogen bond and other weak noncovalent bond such as van der Waals interaction.

NMA-methanol solution (Chemical exchange 1). Time-resolved 2D IR pump–probe spectroscopy of hydrogen-bond chemical exchange dynamics of NMA (N-methylacetamide) in methanol solution was investigated and showed that the two-species model works well in this case (see Chapter 10).[107] Here, the two species are NMA with a single H-bonded MeOD molecule and that with two H-bonded MeOD molecules at the NMA's carbonyl oxygen atom.[108, 109] These two species are denoted as NM_1 and NM_2, respectively. In Figure 12.8, the equilibrium reaction between the two species is shown, that is,

$$NM_1 \underset{k_b}{\overset{k_f}{\rightleftharpoons}} NM_2. \tag{12.19}$$

The H-bond formation and dissociation rate constants are denoted as k_f and k_b, respectively. It should be noted that the amide I frequency of NM_1 is about 20 cm^{-1} larger than that of NM_2, because the latter has two H-bonds at the carbonyl group.[17, 107, 108] Note that a single H-bonding interaction between the amide C=O group and H-bond donor (e.g., water, MeOH) can induce a red-shift of the amide I frequency by about 20 cm^{-1}. Consequently, the amide I IR spectrum of NMA in MeOD is a doublet, and the low- and high-frequency peaks correspond to the amide I transitions of NM_2 and NM_1 species, respectively. Thus, this system is a good example of the chemical exchange processes of anharmonic oscillators, which were discussed in detail in Section 10.3.

Later, detailed heterodyne-detected 2D IR photon echo study for the same composite system with improved time-resolution was performed (see Figure 12.8).[17] At time zero, the 2D IR spectrum exhibits two diagonal peaks, where the upper positive peaks are from the sum of stimulated emission and ground-state bleaching contributions from the two species, and the lower negative peaks are from the excited-state absorption contributions. The two diagonal peaks are diagonally elongated, indicating the presence of short time inhomogeneous solvent environment around the NMA. As the waiting time T increases up to 5 ps, the slopes of the nodal lines decrease to zero, which suggests that the local solvent configuration looks like a homogeneous medium in a timescale longer than 5 ps. However, the more important observation is that the cross-peak amplitudes in the upper-left and lower-right regions increase in time T. This is clear evidence of chemical exchange processes between the two species. Since the amide I vibration is a relatively weak anharmonic oscillator, the corresponding schematic picture directly related to this experiment is Figure 10.4. Consequently, one can immediately find that the cross-peak amplitude rising patterns can provide quantitative information on the conditional probabilities discussed in Section 10.3 and in turn on the H-bond formation and dissociation rate constants. Furthermore, carrying out the same experiments for varying temperature, one can directly measure the reaction enthalpies and entropies associated with the H-bond making and breaking processes.

Acetonitrile-methanol solution (Chemical exchange 2). Another chemical exchange system studied experimentally was CH_3CN in methanol.[110] Again, the CN nitrogen atom can form a single H-bond with CH_3OH molecule. The FT-IR absorption spectrum of the CN stretch in CH_3CN/CH_3OH solution was found to be a doublet at a low temperature, −17°C, with the frequency splitting of 8 cm^{-1}. This indicates

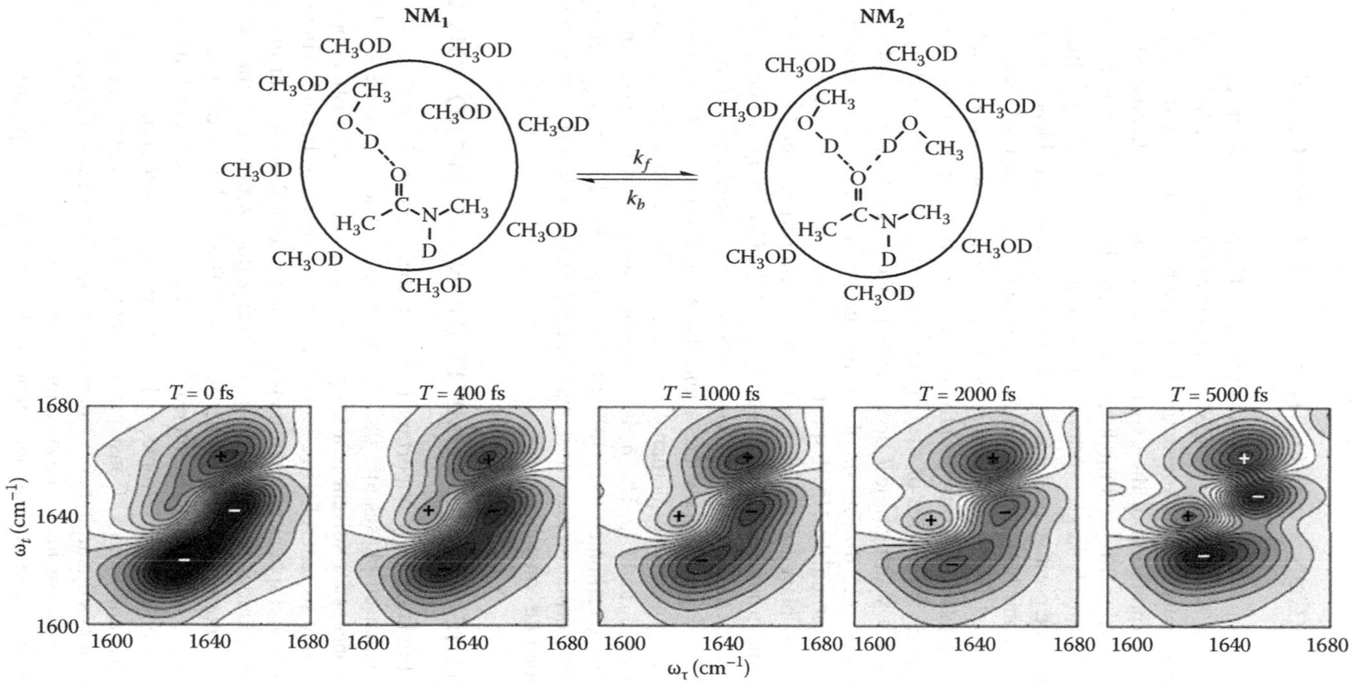

FIGURE 12.8 Two different solvation structures of *N*-methylacetamide in MeOD. These two species are in thermal equilibrium, and the forward and backward reactions are H-bond forming and breaking processes, respectively. The time-resolved 2D IR photon echo spectra are shown in the bottom panel. The waiting time *T* varies from 0 to 5 ps. (From DeCamp, M. F. et al., *Journal of Physical Chemistry B*, 2005, 109, 11016. With permission.)

that there are two different CH_3CN molecules having either zero or one H-bonded CH_3OH molecule around the CN group.

$$H_3C'C\text{æ}N\cdots\cdots H'OCH_3 \underset{k_b}{\overset{k_f}{\rightleftharpoons}} H_3C'C\text{æ}N + CH_3OH$$

Thus, this system is very similar to the NMA/CH_3OH solution, except that the amide I vibration is replaced with CN stretching vibration. Nevertheless, the chemical exchange effects on the experimentally measured 2D IR spectra are quite similar, and the interpretation of the experimental data with the theoretical procedure discussed in Section 10.3 is straightforward. Here, it should be noted that the CN vibration has relatively large overtone anharmonic frequency shift, which is about 19 cm^{-1}. Thus, the positive peaks associated with ground-state bleaching and stimulated emission contributions representing transitions between $v = 0$ and $v = 1$ states are well separated from the negative peaks associated with excited-state absorption from $v = 1$ to $v = 2$. Consequently, this molecular system is a good example of chemical exchange processes of strongly anharmonic oscillators (see Figure 10.3 in Section 10.3). The waiting time T-dependent changes of cross-peak amplitudes were successfully interpreted in terms of conditional probabilities. An interesting point in this case is that, unlike NMR spectroscopy, since the $v = 0 \rightarrow v = 1$ transitions are separately displayed from the $v = 1 \rightarrow v = 2$ transitions, the hydrogen-bonding dynamics of the ground and first excited states of the CN group can be studied separately. The chemical exchange rate constants for the ground-state molecular system were denoted as k_{AB} and k_{BA}, where A and B are the two different species with one and zero hydrogen-bonded methanol, respectively. Those for the first excited state are denoted as k^*_{AB} and k^*_{BA}. The hydrogen-bond dissociation rate constants k_{AB} and k^*_{AB} at 22°C were estimated to be 1.07×10^{10} s^{-1} and 1.27×10^{11} s^{-1}, respectively. The hydrogen-bond formation rate constants could be estimated by using these quantities and relaxation rate constants.

12.7 SOLUTE–SOLVENT COMPLEXATION AND MICRO-SOLVATION

One of the fundamentally important issues in chemistry is the nature of organic solutes in condensed phases and the role of solvents. The homogeneous dielectric continuum concept for solvent is a simple, but quite often unrealistic, approach to the description of solvent roles in chemical reaction dynamics. In simple liquids, due to the isotropic and spherically symmetric properties of intermolecular interactions, the radial distribution function can provide detailed information on the local solvation structure, thermodynamic properties, and diffusive dynamics around a solute molecule. Unlike simple liquids, intermolecular interactions between typical organic solutes and solvents are anisotropic, and their strengths can be comparable to or even larger than thermal energy. Consequently, solute–solvent complexes can exist for finite times, and its dynamic behaviors are without a doubt important in understanding chemical reactions involving such molecules.

In this regard, experimental and theoretical 2D vibrational spectroscopic studies on phenol/benzene/CCl_4 solution showed how such phenomena can be investigated and what quantitative information can be extracted from experimental data.[111–113]

Here, the phenol molecule is the solute, and the solvent is a mixture of benzene and CCl_4. It was known that the phenol can form a complex with a benzene molecule via dispersive interaction, quadrupole–dipole interaction, and so forth. To create equally populated phenol-benzene complex and free phenol in solution, a mixed solvent, benzene+CCl_4, was deliberately used. Here the free phenol represents the case when phenol is in a solvation state without forming van der Waals complex with benzene molecules. The corresponding chemical equilibrium is given by

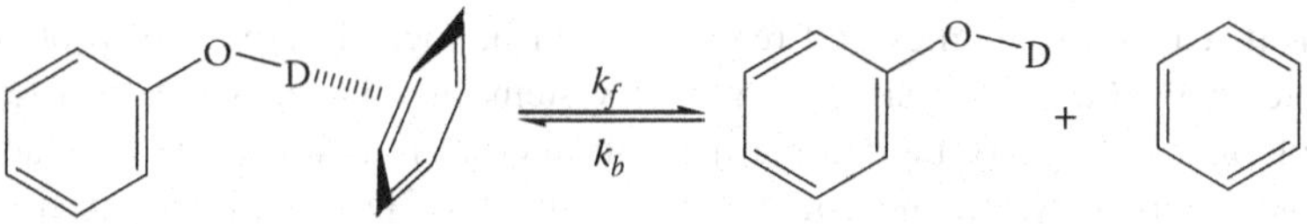

Here, the anharmonic oscillator under spectroscopic investigation is the O-D stretching mode. The IR spectrum of O–D stretch of phenol-D in the mixed solvent is again a doublet, and the low- and high-frequency peaks at 2631 and 2665 cm^{-1} correspond to the O–D vibrational transitions of the phenol-benzene complex form and the free phenol form, respectively. From a number of quantum chemistry calculations using Hartree-Fock, density functional theory, and Møller-Plesset methods, the most stable complex was found to be the T-form structure shown above.[112] Furthermore, the electron correlation effects on the intermolecular interaction are very important so that the Hartree-Fock or density functional theory cannot provide quantitatively reliable potential energy surface in this case.

Again, this molecular system is a good example for chemical exchange of strongly anharmonic oscillator because the overtone anharmonic frequency shift is as large as 91 cm^{-1}. The two species are in equilibrium state so that the time-dependent 2D IR spectra would reveal the underlying chemical exchange processes through the cross-peak amplitude changes. The integrated volumes of the two diagonal and two cross-peaks were estimated as functions of the waiting time T, and such experimental data were successfully used to determine the complex formation and dissociation rate constants. The experimentally measured complex dissociation time was found to be 8 ps. To numerically simulate the 1D and 2D IR spectra, the vibrational Stark effect theory was used to obtain the OD frequency trajectory from MD simulation results. In addition, the transition dipole of the OD stretch were also found to be strongly dependent on the electric field along the OD bond, indicating that the non-Condon effect should not be ignored. The comparisons between theory and experiment were found to be excellent. However, the more important conclusion drawn from the comparative investigation was that the 2D IR spectroscopy of such a complex system can provide detailed information on a local solvation environment and micro-solvation domain formation.[112] Direct evidence on the heterogeneity of solvation environment around a phenol was obtained by examining configurations from the MD trajectories A plausible picture on the dynamic process revealed by this 2D spectroscopy is that the phenol solute undergoes random jumps from one micro-solvation domain to the other, which are reflected by the OD stretch frequency changes. By counting the numbers of benzene and CCl_4 molecules in the vicinity of a phenol, it was found that the local number fraction of benzene molecules is quite different from the mole fraction of bulk benzene/CCl_4 mixed solvent. This suggests that the mixed solvent forms microscopic domains on the molecular level. Furthermore, it was shown that the OD stretch FFCF is directly related to the correlation function of a fluctuating number of benzene molecules in the immediate vicinity of the solute phenol.[112]

12.8 INTERNAL ROTATION

Rotational isomerization around a chemical bond is an important process in the chemical reaction dynamics and reactivity and biological activity of proteins and biomolecules. One of the simplest model systems is ethane, which is a textbook example molecule on isomerization through internal rotation. However, due to the rotational symmetry, ethane could not be used for 2D vibrational spectroscopic investigation. Instead, a 1,2-disubstituted ethane derivative, 1-fluoro-2-isocyanato-ethane (FICE) was chosen for 2D IR spectroscopic study of its rotational isomerization reaction in solution.[114]

Since the FICE contains two different substituents, there are four different conformational isomers. FT-IR spectrum of isocyanate (-NCO) group in FICE/CCl_4 solution shows two peaks at 2265 and 2280 cm^{-1} that correspond to the NCO stretching vibrations of gauche and trans conformers. These two conformers are in equilibrium due to internal rotations as

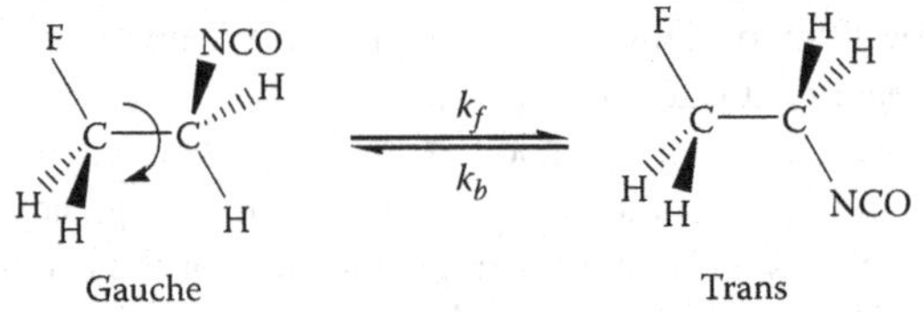

Time-resolved 2D IR spectra were directly used to estimate the internal rotation time constants. Note that this problem is also a chemical exchange process. The integrated volumes of diagonal and cross-peaks were used to extract kinetic constants, and the isomerization time constant was found to be 43 ps. Then, by carrying out density function theory calculations of the barrier heights of FICE, *n*-butane, and ethane, it was even possible to approximately estimate the isomerization time constants of *n*-butane and ethane under the same conditions, which are about 40 and 12 ps, respectively.

12.9 TRANSIENT TWO-DIMENSIONAL IR SPECTROSCOPY: PROTEIN FOLDING AND UNFOLDING

Protein folding, a conformational change of protein as it folds from an ensemble of disordered denatured structures into a compact native structure, has been an important experimental and theoretical research subject. Protein folding or unfolding experiments use a variety of spectroscopic means aimed at measuring kinetics such as rate constants of increasing or decreasing spectroscopic signatures directly reflecting protein's structural changes. From the beginning of the new development of 2D vibrational spectroscopic technique, protein folding study with this novel method has been considered to be one of the most important applications. However, a number of complicating issues such as (1) sensitivity (small signal-to-noise ratio) problems, (2) lack of proper model systems, (3) difficulty of selecting representative marker bands, and so forth made experimental studies quite difficult in reality. Two examples are discussed below.

Ubiquitin unfolding dynamics. Temperature-jump induced by an intense nanosecond pulse with wavelength of 2 μm, which excites OD stretch overtone of the D_2O buffer solution, can trigger protein unfolding processes when the system is initially prepared at a temperature near their melting points. Time-dependent dispersive vibrational echo spectra of ubiquitin protein on nanosecond to millisecond timescales were recorded to elucidate the associated unfolding mechanism.[115] Here, the dispersive vibrational echo spectroscopy is a technically simpler nonlinear IR experiment than the 2D IR photon echo spectroscopy, and its spectrum is identical to the projected 2D IR spectrum onto one frequency axis.[116, 117]

From the temperature-dependent dispersive vibrational echo spectra, the thermal melting temperature of ubiquitin in D_2O was estimated to be about 61°C. The melting curve based on the singular value decomposition analysis of the temperature-dependent dispersive vibrational echo spectra was nicely fitted with a sigmoidal curve, suggesting a simple two-state unfolding kinetics. As the temperature was raised, a concerted blue-shift of the strongly IR-active amide I mode of which transition dipole is perpendicular to the β-sheet strands was observed. In addition, the cross-peak ridges were shrunken, indicating unfolding of β-sheet structure in ubiquitin. To follow the temperature-jump-induced unfolding process, an initial temperature of 58°C was chosen, and the temperature increment induced by the nanosecond 2 μm pulse was about 12°C. The dispersive vibrational echo spectra after temperature-jump were recorded from 20 ns up to 9 ms, and the relative intensity changes at 1621, 1658, and 1677 cm^{-1} were measured to extract information on the unfolding mechanism. Note that a different frequency region of dispersive vibrational echo spectrum represents different types of amide I vibrations that are critically dependent on protein structure. It was found that there are two stages on the course of unfolding, which are separated by timescale. The short-time (tens of microseconds) nonexponential component was attributed to increased configurational flexibility and partial disruptions of antiparallel β-sheet and β-hairpin structures. Nevertheless, it was conjectured that for such a short time the global structure of ubiquitin is still rather close to the nativelike one. The long-time (millisecond) component was then interpreted as a concerted unfolding, exhibiting two-state kinetics.

Transient 2D IR spectroscopy of model β-turn peptide. In order to probe structural changes of proteins, it is necessary to introduce external perturbation to place the system onto a new nonequilibrium state virtually instantaneously in comparison to the timescale of the folding or unfolding process. One of the most popular techniques is the temperature-jump method discussed above. Another popular triggering method is to use a photochemical reaction. In this regard, a disulfide bond has been known as a good UV-vis photo-cleavable site with dissociation energy of about 65 kcal/mol.

By introducing a disulfide bond into a short model peptide (see the molecular structure below), a cyclic disulfide-bridged peptide containing three peptide bonds and two ester groups was synthesized.

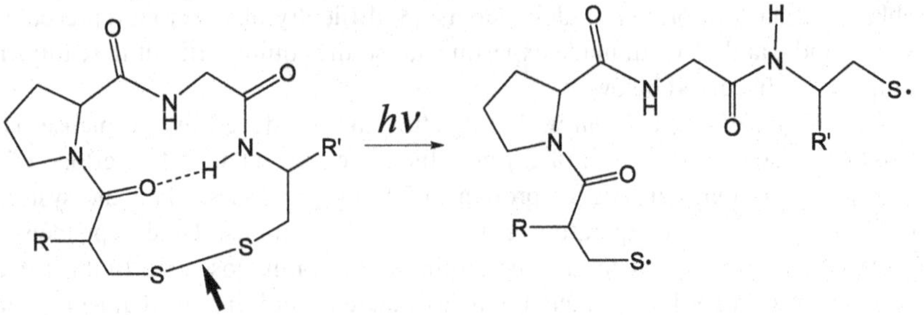

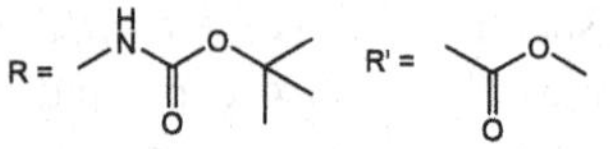

An intense UV-vis pulse can break the disulfide bond to generate linear peptide in a nonequilibrium state. Its subsequent structural change in CD_3CN solution was monitored by using 2D IR spectroscopic technique.[118] Note that the model cyclic peptide studied has a single intramolecular hydrogen bond since the tetrapeptide structure mimics a β-turn motif. Due to this hydrogen-bonding interaction, the amide I local modes of the hydrogen-bond donor and acceptor peptide groups are coupled, which produces corresponding cross-peaks in an equilibrium 2D IR spectrum. After ultrafast photo-cleavage of the disulfide bond, the model peptide unfolds and the hydrogen bond breaks. To obtain the difference 2D IR spectra as a function of the waiting time *T*, two sets of 2D IR spectra had to be recorded simultaneously, one with the ultraviolet pulse switched on, and one with the ultraviolet pulse switched off. Among various peaks reflecting structural changes of the peptide, only the intensity change of the transient cross-peak, which is the characteristic one reporting the hydrogen-bond breaking, was monitored in time *T*. From the MD simulation of the same system, it was found that the hydrogen-bond breaking induces a concomitant opening of the β-turn on a timescale of 160 ps. This experiment is a good example demonstrating the ability of transient 2D IR spectroscopy to directly probe ultrafast changes of local contacts between small groups in biomolecules.

REFERENCES

1. Hamm, P.; Lim, M. H.; Hochstrasser, R. M., Structure of the amide I band of peptides measured by femtosecond nonlinear infrared spectroscopy. *Journal of Physical Chemistry B* 1998, 102, 6123–6138.
2. Park, K.; Cho, M., Time- and frequency-resolved coherent two-dimensional IR spectroscopy: Its complementary relationship with the coherent two-dimensional Raman scattering spectroscopy. *Journal of Chemical Physics* 1998, 109, 10559–10569.
3. Tanimura, Y.; Mukamel, S., Two-dimensional femtosecond vibrational spectroscopy of liquids. *Journal of Chemical Physics* 1993, 99, 9496–9511.
4. Cho, M., Two-dimensional vibrational spectroscopy. In *Advances in multi-photon processes and spectroscopy*, Lin, S. H., Villaeys, A. A., Fujimura, Y., Ed. World Scientific Pulblishing Co.: Singapore, 1999; Vol. 12, pp 229–300.

5. Mukamel, S., Multidimensional femtosecond correlation spectroscopies of electronic and vibrational excitations. *Annual Review of Physical Chemistry* 2000, 51, 691–729.
6. Cho, M., Coherent two-dimensional optical spectroscopy. *Chemical Reviews* 2008, 108, 1331–1418.
7. Khalil, M.; Demirdoven, N.; Tokmakoff, A., Coherent 2D IR spectroscopy: Molecular structure and dynamics in solution. *Journal of Physical Chemistry A.* 2003, 107, 5258–5279.
8. Woutersen, S.; Hamm, P., Nonlinear two-dimensional vibrational spectroscopy of peptides. *Journal of Physics-Condensed Matter* 2002, 14, R1035–R1062.
9. Krimm, S.; Bandekar, J., Vibrational spectroscopy and conformation of peptides, polypeptides, and proteins. *Advances in Protein Chemistry* 1986, 38, 181.
10. Torii, H., Tasumi, M., Theoretical analyses of the amide I infrared bonds of globular proteins. In *Infrared spectroscopy of biomolecules*. Mantsch, H. H., Chapman, D. ed.; Wiley-Liss: New York, 1996; p 1.
11. Torii, H.; Tasumi, M., Model-calculations on the amide-I infrared bands of globular-proteins. *Journal of Chemical Physics* 1992, 96, 3379–3387.
12. Choi, J. H.; Ham, S.; Cho, M., Inter-peptide interaction and delocalization of amide I vibrational excitons in myoglobin and flavodoxin. *Journal of Chemical Physics* 2002, 117, 6821–6832.
13. Choi, J.-H.; Ham, S.; Cho, M., Local amide I mode frequencies and coupling constants in polypeptides. *Journal of Physical Chemistry B* 2003, 107, 9132–9138.
14. Choi, J.-H.; Lee, H.; Lee, K.-K.; Hahn, S.; Cho, M., Computational spectroscopy of ubiquitin: Comparison between theory and experiments. *Journal of Chemical Physics* 2007, 126, 045102.
15. Woutersen, S.; Pfister, R.; Hamm, P.; Mu, Y. G.; Kosov, D. S.; Stock, G., Peptide conformational heterogeneity revealed from nonlinear vibrational spectroscopy and molecular-dynamics simulations. *Journal of Chemical Physics* 2002, 117, 6833–6840.
16. Zanni, M. T.; Asplund, M. C.; Hochstrasser, R. M., Two-dimensional heterodyned and stimulated infrared photon echoes of N-methylacetamide-D. *Journal of Chemical Physics* 2001, 114, 4579.
17. DeCamp, M. F.; DeFlores, L.; McCracken, J. M.; Tokmakoff, A.; Kwac, K.; Cho, M., Amide I vibrational dynamics of N-methylacetamide in polar solvents: The role of electrostatic interactions. *Journal of Physical Chemistry B* 2005, 109, 11016–11026.
18. Kwac, K.; Cho, M., Molecular dynamics simulation study of N-methylacetamide in water. I. Amide I mode frequency fluctuation. *Journal of Chemical Physics* 2003, 119, 2247–2255.
19. Kwac, K.; Cho, M., Molecular dynamics simulation study of N-methylacetamide in water. II. Two-dimensional infrared pump–probe spectra. *Journal of Chemical Physics* 2003, 119, 2256–2263.
20. Schmidt, J. R.; Corcelli, S. A.; Skinner, J. L., Ultrafast vibrational spectroscopy of water and aqueous N-methylacetamide: Comparison of different electronic structure/molecular dynamics approaches. *Journal of Chemical Physics* 2004, 121, 8887.
21. Mikenda, W., Stretching frequency versus bond distance correlation of O-D(H)...Y (Y = N, O, S, Se, Cl, Br, I) hydrogen bonds in solid hydrates. *Journal of Molecular Structure* 1986, 147, 1–15.
22. Scheurer, C.; Piryatinski, A.; Mukamel, S., Signatures of β-peptide unfolding in two-dimensional vibrational echo spectroscopy: A simulation study. *Journal of the American Chemical Society* 2001, 123, 3114.
23. Ham, S.; Kim, J. H.; Lee, H.; Cho, M., Correlation between electronic and molecular structure distortions and vibrational properties. II. Amide I modes of NMA-nD_2O complexes. *Journal of Chemical Physics* 2003, 118, 3491–3498.

24. Bour, P.; Keiderling, T. A., Empirical modeling of the peptide amide I band IR intensity in water solution. *Journal of Chemical Physics* 2003, 119, 11253–11262.
25. Kwac, K.; Cho, M., Two-color pump–probe spectroscopies of two- and three-level systems: 2-dimensional line shapes and solvation dynamics. *Journal of Physical Chemistry A* 2003, 107, 5903–5912.
26. Nibbering, E. T. J.; Elsaesser, T., Ultrafast vibrational dynamics of hydrogen bonds in the condensed phase. *Chemical Reviews* 2004, 104, 1887–1914.
27. Bratos, S.; Gale, G. M.; Gallot, G.; Hache, F.; Lascoux, N.; Leicknam, J. C., Motion of hydrogen bonds in diluted HDO/D_2O solutions: Direct probing with 150 fs resolution. *Physical Review E* 2000, 61, 5211.
28. Gallot, G.; Lascoux, N.; Gale, G. M.; Leicknam, J. C.; Bratos, S.; Pommeret, S., Non-monotonic decay of transient infrared absorption in dilute HDO/D_2O solutions. *Chemical Physics Letters* 2001, 341, 535–539.
29. Laenen, R.; Rauscher, C.; Laubereau, A., Dynamics of local substructures in water observed by ultrafast infrared hole burning. *Physical Review Letters* 1998, 80, 2622–2625.
30. Laenen, R.; Rausch, C.; Laubereau, A., Local substructures of water studied by transient hole-burning spectroscopy in the infrared: Dynamics and temperature dependence. *Journal of Physical Chemistry B.* 1998, 102, 9304–9311.
31. Gaffney, K.; Piletic, I.; Fayer, M. D., Hydrogen bond breaking and reformation in alcohol oligomers following vibrational relaxation of a non-hydrogen bond donating hydroxyl stretch. *Journal of Physical Chemistry A* 2002, 106, 9428–9435.
32. Gaffney, K. J.; Davis, P. H.; Piletic, I. R.; Levinger, N. E.; Fayer, M. D., Hydrogen bond dissociation and reformation in methanol oligomers following hydroxyl stretch relaxation. *Journal of Physical Chemistry A* 2002, 106, 12012–12023.
33. Gaffney, K. J.; Piletic, I. R.; Fayer, M. D., Orientational relaxation and vibrational excitation transfer in methanol–carbon tetrachloride solutions. *Journal of Chemical Physics* 2003, 118, 2270–2278.
34. Asbury, J. B.; Steinel, T.; Stromberg, C.; Gaffney, K. J.; Piletic, I. R.; Goun, A.; Fayer, M. D., Hydrogen bond dynamics probed with ultrafast infrared heterodyne-detected multidimensional vibrational stimulated echoes. *Physical Review Letters* 2003, 91, 237402.
35. Asbury, J. B.; Steinel, T.; Stromberg, C.; Gaffney, K. J.; Piletic, I. R.; Goun, A.; Fayer, M. D., Ultrafast heterodyne detected infrared multidimensional vibrational stimulated echo studies of hydrogen bond dynamics. *Chemical Physics Letters* 2003, 374, 362–371.
36. Kropman, M. F.; Nienhuys, H.-K.; Woutersen, S.; Bakker, H. J., Vibrational relaxation and hydrogen-bond dynamics of HDO:H_2O. *Journal of Physical Chemistry A* 2001, 105, 4622–4626.
37. Woutersen, S.; Bakker, H. J., Resonant intermolecular transfer of vibrational energy in liquid water. *Nature* 1999, 402, 507–509.
38. Woutersen, S.; Emmerichs, U.; Bakker, H. J., Femtosecond mid-IR pump–probe spectroscopy of liquid water: Evidence for a two-component structure. *Science* 1997, 278, 658.
39. Asbury, J. B.; Steinel, T.; Kwak, K.; Corcelli, S. A.; Lawrence, C. P.; Skinner, J. L.; Fayer, M. D., Dynamics of water probed with vibrational echo correlation spectroscopy. *Journal of Chemical Physics* 2004, 121, 12431–12446.
40. Steinel, T.; Asbury, J. B.; Corcelli, S. A.; Lawrence, C. P.; Skinner, J. L.; Fayer, M. D., Water dynamics: Dependence on local structure probed with vibrational echo correlation spectroscopy. *Chemical Physics Letters* 2004, 386, 295–300.
41. Asbury, J. B.; Steinel, T.; Stromberg, C.; Corcelli, S. A.; Lawrence, C. P.; Skinner, J. L.; Fayer, M. D., Water dynamics: Vibrational echo correlation spectroscopy and

comparison to molecular dynamics simulations. *Journal of Physical Chemistry A* 2004, 108, 1107–1119.
42. Eaves, J. D.; Loparo, J. J.; Fecko, C. J.; Roberts, S. T.; Tokmakoff, A.; Geissler, P. L., Hydrogen bonds in liquid water are broken only fleetingly. *Proceedings of the National Academy of Sciences of the USA*. 2005, 102, 13019–13022.
43. Eaves, J. D.; Tokmakoff, A.; Geissler, P. L., Electric field fluctuations drive vibrational dephasing in water. *Journal of Physical Chemistry A*. 2005, 109, 9424–9436.
44. Fecko, C. J.; Eaves, J. D.; Loparo, J. J.; Tokmakoff, A.; Geissler, P. L., Ultrafast hydrogen-bond dynamics in the infrared spectroscopy of water. *Science* 2003, 301, 1698–1702.
45. Loparo, J. J.; Roberts, S. T.; Tokmakoff, A., Multidimensional infrared spectroscopy of water. I. Vibrational dynamics in two-dimensional IR line shapes. *Journal of Chemical Physics* 2006, 125, 194521.
46. Loparo, J. J.; Roberts, S. T.; Tokmakoff, A., Multidimensional infrared spectroscopy of water. II. Hydrogen bond switching dynamics. *Journal of Chemical Physics* 2006, 125, 194522.
47. Hayashi, T.; Jansen, T. L.; Zhuang, W.; Mukamel, S., Collective solvent coordinates for the infrared spectrum of HOD in D_2O based on an ab initio electrostatic map. *Journal of Physical Chemistry A* 2005, 109, (1), 64–82.
48. Lawrence, C. P.; Skinner, J. L., Vibrational spectroscopy of HOD in liquid D_2O. II. Infrared line shapes and vibrational Stokes shift. *Journal of Chemical Physics* 2002, 117, 8847–8854.
49. Cha, S. Y.; Ham, S. H.; Cho, M., Amide I vibrational modes in glycine dipeptide analog: Ab initio calculation studies. *Journal of Chemical Physics* 2002, 117, 740–750.
50. Torii, H.; Tasumi, M., Ab initio molecular orbital study of the amide I vibrational interactions between the peptide groups in di- and tripeptides and considerations on the conformation of the extended helix. *Journal of Raman Spectroscopy* 1998, 29, 81–86.
51. Ham, S.; Cha, S.; Choi, J.-H.; Cho, M., Amide I modes of tripeptides: Hessian matrix reconstruction and isotope effects. *Journal of Chemical Physics* 2003, 119, 1451–1461.
52. Choi, J.-H.; Cho, M., Amide I vibrational circular dichroism of dipeptide: Conformation dependence and fragment analysis. *Journal of Chemical Physics* 2004, 120, 4383–4392.
53. Rubtsov, I. V.; Hochstrasser, R. M., Vibrational dynamics, mode coupling, and structural constraints for acetylproline-NH_2. *Journal of Physical Chemistry B* 2002, 106, 9165–9171.
54. Zanni, M. T.; Gnanakaran, S.; Stenger, J.; Hochstrasser, R. M., Heterodyned two-dimensional infrared spectroscopy of solvent-dependent conformations of acetylproline-NH_2. *Journal of Physical Chemistry B* 2001, 105, 6520–6535.
55. Ge, N. H.; Hochstrasser, R. M., Femtosecond two-dimensional infrared spectroscopy: IR-COSY and THIRSTY. *Phys. Chem. Comm.* 2002, 17–26.
56. Sul, S.; Karaiskaj, D.; Jiang, Y.; Ge, N. H., Conformations of N-acetyl-L-prolinamide by two-dimensional infrared spectroscopy. *Journal of Physical Chemistry B* 2006, 110, 19891–19905.
57. Lee, K.-K.; Hahn, S.; Oh, K.-I.; Choi, J. S.; Joo, C.; Lee, H.; Han, H. Y.; Cho, M., Structure of N-acetylproline amide in liquid water: Experimentally measured and numerically simulated infrared and vibrational circular dichroism spectra. *Journal of Physical Chemistry B* 2006, 110, 18834–18843.
58. Hahn, S.; Lee, H.; Cho, M., Theoretical calculations of infrared absorption, vibrational circular dichroism, and two-dimensional vibrational spectra of acetylproline in liquids water and chloroform. *Journal of Chemical Physics* 2004, 121, 1849–1865.

59. Woutersen, S.; Hamm, P., Structure determination of trialanine in water using polarization sensitive two-dimensional vibrational spectroscopy. *Journal of Physical Chemistry B* 2000, 104, 11316–11320.
60. Woutersen, S.; Hamm, P., Isotope-edited two-dimensional vibrational spectroscopy of trialanine in aqueous solution. *Journal of Chemical Physics* 2001, 114, 2727–2737.
61. Kim, Y. S.; Hochstrasser, R. M., Dynamics of amide I modes of the alanine dipeptide in D_2O. *Journal of Physical Chemistry B* 2005, 109, (14), 6884–6891.
62. Kim, Y. S.; Wang, J. P.; Hochstrasser, R. M., Two-dimensional infrared spectroscopy of the alanine dipeptide in aqueous solution. *Journal of Physical Chemistry B* 2005, 109, 7511–7521.
63. Khalil, M.; Demirdoven, N.; Tokmakoff, A., Vibrational coherence transfer characterized with Fourier-transform 2D IR spectroscopy. *Journal of Chemical Physics* 2004, 121, 362–373.
64. Woutersen, S.; Hamm, P., Time-resolved two-dimensional vibrational spectroscopy of a short α-helix in water. *Journal of Chemical Physics* 2001, 115, 7737–7743.
65. Ham, S.; Hahn, S.; Lee, C.; Kim, T. K.; Kwak, K.; Cho, M., Amide I modes of alpha-helical polypeptide in liquid water: Conformational fluctuation, phase correlation, and linear and nonlinear vibrational spectra. *Journal of Physical Chemistry B* 2004, 108, 9333–9345.
66. Choi, J. H.; Hahn, S.; Cho, M., Amide IIR, VCD, and 2D IR spectra of isotope-labeled α-helix in liquid water: Numerical simulation studies. *International Journal of Quantum Chemistry* 2005, 104, 616–634.
67. Fang, C.; Wang, J.; Kim, Y. S.; Charnley, A. K.; Barber-Armstrong, W.; Smith, A. B., III; Decatur, S. M.; Hochstrasser, R. M., Two-dimensional infrared spectroscopy of isotopomers of an alanine rich α-helix. *Journal of Physical Chemistry B* 2004, 108, 10415–10427.
68. Fang, C.; Hochstrasser, R. M., Two-dimensional infrared spectra of the C^{13}=O^{18} isotopomers of alanine residues in an α-helix. *Journal of Physical Chemistry B* 2005, 109, 18652–18663.
69. Lee, C.; Cho, M., Local amide I mode frequencies and coupling constants in multiple-stranded antiparallel β-sheet polypeptides. *Journal of Physical Chemistry B* 2004, 108, 20397–20407.
70. Cheatum, C. M.; Tokmakoff, A.; Knoester, J., Signatures of β-sheet secondary structures in linear and two-dimensional infrared spectroscopy. *Journal of Chemical Physics* 2004, 120, 8201–8215.
71. Hahn, S.; Kim, S.-S.; Lee, C.; Cho, M., Characteristic two-dimensional IR spectroscopic features of antiparallel and parallel β-sheet polypeptides: Simulation studies. *Journal of Chemical Physics* 2005, 123, 084905.
72. Smith, A. W.; Cheatum, C. M.; Chung, H. S.; Demirdoven, N.; Khalil, M.; Knoester, J.; Tokmakoff, A., Two-dimensional infrared spectroscopy of β-sheet and hairpins. *Biophysical Journal* 2004, 86, 619A.
73. Demirdoven, N.; Cheatum, C. M.; Chung, H. S.; Khalil, M.; Knoester, J.; Tokmakoff, A., Two-dimensional infrared spectroscopy of antiparallel β-sheet secondary structure. *Journal of the American Chemical Society* 2004, 126, 7981–7990.
74. Silva, R. A. G. D.; Sherman, S. A.; Keiderling, T. A., β-hairpin stabilization in a 28-residue peptide derived from the β-subunit sequence of human chorionic gonadotropin hormone. *Biopolymers* 1999, 50, 413–423.
75. Zhao, C.; Polavarapu, P. L.; Das, C.; Balaram, P., Vibrational circular dichroism-hairpin peptides. *Journal of the American Chemical Society* 2000, 122, 8228–8231.
76. Smith, A. W.; Chung, H. S.; Ganim, Z.; Tokmakoff, A., Residual native structure in a thermally denatured β-hairpin. *Journal of Physical Chemistry B* 2005, 109, 17025–17027.

77. Wang, J.; Chen, J.; Hochstrasser, R. M., Local structure of β-hairpin isotopomers by FTIR, 2D IR, and ab initio theory. *Journal of Physical Chemistry B* 2006, 110, 7545–7555.
78. Xu, Y.; Oyola, R.; Gai, F., Infrared study of the stability and folding kinetics of a 15-residue β-hairpin. *Journal of the American Chemical Society* 2003, 125, 15388–15394.
79. Xu, Y.; Wang, T.; Gai, F., Strange temperature dependence of the folding rate of a 16-residue β-hairpin. *Chemical Physics* 2006, 323, 21–27.
80. Searle, M. S.; Platt, G. W.; Bofill, R.; Simpson, S. A.; Ciani, B., Incremental contribution to protein stability from a beta hairpin "finger": Limits on the stability of designed beta hairpin peptides. *Angewandte Chemie-International Edition* 2004, 43, 1991–1994.
81. Wang, T.; Xu, Y.; Du, D. G.; Gai, F., Determining β-sheet stability by Fourier transform infrared difference spectra. *Biopolymers* 2004, 75, 163–172.
82. Toniolo, C.; Benedetti, E., The polypeptide-3(10)-helix. *Trends in Biochemical Sciences* 1991, 16, 350–353.
83. Bolin, K. A.; Millhauser, G. L., alpha and 3(10): The split personality of polypeptide helices. *Accounts of Chemical Research* 1999, 32, 1027–1033.
84. Millhauser, G. L.; Stenland, C. J.; Hanson, P.; Bolin, K. A.; vandeVen, F. J. M., Estimating the relative populations of 3(10)-helix and alpha-helix in Ala-rich peptides: A hydrogen exchange and high field NMR study. *Journal of Molecular Biology* 1997, 267, 963–974.
85. De Guzman, R. N.; Wu, Z. R.; Stalling, C. C.; Pappalardo, L.; Borer, P. N.; Summers, M. F., Structure of the HIV-1 nucleocapsid protein bound to the SL3 {Ψ}-RNA recognition element. *Science* 1998, 279, 384–388.
86. Shea, J. E.; Brooks, C. L., From folding theories to folding proteins: A review and assessment of simulation studies of protein folding and unfolding. *Annual Review of Physical Chemistry* 2001, 52, 499–535.
87. Hahn, S.; Ham, S.; Cho, M., Simulation studies of amide I IR absorption and two-dimensional IR spectra of beta hairpins in liquid water. *Journal of Physical Chemistry B* 2005, 109, 11789–11801.
88. Nagaraj, R.; Balaram, P., Alamethicin, a transmembrane channel. *Accounts of Chemical Research* 1981, 14, 356–362.
89. Gnanakaran, S.; Hochstrasser, R. M.; Garcia, A. E., Nature of structural inhomogeneities on folding a helix and their influence on spectral measurements. *Proceedings of the National Academy of Sciences of the USA* 2004, 101, 9229–9234.
90. Maekawa, H.; Toniolo, C.; Moretto, A.; Broxterman, Q. B.; Ge, N.-H., Different spectral signatures of octapeptide 3(10) and alpha-helices revealed by two-dimensional infrared spectroscopy. *Journal of Physical Chemistry B* 2006, 110, 5834–5837.
91. Maekawa, H.; Toniolo, C.; Broxterman, Q. B.; Ge, N. H., Two-dimensional infrared spectral signatures of 3(10)- and alpha-helical peptides. *Journal of Physical Chemistry B* 2007, 111, 3222–3235.
92. Mukherjee, P.; Krummel, A. T.; Fulmer, E. C.; Kass, I.; Arkin, I. T.; Zanni, M. T., Site-specific vibrational dynamics of the CD3 ζ membrane peptide using heterodyned two-dimensional infrared photon echo spectroscopy. *Journal of Chemical Physics* 2004, 120, (21), 10215–10224.
93. Mukherjee, P.; Kass, I.; Arkin, I. T.; Zanni, M. T., Structural disorder of the CD3 ζ transmembrane domain studied with 2D IR spectroscopy and molecular dynamics simulations. *Journal of Physical Chemistry B* 2006, 110, 24740–24749.
94. Mukherjee, P.; Kass, I.; Arkin, I. T.; Zanni, M. T., Picosecond dynamics of a membrane protein revealed by 2D IR. *Proceedings of the National Academy of Sciences of the USA* 2006, 103, 3528–3533.

95. Torres, J.; Briggs, J. A. G.; Arkin, I. T., Multiple site-specific infrared dichroism of CD3 ζ, a transmembrane helix bundle. *Journal of Molecular Biology* 2002, 316, 365–374.
96. Torres, J.; Briggs, J. A. G.; Arkin, I. T., Convergence of experimental, computational and evolutionary approaches predicts the presence of a tetrameric form for CD3 ζ. *Journal of Molecular Biology* 2002, 316, 375–384.
97. Fang, C.; Senes, A.; Cristian, L.; DeGrado, W. F.; Hochstrasser, R. M., Amide vibrations are delocalized across the hydrophobic interface of a transmembrane helix dimer. *Proceedings of the National Academy of Sciences of the USA* 2006, 103, 16740–16745.
98. Liquier, J., Taillandier, E., Infrared spectroscopy of nucleic acids. In *Infrared spectroscopy of biomolecules*. Mantsch, H. H., Chapman, D. ed.; Wiley-Liss: New York, 1996; p 131.
99. Lee, C.; Park, K. H.; Cho, M., Vibrational dynamics of DNA. I. Vibrational basis modes and couplings. *Journal of Chemical Physics* 2006, 125, (11), 114508.
100. Lee, C.; Cho, M., Vibrational dynamics of DNA. II. Deuterium exchange effects and simulated IR absorption spectra. *Journal of Chemical Physics* 2006, 125, 114509.
101. Lee, C.; Park, K. H.; Kim, J. A.; Hahn, S.; Cho, M., Vibrational dynamics of DNA. III. Molecular dynamics simulations of DNA in water and theoretical calculations of the two-dimensional vibrational spectra. *Journal of Chemical Physics* 2006, 125, 114510.
102. Lee, C.; Cho, M. H., Vibrational dynamics of DNA : IV. Vibrational spectroscopic characteristics of A-, B-, and Z-form DNA's. *Journal of Chemical Physics* 2007, 126, 145102.
103. Krummel, A. T.; Mukherjee, P.; Zanni, M. T., Inter and intrastrand vibrational coupling in DNA studied with heterodyned 2D-IR spectroscopy. *Journal of Physical Chemistry B* 2003, 107, 9165–9169.
104. Krummel, A. T.; Zanni, M. T., DNA vibrational coupling revealed with two-dimensional infrared spectroscopy: Insight into why vibrational spectroscopy is sensitive to DNA structure. *Journal of Physical Chemistry B* 2006, 110, 13991–14000.
105. Reichardt, C., *Solvents and solvent effects in organic chemistry*. Wiley-VCH: Weinheim, 2003.
106. Vinogradov, S. N., Linnell, R. H., *Hydrogen bonding*. Van Nostrand Reinhold: New York, 1971.
107. Woutersen, S.; Mu, Y.; Stock, G.; Hamm, P., Hydrogen-bond lifetime measured by time-resolved 2D-IR spectroscopy: N-methylacetamide in methanol. *Chemical Physics* 2001, 266, 137–147.
108. Kwac, K.; Lee, H.; Cho, M., Non-Gaussian statistics of amide I mode frequency fluctuation of N-methylacetamide in methanol solution: Linear and nonlinear vibrational spectra. *Journal of Chemical Physics* 2004, 120, 1477.
109. Kwac, K.; Cho, M., Hydrogen bonding dynamics and two-dimensional vibrational spectroscopy: N-methylacetamide in liquid methanol. *Journal of Raman Spectroscopy* 2005, 36, 326.
110. Kim, Y. S.; Hochstrasser, R. M., Chemical exchange 2D IR of hydrogen-bond making and breaking. *Proceedings of the National Academy of Sciences of the USA* 2005, 102, 11185–11190.
111. Zheng, J.; Kwak, K.; Asbury, J. B.; Chen, X.; Piletic, I.; Fayer, M. D., Ultrafast dynamics of solute-solvent complexation observed at thermal equilibrium in real time. *Science* 2005, 309, 1338–1343.
112. Kwac, K.; Lee, C.; Jung, Y.; Han, J.; Kwak, K.; Zheng, J. R.; Fayer, M. D.; Cho, M., Phenol-benzene complexation dynamics: Quantum chemistry calculation, molecular dynamics simulations, and two dimensional IR spectroscopy. *Journal of Chemical Physics* 2006, 125, 244508.

113. Zheng, J.; Kwak, K.; Fayer, M. D., Ultrafast 2D IR vibrational echo spectroscopy. *Accounts of Chemical Research* 2007, 40, 75–83.
114. Zheng, J., Kwak, K., Xie, J., Fayer, M. D., Ultrafast carbon-carbon single-bond rotational isomerization in room-temperature solution. *Science* 2006, 313, 1951–1955.
115. Chung, H. S.; Khalil, M.; Smith, A. W.; Ganim, Z.; Tokmakoff, A., Conformational changes during the nanosecond-to-millisecond unfolding of ubiquitin. *Proceedings of the National Academy of Sciences of the USA* 2005, 102, 612.617.
116. Chung, H. S.; Khalil, M.; Tokmakoff, A., Nonlinear infrared spectroscopy of protein conformational change during thermal unfolding. *Journal of Physical Chemistry B* 2004, 108, 15332–15342.
117. Chung, H. S.; Khalil, M.; Tokmakoff, A., Protein denaturing studied with 2D IR and vibrational echo spectroscopy: Equilibrium and temperature-jump measurements. *Biophysical Journal* 2004, 86, 526A.
118. Kolano, C.; Helbing, J.; Kozinski, M.; Sander, W.; Hamm, P., Watching hydrogen-bond dynamics in a β-turn by transient two-dimensional infrared spectroscopy. *Nature* 2006, 444, 469–472.

13 Applications of Two-Dimensional Electronic Spectroscopy

As molecular systems of interest become increasingly complicated, such as photosynthetic complexes, molecular aggregates of quantum dots, or nanoparticles, and so forth, conventional optical spectroscopic methods such as time- or frequency-resolved absorption or spontaneous emission spectroscopy can provide only limited information on the secondary spectroscopic properties such as electronic couplings between chromophores, 3D structures, and excitation and coherence transfers between chromophores or quantum states. For those electronically coupled multi-chromophore systems, the 2D *electronic* spectroscopy based on heterodyne-detected photon echo technique has been found to be of use for extracting far more detailed information from two-dimensionally displayed spectra recorded with respect to the waiting time *T*.[1–4] In the case of electronic systems, except that each electronic chromophore can be approximately modeled as a 2LS in contrast to an effectively three-level anharmonic oscillator, one can use the same theoretical method developed for the amide I vibrations of proteins to numerically calculate the 2D electronic spectra of coupled multi-electronic-chromophore systems.

Electronic photon echo spectroscopy has been extensively used to study ultrafast solvation dynamics and inhomogeneous distribution of electronic transition frequency of chromophore in condensed phase. Furthermore, a fifth-order electronic spectroscopy was theoretically proposed to address the question "Can we separate homogeneous and inhomogeneous contributions to optical spectra?" and shown to be of use in elucidating underlying dynamic inhomogeneity of solute transition frequency in detail.[5] Instead of a simple 2LS, a variety of coupled multi-chromophore complexes, such as photosynthetic protein, semiconductors, DNA, and so on can be studied by using the 2D electronic spectroscopy. Particularly interesting processes would be exciton formation and annihilation, exciton coherence transfer, population relaxation, electron transfer, and the like. These chemical or physical changes of photo-excited states affect diagonal and cross-peak amplitudes and frequencies in time *T*, which reveal detailed spatial correlation and wavefunction overlaps between excitonic states. A few critical examples will be discussed in this chapter.

13.1 APPLICATION TO FENNA–MATTHEWS–OLSON LIGHT-HARVESTING COMPLEX

Photosynthetic light-harvesting complexes containing a few to hundreds of chromophores, such as chlorophylls or bacteriochlorophylls and carotenoids, are important systems that have been investigated by using the heterodyne-detected 2D photon echo method.[1, 2, 6, 7] Electronic interactions between constituent chromophores and chromophore-solvent dynamics play important roles in light absorption of solar radiation, directional excitation transfers from antennae complexes to the reaction center, and dramatic enhancement of trapping efficiency of solar energy.[8] Unfortunately, linear spectroscopy cannot provide sufficiently detailed information to determine the corresponding electronic Hamiltonian, where the diagonal Hamiltonian matrix elements represent site energies of constituent chromophores and the off-diagonal elements are electronic coupling constants. Various models for light-harvesting complexes have been developed, but their validities have been tested by comparing theoretical calculation and simulation results with a few different linear spectra such as absorption, linear dichroism, circular dichroism, and so forth. Despite some successes of such attempts, due to the limited information, contents extractable from linear spectra, exciton dynamics and couplings could not be described in a quantitative manner. In this regard, 2D electronic spectroscopy was shown to be highly useful to extract incisive information on the spatial relationship of the excitonic states. Furthermore, excitation transfer processes within the complex or between two neighboring light-harvesting complexes in real time can be efficiently studied by using this technique.

The first 2D electronic spectroscopy experiment and theory for a coupled multi-chromophore system was reported in 2005, where the Fenna–Matthews–Olson (FMO) pigment protein complex from green sulfur bacterium *Chlorobium tepidum* was considered for the experimental study.[1] The FMO complex is an energy transfer bridge connecting a large peripheral light-harvesting antenna, the chromosome, to the reaction center. Although the FMO complex consists of three protein subunits, the entire photophysics is fully determined by a single unit, and there are seven bacteriochlorophylls (BChl) in it.

Since these seven BChl's are electronically coupled to one another, the corresponding seven one-exciton states ($e_1 - e_7$) are delocalized over a few BChl's.[6] In addition, there are spatially delocalized 21 two-exciton states ($f_1 - f_{21}$). Thus, even without including population or coherence transfer processes, there are quite a number of pathways (polarization diagrams) that contribute to the 2D echo signal.[6, 9] Those third-order photon echo polarizations will produce different signal electric fields with varying phases and temporal amplitudes. The measured signal field is thus a consequence of complicated wave interferences between the signal electric fields. Furthermore, due to the population and coherence transfers in the manifold of seven one-exciton states, the diagonal and cross-peak amplitudes and shapes change in time T.

On the left column of Figure 13.1, the experimentally measured 2D spectra at waiting times 100, 200, 300, 600, and 1,000 fs are shown. Seven vertical and horizontal lines in each spectrum correspond to the one-exciton state energies. At $T = 100$ fs, there are positive diagonal peaks, but due to the spectral congestion the seven diagonal peaks are not fully frequency resolved. However, the lowest diagonal peak associated with $g \leftrightarrow e_1$ transitions is separated from the other diagonal peaks in frequency, and it is produced by the stimulated emission and ground-state bleaching terms:

$$<\boldsymbol{\mu}\xLeftarrow[g\wr \quad e_1\wr]{e_1\wr}|g><g|>, \quad <\boldsymbol{\mu}\xLeftarrow[g\wr e_1\wr]{e_1\wr}|g><g|>. \tag{13.1}$$

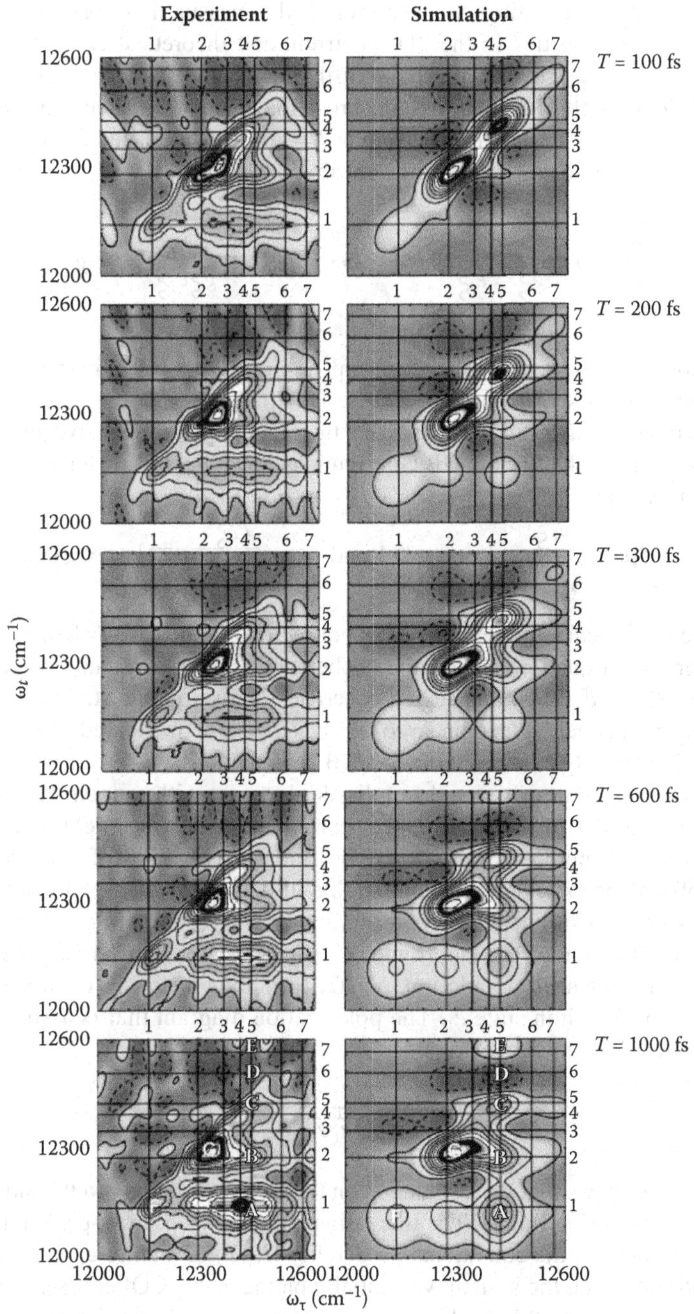

FIGURE 13.1 2D photon echo spectra of FMO light-harvesting complex. The waiting time varies from 100 to 1,000 fs. The five spectra on the left are experimentally measured ones, whereas those on the right are numerically simulated spectra. (From Cho, M., et al., *Journal of Physical Chemistry B*, 2005, 109, 10542. With permission.)

By carefully examining the experimentally measured absorption spectrum, diagonal peak intensities in the 2D spectrum, and theoretical calculation results, it was found that the second, third, and fifth one-exciton states have comparatively large dipole strengths. Nevertheless, the broad diagonally elongated peak centered at around 12,400 cm^{-1} in the 2D spectrum at $T = 100$ fs is produced by the stimulated emission and ground-state bleaching contributions as

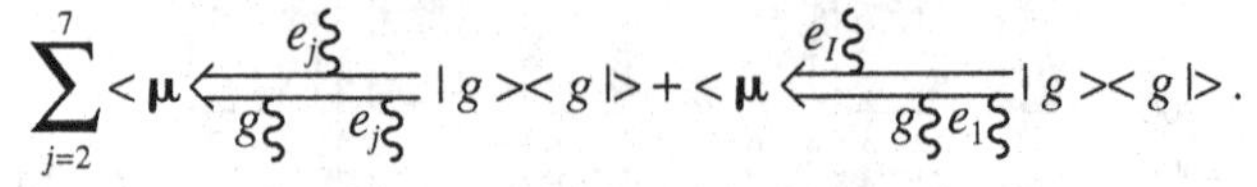

$$\sum_{j=2}^{7} <\mu \overset{e_j}{\underset{g \quad e_j}{\longleftarrow}} |g><g| + <\mu \overset{e_1}{\underset{g e_1}{\longleftarrow}} |g><g|. \tag{13.2}$$

In addition to the diagonal peaks, there appear broad cross-peaks in the lower diagonal region even at short time $T = 100$ fs. This indicates that the seven BChl's are coupled to one another. From the fact that the cross-peaks are positive, one can infer that they are from the SE and GB contributions involving two different one-exciton states, for example, for $j \neq k$

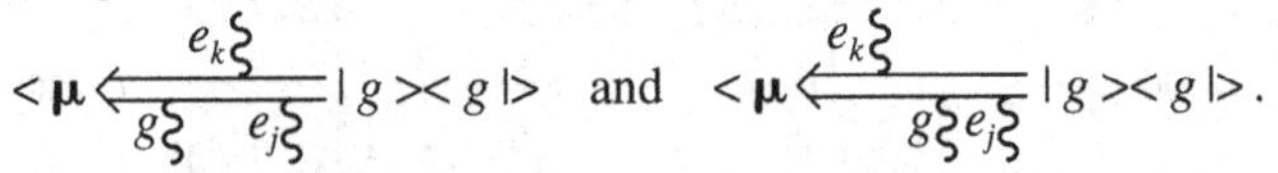

$$<\mu \overset{e_k}{\underset{g \quad e_j}{\longleftarrow}} |g><g| \quad \text{and} \quad <\mu \overset{e_k}{\underset{g e_j}{\longleftarrow}} |g><g|. \tag{13.3}$$

Here, the cross-peaks in the lower diagonal region are the cases when $E_k < E_j$. The first diagram in Equation 13.3 involves coherence oscillation (quantum beat) during T as $\exp(-i\{E_k - E_j\}T/\hbar)$, and such a coherence decays quite fast. The cross-peaks in the upper diagonal region appear to be weak, because the excited-state absorption contributions largely cancel out the SE+GB contributions.

As T increases, all the cross-peak amplitudes increase with concomitant decreases and shape changes of diagonal peaks. Particularly, the cross-peaks in the lower diagonal region increase dramatically in time T. At $T = 1000$ fs, the cross-peak (**A**) amplitude becomes almost comparable to that of the diagonal peak **G**. From the cross-peak position, which is around at $\omega_\tau = \bar{\omega}_{e_4 g}$ and $\omega_t = \bar{\omega}_{e_1 g}$, the time-resolved measurement of the amplitude of the cross-peak **A** provides kinetic information on the downhill population transfer from the fourth one-exciton state e_4 to the lowest one-exciton state e_1. The polarization diagram that is associated with this cross-peak is thus given as

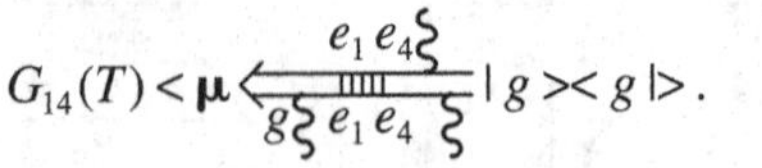

$$G_{14}(T) <\mu \overset{e_1 \, e_4}{\underset{g \, e_1 e_4}{\longleftarrow}} |g><g|. \tag{13.4}$$

This diagram shows that the population on the e_4 state undergoes a transition to that on the e_1 state during time T. The increasing pattern of this cross-peak amplitude is thus determined by the conditional probability $G_{14}(T)$ of finding e_1 state population at time T later when the system was initially on the e_1 state. Of course, there can be more contributions to this peak as long as the corresponding coherence oscillation frequencies during τ and t periods are close to $\bar{\omega}_{e_4 g}$ and $\bar{\omega}_{e_1 g}$. Some of them could be negatively contributing excited-state absorption terms.

Another notable cross-peak is the **B**-peak at $\omega_\tau = \bar{\omega}_{e_4 g}$ or $\bar{\omega}_{e_5 g}$ and $\omega_t = \bar{\omega}_{e_2 g}$ in Figure 13.1. Its amplitude increase is approximately described by the population transfer from e_4 and e_5 states to e_2 state. Thus, one should consider the following diagrams to quantitatively describe its T-dependency,

$$G_{24}(T) < \mu_A \xleftarrow[g \wr e_2 e_4 \wr]{e_2 e_4 \wr} | g >< g | > \quad \text{and} \quad G_{25}(T) < \mu_A \xleftarrow[g \wr e_2 e_5 \wr]{e_2 e_5 \wr} | g >< g | > . \tag{13.5}$$

In addition, one can expect that there should be a population transfer from e_2 to e_1 state as T increases. Indeed, the 2D spectrum at T = 1,000 fs exhibits such a cross-peak at $\omega_\tau = \bar{\omega}_{e_2g}$ and $\omega_t = \bar{\omega}_{e_1g}$. Although only a few cross-peaks have been discussed above, the entire 2D spectrum with respect to T results from complicated kinetic networks of the population transfer processes among the seven one-exciton states. Note that the excitation transfer processes and their effects on the 2D electronic spectra can be considered a seven-species chemical exchange system.

Another interesting observation is that the amplitude of the lowest-energy diagonal peak at $\omega_\tau = \bar{\omega}_{e_1g}$ and $\omega_t = \bar{\omega}_{e_1g}$ remains the same. This can also be easily understood by noting that its time-dependency is determined by the survival probability $G_{11}(T)$. Because the e_1 state is the lowest one-exciton state, once it is excited, the population does not change much because any population transfers from this e_1 state to other states are uphill transitions, which are small.

As emphasized above, the 2D spectrum is a product of complicated interferences between different nonlinear optical transition pathways, but to facilitate analysis of these experimental results, a rather simple theoretical description would be useful and provides the basis for an intuitive understanding of the 2D spectra. To this end, it was necessary to properly parameterize the diagonal and off-diagonal matrix elements, which are the BChl's site energies and coupling constants, respectively, to numerically simulate the time-resolved 2D spectra of the FMO complex (see the spectra on the right column of Figure 13.1).[6] The general trends and spectral changes in the experimentally measured spectra were successfully reproduced by the theoretical calculations. Here, the short-time approximations to the photon echo response functions, which were discussed in detail in Section 5.3, were used, and the modified Redfield theory for the population transfer rate constants was used to obtain the conditional and survival probabilities.[10]

Later, for the same FMO protein complex, another refined 2D electronic spectroscopy experiment was carried out to shed light on coherence transfer processes and underlying excitation migration mechanism within the complex.[2] Since the spectral bandwidth of a femtosecond laser pulse is sufficiently broad enough to cover the transition frequencies of all the seven one-exciton states, the first field-matter interaction can generate an ensemble of multiple electronic coherences, which are superposition states of the electronic ground state and one-exciton states. Then, the second field-matter interaction generates (1) ground-state bleach (hole), (2) populations on the one-exciton states (diagonal density matrix elements), and (3) electronic coherences (off-diagonal density matrix elements in the one-exciton block). The diagrams representing these three cases are, respectively,

$$< \mu \xleftarrow[g \wr e_j \wr]{e_j \wr} | g >< g | >, \; < \mu \xleftarrow[g \wr \;\; e_j \wr]{e_j \wr} | g >< g | >, \; \text{and} \; < \mu \xleftarrow[g \wr \;\; e_j \wr]{e_k \wr} | g >< g | > . \tag{13.6}$$

These third-order polarization components evolve differently during the waiting time T. Time-dependencies of the ground-state bleaching state and the one-exciton population were discussed above, but the coherence evolution and its transition to the other coherence could only be studied by measuring ultrafast (tens of femtosecond) changes of the 2D spectra and by examining quantum beats of the diagonal and off-diagonal peaks in the 2D spectra. Here, a diagrammatic representation of the coherence transfer from $\rho^{(2)}_{e_j e_k}$ to $\rho^{(2)}_{e_j e_l}$ for example is

$G_{jl,jk}(T) < \mu$ 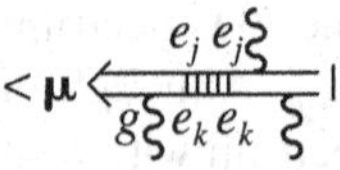 $| g >< g |>$. (13.7)

Again, the conditional probability function describing the above coherence transfer process was denoted as $G_{jl,jk}(T)$. From a series of measured 2D spectra with respect to T, it was shown that the amplitudes of the lowest-energy diagonal peak and the corresponding cross-peak oscillate in time, that is, quantum beating. One can immediately find that they originate from diagrams like

$< \mu$ 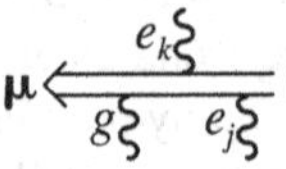 $| g >< g |>$. (13.8)

The power spectrum of oscillating lowest-energy diagonal (at $\omega_\tau = \bar{\omega}_{e_1 g}$ and $\omega_t = \bar{\omega}_{e_1 g}$) peak amplitude showed six different frequency components. This is because, for $j = 1$, there are six different diagrams like Equation 13.8 with $k = 2 \sim 7$. Note that the off-diagonal density matrix element, which describes the time–evolution of the electronic coherence between the jth and kth excitons, is approximately given as $\rho^{(2)}_{jk}(T) \propto \exp\{-i(E_j - E_k)T/\hbar\}$ (note that the superscript "(2)" in $\rho^{(2)}_{jk}(T)$ means that it is a second-order perturbation-expanded density matrix with respect to field-matter interaction Hamiltonian). This suggests that an experimental measurement of the quantum beating pattern of a diagonal peak provides information on the excitonic state energies directly. Furthermore, it was found that the quantum beats of the diagonal and cross-peaks persist even longer than population relaxation times, which is in stark contrast with the notion that the coherences are destroyed quite rapidly in comparison to population relaxation times. It was therefore suggested that chromophore-bath interactions are correlated for different chromophores, that is, a piece of evidence on the breakdown of the independent bath approximation.

In addition, the ratio of the diagonal to antidiagonal widths of the lowest-energy diagonal peak oscillates with the same frequencies of its peak amplitude, but the fluctuation of the diagonal width is anticorrelated with that of the antidiagonal width. This was found to be strong evidence of excitonic quantum coherence. More specifically, direct evidence on coherence transfer was observed by examining the oscillating behavior of the cross-peak between excitons 1 and 3, which is one of the most clearly frequency-resolved cross-peaks. Although from the corresponding power spectrum, all frequency components coupled to either exciton 1 or 3 were identified, the cross-peak amplitude and beating did not appear at time zero. This indicates that the 1–3 coherence was generated at finite time later, that is, coherence transfer from some other coherences to the 1–3 coherence. An interesting suggestion from the analysis of quantum coherences involved in energy transfer was that the generated superposition states are efficient in directing the energy transfer in such a light-harvesting complex, which is analogous to a single quantum computation. This is in contrast with an incoherent hopping mechanism. A further study is required whether a real light-harvesting complex absorbing incoherent sunlight instead of femtosecond coherent laser photons is affected by such effects. In addition, a more refined chromophore-bath interaction model should be developed to address the issue on bath-mediated correlation effects on line broadening and exciton population and coherence transfers.

13.2 APPLICATION TO SEMICONDUCTORS

Two-dimensional electronic spectroscopy has also been applied to semiconductors for studying exciton dynamics, exciton-exciton coupling, and exciton-continuum state coupling.[3, 11, 12] Optical excitation of a direct-gap semiconductor produces electron-hole pairs, which are called excitons because electron and hole pair can result in a bound state due to the Coulomb attraction between the two oppositely charged particles. In the case of GaAs (gallium arsenide) semiconductor heterostructure, excitonic resonance appears at a low temperature because the exciton binding energy is just about 10 meV. In order to study exciton dynamics of which timescale varies from femtosecond to picosecond, a variety of ultrafast spectroscopic means have been used.

The first 2D optical spectroscopy experiment on a semiconductor was performed for GaAs semiconductor quantum wells consisting of 10 periods of 10 nm GaAs well and 10 nm Al-GaAs barrier at 8 K. The heavy-hole and light-hole valence bands were formed, and the two are energetically separated from each other by about 6 meV. In the upper panel of Figure 13.2, the absorption spectrum exhibiting a heavy-hole exciton band, a light-hole exciton band, and continuum band is shown. The spectrum of excitation pulse is also shown in the same figure. Normalized 2D magnitude spectrum shows four well-resolved peaks (see the lower panel in Figure 13.2). Here, it should be mentioned that the x- and y-axes in the 2D spectrum correspond to ω_t and ω_τ, unlike the other 2D spectra shown in this and the previous chapters. First of all, the cross-peaks in this spectrum originate from coherent coupling between the heavy-hole exciton and the light-hole exciton or spatial overlaps of these two excitonic states. Interestingly, the upper left cross-peak intensity appears to be stronger than the two diagonal peaks. It turned out that the excitation-induced dephasing, which is related to incoherent many-body effects, and excitation-induced shift play important roles in couplings. Here, the excitation-induced dephasing means that the effective dephasing rate of the off-diagonal density matrix element for a 2LS contains a term that is linearly proportional to the number density of oscillators. Similarly, the excitation-induced shift means that the resonance frequency is shifted linearly with respect to the number density.

Another notable feature in the 2D spectrum is the presence of two vertical ridges. If the continuum states can be modeled as a collection of inhomogeneously distributed 2LSs, the peaks would appear diagonally elongated, not vertically elongated. From the model simulations, the excitation-induced dephasing was found to play a critical role here, since the characteristic vertically elongated

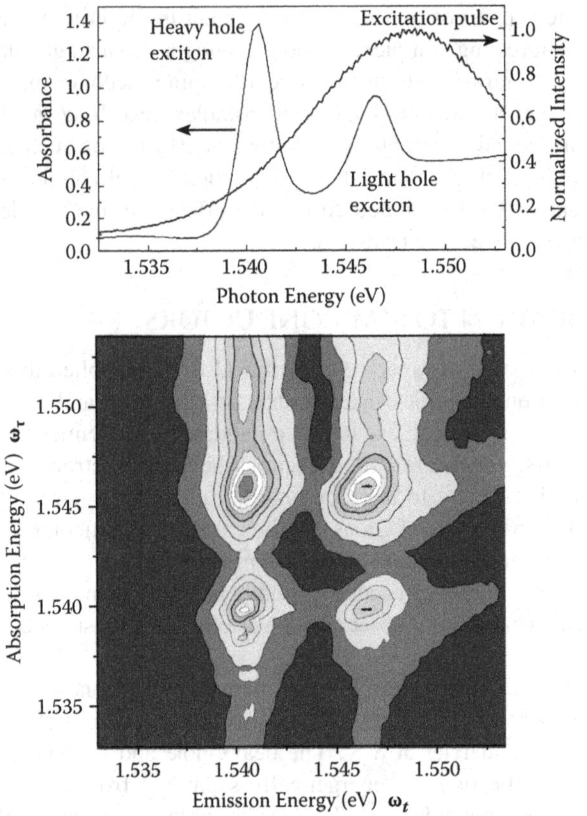

FIGURE 13.2 Absorption spectrum of GaAs quantum wells (upper panel). Also, the excitation pulse spectrum is shown in this figure. 2D magnitude spectrum is shown in the lower panel. (From Borca, C. N., et al., *Chemical Physics Letters*, 2005, 416, 311. With permission.)

cross-peaks appear only when the excitation-induced dephasing is included. This experiment demonstrates that the 2D spectroscopic method can give a critical insight into the microscopic nature of the many-body interactions in semiconductors. From the measurements of the real and imaginary parts of the 2D spectrum, it was even possible to distinguish two different mechanisms, that is, excitation-induced dephasing and excitation-induced shift. The former affects the off-diagonal density matrix amplitude (decoherence), whereas the latter changes its oscillation frequency (spectral diffusion). From these investigations, it was found that the excitation-induced dephasing of the heavy-hole exciton is different from that of the light-hole exciton. This and related experiments demonstrate that the peak-shape analysis of semiconductor 2D electronic spectrum is extremely useful to elucidate the underlying physics of the exciton dynamics induced by many-body interactions, which cannot be easily studied by any other spectroscopic means.

REFERENCES

1. Brixner, T.; Stenger, J.; Vaswani, H. M.; Cho, M.; Blankenship, R. E.; Fleming, G. R., Two-dimensional spectroscopy of electronic couplings in photosynthesis. *Nature* 2005, 434, 625–628.
2. Engel, G. S.; Calhoun, T. R.; Read, E. L.; Ahn, T. K.; Mancal, T.; Cheng, Y. C.; Blankenship, R. E.; Fleming, G. R., Evidence for wavelike energy transfer through quantum coherence in photosynthetic systems. *Nature* 2007, 446, 782–786.
3. Borca, C. N.; Zhang, T. H.; Li, X. Q.; Cundiff, S. T., Optical two-dimensional Fourier transform spectroscopy of semiconductors. *Chemical Physics Letters* 2005, 416, (4–6), 311–315.
4. Hybl, J. D.; Albrecht, A. W.; Gallagher Faeder, S. M.; Jonas, D. M., Two-dimensional electronic spectroscopy. *Chemical Physics Letters* 1998, 297, 307–313.
5. Cho, M.; Fleming, G. R., Fifth-order three-pulse scattering spectroscopy: Can we separate homogeneous and inhomogeneous contributions to optical spectra. *Journal of Physical Chemistry* 1994, 98, (13), 3478–3485.
6. Cho, M.; Vaswani, H. M.; Brixner, T.; Stenger, J.; Fleming, G. R., Exciton analysis in 2D electronic spectroscopy. *Journal of Physical Chemistry B* 2005, 109, 10542–10556.
7. Zigmantas, D.; Read, E. L.; Mancal, T.; Brixner, T.; Gardiner, A. T.; Cogdell, R. J.; Fleming, G. R., Two-dimensional electronic spectroscopy of the B800-B820 light-harvesting complex. *Proceedings of the National Academy of Sciences of the USA* 2006, 103, 12672–12677.
8. van Amerongen, H.; Valkunas, L.; van Grondelle, R., *Photosynthetic excitons*. World Scientific: Singapore, 2000.
9. Cho, M.; Brixner, T.; Stiopkin, I.; Vaswani, H.; Fleming, G. R., Two dimensional electronic spectroscopy of molecular complexes. *Journal of the Chinese Chemical Society* 2006, 53, 15–24.
10. Yang, M.; Fleming, G. R., Influence of phonons on exciton transfer dynamics: comparison of the Redfield, Forster, and modified Redfield equations. *Chemical Physics* 2002, 275, 355–372.
11. Li, X.; Zhang, T.; Borca, C. N.; Cundiff, S. T., Many-body interactions in semiconductors probed by optical two-dimensional Fourier transform spectroscopy. *Physical Review Letters* 2006, 96, 057406.
12. Kuznetsova, I.; Thomas, P.; Meier, T.; Zhang, T.; Li, X.; Mirin, R. P.; Cundiff, S. T., Signatures of many-particle correlations in two-dimensional Fourier-transform spectra of semiconductor nanostructures. *Solid State Communications* 2007, 142, 154–158.

14 Two-Dimensional Second-Order Response Spectroscopy

In Chapter 4, a response function theory for general second-order response spectroscopy was presented and discussed. Here, it will be shown that they can be used as 2D measurement techniques. An essential element for 2D spectroscopy is that radiation–matter interactions cause doubly resonant transitions, and two coherence evolutions should be recorded experimentally. Thus measured 2D signal in time-domain is then doubly Fourier–Laplace transformed to obtain the corresponding 2D spectrum in frequency domain. The second-order response measurement techniques such as time-resolved doubly resonant sum frequency generation, fifth-order Raman scattering, IR–IR-vis four-wave-mixing spectroscopy, and so forth are a few examples that will be considered in this chapter. Note that they all involve two coherence evolutions during the nonlinear optical processes.

Denoting effect operator, two cause operators, and conjugate external fields as $\hat{B}$, $\hat{A}_1$ and $\hat{A}_2$, and $F_1(t)$ and $F_2(t)$, respectively, and using the second-order time-dependent perturbation theory, we showed that

$$\bar{B}(t) = \langle \hat{B}\rho^{(2)}_{A_2A_1}(t)\rangle = \int_0^\infty dt_2 \int_0^\infty dt_1\ \phi_{BA_2A_1}(t_2,t_1)F_2(t-t_2)F_1(t-t_2-t_1), \quad (14.1)$$

where the second-order response function is

$$\phi_{BA_2A_1}(t_2,t_1) = \left(\frac{i}{\hbar}\right)^2 \theta(t_2)\theta(t_1) \langle [[\hat{B}(t_2+t_1), \hat{A}_2(t_1)], \hat{A}_1(0)]\rho(-\infty)\rangle. \quad (14.2)$$

Expanding the two commutators in Equation 14.2, one can rewrite it as

$$\begin{aligned}\phi_{BA_2A_1}(t_2,t_1) = \left(\frac{i}{\hbar}\right)^2 \theta(t_2)\theta(t_1)\{&\langle \hat{B}(t_2+t_1)\hat{A}_2(t_1)\hat{A}_1(0)\rho(-\infty)\rangle \\ &- \langle \hat{A}_2(t_1)\, \hat{B}(t_2+t_1)\, \hat{A}_1(0)\, \rho(-\infty)\rangle \\ &- \langle \hat{A}_1(0)\, \hat{B}(t_2+t_1)\, \hat{A}_2(t_1)\, \rho(-\infty)\rangle \\ &+ \langle \hat{A}_1(0)\, \hat{A}_2(t_1)\, \hat{B}(t_2+t_1)\, \rho(-\infty)\rangle\}. \end{aligned} \quad (14.3)$$

Detailed expressions for the effect operator and effective radiation–matter interaction Hamiltonian should be properly chosen to describe a given experimental result or nonlinear optical process of interest.

In the present chapter, we will focus on a few different 2D second-order response spectroscopic techniques. Although there are a number of possible and potentially useful second-order 2D spectroscopic methods in general, only a few simple cases will be discussed in detail. Nevertheless, one can easily explore other possibilities and experimental feasibilities by using the general theoretical framework presented and discussed in this book.

14.1 TWO-DIMENSIONAL SUM FREQUENCY GENERATION

One of the most widely used second-order nonlinear optical spectroscopic methods is the sum frequency generation (SFG), including second-harmonic generation.[1] SFG has been extensively used to study molecular dynamics, chemical reaction, molecular orientation, and various material properties of molecules and composite systems on surface or at interface. The SFG and difference frequency generation (DFG) signals are nonzero for those samples having no centrosymmetry, and they are the lowest-order nonlinear optical processes. The SFG signal from molecules in an isotropic medium such as solution vanishes because the rotational average of typical third-rank tensorial response function over randomly oriented molecules usually vanishes. However, it was shown that polarization-controlled SFG or DFG of molecules in solution can be detected when each optical chromophore is chiral and when the solution sample is not racemic.[2–8] This suggests that the SFG technique is a useful nonlinear *optical activity* spectroscopy.

A general theory of SFG was discussed in Chapter 4. Two electric fields propagating in the directions of $\mathbf{k}_1$ and $\mathbf{k}_2$ interact with the matter, and two consecutive absorptive interactions induce a sequence of optical transitions from g to e to f. Then, thus created coherence $\rho_{fg}^{(2)}$ corresponds to a collection of oscillating dipoles and radiates electric field whose frequency is the sum of the $\mathbf{E}_1$ and $\mathbf{E}_2$ field frequencies. Thus, the two cause operators and the effect operator are all $\boldsymbol{\mu}$, and the two conjugate external fields are $\mathbf{E}_1$ and $\mathbf{E}_2$:

$$\hat{A}_1 F_1(t) = \boldsymbol{\mu} \cdot \mathbf{e}_1 E_1(t) e^{i\mathbf{k}_1 \cdot \mathbf{r} - i\omega_1 t}$$

$$\hat{A}_2 F_2(t) = \boldsymbol{\mu} \cdot \mathbf{e}_2 E_2(t) e^{i\mathbf{k}_2 \cdot \mathbf{r} - i\omega_2 t}$$

$$\hat{B} = \boldsymbol{\mu} \cdot \qquad (14.4)$$

Here, we considered the transverse electric field component travelling in the direction of $\mathbf{k}_j$ (for $j = 1$ and 2) not $-\mathbf{k}_j$, since they are involved in absorptive radiation–matter interactions in the present case.

The second-order SFG polarization is the expection value of the above effect-operator over the second-order perturbation-expanded density matrix, and its diagram representation is

$$\langle \boldsymbol{\mu} \overset{\boldsymbol{\mu}\mathbf{E}_2 \;\; \boldsymbol{\mu}\mathbf{E}_1}{\underset{f \;\;\;\;\; e}{\Longleftarrow\!=\!=\!=\!=}} | g \rangle\langle g | \rangle . \qquad (14.5)$$

The SFG polarization is then given as

$$\mathbf{P}_{SFG}(\mathbf{r},t) = e^{i(\mathbf{k}_1+\mathbf{k}_2)\cdot\mathbf{r}-i(\omega_1+\omega_2)t} \int_0^\infty dt_2 \int_0^\infty dt_1\ \phi_{\mu\mu\mu}(t_2,t_1) : \mathbf{e}_2\mathbf{e}_1 E_2(t-t_2)E_1(t-t_2-t_1)$$
$$\times e^{i(\omega_1+\omega_2)t_2+i\omega_1 t_1}, \qquad (14.6)$$

where the third-rank tensorial all-electric-dipole response function is defined as

$$\phi_{\mu\mu\mu}(t_2,t_1) = \left(\frac{i}{\hbar}\right)^2 \theta(t_2)\theta(t_1) < [[\boldsymbol{\mu}(t_2+t_1), \boldsymbol{\mu}(t_1)], \boldsymbol{\mu}(0)]\rho(-\infty) >. \qquad (14.7)$$

Although the second-order response function above describes all the possible second-order optical processes, we will specifically consider the case when the two excited states |e> and |f> are real quantum states, not virtual states, and when the two incident beams radiations with frequencies of ω_1 and ω_2 are *doubly resonant* with transitions between g and e states and between e and f states, respectively.[9] In this case of the doubly resonant SFG, for $E_f > E_e > E_g$, we have $\omega_1 + \omega_2 \simeq \bar{\omega}_{fg}$ and $\omega_1 \simeq \bar{\omega}_{eg}$. Then, among the four terms in Equation 14.3, only the first plays an important role and resonates with the external fields. From the Maxwell equation with SFG polarization given in Equation 14.6, one can find that the radiated SFG field is given as

$$\mathbf{E}_{SFG}(\mathbf{r},t) = -i\omega_s\, e^{i(\mathbf{k}_1+\mathbf{k}_2)\cdot\mathbf{r}-i(\omega_1+\omega_2)t} \boldsymbol{\mu}_{gf}\boldsymbol{\mu}_{fe}\boldsymbol{\mu}_{eg} : \mathbf{e}_2\mathbf{e}_1 \int_0^\infty dt_2 \int_0^\infty dt_1 \frac{1}{\hbar^2} G_1(t_2,t_1)$$
$$\times E_2(t-t_2)E_1(t-t_2-t_1)e^{i(\omega_1+\omega_2-\bar{\omega}_{fg})t_2+i(\omega_1-\bar{\omega}_{eg})t_1}. \qquad (14.8)$$

where the line-shape function G_1 is

$$G_1(t_2,t_1) = < \exp_+\left[-\frac{i}{\hbar}\int_0^{t_2} d\tau U_{fg}(\tau)\right]\exp_-\left[-\frac{i}{\hbar}\int_0^{t_1} d\tau U_{eg}(-\tau)\right] >_B. \qquad (14.9)$$

This line shape function can often be approximately written as

$$G_1(t_2,t_1) = \exp\{-\gamma_{ff}t_2 - \gamma_{ee}t_1\} \qquad (14.10)$$

or

$$G_1(t_2,t_1) = \exp\left\{-\frac{1}{2}\Delta_{ff}^2 t_2^2 - \frac{1}{2}\Delta_{ee}^2 t_1^2\right\}. \qquad (14.11)$$

The former (Equation 14.10) corresponds to the Markovian limit (optical Bloch approximation) expression and gives 2D Lorentzian peak shape, and the latter

(Equation 14.11) is the case of short-time approximation to the line-broadening function $g(t)$ or of large inhomogeneous broadening limit and gives 2D Gaussian peak shape.

Note that the SFG field in Equation 14.8 is a function of experimentally controllable frequencies ω_1 and ω_2. Thus, the homodyne-detected SFG intensity or the heterodyne-detected SFG amplitude is essentially a 2D function in frequency domain. A straightforward application of the doubly-resonant 2D SFG is to study optical chromophores adsorbed on surface with anisotropic orientational distribution. In this case, the rotational average of the third-rank tensor $\boldsymbol{\mu}_{gf}\boldsymbol{\mu}_{fe}\boldsymbol{\mu}_{eg}$ should be properly performed. We will not, however, provide any further discussion along this line, because this subject has been extensively studied before, not just experimentally, but also theoretically. In this chapter, we will focus on the case of chiral molecules in solution.[9]

14.2 TWO-DIMENSIONAL SUM FREQUENCY GENERATION OF SOLUTION SAMPLE

For solution samples, three-wave-mixing techniques have not been widely used because signals vanish or are quite small. Note that the only rotationally invariant isomer, which is a third-rank tensor, is the Levi–Civita tensor. Note that $\varepsilon_{XYZ} = \varepsilon_{YZX} = \varepsilon_{ZXY} = -\varepsilon_{XZY} = -\varepsilon_{YXZ} = -\varepsilon_{ZYX} = 1$. Thus, the case when the three beam polarization directions are mutually orthogonal to one another will be specifically considered in this section. By using the theoretical results in Section 3.3, the rotational average of the all-electric-dipole transition strength, $[\overline{\boldsymbol{\mu}_{gf}\boldsymbol{\mu}_{fe}\boldsymbol{\mu}_{eg}}]_{ijk}$, can be rewritten as, in terms of transition dipole matrix elements in a molecule-fixed frame,

$$[\overline{\boldsymbol{\mu}_{gf}\boldsymbol{\mu}_{fe}\boldsymbol{\mu}_{eg}}]_{ijk} = \frac{1}{6}\varepsilon_{ijk}\sum_{\lambda,\mu,\nu}\varepsilon_{\lambda\mu\nu}\left[\boldsymbol{\mu}_{gf}^{M}\right]_{\lambda}\left[\boldsymbol{\mu}_{fe}^{M}\right]_{\mu}\left[\boldsymbol{\mu}_{eg}^{M}\right]_{\nu}. \tag{14.12}$$

Here, the indices i, j, and k represent the axes in a space-fixed frame, and λ, μ, and ν are those in a molecule-fixed frame. Equation 14.12 can also be rewritten as

$$[\overline{\boldsymbol{\mu}_{gf}\boldsymbol{\mu}_{fe}\boldsymbol{\mu}_{eg}}]_{ijk} = \frac{1}{6}\varepsilon_{ijk}\boldsymbol{\mu}_{gf}^{M}\cdot\left(\boldsymbol{\mu}_{fe}^{M}\times\boldsymbol{\mu}_{eg}^{M}\right) = \frac{1}{6}\varepsilon_{ijk}\left(\boldsymbol{\mu}_{gf}^{M}\times\boldsymbol{\mu}_{fe}^{M}\right)\cdot\boldsymbol{\mu}_{eg}^{M}. \tag{14.13}$$

This suggests that, when the three transition dipole vectors $\boldsymbol{\mu}_{gf}^{M}$, $\boldsymbol{\mu}_{fe}^{M}$, and $\boldsymbol{\mu}_{eg}^{M}$ in a molecule-fixed frame do not lie on a common plane and when the angles between $\boldsymbol{\mu}_{fe}^{M}$ and $\boldsymbol{\mu}_{eg}^{M}$ and between $\boldsymbol{\mu}_{gf}^{M}$ and $\boldsymbol{\mu}_{fe}^{M}$ are neither 0 nor π, $\boldsymbol{\mu}_{gf}^{M}\cdot(\boldsymbol{\mu}_{fe}^{M}\times\boldsymbol{\mu}_{eg}^{M})$ does not vanish. This is an important selection rule for the nonzero SFG signal from molecules in an isotropic medium. In addition, from the property of the Levi–Civita epsilon, ε_{ijk}, the SFG signal field polarization direction should be orthogonal to both of the two incident beam polarization directions as well as $\mathbf{e}_1 \perp \mathbf{e}_2$. This is an experimental requirement for the doubly-resonant three-wave-mixing measurements. Hereafter, without any loss of generality, we will consider the [*XYZ*] tensor element of $[\overline{\boldsymbol{\mu}_{gf}\boldsymbol{\mu}_{fe}\boldsymbol{\mu}_{eg}}]$, which is given as

$$[\overline{\boldsymbol{\mu}_{gf}\boldsymbol{\mu}_{fe}\boldsymbol{\mu}_{eg}}]_{XYZ} = \frac{1}{6}\boldsymbol{\mu}_{gf}^{M}\cdot\left(\boldsymbol{\mu}_{fe}^{M}\times\boldsymbol{\mu}_{eg}^{M}\right). \tag{14.14}$$

From Equations 14.8 and 14.14, one can find that the rotationally averaged SFG signal field is finally given as

$$\hat{\mathrm{E}}_{XYZ}^{SFG}(t,\omega_2+\omega_1,\omega_1) = -\frac{i\omega_s}{6}\mathrm{e}^{i(\mathbf{k}_1+\mathbf{k}_2)\cdot\mathbf{r}-i(\omega_1+\omega_2)t}\boldsymbol{\mu}_{gf}^{M}\cdot(\boldsymbol{\mu}_{fe}^{M}\times\boldsymbol{\mu}_{eg}^{M})\int_0^{\infty}dt_2\int_0^{\infty}dt_1\frac{1}{\hbar^2}G_1(t_2,t_1)$$
$$\times E_2(t-t_2)E_1(t-t_2-t_1)\mathrm{e}^{i(\omega_1+\omega_2-\bar{\omega}_{fg})t_2+i(\omega_1-\bar{\omega}_{eg})t_1}. \tag{14.15}$$

Hereafter, we shall focus on the time-resolved measurement utilizing ultrashort laser pulses. The first two pulses are assumed to be centered at $t = -T - \tau$ and $t = -T$ in time domain. This means that the delay time between the two pulses is τ and that the electric field amplitude after time T from the second pulse is measured at $t = 0$ by using a heterodyne-detection method. Then, in the impulsive limit, the electric field amplitude thus measured is linearly proportional to the corresponding line-shape function as

$$\hat{\mathrm{E}}_{XYZ}^{SFG}(t,T,\tau) = -\frac{i\omega_s}{6\hbar^2}e^{i\mathbf{k}_s\cdot\mathbf{r}-i\omega_s t}\boldsymbol{\mu}_{gf}^{M}\cdot\left(\boldsymbol{\mu}_{fe}^{M}\times\boldsymbol{\mu}_{eg}^{M}\right)G_1(t+T,\tau)\mathrm{e}^{i(\omega_1+\omega_2-\bar{\omega}_{fg})T+i(\omega_1-\bar{\omega}_{eg})\tau}. \tag{14.16}$$

In order to measure the above signal field, one can use a local oscillator field $\mathbf{E}_{LO}(\mathbf{r},t) = \mathbf{E}_{LO}^{*}(t)e^{-i\mathbf{k}_s\cdot\mathbf{r}+i\omega_s t}$, and its pulse envelope $E_{LO}(t)$ is also assumed to be close to a Dirac delta function at $t = 0$ to achieve time-resolved measurement of the SFG field amplitude and phase for varying time T. Then, the measured signal is Fourier–Laplace transformed as

$$\tilde{\mathrm{E}}_{XYZ}^{SFG}(\bar{\omega}_T,\bar{\omega}_\tau) = \int_0^{\infty}dT\int_0^{\infty}d\tau\,\hat{\mathrm{E}}_{ZYX}^{SFG}(T,\tau)\exp(i\bar{\omega}_T T + i\bar{\omega}_\tau\tau). \tag{14.17}$$

For the sake of notational simplicity, let us define two frequency variables as

$$\omega_T = \omega_1 + \omega_2 + \bar{\omega}_T$$
$$\omega_\tau = \omega_1 + \bar{\omega}_\tau. \tag{14.18}$$

Using the two dephasing models in Equations 14.10 and 14.11, one finds that the 2D SFG spectra are

$$\tilde{E}^{SFG}_{XYZ}(\omega_T,\omega_\tau) = -\frac{i\omega_s}{6\hbar^2}\mu^M_{gf}\cdot\left(\mu^M_{fe}\times\mu^M_{eg}\right)L(\bar{\omega}_{fg},\gamma_{ff},\bar{\omega}_{eg},\gamma_{ee}) \tag{14.19}$$

$$\tilde{E}^{SFG}_{XYZ}(\omega_T,\omega_\tau) = -\frac{i\omega_s}{6\hbar^2}\mu^M_{gf}\cdot\left(\mu^M_{fe}\times\mu^M_{eg}\right)\Gamma\left(\bar{\omega}_{fg},\Delta^2_{ff},\bar{\omega}_{eg},\Delta^2_{ee}\right). \tag{14.20}$$

The 2D Lorentzian and Gaussian peak shape functions were defined in Chapter 7, but for the sake of completeness, they are rewritten here:

$$L(\bar{\omega}_{fg},\gamma_{ff},\bar{\omega}_{eg},\gamma_{ee}) = \frac{1}{(\omega_T-\bar{\omega}_{fg}+i\gamma_{ff})(\omega_\tau-\bar{\omega}_{eg}-i\gamma_{ee})} \tag{14.21}$$

$$\Gamma\left(\bar{\omega}_{fg},\Delta^2_{ff},\bar{\omega}_{eg},\Delta^2_{ee}\right) = \frac{\pi}{\Delta_{ee}\Delta_{ff}}\exp\left(-\frac{(\omega_\tau-\bar{\omega}_{eg})^2}{2\Delta^2_{ee}}\right)$$
$$\times\left\{\exp\left(-\frac{(\omega_T-\bar{\omega}_{fg})^2}{2\Delta^2_{ff}}\right)+\frac{2i}{\sqrt{\pi}}F\left(\frac{\omega_T-\bar{\omega}_{fg}}{\sqrt{2}\Delta_{ff}}\right)\right\}. \tag{14.22}$$

The above results, Equations 14.19 and 14.20, were obtained for a three-level system. However, for a coupled multi-chromophore system, there are manifolds of singly and doubly excited states, and in that case the 2D SFG spectrum can be written as a sum of all independent contributions as

$$\tilde{E}^{SFG}_{XYZ}(\omega_T,\omega_\tau) = -\frac{i\omega_s}{6\hbar^2}\sum_e\sum_f\mu^M_{gf}\cdot\left(\mu^M_{fe}\times\mu^M_{eg}\right)\Gamma\left(\bar{\omega}_{fg},\Delta^2_{ff},\bar{\omega}_{eg},\Delta^2_{ee}\right). \tag{14.23}$$

This result indicates that the resultant SFG spectrum is the product of wave interferences. Hereafter, the factor $\omega_s/6\hbar^2$ in Equations 14.19 and 14.23 will be omitted for the sake of notational simplicity. In the following sections, we will consider a few simple coupled dimer systems to show what information can be extracted from the 2D SFG spectrum.

14.3 TWO-DIMENSIONAL SUM FREQUENCY GENERATION OF COUPLED TWO-LEVEL SYSTEM DIMER

In Section 9.1, the model Hamiltonian for coupled 2LS dimer was presented and discussed in detail. It was shown that there are two singly excited states e_1 and e_2 and a doubly excited state f. Therefore, there are two different SFG diagrams in this case, and they are

$$<\mu\overset{\mu E_2\ \ \mu E_1}{\xLeftarrow{\ f\ \ \ e_1\ }}|g><g| \quad \text{and} \quad <\mu\overset{\mu E_2\ \ \mu E_1}{\xLeftarrow{\ f\ \ \ e_2\ }}|g><g|. \tag{14.24}$$

The SFG fields associated with the two polarizations in Equation 14.24 interfere with each other to produce the total SFG field. Fourier-Laplace transformation of the time-resolved heterodyne-detected SFG signal gives us the 2D SFG spectrum, that is,

$$\tilde{E}^{SFG}_{XYZ}(\omega_T,\omega_\tau) = -i\boldsymbol{\mu}^M_{gf}\cdot\left(\boldsymbol{\mu}^M_{fe_1}\times\boldsymbol{\mu}^M_{e_1g}\right)\Gamma\left(\bar{\omega}_{fg},\Delta^2_{ff},\bar{\omega}_{e_1g},\Delta^2_{e_1e_1}\right)$$
$$-i\boldsymbol{\mu}^M_{gf}\cdot\left(\boldsymbol{\mu}^M_{fe_2}\times\boldsymbol{\mu}^M_{e_2g}\right)\Gamma\left(\bar{\omega}_{fg},\Delta^2_{ff},\bar{\omega}_{e_2g},\Delta^2_{e_2e_2}\right), \qquad (14.25)$$

where the 2D Gaussian peak shape approximation was used.

Now, the next step is to calculate the transition dipole matrix elements in Equation 14.25. From Equations 9.11 and 9.12, one can find the following relationships,

$$\boldsymbol{\mu}^M_{e_1g} = \boldsymbol{\mu}^M_{fe_2} \quad \text{and} \quad \boldsymbol{\mu}^M_{e_2g} = \boldsymbol{\mu}^M_{fe_1}. \qquad (14.26)$$

The transition dipoles in the above equation are all associated with one-quantum transitions. However, the more important factor determining the SFG of solution sample is the transition amplitude from the doubly excited state to the ground state, $\boldsymbol{\mu}^M_{gf}$ (=<0, 0|$\hat{\boldsymbol{\mu}}^M$|1,1>). This two-quantum transition dipole matrix element can be calculated by considering the following expanded electric dipole operator,

$$\hat{\boldsymbol{\mu}} = \hat{\boldsymbol{\mu}}_1 + \hat{\boldsymbol{\mu}}_2 + \hat{\boldsymbol{\mu}}_1\mathbf{T}_{12}\hat{\boldsymbol{\alpha}}_2 + \hat{\boldsymbol{\mu}}_2\mathbf{T}_{21}\hat{\boldsymbol{\alpha}}_1 + \cdots \qquad (14.27)$$

where $\hat{\boldsymbol{\mu}}_j$ and $\hat{\boldsymbol{\alpha}}_j$ are the electric dipole and molecular polarizability operators of the *j*th chromophore. $\mathbf{T}_{12}$ is the second-rank dipole-dipole interaction tensor (see Equation 9.2). The third and fourth terms on the right-hand side of Equation 14.27 are the induced dipole operators, and they are responsible for making the two-quantum transition dipole matrix element $\boldsymbol{\mu}^M_{gf}$ nonzero. Inserting Equation 14.27 into $<0,0\,|\,\hat{\boldsymbol{\mu}}^M|\,1,1>$, one can find that $\boldsymbol{\mu}^M_{gf}$ is approximately given as

$$\boldsymbol{\mu}^M_{gf} \cong \mathbf{d}_1\mathbf{T}_{12}\boldsymbol{\alpha}_2 + \mathbf{d}_2\mathbf{T}_{21}\boldsymbol{\alpha}_1, \qquad (14.28)$$

where $\mathbf{d}_1 = <0,0|\hat{\boldsymbol{\mu}}^M_1|1,0>$, $\mathbf{d}_2 = <0,0\,|\,\hat{\boldsymbol{\mu}}^M_2|\,0,1>$, $\boldsymbol{\alpha}_1 =< 0,0|\hat{\boldsymbol{\alpha}}^M_1|1,0>$, and $\boldsymbol{\alpha}_2 = <0,0\,|\,\hat{\boldsymbol{\alpha}}^M_2|\,0,1>$. Note that these four transition matrix elements are all defined in a molecule-fixed frame. The physical meaning of Equation 14.28 is that the electric dipole transition of one chromophore in the doubly excited dimer can stimulate a transition of its neighboring chromophore through the transition dipole-dipole interaction. These two transitions occur simultaneously to allow the two-quantum transition from *f* to *g*.

Inserting Equation 14.28 into 14.25 and using the relationships in Equation 14.26, we get

$$\tilde{E}^{SFG}_{ZYX}(\omega_T,\omega_\tau) = -i(\mathbf{d}_1\mathbf{T}_{12}\boldsymbol{\alpha}_2 + \mathbf{d}_2\mathbf{T}_{21}\boldsymbol{\alpha}_1)\cdot(\mathbf{d}_2\times\mathbf{d}_1)\left\{\Gamma\left(\bar{\omega}_{fg},\Delta^2_{ff},\bar{\omega}_{e_1g},\Delta^2_{e_1e_1}\right)\right.$$
$$\left.-\Gamma\left(\bar{\omega}_{fg},\Delta^2_{ff},\bar{\omega}_{e_2g},\Delta^2_{e_2e_2}\right)\right\}. \qquad (14.29)$$

This is an interesting result for the 2D SFG of a chiral coupled 2LS dimer in solution.[9] First of all, the SFG signal does not vanish when the three vectors, (1) $\mathbf{d}_1\tilde{\mathbf{T}}_{12}\boldsymbol{\alpha}_2 + \mathbf{d}_2\tilde{\mathbf{T}}_{21}\boldsymbol{\alpha}_1$, (2) $\mathbf{d}_2$, and (3) $\mathbf{d}_1$, are not on a common plane in a molecule-fixed frame. Chiral dimer and molecular complex are good examples. Secondly, because the dipole–dipole interaction tensor is proportional to $1/R^3$ with R being the intermolecular distance, as the two chromophores become separated far apart, the overall signal amplitude or intensity decreases as $1/R^3$ in the case of the heterodyne measurement or as $1/R^6$ in the case of the homodyne measurement. The above selection rules suggest that the doubly resonant three-wave-mixing measurement technique is possibly an optical activity spectroscopy probing molecular chirality originating from the dimer conformation and electronic coupling. Thirdly, it should be noted that the two terms in Equation 14.29 have the same transition strength with opposite signs. Thus, if the dimer is a homodimer and if the coupling constant is small, we have $\bar{\omega}_{e_1g} = \bar{\omega}_{e_2g}$, and the two terms on the right-hand side of Equation 14.29 cancel out exactly. This is why the SFG signal vanishes for completely uncoupled chromophores in solution, when each chromophore is modeled as a 2LS and the incident beam is resonant with its transition. A lack of complete cancellation (destructive interference) of the two resonant optical transition pathways is required for the nonzero SFG signals from a coupled 2LS dimer. Here, it is noted that both the electronic coupling constant and the induced transition dipole in Equation 14.28 are functions of inter-chromophore distance R. As R increases, both decrease as approximately $1/R^3$.

The 2D SFG technique has a certain advantage in frequency resolution, in comparison with the other linear spectroscopies. The absorption spectrum is for example given by a sum of two terms associated with $g \leftrightarrow e_1$ and $g \leftrightarrow e_2$ transitions as

$$\kappa_a(\omega) \propto |\boldsymbol{\mu}_{ge_1}|^2 f(\omega - \bar{\omega}_{e_1g}) + |\boldsymbol{\mu}_{ge_2}|^2 f(\omega - \bar{\omega}_{e_2g}) \tag{14.30}$$

where $f(\omega - \bar{\omega}_{e_1g})$ is an appropriate line-shape function. Note that the two terms in Equation 14.30 are positive and add together to produce the absorption spectrum. Therefore, if each spectral bandwidth is comparable or larger than the frequency-splitting magnitude $\bar{\omega}_{e_2e_1}$, the absorption spectrum will appear as a singlet. This is the so-called spectral congestion problem, and thus 1D absorption spectroscopy is inevitably a low-resolution technique. However, even in that case of spectrally congested dimer system, the present 2D SFG method is better in frequency resolution than 1D method. Since the two peaks in the 2D SFG spectrum have opposite signs, the spectrum will appear as a positive–negative couplet, and its frequency splitting magnitude, that is, peak-to-peak frequency difference, is related to the coupling constant J. If J is much larger than the spectral bandwidth, the positive-peak to negative-peak frequency difference becomes simply identical to $2J$. However, if J is comparable or even smaller than the spectral bandwidth, the peak-to-peak frequency difference could be largely determined by the dephasing constant or bandwidth (see the peak shape analysis of 2D pump–probe spectrum given in Section 6.3).

EXERCISE 14.1

Even for a dilute solution of 2LS chromophores, one can create a large fraction of chromophores in their excited states with an intense laser pulse. Then, is it possible to radiate second harmonic field by a simultaneous de-excitation of two excited-state chromophores? If not, why? If yes, what are the requirements?

14.4 TWO-DIMENSIONAL SUM FREQUENCY GENERATION OF COUPLED ANHARMONIC OSCILLATORS

In Section 9.6, the model Hamiltonian of coupled anharmonic oscillators was presented. After diagonalizing the corresponding Hamiltonian matrices, one can obtain the eigenfunctions and eigenvalues of singly and doubly excited states. In this case, there are two singly excited states e_1 and e_2 that are delocalized over the two oscillators, and also there are three doubly excited states $f_1 - f_3$, which are either combination or overtone states. Due to the presence of three doubly excited states, the number of diagrams contributing to the 2D SFG signal field is six:

$$
\langle \mu \xleftarrow[f_1 \ \ e_1]{\mu E_2 \ \mu E_1} | g \rangle \langle g |, \quad
\langle \mu \xleftarrow[f_1 \ \ e_2]{\mu E_2 \ \mu E_1} | g \rangle \langle g |,
$$

$$
\langle \mu \xleftarrow[f_2 \ \ e_1]{\mu E_2 \ \mu E_1} | g \rangle \langle g |, \quad
\langle \mu \xleftarrow[f_2 \ \ e_2]{\mu E_2 \ \mu E_1} | g \rangle \langle g |,
$$

$$
\langle \mu \xleftarrow[f_3 \ \ e_1]{\mu E_2 \ \mu E_1} | g \rangle \langle g |, \quad \text{and} \quad
\langle \mu \xleftarrow[f_3 \ \ e_2]{\mu E_2 \ \mu E_1} | g \rangle \langle g |. \tag{14.31}
$$

From Equation 14.31, we have

$$
\begin{aligned}
\tilde{E}_{ZYX}^{SFG}(\omega_T,\omega_\tau) = &-i\mu_{gf_1}^M \cdot \left(\mu_{f_1 e_1}^M \times \mu_{e_1 g}^M \right) \Gamma\left(\overline{\omega}_{f_1 g}, \Delta_{f_1 f_1}^2, \overline{\omega}_{e_1 g}, \Delta_{e_1 e_1}^2 \right) \\
&-i\mu_{gf_1}^M \cdot \left(\mu_{f_1 e_2}^M \times \mu_{e_2 g}^M \right) \Gamma\left(\overline{\omega}_{f_1 g}, \Delta_{f_1 f_1}^2, \overline{\omega}_{e_2 g}, \Delta_{e_2 e_2}^2 \right) \\
&-i\mu_{gf_2}^M \cdot \left(\mu_{f_2 e_1}^M \times \mu_{e_1 g}^M \right) \Gamma\left(\overline{\omega}_{f_2 g}, \Delta_{f_2 f_2}^2, \overline{\omega}_{e_1 g}, \Delta_{e_1 e_1}^2 \right) \\
&-i\mu_{gf_2}^M \cdot \left(\mu_{f_2 e_2}^M \times \mu_{e_2 g}^M \right) \Gamma\left(\overline{\omega}_{f_2 g}, \Delta_{f_2 f_2}^2, \overline{\omega}_{e_2 g}, \Delta_{e_2 e_2}^2 \right) \\
&-i\mu_{gf_3}^M \cdot \left(\mu_{f_3 e_1}^M \times \mu_{e_1 g}^M \right) \Gamma\left(\overline{\omega}_{f_3 g}, \Delta_{f_3 f_3}^2, \overline{\omega}_{e_1 g}, \Delta_{e_1 e_1}^2 \right) \\
&-i\mu_{gf_3}^M \cdot \left(\mu_{f_3 e_2}^M \times \mu_{e_2 g}^M \right) \Gamma\left(\overline{\omega}_{f_3 g}, \Delta_{f_3 f_3}^2, \overline{\omega}_{e_2 g}, \Delta_{e_2 e_2}^2 \right).
\end{aligned} \tag{14.32}
$$

All the transition dipole matrix elements for a general coupled multi-chromophore system were already presented in Equation 9.81. The one-quantum transition dipole matrix elements are identical to those of a coupled 2LS dimer. In order to obtain the expressions for the other transition dipole matrix elements involving transitions to and from the doubly excited states in Equation 14.32, one should have the eigenvectors of the three doubly excited states. With the basis set of the doubly excited states, {|2,0>, |0,2>, |1,1>}, the eigenvector elements of the jth doubly excited state f_j were denoted as c_{j1}, c_{j2}, and c_{j3} (see Equation 9.76). To approximately calculate the transition dipole matrix elements between g and f_j states and between e_j and f_k states, it is useful to expand the electric dipole operator in terms of the coordinates of *local* oscillators as

$$\boldsymbol{\mu} = \boldsymbol{\mu}^{(0)} + \boldsymbol{\mu}_1^{(1)} q_1 + \boldsymbol{\mu}_2^{(1)} q_2 + \frac{1}{2}\boldsymbol{\mu}_1^{(2)} q_1^2 + \frac{1}{2}\boldsymbol{\mu}_2^{(2)} q_2^2 + \boldsymbol{\mu}_{12}^{(2)} q_1 q_2 + \cdots, \qquad (14.33)$$

where q_1 and q_2 are the two local oscillator coordinates and $\boldsymbol{\mu}_j^{(1)} = (\partial\boldsymbol{\mu}/\partial q_j)_0$, $\boldsymbol{\mu}_j^{(2)} = (\partial^2\boldsymbol{\mu}/\partial q_j^2)_0$, and $\boldsymbol{\mu}_{jk}^{(2)} = (\partial^2\boldsymbol{\mu}/\partial q_j \partial q_k)_0$. The second-order expansion terms in Equation 14.33 have been referred to as the electric anharmonicity.

Then, in addition to the two transition dipole matrix elements $\boldsymbol{\mu}_{e_1 g}^M$ and $\boldsymbol{\mu}_{e_2 g}^M$, the remaining matrix elements required for the calculation of Equation 14.32 are found to be

$$\begin{aligned}
\boldsymbol{\mu}_{f_1 e_1}^M &= \left(\sqrt{2}c_{11}\cos\theta + c_{13}\sin\theta\right)\boldsymbol{\mu}_1^{(1)} + \left(c_{13}\cos\theta + \sqrt{2}c_{12}\sin\theta\right)\boldsymbol{\mu}_2^{(1)} \\
\boldsymbol{\mu}_{f_2 e_1}^M &= \left(\sqrt{2}c_{21}\cos\theta + c_{23}\sin\theta\right)\boldsymbol{\mu}_1^{(1)} + \left(c_{23}\cos\theta + \sqrt{2}c_{22}\sin\theta\right)\boldsymbol{\mu}_2^{(1)} \\
\boldsymbol{\mu}_{f_1 e_2}^M &= \left(-\sqrt{2}c_{11}\sin\theta + c_{13}\cos\theta\right)\boldsymbol{\mu}_1^{(1)} + \left(-c_{13}\sin\theta + \sqrt{2}c_{12}\cos\theta\right)\boldsymbol{\mu}_2^{(1)} \\
\boldsymbol{\mu}_{f_2 e_2}^M &= \left(-\sqrt{2}c_{21}\sin\theta + c_{23}\cos\theta\right)\boldsymbol{\mu}_1^{(1)} + \left(-c_{23}\sin\theta + \sqrt{2}c_{22}\cos\theta\right)\boldsymbol{\mu}_2^{(1)} \\
\boldsymbol{\mu}_{f_3 e_1}^M &= \left(\sqrt{2}c_{31}\cos\theta + c_{33}\sin\theta\right)\boldsymbol{\mu}_1^{(1)} + \left(c_{33}\cos\theta + \sqrt{2}c_{32}\sin\theta\right)\boldsymbol{\mu}_2^{(1)} \\
\boldsymbol{\mu}_{f_3 e_2}^M &= \left(-\sqrt{2}c_{31}\sin\theta + c_{33}\cos\theta\right)\boldsymbol{\mu}_1^{(1)} + \left(-c_{33}\sin\theta + \sqrt{2}c_{32}\cos\theta\right)\boldsymbol{\mu}_2^{(1)} \\
\boldsymbol{\mu}_{f_1 g}^M &= c_{11}\boldsymbol{\mu}_1^{(2)} + c_{12}\boldsymbol{\mu}_2^{(2)} + c_{13}\boldsymbol{\mu}_{12}^{(2)} \\
\boldsymbol{\mu}_{f_2 g}^M &= c_{21}\boldsymbol{\mu}_1^{(2)} + c_{22}\boldsymbol{\mu}_2^{(2)} + c_{23}\boldsymbol{\mu}_{12}^{(2)} \\
\boldsymbol{\mu}_{f_3 g}^M &= c_{31}\boldsymbol{\mu}_1^{(2)} + c_{32}\boldsymbol{\mu}_2^{(2)} + c_{33}\boldsymbol{\mu}_{12}^{(2)}.
\end{aligned} \qquad (14.34)$$

One can calculate the first and second derivatives of dipole moment with respect to a given *local* oscillator coordinate by using a variety of quantum chemistry calculation methods with employing a finite difference method. However, the second derivatives such as $\boldsymbol{\mu}_{12}^{(2)}$ are strongly dependent on detailed structures of chiral molecules like dipeptides so that one should carry out quite a number of numerical calculations for varying conformations. Thus, the following approximate relationship between $\boldsymbol{\mu}_{12}^{(2)}$ and first derivative was found to be quite useful:

$$\left(\frac{\partial^2\boldsymbol{\mu}}{\partial q_1\partial q_2}\right)\approx\left(\frac{\partial\boldsymbol{\mu}}{\partial q_1}\right)\mathbf{T}\left(\frac{\partial\alpha}{\partial q_2}\right)+\left(\frac{\partial\alpha}{\partial q_1}\right)\mathbf{T}\left(\frac{\partial\boldsymbol{\mu}}{\partial q_2}\right), \quad (14.35)$$

where the transition polarizability denoted as $(\partial\alpha/\partial q_j)_0$, which is a second-rank tensor, can be readily calculated. Here, $\mathbf{T}$ is again the dipole-dipole interaction tensor. Note that $\boldsymbol{\mu}_{12}^{(2)}$ is a complicated function of the transition dipole vectors and polarizability tensors of the two local oscillators as well as of relative distance and orientation between the two.

Using the above transition dipole matrix elements, one can obtain the transition strengths for the six terms in Equation 14.32, which essentially determine the amplitude of each individual peak in the experimentally measured 2D SFG spectrum. For the coupled anharmonic oscillators, one can find the following three relationships,

$$\begin{aligned}
&\boldsymbol{\mu}_{gf_1}^M\cdot\left(\boldsymbol{\mu}_{f_1e_1}^M\times\boldsymbol{\mu}_{e_1g}^M\right)=-\boldsymbol{\mu}_{gf_1}^M\cdot\left(\boldsymbol{\mu}_{f_1e_2}^M\times\boldsymbol{\mu}_{e_2g}^M\right)\\
&\boldsymbol{\mu}_{gf_2}^M\cdot\left(\boldsymbol{\mu}_{f_2e_1}^M\times\boldsymbol{\mu}_{e_1g}^M\right)=-\boldsymbol{\mu}_{gf_2}^M\cdot\left(\boldsymbol{\mu}_{f_2e_2}^M\times\boldsymbol{\mu}_{e_2g}^M\right)\\
&\boldsymbol{\mu}_{gf_3}^M\cdot\left(\boldsymbol{\mu}_{f_3e_1}^M\times\boldsymbol{\mu}_{e_1g}^M\right)=-\boldsymbol{\mu}_{gf_3}^M\cdot\left(\boldsymbol{\mu}_{f_3e_2}^M\times\boldsymbol{\mu}_{e_2g}^M\right).
\end{aligned} \quad (14.36)$$

Therefore, there will appear three positive-negative couplets with frequency splitting of $\omega_{e_2e_1}$. Furthermore, the three terms in Equation 14.36 are found to be

$$\begin{aligned}
&\boldsymbol{\mu}_{gf_1}^M\cdot\left(\boldsymbol{\mu}_{f_1e_1}^M\times\boldsymbol{\mu}_{e_1g}^M\right)=A_1\left(c_{11}\boldsymbol{\mu}_1^{(2)}+c_{12}\boldsymbol{\mu}_2^{(2)}+c_{13}\boldsymbol{\mu}_{12}^{(2)}\right)\cdot\left(\boldsymbol{\mu}_1^{(1)}\times\boldsymbol{\mu}_2^{(1)}\right)\\
&\boldsymbol{\mu}_{gf_2}^M\cdot\left(\boldsymbol{\mu}_{f_2e_1}^M\times\boldsymbol{\mu}_{e_1g}^M\right)=A_2\left(c_{21}\boldsymbol{\mu}_1^{(2)}+c_{22}\boldsymbol{\mu}_2^{(2)}+c_{23}\boldsymbol{\mu}_{12}^{(2)}\right)\cdot\left(\boldsymbol{\mu}_1^{(1)}\times\boldsymbol{\mu}_2^{(1)}\right)\\
&\boldsymbol{\mu}_{gf_3}^M\cdot\left(\boldsymbol{\mu}_{f_3e_1}^M\times\boldsymbol{\mu}_{e_1g}^M\right)=A_3\left(c_{31}\boldsymbol{\mu}_1^{(2)}+c_{32}\boldsymbol{\mu}_2^{(2)}+c_{33}\boldsymbol{\mu}_{12}^{(2)}\right)\cdot\left(\boldsymbol{\mu}_1^{(1)}\times\boldsymbol{\mu}_2^{(1)}\right),
\end{aligned} \quad (14.37)$$

where $A_j=\sqrt{2}(c_{j1}-c_{j2})\cos\theta\sin\theta-c_{j3}\cos 2\theta$. From this result, one can deduce a set of selection rules for doubly resonant 2D SFG spectroscopy of coupled anharmonic oscillators. First of all, at least one of the three quantities, $\boldsymbol{\mu}_1^{(2)}\cdot(\boldsymbol{\mu}_1^{(1)}\times\boldsymbol{\mu}_2^{(1)})$, $\boldsymbol{\mu}_2^{(2)}\cdot(\boldsymbol{\mu}_1^{(1)}\times\boldsymbol{\mu}_2^{(1)})$, and $\boldsymbol{\mu}_{12}^{(2)}\cdot(\boldsymbol{\mu}_1^{(1)}\times\boldsymbol{\mu}_2^{(1)})$, should be nonzero. Secondly, the corresponding coefficient, such as A_1c_{11} that is the coefficient of $\boldsymbol{\mu}_1^{(2)}\cdot(\boldsymbol{\mu}_1^{(1)}\times\boldsymbol{\mu}_2^{(1)})$ in the expression for $\boldsymbol{\mu}_{gf_1}^M\cdot(\boldsymbol{\mu}_{f_1e_1}^M\times\boldsymbol{\mu}_{e_1g}^M)$, should be nonzero. Let us consider the zero coupling limit, that is, uncoupled anharmonic oscillators. In this case, one can show that $A_j=0$ for all j (= 1 ~ 3). As a result, nonzero coupling is a requirement for the doubly resonant 2D SFG. Thirdly, in addition to nonzero transition dipoles of the two local oscillators, the second-derivatives of dipole moment with respect to the vibrational coordinates, such as $\boldsymbol{\mu}_1^{(2)}$, $\boldsymbol{\mu}_2^{(2)}$, and $\boldsymbol{\mu}_{12}^{(2)}$, should be finite, that is, nonzero electric anharmonicities.

In the case of the coupled 2LS dimer discussed in Section 14.3, the doubly excited state is just a product of excited state wavefunctions of the 2LS chromophores. However, due to the potential anharmonicities of the coupled anharmonic oscillators, the transition dipole matrix elements between g and f_j states can be nonzero even in the limiting case when the second derivatives of the electric dipole with respect to vibrational coordinates, which are $\boldsymbol{\mu}_1^{(2)}$, $\boldsymbol{\mu}_2^{(2)}$, and $\boldsymbol{\mu}_{12}^{(2)}$, are vanishingly small. In Equation 14.37, the two-quantum transition dipole matrix element representing the amplitude of transition between f_j and g states is, in this case of vanishingly small electric anharmonicity, given by

$$< f_j | \boldsymbol{\mu} | g > = < f_j | \boldsymbol{\mu}_1^{(1)} q_1 + \boldsymbol{\mu}_2^{(1)} q_2 | g > = \boldsymbol{\mu}_1^{(1)} < f_j | q_1 | g > + \boldsymbol{\mu}_2^{(1)} < f_j | q_2 | g > . \quad (14.38)$$

The above quantity vanishes if the ground- and doubly-excited states are harmonic oscillator wavefunctions. In reality, they are nonzero due to the potential (mechanical) anharmonicity. Using the Rayleigh-Schrödinger perturbation theory and treating the anharmonic potential as perturbation Hamiltonian, one can express the doubly excited state f_j as a linear combination of product states of harmonic oscillator wavefunctions. However, the two-quantum transition dipole contributions from mechanical anharmonicity may not be important in the 2D SFG or DFG, because $\boldsymbol{\mu}_1^{(1)}$ and $\boldsymbol{\mu}_2^{(1)}$ are orthogonal to $\boldsymbol{\mu}_1^{(1)} \times \boldsymbol{\mu}_2^{(1)}$ vector. However, any deviation from the above approximation, Equation 14.38, can make the mechanical anharmonicity-induced contribution to $\boldsymbol{\mu}_{f_j g}$ non-negligible.

In the previous section, an enhancement of frequency resolution via 2D SFG measurement for a coupled 2LS dimer was discussed. Similarly, one can expect the same frequency-resolution enhancement of 2D SFG for coupled anharmonic oscillators. The IR absorption spectroscopy is essentially determined by the two independent one-quantum transition processes between g and e_1 and between g and e_2 states. Thus, even in the case when the 1D spectrum is spectrally congested, the 2D SFG spectrum of coupled anharmonic oscillators could exhibit six different frequency-resolved peaks. Particularly, there will appear three positive-negative dual peaks (couplets), where the frequency difference between the positive and negative peaks in a given couplet is related to the transition frequency difference between the two singly excited states e_1 and e_2. Furthermore, the relative energies of f_j states can be determined by examining the 2D SFG spectrum. Noting that the frequency splits in the manifold of singly excited states and those of doubly excited states are highly sensitive to the detailed structure of the coupled system, the time-resolved 2D SFG spectroscopy of coupled multi-chromophore system in solution can be a useful tool for studying structure and dynamics of complex molecules. For such a multilevel system, the expression for the 2D SFG spectrum in Equation 14.23 can be used to numerically calculate or to find a proper way to interpret the experimentally measured spectrum.

EXERCISE 14.2

The second selection rule for doubly resonant 2D SFG of coupled anharmonic oscillators is that the coupling J should be nonzero. Why do all A_j values in Equation 14.37 vanish in the zero coupling limit?

14.5 TWO-DIMENSIONAL DIFFERENCE FREQUENCY GENERATION

In the previous sections, only the 2D SFG spectroscopy was considered for both coupled 2LS dimer and coupled anharmonic oscillators. However, it is a straightforward exercise to develop a theory for the 2D DFG spectroscopy. DFG is another three-wave-mixing process involving two electric dipole interactions with external field. Similar to the SFG, the first interaction of matter with $\mathbf{E}_1$ electric field propagating in the $\mathbf{k}_1$-direction induces an absorptive transition from g to f, and the second one with $\mathbf{E}_2$ electric field component traveling in the direction of $-\mathbf{k}_2$ induces a stimulated emissive transition from f to e. Here, it is assumed that $E_f > E_e > E_g$. Then, thus created coherence $\rho_{eg}^{(2)}$ radiates a coherent electric field whose frequency is the difference of the $\mathbf{E}_1$ and $\mathbf{E}_2$ field frequencies. In this case of DFG, the effective radiation–matter interactions and effect operator are

$$\hat{A}_1 F_1(t) = \boldsymbol{\mu} \cdot \mathbf{e}_1 E_1(t) e^{i k_1 \cdot \mathbf{r} - i \omega_1 t}$$

$$\hat{A}_2 F_2(t) = \boldsymbol{\mu} \cdot \mathbf{e}_2^* E_2^*(t) e^{-i k_2 \cdot \mathbf{r} + i \omega_2 t}$$

$$\hat{B} = \boldsymbol{\mu} \cdot \tag{14.39}$$

The polarization components that are associated with this DFG are then diagrammatically represented as

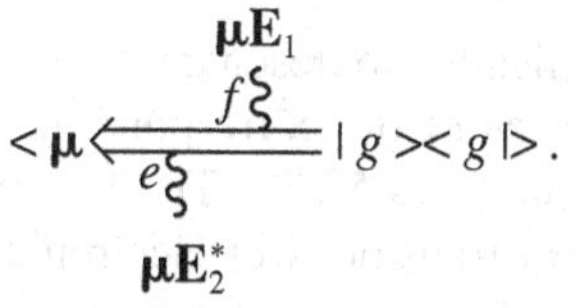

$$\begin{matrix} & \mu E_1 \\ & f \gtrless \\ <\mu \Longleftarrow & \overline{} | g > < g | > . \\ & e \gtrless \\ & \mu E_2^* \end{matrix} \tag{14.40}$$

Using the second-order response function theory with the above cause- and effect-operators with conjugate external fields, one can find that the second-order DFG polarization is given as

$$\mathbf{P}_{DFG}(\mathbf{r},t) = e^{i(\mathbf{k}_1 - \mathbf{k}_2) \cdot \mathbf{r} - i(\omega_1 - \omega_2)t} \int_0^\infty dt_2 \int_0^\infty dt_1 \ \phi_{\mu\mu\mu}(t_2, t_1) : \mathbf{e}_2^* \mathbf{e}_1 E_2^*(t - t_2)$$

$$\times E_1(t - t_2 - t_1) e^{i(\omega_1 - \omega_2)t_2 + i\omega_1 t_1} . \tag{14.41}$$

Note that the second-order DFG polarization propagates in the direction of $\mathbf{k}_1 - \mathbf{k}_2$ and oscillates with frequency of $\omega_1 - \omega_2$. Instead of electronically nonresonant DFG, which has been extensively used to generate different color radiation and also to study electronic and optical properties of molecules on surface or at interface, we shall consider the doubly resonant DFG,

$$\hat{\mathbf{E}}_{DFG}(t) = \frac{i\omega_s}{\hbar^2} e^{i(\mathbf{k}_1-\mathbf{k}_2)\cdot\mathbf{r}-i(\omega_1-\omega_2)t} \boldsymbol{\mu}_{ge}\boldsymbol{\mu}_{ef}\boldsymbol{\mu}_{fg} : \mathbf{e}_2^*\mathbf{e}_1 \int_0^\infty dt_2 \int_0^\infty dt_1 \{G_1(t_2,t_1)e^{i(\omega_1-\omega_2-\bar{\omega}_{eg})t_2+i(\omega_1-\bar{\omega}_{fg})t_1}$$

$$-G_2(t_2,t_1)e^{i(\omega_1-\omega_2-\bar{\omega}_{fe})t_2+i(\omega_1-\bar{\omega}_{fg})t_1}\}E_2^*(t-t_2)E_1(t-t_2-t_1) \tag{14.42}$$

where the line-shape function $G_1(t_2\ t_1)$ is identical to Equation 14.9 except that e and f are exchanged.

Now, similar to the SFG, one can use this DFG method to study molecular chirality too. Focusing on the XYZ-tensor element of the DFG response function, one can find that the 2D DFG spectrum within the 2D Gaussian peak shape approximation is given as

$$\tilde{\mathrm{E}}_{XYZ}^{DFG}(\omega_T,\omega_\tau) = -\frac{i\omega_s}{6\hbar^2}\boldsymbol{\mu}_{ge}^M \cdot \left(\boldsymbol{\mu}_{ef}^M \times \boldsymbol{\mu}_{fg}^M\right)\{\Gamma\left(\bar{\omega}_{eg},\Delta_{ee}^2,\bar{\omega}_{fg},\Delta_{ff}^2\right) - \Gamma\left(\bar{\omega}_{fe},\Delta_{ff}^2+\Delta_{ee}^2,\bar{\omega}_{fg},\Delta_{ff}^2\right)\} \tag{14.43}$$

For the coupled 2LS dimer and coupled anharmonic oscillators, by following the same procedures in Section 14.4, detailed theoretical expressions for the doubly resonant 2D DFG spectra can be obtained. This task will be left for the readers.

EXERCISE 14.3

Obtain the expressions for the 2D DFG spectra of coupled 2LS dimer and of coupled anharmonic oscillators, which should be similar to Equations 14.25 and 14.32. Provide a discussion on selection rules from the resulting expressions.

14.6 IR–IR-VIS SUM FREQUENCY GENERATION AND DIFFERENCE FREQUENCY GENERATION

In Section 4.5, the electronically nonresonant IR-IR-vis (IIV) four-wave-mixing process was described in terms of the corresponding second-order response function $\phi_{\alpha\mu\mu}(t_2,t_1)$ defined in Equation 4.57.[10, 11] The first two IR beams induce doubly resonant-enhanced vibrational transitions of electronically ground-state molecules. Then, the visible beam whose frequency is far from any of electronic transition frequencies is used to induce a Raman scattering process to generate coherently emitted IIV four-wave-mixing signal field.[10, 12–14] One practical advantage of this IIV-SFG or IIV-DFG over the other 2D vibrational spectroscopic techniques is that the detected signal field is visible and electronically nonresonant. Therefore, the signal field is not reabsorbed by the molecular system, whereas the photon echo signal field is reabsorbed by the sample so that it usually requires a narrow sample thickness and low optical density. In this particular case of IIV-SFG or IIV-DFG, the two cause operators are electric dipole operators and the effect operator is the dipole induced by a single radiation–matter interaction with electronically nonresonant visible electric field.

The model system considered here consists of three vibrational states, g, e, and f, with a single virtual state. Here, the virtual state is needed just as an intermediate state for the Raman process. As shown in Section 4.5, the two radiation–matter interactions and effect operator that are relevant to the IIV-SFG are given as

$$\hat{A}_1 F_1(t) = \boldsymbol{\mu} \cdot \mathbf{e}_{IR1} E_{IR1}(t)\, e^{i\mathbf{k}_{IR1}\cdot\mathbf{r} - i\omega_{IR1}t}$$

$$\hat{A}_2 F_2(t) = \boldsymbol{\mu} \cdot \mathbf{e}_{IR2} E_{IR2}(t)\, e^{i\mathbf{k}_{IR2}\cdot\mathbf{r} - i\omega_{IR2}t}$$

$$\hat{B} = \boldsymbol{\mu}_{ind}(\mathrm{r},t) = \boldsymbol{\alpha} \cdot \mathbf{E}_{vis}(t)\, e^{i\mathbf{k}_{vis}\cdot\mathbf{r} - i\omega_{vis}t}. \tag{14.44}$$

On the other hand, for the IIV-DFG, the corresponding interaction Hamiltonians and effect operator are

$$\hat{A}_1 F_1(t) = \boldsymbol{\mu} \cdot \mathbf{e}_{IR1} E_{IR1}(t)\, e^{i\mathbf{k}_{IR1}\cdot\mathbf{r} - i\omega_{IR1}t}$$

$$\hat{A}_2 F_2(t) = \boldsymbol{\mu} \cdot \mathbf{e}^*_{IR2} E^*_{IR2}(t)\, e^{-i\mathbf{k}_{IR2}\cdot\mathbf{r} + i\omega_{IR2}t}$$

$$\hat{B} = \boldsymbol{\mu}_{ind}(\mathrm{r},t) = \boldsymbol{\alpha} \cdot \mathbf{e}_{vis} E_{vis}(t)\, e^{i\mathbf{k}_{vis}\cdot\mathbf{r} - i\omega_{vis}t}. \tag{14.45}$$

Since the theoretical result for the IIV-DFG is essentially identical to that for the IIV-SFG, we shall focus on the IIV-SFG process only.

The diagram representation of the IIV-SFG polarization is given as

$$< \alpha \mathrm{E}_{vis} \xleftarrow[\;]{\; \boldsymbol{\mu}\mathbf{E}_{\mathrm{IR2}}\ \boldsymbol{\mu}\mathbf{E}_{\mathrm{IR1}} \atop f\,\xi \quad e\,\xi \;} | g >< g |, \tag{14.46}$$

which is

$$\mathbf{P}_{IIV-SFG}(\mathbf{r},t) = e^{i(\mathbf{k}_{IR1}+\mathbf{k}_{IR2}+\mathbf{k}_{vis})\cdot\mathbf{r} - i(\omega_{IR1}+\omega_{IR2}+\omega_{vis})t}$$
$$\times E_{vis}(t) \int_0^\infty dt_2 \int_0^\infty dt_1\ \phi_{\alpha\mu\mu}(t_2,t_1) \vdots \mathbf{e}_{vis}\mathbf{e}_{IR2}\mathbf{e}_{IR1} E_{IR2}(t-t_2)$$
$$\times E_{IR1}(t-t_2-t_1)\, e^{i(\omega_{IR1}+\omega_{IR2})t_2 + i\omega_{IR1}t_1}. \tag{14.47}$$

The second-order response function $\phi_{\alpha\mu\mu}(t_2,t_1)$ is

$$\phi_{\alpha\mu\mu}(t_2,t_1) = \left(\frac{i}{\hbar}\right)^2 \theta(t_2)\theta(t_1) < [[\boldsymbol{\alpha}(t_2+t_1), \boldsymbol{\mu}(t_1)], \boldsymbol{\mu}(0)]\rho(-\infty) >. \tag{14.48}$$

For a three-level system with $E_f > E_e > E_g$, we have $\omega_{IR1} + \omega_{IR2} \simeq \bar{\omega}_{fg}$, and $\omega_{IR1} \simeq \bar{\omega}_{eg}$. Then, considering the doubly resonant term in the second-order response function components, one can find that the IIV-SFG signal field is approximately given as

$$\mathbf{E}_{IIV-SFG}(\mathbf{r},t) = -\frac{i\omega_s}{\hbar^2} e^{i\mathbf{k}_s\cdot\mathbf{r}-i\omega_s t}\, \boldsymbol{\alpha}_{gf}\boldsymbol{\mu}_{fe}\boldsymbol{\mu}_{eg} \vdots\, \mathbf{e}_{vis}\mathbf{e}_{IR2}\mathbf{e}_{IR1}E_{vis}(t)\int_0^\infty dt_2 \int_0^\infty dt_1\, G_1(t_2,t_1)$$
$$\times E_{IR2}(t-t_2)E_{IR1}(t-t_2-t_1)\, e^{i(\omega_{IR1}+\omega_{IR2}-\bar{\omega}_{fg})t_2 + i(\omega_{IR1}-\bar{\omega}_{eg})t_1}. \quad (14.49)$$

Assuming that the two IR pulse amplitudes peak at $t = -T - \tau$ and $t = -T$ and that they are impulsive, we have

$$\mathbf{E}_{IIV-SFG}(\mathbf{r},t) \propto -\frac{i\omega_s}{\hbar^2} e^{i\mathbf{k}_s\cdot\mathbf{r}-i\omega_s t}\, \boldsymbol{\alpha}_{gf}\boldsymbol{\mu}_{fe}\boldsymbol{\mu}_{eg} \vdots\, \mathbf{e}_{vis}\mathbf{e}_{IR2}\mathbf{e}_{IR1}E_{vis}(t)G_1(t+T,\tau)$$
$$\times\, e^{i(\omega_{IR1}+\omega_{IR2}-\bar{\omega}_{fg})T + i(\omega_{IR1}-\bar{\omega}_{eg})\tau}. \quad (14.50)$$

This signal electric field is allowed to interfere with an independent local oscillator whose frequency is identical to that of the signal field. Here, the local oscillator field is also assumed to be impulsive. Then, the measured signal is Fourier–Laplace transformed to obtain the corresponding 2D IIV-SFG spectrum. Using the 2D Gaussian peak shape approximation, we get

$$\tilde{\mathbf{E}}_{IIV-SFG}(\omega_T,\omega_\tau) = -\frac{i\omega_s}{\hbar^2} \boldsymbol{\alpha}_{gf}\boldsymbol{\mu}_{fe}\boldsymbol{\mu}_{eg} \vdots\, \mathbf{e}_{vis}\mathbf{e}_{IR2}\mathbf{e}_{IR1}\Gamma\left(\bar{\omega}_{fg},\Delta^2_{ff},\bar{\omega}_{eg},\Delta^2_{ee}\right). \quad (14.51)$$

This result can be easily generalized to a multistate system. For N-coupled multichromophore systems, where each chromophore is a 2LS (3LS), there are N singly excited states $\{e_j\}$ and $N(N-1)/2$ ($N(N+1)/2$) doubly excited states. In that case, Equation 14.51 should be rewritten as the sum over all possible contributions,

$$\tilde{\mathbf{E}}_{IIV-SFG}(\omega_T,\omega_\tau) = -\frac{i\omega_s}{\hbar^2}\sum_j\sum_k \boldsymbol{\alpha}_{gf_k}\boldsymbol{\mu}_{f_ke_j}\boldsymbol{\mu}_{e_jg} \vdots\, \mathbf{e}_{vis}\mathbf{e}_{IR2}\mathbf{e}_{IR1}\Gamma\left(\bar{\omega}_{f_kg},\Delta^2_{f_kf_k},\bar{\omega}_{e_jg},\Delta^2_{e_je_j}\right). \quad (14.52)$$

Note that the measured 2D spectrum results from interferences of different pathways contributing to IIV-SFG at amplitude level. Now, from Equation 14.52, it becomes possible to deduce the selection rules for IIV-SFG. Firstly, the two vibrational modes (transitions) should be IR-active. The last vibrational transition from f to g is a Raman transition process so that it should be Raman-allowed. Unlike other three-wave-mixing processes, the IIV-SFG is a four-wave-mixing process so that it is readily applicable to isotropic solution sample.

The next step is to calculate the rotational average of the IIV-SFG field over randomly oriented molecules in an isotropic medium. Assume that the three incident beam propagation directions are *almost* parallel to the Z-axis in a space-fixed frame and that they are linearly polarized in the direction parallel to the X-axis. Then, if the X-component of the IIV-SFG field vector is detected, the 2D IIV-SFG spectrum is found to be

$$\tilde{E}_X^{IIV-SFG}(\omega_T,\omega_\tau) = -\frac{i\omega_s}{\hbar^2}\sum_j\sum_k[\boldsymbol{\alpha}_{gf_k}\boldsymbol{\mu}_{f_ke_j}\boldsymbol{\mu}_{e_jg}]_{XXXX}\Gamma\left(\bar{\omega}_{f_kg},\Delta^2_{f_kf_k},\bar{\omega}_{e_jg},\Delta^2_{e_je_j}\right)$$

$$= -\frac{i\omega_s}{15\hbar^2}\sum_j\sum_k\Gamma\left(\bar{\omega}_{f_kg},\Delta^2_{f_kf_k},\bar{\omega}_{e_jg},\Delta^2_{e_je_j}\right)$$

$$\times \sum_{m_1,m_2,m_3,m_4=x,y,z}(\delta_{m_1m_2}\delta_{m_3m_4}+\delta_{m_1m_3}\delta_{m_2m_4}+\delta_{m_1m_4}\delta_{m_2m_3})$$

$$\times[\boldsymbol{\alpha}_{gf_k}\boldsymbol{\mu}_{f_ke_j}\boldsymbol{\mu}_{e_jg}]^M_{m_1m_2m_3m_4}. \qquad (14.53)$$

Here, the transition polarizability and dipole matrix elements in the square bracket $[\ldots]^M$ in Equation 14.53 are those in a molecule-fixed frame. The IIV-SFG spectrum displayed in the 2D frequency space spanned by ω_τ and ω_T could exhibit cross-peaks, and their amplitudes are critically dependent on electronic structure via both electric and mechanical anharmonicities. Particularly, these anharmonicities are secondary spectroscopic properties and highly sensitive functions of molecular conformation.[11, 15, 16] Thus, establishing relationships between cross-peak amplitudes and various anharmonic properties is invaluable for quantitative analysis of experimentally measured 2D IIV-SFG spectrum to eventually extract information on molecular structure and dynamics of complex molecules in condensed phases.

We next consider the transition dipole and polarizability matrix elements for weakly anharmonic oscillators more in detail. Without loss of generality, it is assumed that the first transition from g to e corresponds to the vibrational transition of q_1-mode. The second transition from e to f state corresponds to the vibrational transition of q_2-mode. Then, the ground state, singly excited state, and doubly excited state can be written in terms of the vibrational quantum numbers of the two modes as

$$|g\rangle = |0_1,0_2\rangle$$

$$|e\rangle = |1_1,0_2\rangle$$

$$|f\rangle = |1_1,1_2\rangle. \qquad (14.54)$$

Here, n_1 and n_2 in $|n_1, n_2\rangle$ are the corresponding vibrational quantum numbers. For anharmonic oscillators, by using the first-order Rayleigh-Schrödinger perturbation theory, it is possible to expand the anharmonic wavefunctions in Equation 14.54 as

$$|0_1,0_2\rangle = |0_1,0_2\rangle^{(0)} + |0_1,0_2\rangle^{(1)}, \qquad (14.55)$$

where the zero-order term $|0_1, 0_2>^{(0)}$ is just the product state of harmonic oscillator wavefunctions, and the first-order correction term $|0_1, 0_2>^{(1)}$ is given as

$$|0_1,0_2>^{(1)}=\sum_{K\neq|0_1,0_2>^{(0)}}\frac{^{(0)}<K|V_{anh}|0_1,0_2>^{(0)}}{-\hbar\omega_K}|K>^{(0)}. \tag{14.56}$$

Here, the summation is over all possible product states of harmonic oscillator wavefunctions, except for $|0_1, 0_2>^{(0)}$. Similarly, the combination state f is expanded as

$$|1_1,1_2>=|1_1,1_2>^{(0)}+|1_1,1_2>^{(1)}, \tag{14.57}$$

where

$$|1_1,1_2>^{(1)}=\sum_{M\neq|1_1,1_2>^{(0)}}\frac{^{(0)}<M|V_{anh}|1_1,1_2>^{(0)}}{\hbar(\omega_1+\omega_2-\omega_M)}|M>^{(0)}. \tag{14.58}$$

In Equations 14.56 and 14.58, V_{anh} is the anharmonic part of the potential function, that is,

$$\begin{aligned}V_{anh}(\mathbf{q})&=\frac{1}{3!}\sum_{ijk}\left(\frac{\partial^3 V}{\partial q_i\partial q_j\partial q_k}\right)_0 q_iq_jq_k+\frac{1}{4!}\sum_{ijkl}\left(\frac{\partial^4 V}{\partial q_i\partial q_j\partial q_k\partial q_l}\right)_0 q_iq_jq_kq_l+\cdots\\&=\sum_{i\le j\le k}v_{ijk}^{(3)}q_iq_jq_k+\sum_{i\le j\le k\le l}v_{ijkl}^{(3)}q_iq_jq_kq_l+\cdots.\end{aligned} \tag{14.59}$$

Now, the transition dipole matrix elements determining the transition strength of the IIV-SFG process are associated with one-quantum vibrational transitions that are allowed for harmonic oscillators, that is,

$$<e|\hat{\boldsymbol{\mu}}|g>\cong\boldsymbol{\mu}_1^{(1)}<e|q_1|g>\cong\boldsymbol{\mu}_1^{(1)}\,^{(0)}<1_1,0_2|q_1|0_1,0_2>^{(0)}=\sqrt{\frac{\hbar}{2m_1\omega_1}}\boldsymbol{\mu}_1^{(1)}$$

$$<f|\hat{\boldsymbol{\mu}}|e>\cong\boldsymbol{\mu}_2^{(1)}<f|q_2|e>\cong\boldsymbol{\mu}_2^{(1)}\,^{(0)}<1_1,1_2|q_2|1_1,0_2>^{(0)}=\sqrt{\frac{\hbar}{2m_2\omega_2}}\boldsymbol{\mu}_2^{(1)}, \tag{14.60}$$

where $\boldsymbol{\mu}_j^{(1)}\equiv(\partial\boldsymbol{\mu}/\partial q_j)_0$ and m_j and ω_j are the reduced mass and angular frequency of the jth oscillator.

Next, let us consider the two-quantum transition polarizability matrix element $\boldsymbol{\alpha}_{gf}$, defined as $\boldsymbol{\alpha}_{gf}=<g|\hat{\boldsymbol{\alpha}}|f>$. Again, in order to calculate this matrix element, it is necessary to expand the polarizability operator in terms of vibrational coordinates as

$$\hat{\boldsymbol{\alpha}}=\boldsymbol{\alpha}^{(0)}+\sum_j\boldsymbol{\alpha}_j^{(1)}q_j+\frac{1}{2}\sum_{j,k}\boldsymbol{\alpha}_{jk}^{(2)}q_jq_k+\cdots \tag{14.61}$$

where $\boldsymbol{\alpha}_j^{(1)} \equiv (\partial\boldsymbol{\alpha}/\partial q_j)_0$ and $\boldsymbol{\alpha}_{jk}^{(2)} \equiv (\partial^2\boldsymbol{\alpha}/\partial q_j \partial q_k)_0$. Then, $\boldsymbol{\alpha}_{gf}$ is given as the sum of two distinctively different terms,[17]

$$\boldsymbol{\alpha}_{gf} = <0_1,0_2 \,|\, \hat{\boldsymbol{\alpha}} \,|\, 1_1,1_2> = \boldsymbol{\alpha}_{gf}^{elec} + \boldsymbol{\alpha}_{gf}^{mech} \tag{14.62}$$

where $\boldsymbol{\alpha}_{gf}^{elec}$ and $\boldsymbol{\alpha}_{gf}^{mech}$ are the contributions associated with electric and mechanical anharmonicities, respectively:

$$\boldsymbol{\alpha}_{gf}^{elec} = {}^{(0)}\!<0_1,0_2 \,|\, q_1 q_2 \,|\, 1_1,1_2>^{(0)} \boldsymbol{\alpha}_{12}^{(2)} = \frac{\hbar}{2\sqrt{m_1\omega_1 m_2\omega_2}} \boldsymbol{\alpha}_{12}^{(2)} \tag{14.63}$$

and

$$\boldsymbol{\alpha}_{gf}^{mech} = \sum_j c_j \boldsymbol{\alpha}_j^{(1)} \tag{14.64}$$

with

$$c_j = {}^{(0)}\!<0_1,0_2 \,|\, q_j \,|\, 1_1,1_2>^{(1)} + {}^{(1)}\!<0_1,0_2 \,|\, q_j \,|\, 1_1,1_2>^{(0)}. \tag{14.65}$$

Note that c_j values vanish for perfect harmonic oscillators. Inserting the first-order wavefunction corrections $|\, 1_1,1_2>^{(1)}$ and ${}^{(1)}\!<0_1,0_2 \,|$ into Equation 14.65 above, we get

$$c_j = \frac{\hbar}{4\sqrt{m_1\omega_1 m_2\omega_2}} \frac{v_{12j}^{(3)}}{m_j\omega_j(\omega_1+\omega_2-\omega_j)}. \tag{14.66}$$

Here, the definition of $v_{12j}^{(3)}$ was given in Equation 14.59. In Equation 14.64, two important terms are those for j = 1 and 2 because the diagonal cubic anharmonic coefficients $v_{112}^{(3)}$ and $v_{122}^{(3)}$ are usually larger than any other coefficients $v_{12j}^{(3)}$ (for $j \neq 1$ and 2).[11] However, if there is a mode j with large $v_{12j}^{(3)}$ (for $j \neq 1$ and 2) and/or if the sum of ω_1 and ω_2 is close to its frequency ω_j as $\omega_j \approx \omega_1 + \omega_2$, it acts like a promoting mode that makes the resonant-enhanced anharmonic coupling between the two modes 1 and 2 sizable.[17] For example, if the two modes are the same, that is, $\omega_1 = \omega_2$, so that the doubly excited state is just its overtone state, the resonantly enhanced anharmonic coupling induced by the other promoting mode whose frequency is approximately twice of the target mode frequency is known as the 1:2 Fermi resonance coupling.[18] Now, the above results on mechanical couplings suggest that the anharmonic couplings between the two modes via $v_{112}^{(3)} q_1^2 q_2$ and $v_{122}^{(3)} q_1 q_2^2$ or the presence of promoting modes that are involved in an anharmonic coupling between q_1 and q_2 modes are critical in making the mechanical anharmonicity-induced IIV-SFG process.

Combining the results for the electric and mechanical anharmonicity contributions to the two-quantum transition polarizability matrix element, we have

$$\boldsymbol{\alpha}_{gf}\boldsymbol{\mu}_{fe}\boldsymbol{\mu}_{eg} \cong \frac{\hbar}{2\sqrt{m_1\omega_1 m_2\omega_2}}\left\{\boldsymbol{\alpha}_{12}^{(2)}\boldsymbol{\mu}_1^{(1)}\boldsymbol{\mu}_1^{(1)} + \sum_j \frac{v_{12j}^{(3)}}{2m_j\omega_j(\omega_1+\omega_2-\omega_j)}\boldsymbol{\alpha}_j^{(1)}\boldsymbol{\mu}_1^{(1)}\boldsymbol{\mu}_1^{(1)}\right\}. \tag{14.67}$$

Note that this quantity determines the amplitude of the cross peak at $\omega_\tau = \omega_1$ and $\omega_T = \omega_1 + \omega_2 - \Delta_{12}$, where Δ_{12} is the combination anharmonic frequency shift. In summary, the cross peaks in a given 2D IIV-SFG spectrum are produced by two different coupling mechanisms. The first coupling mechanism originates from nonzero electric anharmonicity, which originates from nonlinear dependency of polarizability operator (or electric dipole operator) with respect to vibrational coordinates. The second coupling mechanism is from the mechanical anharmonicity. Two different modes are coupled to each other due to finite potential anharmonicity. Sometimes, a third mode participates in an enhancement of the mechanical coupling between the two, if the corresponding cubic anharmonic coefficient is large and the Fermi-type resonance enhancement factor of $(\omega_1 + \omega_2 - \omega_j)^{-1}$ is large. Thus, an experimental observation of cross-peak at $\omega_\tau = \omega_1$ and $\omega_T = \omega_1 + \omega_2$ means that the corresponding two modes are coupled via one or both of the above coupling mechanisms.

EXERCISE 14.4

In the main context and Equation 14.66, we only considered cubic anharmonicity for the possible mechanical coupling processes. Thus, the Fermi resonance enhancement of the anharmonic coupling was discussed. However, if the quartic terms in the anharmonically expanded potential function are included in Equations 14.65 and 14.66, there will be more terms contributing to the mechanical coupling. In particular, the Darling-Dennison resonance enhancement of the mechanical coupling is expected to be very large. Discuss this possibility and obtain the expression for $\boldsymbol{\alpha}_{gf}^{mech}$.

An early IIV four-wave-mixing experiment was performed to measure the cross-peak between CC stretch and CN stretch modes in CH_3CN molecule.[12, 13] Instead of IIV-SFG, the IIV-DFG method in frequency domain was used to obtain the corresponding 2D spectrum, where the first IR radiation–matter interaction induces transition from g to f, where the f state is the combination state of the CC and CN stretch modes. To determine the absolute magnitude of the corresponding IIV-DFG cross peak, *ab initio* calculations of all the required vibrational properties including harmonic frequencies, reduced masses, transition dipole and polarizability matrix elements $\boldsymbol{\mu}_j^{(1)}$ and $\boldsymbol{\alpha}_j^{(1)}$, cubic anharmonic coefficients, $v_{ijk}^{(3)}$, and electric anharmonicities of dipole moments, $\boldsymbol{\mu}_{jk}^{(2)}$, were performed.[17] Note that the IIV-DFG involves a two-quantum dipole transition from g to f instead of two-quantum polarizability transition. Thus, the second derivatives of dipole moment such as $\boldsymbol{\mu}_{jk}^{(2)}$ were needed instead of $\boldsymbol{\alpha}_{jk}^{(2)}$. It turned out that, in the case of the IIV-DFG cross-peak between the CC and CN stretching vibrations, both electric and mechanical anharmonic contributions, which are $\boldsymbol{\mu}_{gf}^{elec}$ and $\boldsymbol{\mu}_{gf}^{mech}$, are comparable in magnitude.

If two oscillators are not directly connected to each other via chemical bonds, the contribution from mechanical anharmonicity-induced coupling can be small in comparison to that from electric anharmonicity-induced coupling. The former can be considered a through-bond coupling and the latter a through-space coupling. If the electric anharmonic coupling is the dominant contribution, the signal amplitude (intensity) is linearly proportional to $\boldsymbol{\alpha}_{12}^{(2)}$ ($[\boldsymbol{\alpha}_{12}^{(2)}]^2$). Noting that $\boldsymbol{\alpha}_{12}^{(2)}$ can be approximately written as $2\boldsymbol{\alpha}_1^{(1)}\mathbf{T}_{12}\boldsymbol{\alpha}_2^{(1)}$ and that $\mathbf{T}_{12}$ is inversely proportional to $1/R^3$, one finds that the signal amplitude (intensity) decays as $1/R^3$ ($1/R^6$). Furthermore, $\boldsymbol{\alpha}_{12}^{(2)}$ approximated as above strongly depends on the relative orientations of the two modes via $2\boldsymbol{\alpha}_1^{(1)}\mathbf{T}_{12}\boldsymbol{\alpha}_2^{(1)}$. Thus, the IIV four-wave-mixing signal amplitude (intensity) can provide information on distance and geometry of the two oscillators.

It is interesting to compare the present 2D spectroscopy probing molecular second-order response with the third-order response 2D vibrational spectroscopy, for example, 2D photon echo.[19] In the latter case, the vibrational couplings at the level of harmonic oscillator wavefunctions are important in producing nonzero cross peaks. On the other hand, the IIV-SFG, for example, requires different types of couplings originating from mechanical and electric anharmonicities. Thus, the extracted information from the 2D vibrational spectroscopy based on the second-order response measurement is distinctively different from that with the photon echo–type 2D vibrational spectroscopy. Thus, the 2D second-order response spectroscopy should be considered a complementary method capable of extracting another class of secondary spectroscopic properties of coupled multi-chromophore systems and polyatomic molecules.

14.7 OTHER IR–IR-VIS FOUR-WAVE-MIXINGS

The time-resolved IIV-SFG and -DFG spectroscopy utilizes two infrared pulses to create consecutive vibrational coherences (or 2D vibrational transient grating), and then radiated signal field by oscillating induced-dipoles is detected. Since the third radiation–matter interaction can be effectively described by an electronically nonresonant Raman process, the corresponding second-order response function is in essence two-time correlation function, $\phi_{\alpha\mu\mu}(t_2, t_1)$.[10, 18] The sequence of involved radiation–matter interactions is thus IR-excitation, IR-excitation, and Raman transition. However, one can create such 2D vibrational coherences in the sample via IR-excitation + Raman-excitation or Raman-excitation + IR-excitation.[20, 21] In these cases, the emitted signal field is in the IR frequency range, but still the entire nonlinear optical processes are four-wave-mixing.

In Figure 14.1, the energy level diagram of the IIV-SFG is shown, where it is also denoted as IR–IR-Raman method because of the corresponding time-ordered interaction sequence. The energy level diagram in the middle of Figure 14.1 describes another type of IR-vis four-wave-mixing process. The first IR radiation–matter interaction induces a vibrational transition from g to e. Then, the two visible pulses with wavevectors of $\mathbf{k}_{vis1}$ and $\mathbf{k}_{vis2}$, which simultaneously propagate in time and overlap at the sample in space, are used to create the second vibrational coherence between g and f via a Raman process. Then, the vibrational coherence oscillating with frequency $\bar{\omega}_{fg}$ radiates IR signal field. From the sequence of vibrational transitions

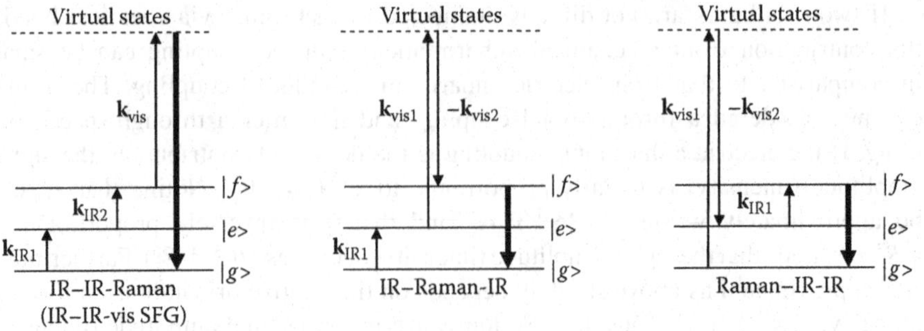

FIGURE 14.1 Three different IR-visible four-wave-mixing spectroscopic methods. Depending on the sequence of radiation–matter interactions, one can create different 2D vibrational transient grating in the sample.

involved in this case, it is named as the IR–Raman-IR spectroscopy. In this particular case, we find that the corresponding cause operators, conjugate fields, and effect operator are given as

$$\hat{A}_1 F_1(t) = \boldsymbol{\mu}\cdot\mathbf{e}_{IR} E_{IR}(t)\, e^{i\mathbf{k}_{IR}\cdot\mathbf{r}-i\omega_{IR}t}$$

$$\hat{A}_2 F_2(t) = \boldsymbol{\alpha}\cdot\mathbf{E}^*_{vis2}(t)\mathbf{E}_{vis1}(t)\, e^{-i\mathbf{k}_{vis2}\cdot\mathbf{r}+i\omega_{vis2}t}\, e^{i\mathbf{k}_{vis1}\cdot\mathbf{r}-i\omega_{vis1}t}$$

$$\hat{B} = \boldsymbol{\mu}. \tag{14.68}$$

Then, the diagram representation of this IR–Raman-IR polarization is

$$\begin{array}{c} \boldsymbol{\alpha}\mathbf{E}^*_{v2}\mathbf{E}_{v1} \quad \boldsymbol{\mu}\mathbf{E}_{IR} \\ <\boldsymbol{\mu} \xLeftarrow{\;f\wr \quad e\wr\;} |\, g><g\,|>. \end{array} \tag{14.69}$$

It is straightforward to obtain the expression for this polarization in terms of second-order response function, and it is given as

$$\begin{aligned} \mathbf{P}_{IR-Raman-IR}(\mathbf{r},t) &= e^{i(\mathbf{k}_{IR}+\mathbf{k}_{vis1}-\mathbf{k}_{vis2})\cdot\mathbf{r}-i(\omega_{IR}+\omega_{vis1}-\omega_{vis2})t}\int_0^\infty dt_2 \int_0^\infty dt_1\; \phi_{\mu\alpha\mu}(t_2,t_1)\vdots\mathbf{e}^*_{vis2}\mathbf{e}_{vis1}\mathbf{e}_{IR} \\ &\times E^*_{vis2}(t-t_2)E_{vis1}(t-t_2)E_{IR}(t-t_2-t_1)\,e^{i(\omega_{IR}+\omega_{vis1}-\omega_{vis2})t_2+i\omega_{IR}t_1}, \end{aligned} \tag{14.70}$$

where the second-order response function is defined as

$$\phi_{\mu\alpha\mu}(t_2,t_1) = \left(\frac{i}{\hbar}\right)^2 \theta(t_2)\theta(t_1) < [[\boldsymbol{\mu}(t_2+t_1),\boldsymbol{\alpha}(t_1)],\boldsymbol{\mu}(0)]\rho(-\infty) >. \tag{14.71}$$

The differences between the IIV-SFG (or IR–IR-Raman) and the present IR–Raman-IR are (1) the time-orders of the last three radiation–matter interactions, (2) the nature of created 2D vibrational coherence, and (3) the frequency range of emitted signal field. However, the second-order response function for the IR-Raman-IR $\phi_{\mu\alpha\mu}(t_2,t_1)$ is very similar to that of IR–IR-Raman response function $\phi_{\alpha\mu\mu}(t_2,t_1)$. Consequently, one can use the same theoretical procedure to calculate the amplitude of the IR–Raman-IR signal field so that any further discussion on the relationship between the signal and transition matrix elements in terms of electric and mechanical anharmonicities for the IR–Raman-IR spectroscopy will not be presented here. Nevertheless, from Equation 14.70, it is possible to obtain the corresponding 2D IR–Raman-IR spectrum, for a multilevel system,

$$\tilde{\mathbf{E}}_{IR-Raman-IR}(\omega_T,\omega_\tau) = -\frac{i\omega_s}{\hbar^2}\sum_j\sum_k \boldsymbol{\mu}_{gf_k}\boldsymbol{\alpha}_{f_ke_j}\boldsymbol{\mu}_{e_jg} \vdots \mathbf{e}^*_{vis2}\mathbf{e}_{vis1}\mathbf{e}_{IR}$$

$$\times\Gamma\left(\bar{\omega}_{f_kg},\Delta^2_{f_kf_k},\bar{\omega}_{e_jg},\Delta^2_{e_je_j}\right). \tag{14.72}$$

Since the selection rules for the IR–Raman-IR spectroscopy are different from those for IR–IR-Raman spectroscopy, the vibrational properties extracted from the IR–Raman-IR spectroscopy should be complementary.

EXERCISE 14.5

Considering both electric and mechanical anharmonic coupling mechanisms, one can obtain the theoretical expressions for the 2D IR-Raman-IR spectra of a three-level system, coupled 2LS dimer, and coupled anharmonic oscillators. Can you provide discussions on the set of selection rules as well as on how the 2D spectra are related to detailed molecular conformation?

The third energy-level diagram in Figure 14.1 is yet another type of IR-vis four-wave-mixing process. The first effective radiation–matter interaction between molecular polarizability and visible pulses induces a vibrational transition from g to e. The second vibrational transition from e to f is then induced by a time-delayed IR pulse. Finally, the vibrational coherence between g and f radiates the IR signal field. Therefore, this particular experimental scheme will be called Raman–IR-IR spectroscopy. The corresponding cause operators, conjugate fields, and effect operator are given as

$$\hat{A}_1F_1(t) = \boldsymbol{\alpha}\cdot\mathbf{E}^*_{vis2}(t)\mathbf{E}_{vis1}(t)\,e^{-i\mathbf{k}_{vis2}\cdot\mathbf{r}+i\omega_{vis2}t}\,e^{i\mathbf{k}_{vis1}\cdot\mathbf{r}-i\omega_{vis1}t}$$

$$\hat{A}_2F_2(t) = \boldsymbol{\mu}\cdot\mathbf{e}_{IR}E_{IR}(t)\,e^{i\mathbf{k}_{IR}\cdot\mathbf{r}-i\omega_{IR}t}$$

$$\hat{B} = \boldsymbol{\mu}\cdot \tag{14.73}$$

The diagram representation of this IR-Raman-IR polarization is

$$<\mu \xleftarrow[\quad f \wr \qquad e \wr \quad]{\boldsymbol{\mu}\mathbf{E}_{\mathrm{IR}} \quad \boldsymbol{\alpha}\mathbf{E}^*_{\mathrm{v2}}\mathbf{E}_{\mathrm{v1}}} | g >< g |>. \tag{14.74}$$

From this, one can immediately find that the polarization is expressed as

$$\mathbf{P}_{Raman-IR-IR}(\mathbf{r},t) = e^{i(\mathbf{k}_{vis1}-\mathbf{k}_{vis2}+\mathbf{k}_{IR})\cdot\mathbf{r}-i(\omega_{vis1}-\omega_{vis2}+\omega_{IR})t}\int_0^\infty dt_2 \int_0^\infty dt_1 \phi_{\mu\mu\alpha}(t_2,t_1) \vdots \mathbf{e}_{IR}\mathbf{e}^*_{vis2}\mathbf{e}_{vis1}$$
$$\times E_{IR}(t-t_2)E^*_{vis2}(t-t_2-t_1)E_{vis1}(t-t_2-t_1)\, e^{i(\omega_{IR}+\omega_{vis1}-\omega_{vis2})t_2+i(\omega_{vis1}-\omega_{vis2})t_1}, \tag{14.75}$$

where the associated second-order response function is defined as

$$\phi_{\mu\mu\alpha}(t_2,t_1) = \left(\frac{i}{\hbar}\right)^2 \theta(t_2)\theta(t_1) < [[\boldsymbol{\mu}(t_2+t_1),\boldsymbol{\mu}(t_1)],\boldsymbol{\alpha}(0)]\rho(-\infty) >. \tag{14.76}$$

When f is one of the combination states, the last transition is a two-quantum process. Except for a few minor differences, the underlying physics are identical to those of the IR–IR-Raman spectroscopy. The 2D Raman–IR-IR spectrum for a multilevel system can then be found to be

$$\tilde{\mathbf{E}}_{Raman-IR-IR}(\omega_T,\omega_\tau) = -\frac{i\omega_s}{\hbar^2}\sum_j\sum_k \boldsymbol{\mu}_{gf_k}\boldsymbol{\mu}_{f_k e_j}\boldsymbol{\alpha}_{e_j g} \vdots \mathbf{e}_{IR}\mathbf{e}^*_{vis2}\mathbf{e}_{vis1}$$
$$\times \Gamma\left(\bar{\omega}_{f_k g},\Delta^2_{f_k f_k},\bar{\omega}_{e_j g},\Delta^2_{e_j e_j}\right). \tag{14.77}$$

A detailed discussion on how to calculate the transition dipole and polarizability matrix elements will not be presented here, but again this method can provide complementary information on secondary vibrational spectroscopic properties of complicated molecular systems.

14.8 FIFTH-ORDER RAMAN SCATTERING

As discussed in Section 3.5, time-resolved coherent Raman scattering (CRS) spectroscopy requires three incident beams in the most general case. Two pump pulses with center frequencies ω_1 and ω_2 and wavevectors $\mathbf{k}_1$ and $\mathbf{k}_2$ are used to create transient spatial grating in the sample with wavevector $\mathbf{k}_1 - \mathbf{k}_2$ and frequency $\omega_1 - \omega_2$. After a finite delay time τ, a third pulse with frequency ω_3 and wavevector $\mathbf{k}_3$ is injected into the sample to stimulate a scattering process by the grating. The CRS signal field with wavevector $\mathbf{k}_1 - \mathbf{k}_2 + \mathbf{k}_3$ is then detected. The CRS is an optical process whose signal amplitude is *not* linear with respect to the external field amplitude. However, treating the first two radiation–matter interactions as a single effective interaction

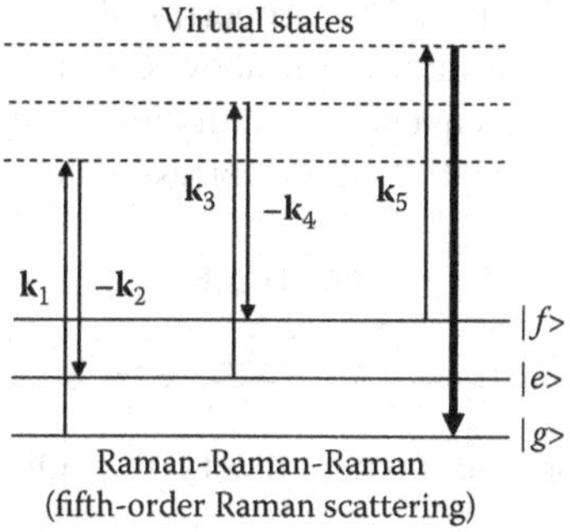

FIGURE 14.2 Fifth-order Raman scattering (FORS) spectroscopy. A critical difference of the present FORS from the 2D IR-IR-Raman spectroscopy in Figure 14.1 is that the 2D vibrational transient grating is created by two time-separated coherent Raman excitations.

between molecular polarizability and $\mathbf{E}^2(\mathbf{r},t)$, one can still use the linear response theory to describe this third-order CRS process with respect to the external electric field intensity.

Now, let us consider fifth-order Raman scattering (FORS) with electronically nonresonant beams,[22] even though its fully resonant version was also theoretically discussed in a literature.[23] The most general FORS experiment would be to use five different beams. The first two pulses propagate in two different directions $\mathbf{k}_1$ and $\mathbf{k}_2$, but they are overlapped in time. These two pulses are used to create the first transient grating in the sample. Secondly, after a finite delay time τ later, the second and third pulses that also overlap in the sample in time and space are used to create the second transient grating, whose frequency and wavevector are then $\omega_1 - \omega_2 + \omega_3 - \omega_4$ and $\mathbf{k}_1 - \mathbf{k}_2 + \mathbf{k}_3 - \mathbf{k}_4$, respectively. Note that only those chromophores that interact with all these four pulses are considered. After the second delay time T, the fifth pulse whose frequency and wavevector are ω_5 and $\mathbf{k}_5$, respectively, interacts with thus created 2D transient grating to generate coherent FORS field (see Figure 14.2). From the phase-matching condition, the frequency and wavevector of the FORS signal field are $\omega_s = \omega_1 - \omega_2 + \omega_3 - \omega_4 + \omega_5$ and $\mathbf{k}_s = \mathbf{k}_1 - \mathbf{k}_2 + \mathbf{k}_3 - \mathbf{k}_4 + \mathbf{k}_5$, respectively. Since five electric dipole–electric field interactions are involved, it was called the fifth-order spectroscopy.[22] However, as will be shown below, in the case of electronically nonresonant limit, the entire molecular response can be described by considering the second-order polarizability response function. The cause operators, their conjugated external fields, and effect operator for this coherent FORS experiment are given as

$$(1)\quad \hat{A}_1 = \boldsymbol{\alpha}\cdot\mathbf{E}_1(t+T+\tau)e^{i\mathbf{k}_1\cdot\mathbf{r}-i\omega_1 t} \quad \text{and} \quad F_1 = \mathbf{E}_2^*(t+T+\tau)e^{-i\mathbf{k}_2\cdot\mathbf{r}+i\omega_2 t}$$

$$(2)\quad \hat{A}_2 = \boldsymbol{\alpha}\cdot\mathbf{E}_3(t+T)e^{i\mathbf{k}_3\cdot\mathbf{r}-i\omega_3 t} \quad \text{and} \quad F_2 = \mathbf{E}_4^*(t+T)e^{-i\mathbf{k}_4\cdot\mathbf{r}+i\omega_4 t}$$

$$(3)\quad \hat{B} = \boldsymbol{\alpha}\cdot\mathbf{E}_5(t)e^{i\mathbf{k}_5\cdot\mathbf{r}-i\omega_5 t}. \tag{14.78}$$

The FORS signal field is then linearly proportional to the fifth-order polarization that is given as the expectation value of the above effect operator at time t only when the matter experienced the sequence of radiation–matter interactions described above. Diagrammatic representation of the corresponding fifth-order polarization is given as

$$<\boldsymbol{\alpha}\mathbf{E}_5 \overset{\boldsymbol{\alpha}\mathbf{E}_4^*\mathbf{E}_3 \quad \boldsymbol{\alpha}\mathbf{E}_2^*\mathbf{E}_1}{\overset{f\wr \qquad e\wr}{\Longleftarrow\!=\!=\!=\!=}} |g><g|. \quad (14.79)$$

From the second-order response function theory, the FORS polarization is given as

$$\mathbf{P}_{FORS}(\mathbf{r},t) = e^{i\mathbf{k}_s\cdot\mathbf{r}-i\omega_s t} E_5(t)\int_0^\infty dt_2 \int_0^\infty dt_1\, \phi_{\alpha\alpha\alpha}(t_2,t_1) \otimes \mathbf{e}_5\mathbf{e}_4^*\mathbf{e}_3\mathbf{e}_2^*\mathbf{e}_1$$
$$\times E_4^*(t-t_2+T)E_3(t-t_2+T)E_2^*(t-t_2-t_1+T+\tau)$$
$$\times E_1(t-t_2-t_1+T+\tau)e^{i(\omega_1-\omega_2+\omega_3-\omega_4)t_2}\, e^{i(\omega_1-\omega_2)t_1}. \quad (14.80)$$

Here, the FORS response function, which is a sixth-rank tensor, is given as

$$\phi_{\alpha\alpha\alpha}(t_2,t_1) \equiv \left(\frac{i}{\hbar}\right)^2 \theta(t_2)\theta(t_1) < [[\boldsymbol{\alpha}(t_2+t_1),\boldsymbol{\alpha}(t_1)],\boldsymbol{\alpha}(0)]\rho(-\infty)>. \quad (14.81)$$

An early experimental attempt was to use femtosecond laser pulses to study intermolecular vibrations of liquids such as CS_2.[24–27] In that case, the five pulses are degenerate so that their center frequencies are all the same, that is, $\omega_1 = \omega_2 = \omega_3 = \omega_4 = \omega_5 = \omega$. In this limiting case, the FORS polarization in Equation 14.80 is simplified as

$$\mathbf{P}_{FORS}(\mathbf{r},t) = e^{i\mathbf{k}_s\cdot\mathbf{r}-i\omega t} E_5(t)\int_0^\infty dt_2 \int_0^\infty dt_1\, \phi_{\alpha\alpha\alpha}(t_2,t_1) \otimes \mathbf{e}_5\mathbf{e}_4^*\mathbf{e}_3\mathbf{e}_2^*\mathbf{e}_1$$
$$\times E_4^*(t-t_2+T)E_3(t-t_2+T)E_2^*(t-t_2-t_1+T+\tau)E_1(t-t_2-t_1+T+\tau). \quad (14.82)$$

If the incident beams are all impulsive so that each pulse has broad spectral bandwidth, a manifold Raman-active vibrational mode can be excited via these coherent Raman processes. Two consecutive vibrational excitations are thus created, and the resultant 2D vibrational transient grating scatters the fifth visible pulse toward the direction of $\mathbf{k}_s$. Then, the scattering field intensity is measured with respect to the two delay times τ and T. In this impulsive limit, the FORS polarization is simply proportional to the second-order polarizability-polarizability-polarizability response function as

$$\mathbf{P}_{FORS}(\mathbf{r},t) \propto e^{i\mathbf{k}_s\cdot\mathbf{r}-i\omega t} E_5(t)\phi_{\alpha\alpha\alpha}(t+T,\tau) \otimes \mathbf{e}_5\mathbf{e}_4^*\mathbf{e}_3\mathbf{e}_2^*\mathbf{e}_1. \quad (14.83)$$

Then, the radiated FORS electric field amplitude becomes

$$\mathbf{E}_{FORS}(t) \propto i\omega E_5(t)\phi_{\alpha\alpha\alpha}(t+T,\tau) \otimes \mathbf{e}_5\mathbf{e}_4^*\mathbf{e}_3\mathbf{e}_2^*\mathbf{e}_1. \quad (14.84)$$

If the above FORS signal field is homodyne detected, the measured signal is given as

$$S_{FORS}(T,\tau) \propto \int dt \, | E_s^{(5)}(t) |^2 \propto | \phi_{\alpha\alpha\alpha}(T,\tau) \otimes \mathbf{e}_s^* \mathbf{e}_5 \mathbf{e}_2^* \mathbf{e}_3 \mathbf{e}_2^* \mathbf{e}_1 |^2, \tag{14.85}$$

where the unit vector of the measured signal field vector is denoted as $\mathbf{e}_s$.

Unfortunately, however, the cascading contribution to the measured signal was found to be large in the electronically nonresonant FORS case, and sometimes it is even dominant so that a direct measurement of the FORS signal without any contamination from the two third-order cascading background signal was found to be extremely difficult in practice.[28, 29] Nevertheless, there was a theoretical proposition that the direct FORS signal field can be selectively measured by noting that the phase of the cascading fifth-order signal field is different from the direct FORS signal field.[30] Secondly, if the incident beams are close to resonances with electronic transitions, the cascading contribution to the fifth-order signal is likely to be smaller than the direct fifth-order term.

Much like the time-and-frequency-resolved CRS spectroscopy, one can also develop a nondegenerate FORS technique to study 2D Raman responses from high-frequency intramolecular vibrations. Consider the case when one can experimentally control the frequency differences $\Omega_1 = \omega_1 - \omega_2$ and $\Omega_2 = \omega_3 - \omega_4$. If these two frequencies Ω_1 and Ω_2 are close to vibrational frequencies of q_1 and q_2 modes, doubly resonant vibrational enhancement of the FORS process becomes possible.

Using the new notations for the two frequency differences Ω_1 and Ω_2 and from Equation 14.82, one can find that the generated FORS electric field amplitude is given as

$$\mathbf{E}_{FORS}(t) = i\omega_s E_5(t) \int_0^\infty dt_2 \int_0^\infty dt_1 \, \phi_{\alpha\alpha\alpha}(t_2,t_1) \otimes \mathbf{e}_5 \mathbf{e}_4^* \mathbf{e}_3 \mathbf{e}_2^* \mathbf{e}_1 E_4^*(t-t_2+T) E_3(t-t_2+T)$$
$$\times E_2^*(t-t_2-t_1+T+\tau) E_1(t-t_2-t_1+T+\tau) e^{i(\Omega_1+\Omega_2)t_2} e^{i\Omega_1 t_1}. \tag{14.86}$$

This result is formally identical to that of IIV-SFG, except that the second-order response function $\phi_{\alpha\mu\mu}(t_2,t_1)$ in Equation 14.47 is replaced with $\phi_{\alpha\alpha\alpha}(t_2,t_1)$.[10, 18, 20] In order to present a detailed theoretical description on the FORS, let us consider the same three-level system considered above for the IIV-SFG. Assuming that the incident beams are impulsive, one can approximately rewrite Equation 14.86 as

$$\mathbf{E}_{FORS}(t) \propto -\frac{i\omega_s}{\hbar^2} \boldsymbol{\alpha}_{gf} \boldsymbol{\alpha}_{fe} \boldsymbol{\alpha}_{eg} \otimes \mathbf{e}_5 \mathbf{e}_4^* \mathbf{e}_3 \mathbf{e}_2^* \mathbf{e}_1 E_5(t) G_1(t+T,\tau) e^{i(\Omega_1+\Omega_2-\bar{\omega}_{fg})T + i(\Omega_1-\bar{\omega}_{eg})\tau}. \tag{14.87}$$

The heterodyne-detected signal, which is a function of both τ and T, is then Fourier-Laplace transformed to obtain the corresponding 2D FORS spectrum. The 2D Gaussian peak shape approximation gives us

$$\tilde{\mathbf{E}}_{FORS}(\omega_T,\omega_\tau) = -\frac{i\omega_s}{\hbar^2} \boldsymbol{\alpha}_{gf} \boldsymbol{\alpha}_{fe} \boldsymbol{\alpha}_{eg} \otimes \mathbf{e}_5 \mathbf{e}_4^* \mathbf{e}_3 \mathbf{e}_2^* \mathbf{e}_1 \Gamma\left(\bar{\omega}_{fg}, \Delta_{ff}^2, \bar{\omega}_{eg}, \Delta_{ee}^2\right). \tag{14.88}$$

For a multilevel system, we have

$$\tilde{\mathbf{E}}_{FORS}(\omega_T,\omega_\tau) = -\frac{i\omega_s}{\hbar^2}\sum_j\sum_k \boldsymbol{\alpha}_{gf_k}\boldsymbol{\alpha}_{f_k e_j}\boldsymbol{\alpha}_{e_j g} \otimes \mathbf{e}_5\mathbf{e}_4^*\mathbf{e}_3\mathbf{e}_2^*\mathbf{e}_1\Gamma\left(\bar{\omega}_{f_k g},\Delta^2_{f_k f_k},\bar{\omega}_{e_j g},\Delta^2_{e_j e_j}\right). \tag{14.89}$$

Now, for the sake of simplicity, let us consider the *XXXXXX*-measurement, where all polarization directions including that of the FORS signal field are parallel to the *X*-axis in a space-fixed frame. In addition, considering the two coupling mechanisms that originate from electric and mechanical (cubic) anharmonic couplings,[31] the 2D FORS spectrum of the cross-peak at $\omega_\tau = \omega_1$ and $\omega_T = \omega_1 + \omega_2 - \Delta_{12}$ can be written as

$$\tilde{\mathrm{E}}_{FORS}(\omega_T = \omega_1+\omega_2,\omega_\tau=\omega_1) \cong -\frac{i\omega_s}{\hbar^2}\frac{\hbar}{2\sqrt{m_1\omega_1 m_2\omega_2}}\Gamma\left(\bar{\omega}_{fg},\Delta^2_{ff},\bar{\omega}_{eg},\Delta^2_{ee}\right)$$

$$\times\left\{\left[\boldsymbol{\alpha}^{(2)}_{12}\boldsymbol{\alpha}^{(1)}_{1}\boldsymbol{\alpha}^{(1)}_{1}\right]_{XXXXXX} + \sum_j \frac{V^{(3)}_{12j}}{2m_j\omega_j(\omega_1+\omega_2-\omega_j)}\left[\boldsymbol{\alpha}^{(1)}_{j}\boldsymbol{\alpha}^{(1)}_{1}\boldsymbol{\alpha}^{(1)}_{1}\right]_{XXXXXX}\right\}. \tag{14.90}$$

Here, it is again noted that the quartic anharmonic couplings were ignored in the above derivation for the sake of simplicity, but, as mentioned in Exercise 14.4, the Darling-Dennison-type resonance enhancement of mechanical coupling induced by quartic anharmonicities could play an important role in some cases, depending on the symmetry of molecule.

Overall, the results for FORS discussed here differ from the case of IIV-SFG by the associated selection rules. In the present case, the vibrational modes 1 and 2 should be Raman-active. In addition, the two modes should be coupled to each other via either electric or mechanical couplings. Again, the Fermi-type (and possibly Darling-Dennison) resonance enhancement of mechanical coupling is also expected in this case.

REFERENCES

1. Shen, Y. R., *The principles of nonlinear optics*. John Wiley & Sons: New York, 1984.
2. Belkin, M. A.; Kulakov, T. A.; Ernst, K.-H.; Yan, L.; Shen, Y. R., Sum frequency vibrational spectroscopy on chiral liquids: A novel technique to probe molecular chirality. *Physical Review Letters* 2000, 85, 4474.
3. Belkin, M. A.; Han, S. H.; Wei, X.; Shen, Y. R., Sum frequency generation in chiral liquids near electronic resonance. *Physical Review Letters* 2001, 87, 113001.
4. Belkin, M. A.; Shen, Y. R., Doubly resonant IR-UV sum frequency vibrational spectroscopy on molecular chirality. *Physical Review Letters* 2003, 91, 213907.
5. Belkin, M. A.; Shen, Y.-R.; Harris, R. A., Sum frequency vibrational spectroscopy of chiral liquids off and close to electronic resonance and the antisymmetric Raman tensor. *Journal of Chemical Physics* 2004, 120, 10118–10126.
6. Cho, M., Time-resolved vibrational optical activity measurement by the infrared-visible sum frequency-generation with circularly polarized infrared light. *Journal of Chemical Physics* 2002, 116, 1562–1570.

7. Cheon, S.; Cho, M., Circularly polarized infrared and visible sum frequency-generation spectroscopy: Vibrational optical activity measurement. *Physical Review A* 2005, 71, 013808.
8. Fischer, P.; Hache, F., Nonlinear optical spectroscopy of chiral molecules. *Chirality* 2005, 17, 421–437.
9. Cheon, S.; Lee, H.; Choi, J. H.; Cho, M., Doubly resonant three-wave-mixing spectroscopy of a chiral coupled-chromophore system in solution: Coherent two-dimensional optical activity spectroscopy. *Journal of Chemical Physics* 2007, 126, 054505.
10. Park, K.; Cho, M., Time- and frequency-resolved coherent two-dimensional IR spectroscopy: Its complementary relationship with the coherent two-dimensional Raman scattering spectroscopy. *Journal of Chemical Physics* 1998, 109, 10559–10569.
11. Cho, M., Theoretical description of two-dimensional vibrational spectroscopy by infrared-infrared-visible sum frequency generation. *Physical Review A* 2000, 6102, 023406.
12. Zhao, W.; Wright, J. C., Measurement of $\chi^{(3)}$ for doubly vibrationally enhanced four wave mixing spectroscopy. *Physical Review Letters* 1999, 83, 1950–1953.
13. Zhao, W.; Wright, J. C., Spectral simplification in vibrational spectroscopy using doubly vibrationally enhanced infrared four wave mixing. *Journal of the American Chemical Society* 1999, 121, 10994–10998.
14. Zhao, W.; Wright, J. C., Doubly vibrationally enhanced four wave mixing: The optical analog to 2D NMR. *Physical Review Letters* 2000, 84, 1411–1414.
15. Okumura, K.; Tokmakoff, A.; Tanimura, Y., Structural information from two-dimensional fifth-order Raman spectroscopy. *Journal of Chemical Physics* 1999, 111, 492–503.
16. Hahn, S.; Kwak, K.; Cho, M., Two-dimensional vibrational spectroscopy. IV. Relationship between through-space vibrational coupling and intermolecular distance. *Journal of Chemical Physics* 2000, 112, 4553–4556.
17. Kwak, K.; Cha, S.; Cho, M. H.; Wright, J. C., Vibrational interactions of acetonitrile: Doubly vibrationally resonant IR-IR-visible four-wave-mixing spectroscopy. *Journal of Chemical Physics* 2002, 117, 5675–5687.
18. Park, K.; Cho, M. H.; Hahn, S.; Kim, D., Two-dimensional vibrational spectroscopy. II. Ab initio calculation of the coherent 2D infrared response function of $CHCl_3$ and comparison with the 2D Raman response function. *Journal of Chemical Physics* 1999, 111, 4131–4139.
19. Cho, M., Coherent two-dimensional optical spectroscopy. *Chemical Reviews* 2008, 108, 1331–1418.
20. Cho, M., Two-dimensional vibrational spectroscopy. In *Advances in multi-photon processes and spectroscopy*, Lin, S. H., Villaeys, A. A., Fujimura, Y., Ed. World Scientific Pulblishing Co.: Singapore, 1999; Vol. 12, pp 229–300.
21. Cho, M., Two-dimensional vibrational spectroscopy. III. Theoretical description of the coherent two-dimensional IR-Raman spectroscopy for the investigation of the coupling between both IR- and Raman-active vibrational modes. *Journal of Chemical Physics* 1999, 111, 4140–4147.
22. Tanimura, Y.; Mukamel, S., Two-dimensional femtosecond vibrational spectroscopy of liquids. *Journal of Chemical Physics* 1993, 99, 9496–9511.
23. Cho, M., On the resonant coherent two-dimensional Raman scattering. *Journal of Chemical Physics* 1998, 109, 5327–5337.
24. Tominaga, K.; Yoshihara, K., 5th order optical-response of liquid CS_2 observed by ultrafast nonresonant six-wave mixing. *Physical Review Letters* 1995, 74, 3061–3064.
25. Tominaga, K.; Yoshihara, K., Fifth-order nonlinear spectroscopy on the low-frequency modes of liquid CS_2. *Journal of Chemical Physics* 1996, 104, 4419–4426.

26. Tokmakoff, A.; Fleming, G. R., Two-dimensional Raman spectroscopy of the intermolecular modes of liquid CS_2. *Journal of Chemical Physics* 1997, 106, 2569–2582.
27. Tokmakoff, A.; Lang, M. J.; Larsen, D. S.; Fleming, G. R.; Chernyak, V.; Mukamel, S., Two-dimensional raman spectroscopy of vibrational interactions in liquids. *Physical Review Letters* 1997, 79, 2702–2705.
28. Blank, D. A.; Kaufman, L. J.; Fleming, G. R., Fifth-order two-dimensional Raman spectra of CS_2 are dominated by third-order cascades. *Journal of Chemical Physics* 1999, 111, 3105–3114.
29. Blank, D. A.; Kaufman, L. J.; Fleming, G. R., Direct fifth-order electronically nonresonant Raman scattering from CS_2 at room temperature. *Journal of Chemical Physics* 2000, 113, 771–778.
30. Kaufman, L. J.; Heo, J. Y.; Fleming, G. R.; Sung, J. Y.; Cho, M., Fifth-order electronically non-resonant Raman scattering: two-dimensional Fourier deconvolution. *Chemical Physics* 2001, 266, 251–271.
31. Okumura, K.; Tanimura, Y., Femtosecond two-dimensional spectroscopy from anharmonic vibrational modes of molecules in the condensed phase. *Journal of Chemical Physics* 1997, 107, 2267–2283.

15 Linear Optical Activity Spectroscopy

Since optical activity is manifested by almost all natural products, a better understanding of chiro-optical properties is critical for studies of the molecular basis of biological activity.[1] By definition, optical activity (OA) is related to the *differential interaction of a chiral molecule with left and right circularly polarized radiation during quantum excitation*. This, however, does not mean that the optical activity of a chiral molecule should always be measured by using left and right circularly polarized (LCP and RCP) lights. Note that the LCP and RCP lights are linear combinations of two orthogonal linearly polarized lights with a certain phase difference, that is, $\mathbf{e}_L = (\mathbf{e}_1 + i\mathbf{e}_2)/\sqrt{2}$ and $\mathbf{e}_R = (\mathbf{e}_1 - i\mathbf{e}_2)/\sqrt{2}$. Therefore, any linearly polarized light can be written as a linear combination of LCP and RCP. Thus, depending on the optical activity property of interest, one can use LCP and RCP lights or just linearly polarized light. For example, circular dichroism (CD) spectroscopy is to measure the differential absorption of LCP and RCP lights by any object with a chiral structure (see the upper panel of Figure 15.1).[1] It has been applied to structural analyses for a wide range of chemical and biological systems in condensed phases. Optical rotatory dispersion (ORD) is to measure the rotation angle of the transmitted electric field polarization direction in comparison with the incident beam polarization direction (the lower panel of Figure 15.1). The CD and ORD spectra are related to the imaginary and real parts of the linear optical activity susceptibility, which is defined as the difference between the two linear susceptibilities measured with LCP and RCP lights.

Typically, the optical activity is a notoriously weak effect since it involves an interaction of magnetic dipole with external magnetic field. This renders the time-resolved optical activity (CD and ORD) spectroscopy experimentally difficult, even though the time-resolved CD or ORD spectroscopy is capable of providing crucial information on the structural changes of biomolecules in the processes of their functions. In the vibrational frequency domain, two important optical activity measurement methods have been used. The first is an infrared analog of electronic CD, which has been called the vibrational CD (VCD).[2,3] The second is the Raman optical activity (ROA), which is an optical activity version of Raman scattering spectroscopy.[1,4,5] Much like the relationship between IR absorption and Raman scattering, the VCD and ROA techniques are complementary to each other. In addition to these two vibrational OA measurement methods, one can also use singly vibrationally resonant nonlinear optical spectroscopy to study chiral nature of molecules in solution, as will be discussed later in this chapter. All these optical activity measurement methods can be considered as a particular class of linear response spectroscopy, and the corresponding linear response functions averaged

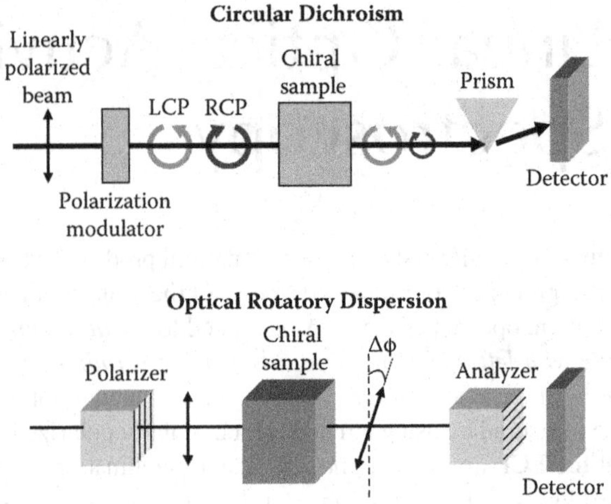

FIGURE 15.1 Experimental schemes of circular dichroism and optical rotatory dispersion measurements. In the case of circular dichroism, the linearly polarized beam polarization is modulated to convert it into either LCP or RCP beams. Since chiral molecules can absorb LCP and RCP beams differently, the differential absorption provides information on molecular chirality and stereochemistry. The optical rotatory dispersion measurement uses a linearly polarized beam. Since the refractive indexes for LCP and RCP are different for chiral sample, the incident beam polarization direction rotates and then the rotation angle is measured.

over randomly oriented chiral molecules in solutions will be presented and discussed here.

15.1 RADIATION–MATTER INTERACTION HAMILTONIAN AND POLARIZATION

For a theoretical description of the relevant linear response function and the corresponding optical activity susceptibility, we need to consider the following radiation–matter interaction Hamiltonian,

$$\begin{aligned} H_{rad-mat} &= -\boldsymbol{\mu}\cdot\mathbf{E}(\mathbf{r},t) - \mathbf{m}\cdot\mathbf{B}(\mathbf{r},t) - (1/2)\mathbf{Q}:\nabla\mathbf{E}(\mathbf{r},t) \\ &= -\mu_j E_j(\mathbf{r},t) - m_j B_j(\mathbf{r},t) - (1/2)Q_{kj}\nabla_k E_j(\mathbf{r},t). \end{aligned} \tag{15.1}$$

Here, we again used the Einstein summation convention, where the repeated index means summation over the index ($j = x, y, z$). Typically, the last two terms are two to three orders of magnitude smaller than the electric dipole-electric field interaction energy, which is the first term. Therefore, in Section 3.4, only the first term on the right-hand side of Equation 15.1 was taken into consideration for calculating the light-absorption process.

The radiation–matter interaction Hamiltonian in Equation 15.1 was written in terms of electric field, magnetic field, and gradient of electric field to describe three different interactions. However, using the relationship between **E** and **B** via the vector potential **A** in Coulomb gauge, that is, $\mathbf{E} = -(1/c)(\partial\mathbf{A}/\partial t)$ and $\mathbf{B} = \nabla \times \mathbf{A}$, and taking the spatial gradient of the transverse electric field, one can rewrite Equation 15.1 as

$$
\begin{aligned}
H_{rad-mat} &= -\{\mu_j + (\mathbf{m}\times\hat{\mathbf{k}})_j + (i/2)Q_{kj}k_k\}E_j(t)\,e^{i\mathbf{k}\cdot\mathbf{r}-i\omega t} \\
&\quad - \{\mu_j + (\mathbf{m}\times\hat{\mathbf{k}})_j - (i/2)Q_{kj}k_k\}E_j^*(t)\,e^{-i\mathbf{k}\cdot\mathbf{r}+i\omega t} \\
&= -\{\boldsymbol{\mu} + (\mathbf{m}\times\hat{\mathbf{k}}) + (i/2)\mathbf{k}\cdot\mathbf{Q}\}\cdot\mathbf{e}E(t)\mathbf{e}^{i\mathbf{k}\cdot\mathbf{r}-i\omega t} \\
&\quad - \{\boldsymbol{\mu} + (\mathbf{m}\times\hat{\mathbf{k}}) - (i/2)\mathbf{k}\cdot\mathbf{Q}\}\cdot\mathbf{e}^*E^*(t)\mathbf{e}^{-i\mathbf{k}\cdot\mathbf{r}+i\omega t}.
\end{aligned}
\tag{15.2}
$$

Consequently, the first-order expanded dipole operator with respect to the wavevector **k**, which is valid beyond the electric dipole approximation, can be defined as

$$
\boldsymbol{\mu}^{(+\mathbf{k})} = \boldsymbol{\mu} + (\mathbf{m}\times\hat{\mathbf{k}}) + (i/2)\mathbf{k}\cdot\mathbf{Q} \quad \text{and} \quad \boldsymbol{\mu}^{(-\mathbf{k})} = \boldsymbol{\mu} + (\mathbf{m}\times\hat{\mathbf{k}}) - (i/2)\mathbf{k}\cdot\mathbf{Q} \tag{15.3}
$$

where $\hat{\mathbf{k}}$ is the unit vector of **k**. The first radiation–matter interaction term in Equation 15.2 describes an absorptive process, whereas the second describes a stimulated emissive interaction. The electric dipole (or long wavelength) approximation is based on the assumption that the last two terms in Equation 15.3, which are associated with the magnetic dipole and electric quadrupole operators, are negligibly small because the molecular dimension (size) is much smaller than the wavelength of the field. Thus, if one is interested in the optical activity properties that are determined by the magnetic dipole–magnetic field and electric quadrupole–electric field interactions, the polarization, which is defined as the expectation value of the electric dipole operator, should be generalized as

$$
\begin{aligned}
\mathbf{P}^{(n)}(\mathbf{r},t) &= \langle \boldsymbol{\mu}\rho^{(n)}(\mathbf{r},t)\rangle + \langle (\mathbf{m}\times\hat{\mathbf{k}})\rho^{(n)}(\mathbf{r},t)\rangle - (i/2)\langle (\mathbf{k}\cdot\mathbf{Q})\rho^{(n)}(\mathbf{r},t)\rangle \\
&= \bar{\boldsymbol{\mu}}^{(n)}(\mathbf{r},t) + \bar{\mathbf{m}}^{(n)}(\mathbf{r},t)\times\hat{\mathbf{k}} - (i/2)\mathbf{k}\cdot\bar{\mathbf{Q}}^{(n)}(\mathbf{r},t).
\end{aligned}
\tag{15.4}
$$

Here, the wavevector **k** is that of the radiated electric field. The first term in the above equation was only considered in the descriptions of a number of linear and nonlinear spectroscopies in the previous chapters. The second and third terms in Equation 15.4 are the contributions from the nonequilibrium magnetic dipole and electric quadrupole. The definition of polarization in Equation 15.4, which includes the lowest-order contributions from the magnetic dipole and electric quadrupole, is valid for not only linear but also nonlinear optical activity spectroscopy in general. If the density operator $\rho^{(n)}(\mathbf{r},t)$ is the nth-order perturbation-expanded one, Equation 15.4 is the nth-order polarization. Also, it should be noted that the negative sign for the nonequilibrium electric quadrupole term in Equation 15.4 should be chosen because the last matter interaction is with vacuum field and is an emissive process in nature. Within the linear response theory, the latter two terms can also be calculated by using the corresponding linear response functions, as will be shown below.

15.2 CIRCULAR DICHROISM AND OPTICAL ROTATORY DISPERSION

There are a few different optical activity measurement techniques widely used, such as CD, ORD, linear birefringence, chiral luminescence, ROA, and so forth. However, only the CD and ORD will be considered in detail in the present section. The circular dichroism is to measure the differential absorption of LCP and RCP lights by chiral molecules, whereas the ORD is to measure the rotation angle of a linearly polarized beam by chiral molecules. CD is connected to ORD by the well-known Kramers–Kronig transformation (see Equations 3.16 and 3.17).

Using the radiation–matter interaction Hamiltonian in Equation 15.2 and the generalized linear polarization defined in Equation 15.4, one can obtain theoretical descriptions of CD and ORD. Here, we consider the case when the *electric field* created by the polarization induced by the above radiation–matter interaction Hamiltonian in Equation 15.2 is detected. Now, there are three cause operators and three effect operators to be considered (see Equation 15.2). Thus, up to the first-order radiation–matter interactions with respect to wavevector **k**, one needs to consider nine different contributions to the total linear polarization $\mathbf{P}^{(1)}(\mathbf{r},t)$. However, since the magnetic dipole–magnetic field and electric quadrupole–electric field interactions are two to three orders of magnitude smaller than the electric dipole–electric field interaction, only those contributions that are linear with respect to **m** or **Q** will be taken into account. Then, only five combinations of cause-and-effect operators are to be considered, and they are

$$(1)\quad \hat{A}=\boldsymbol{\mu},\ F=\mathbf{E}(\mathbf{r},t),\quad \text{and}\quad \hat{B}=\boldsymbol{\mu}$$

$$(2)\quad \hat{A}=(\mathbf{m}\times\hat{\mathbf{k}}),\ F=\mathbf{E}(\mathbf{r},t)\quad \text{and}\quad \hat{B}=\boldsymbol{\mu}$$

$$(3)\quad \hat{A}=(i/2)\mathbf{k}\cdot\mathbf{Q},\ F=\mathrm{E}(\mathrm{r},t),\quad \text{and}\quad \hat{B}=\boldsymbol{\mu}$$

$$(4)\quad \hat{A}=\boldsymbol{\mu},\ F=\mathbf{E}(\mathbf{r},t),\quad \text{and}\quad \hat{B}=(\mathbf{m}\times\hat{\mathbf{k}})$$

$$(5)\quad \hat{A}=\boldsymbol{\mu},\ F=\mathbf{E}(\mathbf{r},t),\quad \text{and}\quad \hat{B}=-(i/2)\mathbf{k}\cdot\mathbf{Q}. \qquad (15.5)$$

The expectation value of the effect operator $\boldsymbol{\mu}^{(-k)}$ in Equation 15.3, which is the linear polarization, is thus given as the sum of five distinctively different contributions as

$$\mathbf{P}^{(1)}(\mathbf{r},t) = \langle \boldsymbol{\mu} \overset{\boldsymbol{\mu}\mathbf{E}}{\Longleftarrow} \rho(t_0) \rangle + \langle \boldsymbol{\mu} \overset{\mathbf{m}\mathbf{B}}{\Longleftarrow} \rho(t_0) \rangle + \langle \boldsymbol{\mu} \overset{(1/2)\,\mathbf{Q}\nabla\mathbf{E}}{\Longleftarrow} \rho(t_0) \rangle$$

$$+ \langle \mathbf{m} \times \hat{\mathbf{k}} \overset{\boldsymbol{\mu}\mathbf{E}}{\Longleftarrow} \rho(t_0) \rangle - \langle (i/2)\mathbf{k} \cdot \mathbf{Q} \overset{\boldsymbol{\mu}\mathbf{E}}{\Longleftarrow} \rho(t_0) \rangle$$

$$= \int_0^\infty d\tau \{\phi_{\mu\mu}(\tau) + \phi_{\mu m}(\tau) + (i/2)\phi_{\mu Q}(\tau) + \phi_{m\mu}(\tau) - (i/2)\phi_{Q\mu}(\tau)\} \cdot \mathbf{e}E(\mathbf{r}, t-\tau), \tag{15.6}$$

where the dipole–dipole linear response function $\phi_{\mu\mu}(\tau)$ was already defined in Equation 3.79 and the other linear response functions in Equation 15.6 are defined as

$$\phi_{\mu m}(\tau) \equiv \frac{i}{\hbar}\theta(\tau) \langle [\boldsymbol{\mu}(\tau), \mathbf{m}(0) \times \hat{\mathbf{k}}]\rho(-\infty) \rangle$$

$$\phi_{\mu Q}(\tau) \equiv \frac{i}{\hbar}\theta(\tau) \langle [\boldsymbol{\mu}(\tau), \mathbf{k} \cdot \mathbf{Q}(0)]\rho(-\infty) \rangle$$

$$\phi_{m\mu}(\tau) \equiv \frac{i}{\hbar}\theta(\tau) \langle [\mathbf{m}(\tau) \times \hat{\mathbf{k}}, \boldsymbol{\mu}(0)]\rho(-\infty) \rangle$$

$$\phi_{Q\mu}(\tau) \equiv \frac{i}{\hbar}\theta(\tau) \langle [\mathbf{k} \cdot \mathbf{Q}(\tau), \boldsymbol{\mu}(0)]\rho(-\infty) \rangle. \tag{15.7}$$

The energy level diagrams corresponding to the five terms in Equation 15.6 are shown in Figure 15.2. The first three cases in Equation 15.6 or in Figure 15.2 describe the linear processes when the free-induction-decay (FID) field is generated by an electric dipole–electric field interaction. On the other hand, the fourth and fifth ones in Equation 15.6 are the cases when the generated FID is produced by the magnetic dipole–magnetic field and electric quadrupole–electric field interactions, respectively. Note that the FID is usually defined as the electric field radiated by a collection of dipoles. However, as shown above, the FID field beyond the electric dipole approximation should include contributions from the magnetic dipole and electric quadrupole terms too. Equation 15.6 is a quite general expression for the linear optical activity polarization, which is valid for either solution sample or systems on surface or at interface. In the present section, we shall consider the solution sample containing chiral molecules.

Differential optical activity measurement. Hereafter, without loss of generality, the beam propagation direction is assumed to be along the Z-axis in a space-fixed frame so that $\hat{\mathbf{k}} = \hat{Z}$. Then, the X-component of the signal field produced by

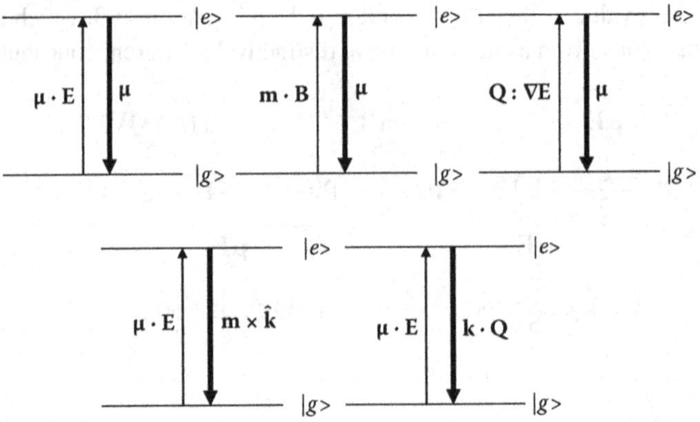

FIGURE 15.2 Five different energy-level diagrams associated with each term in Equation 15.6. The first three are the cases when the last radiation–matter interaction for generating free-induction decay is between electric dipole and vacuum electric field. On the other hand, the fourth and fifth ones are the cases when the free-induction decay is generated by the magnetic dipole–magnetic field and electric quadrupole–electric field interactions, respectively.

the above linear polarization is detected by employing either heterodyne or homodyne detection method. In this case, the polarization directions of the LCP and RCP beams are

$$\mathbf{e}_{LCP} = (\hat{X} + i\hat{Y})/\sqrt{2}$$

$$\mathbf{e}_{RCP} = (\hat{X} - i\hat{Y})/\sqrt{2}. \tag{15.8}$$

Then, for the LCP and RCP beams, the corresponding X-components of the linear polarizations are

$$\begin{aligned} P^X_{LCP}(\mathbf{r},t) &= \frac{i}{\hbar\sqrt{2}}\int_0^\infty d\tau < [\mu_X(\tau), \mu_X(0) + i\mu_Y(0)]\rho(-\infty) > E(\mathbf{r},t-\tau) \\ &+ \frac{i}{\hbar\sqrt{2}}\int_0^\infty d\tau < [\mu_X(\tau), m_Y(0) - im_X(0)]\rho(-\infty) > E(\mathbf{r},t-\tau) \\ &+ \frac{ik}{2\sqrt{2}}\left(\frac{i}{\hbar}\right)\int_0^\infty d\tau < [\mu_X(\tau), Q_{XZ}(0) + iQ_{YZ}(0)]\rho(-\infty) > E(\mathbf{r},t-\tau) \\ &+ \frac{i}{\hbar\sqrt{2}}\int_0^\infty d\tau < [m_Y(\tau), \mu_X(0) + i\mu_Y(0)]\rho(-\infty) > E(\mathbf{r},t-\tau) \\ &- \frac{ik}{2\sqrt{2}}\left(\frac{i}{\hbar}\right)\int_0^\infty d\tau < [Q_{XZ}(\tau), \mu_X(0) + i\mu_Y(0)]\rho(-\infty) > E(\mathbf{r},t-\tau) \end{aligned} \tag{15.9}$$

$$P_{RCP}^{X}(\mathbf{r},t)=\frac{i}{\hbar\sqrt{2}}\int_{0}^{\infty}d\tau<[\mu_X(\tau),\mu_X(0)-i\mu_Y(0)]\rho(-\infty)>E(\mathbf{r},t-\tau)$$

$$+\frac{i}{\hbar\sqrt{2}}\int_{0}^{\infty}d\tau<[\mu_X(\tau),m_Y(0)+im_X(0)]\rho(-\infty)>E(\mathbf{r},t-\tau)$$

$$+\frac{ik}{2\sqrt{2}}\left(\frac{i}{\hbar}\right)\int_{0}^{\infty}d\tau<[\mu_X(\tau),Q_{XZ}(0)-iQ_{YZ}(0)]\rho(-\infty)>E(\mathbf{r},t-\tau)$$

$$+\frac{i}{\hbar\sqrt{2}}\int_{0}^{\infty}d\tau<[m_Y(\tau),\mu_X(0)-i\mu_Y(0)]\rho(-\infty)>E(\mathbf{r},t-\tau)$$

$$-\frac{ik}{2\sqrt{2}}\left(\frac{i}{\hbar}\right)\int_{0}^{\infty}d\tau<[Q_{XZ}(\tau),\mu_X(0)-i\mu_Y(0)]\rho(-\infty)>E(\mathbf{r},t-\tau). \quad (15.10)$$

The next step is to perform rotational averaging of $P^X(t)$'s for randomly oriented chiral molecules in an isotropic medium. Note that the only rotationally invariant second- and third-rank tensors are the Kronecker delta and Levi–Civita epsilon, respectively. The rotationally averaged $<[\mu_X(\tau),i\mu_Y(0)]\rho(-\infty)>$ term for example vanishes due to $\delta_{XY}=0$. In addition, the third and fifth terms in Equations 15.9 and 15.10 also vanish because the Levi–Civita epsilon is antisymmetric with respect to any change of two indexes, that is, $\varepsilon_{xyz}=-\varepsilon_{xzy}$, whereas the quadrupole tensor is symmetric, that is, $Q_{yz}=Q_{zy}$.[6] Here, x, y, and z are the three Cartesian coordinates in a molecule-fixed frame. The rotationally averaged polarizations are then

$$\widehat{P}_{LCP}^{X}(\mathbf{r},t)=\frac{i}{\hbar\sqrt{2}}\int_{0}^{\infty}d\tau<[\mu_X(\tau),\mu_X(0)]\rho(-\infty)>E(\mathbf{r},t-\tau)$$

$$+\frac{i}{\hbar\sqrt{2}}\int_{0}^{\infty}d\tau<[\mu_X(\tau),-im_X(0)]\rho(-\infty)>E(\mathbf{r},t-\tau)$$

$$+\frac{i}{\hbar\sqrt{2}}\int_{0}^{\infty}d\tau<[m_Y(\tau),i\mu_Y(0)]\rho(-\infty)>E(\mathbf{r},t-\tau) \quad (15.11)$$

$$\widehat{P}_{RCP}^{X}(\mathbf{r},t)=\frac{i}{\hbar\sqrt{2}}\int_{0}^{\infty}d\tau<[\mu_X(\tau),\mu_X(0)]\rho(-\infty)>E(\mathbf{r},t-\tau)$$

$$+\frac{i}{\hbar\sqrt{2}}\int_{0}^{\infty}d\tau<[\mu_X(\tau),im_X(0)]\rho(-\infty)>E(\mathbf{r},t-\tau)$$

$$+\frac{i}{\hbar\sqrt{2}}\int_{0}^{\infty}d\tau<[m_Y(\tau),-i\mu_Y(0)]\rho(-\infty)>E(\mathbf{r},t-\tau). \quad (15.12)$$

In Equations 15.11 and 15.12, the first terms are identical to the usual electric dipole–electric dipole response function discussed in Section 3.4. The second and third terms in these equations are related to the optical activity (CD and ORD). Equations 15.11 and 15.12 can be further simplified by considering a property of quantum correlation function:

$$<[A(\tau),B(0)]\rho(-\infty)> = -<[B^*(\tau),A^*(0)]\rho(-\infty)>^* \tag{15.13}$$

where $A(\tau)=e^{iH\tau/\hbar}A(0)e^{-iH\tau/\hbar}$ and $B^*(\tau)=e^{iH\tau/\hbar}B^*(0)e^{-iH\tau/\hbar}$. Then, Equations 15.11 and 15.12 can be rewritten as

$$\hat{P}^X_{LCP}(\mathbf{r},t)=\frac{i}{\hbar\sqrt{2}}\int_0^\infty d\tau<[\mu_X(\tau),\mu_X(0)]\rho(-\infty)>E(\mathbf{r},t-\tau)$$

$$+\frac{\sqrt{2}i}{\hbar}\int_0^\infty d\tau\,\mathrm{Im}[<[\mu_X(\tau),m_X(0)]\rho(-\infty)>]E(\mathbf{r},t-\tau) \tag{15.14}$$

$$\hat{P}^X_{RCP}(\mathbf{r},t)=\frac{i}{\hbar\sqrt{2}}\int_0^\infty d\tau<[\mu_X(\tau),\mu_X(0)]\rho(-\infty)>E(\mathbf{r},t-\tau)$$

$$-\frac{\sqrt{2}i}{\hbar}\int_0^\infty d\tau\,\mathrm{Im}[<[\mu_X(\tau),m_X(0)]\rho(-\infty)>]E(\mathbf{r},t-\tau). \tag{15.15}$$

Here, we used the following properties, $\mu^*=\mu$, $m^*=-m$, and $<[\mu_X(\tau),m_X(0)]\times\rho(-\infty)> = <[\mu_Y(\tau),m_Y(0)]\rho(-\infty)>$. The first term in the expression for $\hat{P}^X_{LCP}(\mathbf{r},t)$ is identical to that for $\hat{P}^X_{RCP}(\mathbf{r},t)$. Thus, the difference polarization defined as $\Delta\hat{P}^X(\mathbf{r},t)=\hat{P}^X_{LCP}(\mathbf{r},t)-\hat{P}^X_{RCP}(\mathbf{r},t)$ is determined by the magnetic dipole–electric dipole (chiral) response function term, $(i/\hbar)\,\mathrm{Im}[<[\mu_X(\tau),m_X(0)]\rho(-\infty)>]$.

Inserting Equations 15.14 and 15.15 into the Maxwell equation (Equation 3.80) and following the same procedure described in Section 3.4, one can obtain the absorption coefficients of a given molecular system for LCP and RCP lights. Then, the difference of the two absorption coefficients obtained, which is the definition of the CD, is found to be

$$\Delta\kappa_a(\omega)=\frac{4\pi\omega}{n(\omega)c}\left(\chi''_{LCP}(\omega)-\chi''_{RCP}(\omega)\right)=\frac{4\pi\omega}{n(\omega)c}\Delta\chi''(\omega), \tag{15.16}$$

where the optical activity susceptibility, which is a complex function, is

$$\Delta\chi(\omega)=\frac{2\sqrt{2}i}{\hbar}\int_0^\infty dt\,\mathrm{Im}[<[\mu_X(t),m_X(0)]\rho(-\infty)>]e^{i\omega t}. \tag{15.17}$$

For a 2LS, after rotational average, one can find that the CD spectrum can then be calculated by

$$\Delta\kappa_a(\omega)=\frac{8\sqrt{2}\pi\omega}{3n(\omega)c}\mathrm{Im}[\boldsymbol{\mu}_{ge}\cdot\mathbf{m}_{eg}]\mathrm{Re}[\int_0^\infty dt\{e^{-i\bar{\omega}_{eg}t-g(t)}+e^{i\bar{\omega}_{eg}t-g^*(t)}\}e^{i\omega t}]. \tag{15.18}$$

Here, it is noted that the rotationally averaged quantity $\text{Im}[(\boldsymbol{\mu}_{ge})_x(\mathbf{m}_{eg})_x]$ is identical to $(1/3)\,\text{Im}[\boldsymbol{\mu}_{ge}\cdot\mathbf{m}_{eg}]$. As can be seen in Equation 15.18, the CD intensity is determined by the corresponding rotatory strength $\text{Im}[\boldsymbol{\mu}_{ge}\cdot\mathbf{m}_{eg}]$ for a given transition.[1] In addition to the CD, the ORD spectrum is related to the real part of the optical activity susceptibility in Equation 15.17, and it is in principle connected to the CD spectrum by the Kramers–Kronig transformation. One can further develop a theory for vibrational CD using the results presented here.

EXERCISE 15.1

The ORD spectrum is related to the refractive index difference defined as $\Delta n(\omega) = n_L(\omega) - n_R(\omega)$. More specifically, the ORD spectrum $\Delta\varphi(\omega)$ is defined as $\Delta\varphi(\omega) \equiv \Delta n(\omega)\omega L/2c$. Then, find the relationship between $\Delta n(\omega)$ and the real part of the optical activity susceptibility in Equation 15.17.

Cross-polarization optical activity measurement. In the above, we considered the case when the CD spectrum is measured by taking the difference between the absorbances with LCP and RCP beams or pulses, which is the conventional method. However, it is possible to measure the chiral susceptibility associated with the magnetic dipole–electric dipole response function by properly controlling the incident beam and detected FID polarization directions.[7] Instead of circularly polarized beams, let us consider the case when the incident beam is linearly polarized along the X-direction and the beam propagation direction is along the Z-axis. Then, after rotational averaging of the linear polarization over randomly oriented molecules, one can find that the X- and Y-components of the linear polarization vector are given as

$$\hat{P}_X(\mathbf{r},t) = \frac{i}{\hbar}\int_0^\infty d\tau < [\mu_X(\tau),\mu_X(0)]\rho(-\infty) > E(\mathbf{r},t-\tau)$$

$$\hat{P}_Y(\mathbf{r},t) = -\frac{2}{\hbar}\int_0^\infty d\tau\, \text{Im}[< [\mu_Y(\tau),m_Y(0)]\rho(-\infty) >]E(\text{r},t-\tau). \quad (15.19)$$

Note that $\hat{P}_X(\mathbf{r},t)$ and $\hat{P}_Y(\mathbf{r},t)$ are responsible for generating free-induction-decay fields. Here, the electric dipole–electric quadrupole response function contribution vanishes in the Y-component of the polarization vector. Consequently, if one selectively measures the Y-component of the FID field that is generated by the linear polarization $\hat{P}_Y(\mathbf{r},t)$ whose direction is perpendicular to the incident beam polarization direction, it will be possible to measure the magnetic dipole–electric dipole response function or the corresponding chiral susceptibility containing information on both the CD and ORD of chiral molecules in solution.[7]

The polarizations $\hat{P}_X(\mathbf{r},t)$ and $\hat{P}_Y(\mathbf{r},t)$, of which Fourier transforms are related to the absorption and refractive index and CD and ORD spectra, respectively, are the sources of radiated FID fields, and they should obey the Maxwell equation. For the transverse component of the emitted signal electric field $\mathbf{E}_s(Z,t)$ propagating along the Z-direction, the Maxwell equation is given as

$$\nabla^2\mathbf{E}_s(Z,t) - \frac{1}{c^2}\frac{\partial^2}{\partial t^2}\mathbf{E}_s(Z,t) = \frac{4\pi}{c^2}\frac{\partial^2}{\partial t^2}\mathbf{P}^{(1)}(Z,t). \quad (15.20)$$

Since there are X and Y components of the signal electric field and polarization vectors, we have

$$\mathbf{E}_s(Z,t) = E_s^X(Z,t)\hat{X} + E_s^Y(Z,t)\hat{Y} \tag{15.21}$$

$$\mathbf{P}^{(1)}(Z,t) = \widehat{P}_X(Z,t)\hat{X} + \widehat{P}_Y^{(1)}(Z,t)\hat{Y}. \tag{15.22}$$

Inserting Equations 15.21 and 15.22 into 15.20, we get the coupled Maxwell equations,

$$\nabla^2 E_s^X(Z,t) - \frac{1}{c^2}\frac{\partial^2}{\partial t^2}E_s^X(Z,t) \cong \frac{4\pi}{c^2}\frac{\partial^2}{\partial t^2}\int_{-\infty}^{t} d\tau[\phi_{\mu\mu}(t-\tau)]_{XX}E_s^X(Z,\tau) \tag{15.23}$$

$$\nabla^2 E_s^Y(Z,t) - \frac{1}{c^2}\frac{\partial^2}{\partial t^2}E_s^Y(Z,t)$$

$$= \frac{4\pi}{c^2}\frac{\partial^2}{\partial t^2}\left[\int_{-\infty}^{t} d\tau[\phi_{\mu\mu}(t-\tau)]_{YY}E_s^Y(Z,\tau) - \int_{-\infty}^{t} d\tau[\phi_{\mu m}(t-\tau)]_{YY}E_s^X(Z,\tau)\right]. \tag{15.24}$$

Here, the shorthand notations of the response functions, $[\phi_{\mu\mu}(t-\tau)]_{XX}$ and $[\phi_{\mu m}(t-\tau)]_{YY}$, were used, and their definitions are

$$[\phi_{\mu\mu}(t-\tau)]_{XX} = \frac{i}{\hbar} < [\mu_X(t-\tau), \mu_X(0)]\rho(-\infty) > \tag{15.25}$$

$$[\phi_{\mu m}(t-\tau)]_{YY} = \frac{2}{\hbar}\mathrm{Im}[< [\mu_Y(t-\tau), m_Y(0)]\rho(-\infty) >]. \tag{15.26}$$

Equation 15.23 is just the Maxwell equation of the absorptive (lossy) medium, and the susceptibility $\chi_{\mu\mu}(\omega)$ associated with the dipole-dipole response function was discussed in detail in Section 3.4. The electric field $E_s^X(Z,t)$, obtained from Equation 15.23, is the usual FID field radiated by a collection of oscillating electric dipoles.

In order to solve the coupled Maxwell equation in Equation 15.24, we first obtain the solution for $E_s^X(Z,\omega)$ in frequency domain. Taking the Fourier transform of Equation 15.23 and using the slowly-varying-amplitude approximation, we have

$$E_s^X(Z,\omega) \cong E_s^X(0,\omega)\exp(ik'Z) \tag{15.27}$$

where

$$E_s^X(0,\omega) = \int_0^{\infty} dt\, E(t)e^{i(\omega-\omega_c)t} \tag{15.28}$$

$$k'(\omega) = \frac{\omega}{c}[1 + 4\pi\chi_{\mu\mu}(\omega)]^{1/2}. \tag{15.29}$$

Here, $\chi_{\mu\mu}(\omega)$ is just the linear susceptibility associated with the electric dipole–electric dipole response function. To obtain the Y-component of the radiated signal electric field $E_s^Y(Z,t)$ at position Z, which corresponds to the optical activity FID field, we again invoke the slowly varying amplitude approximation to the temporal envelope and also assume that the energy transfer among waves is significantly large only after the waves travel over a distance longer than their wavelengths. Then, inserting the solution for $E_s^X(Z,\omega)$ into Equation 15.24 and taking Fourier transform of Equation 15.24, we have

$$ik'\frac{\partial}{\partial z}E_s^Y(Z,\omega) \cong \frac{2\pi\omega^2}{c^2}\chi_{\mu m}(\omega)E_s^X(Z,\omega), \tag{15.30}$$

where

$$\chi_{\mu m}(\omega) = \int_0^\infty dt[\phi_{\mu m}(t)]_{YY}e^{i\omega t}. \tag{15.31}$$

In order to obtain Equation 15.30, we assumed that $1+4\pi\chi'_{\mu\mu}(\omega) \gg \chi''_{\mu\mu}(\omega)$. Noting that the relationship between the optical activity susceptibility $\Delta\chi(\omega)$ given in Equation 15.17 and $\chi_{\mu m}(\omega)$ in Equation 15.31, is,

$$\chi_{\mu m}(\omega) = -\frac{i}{\sqrt{2}}\Delta\chi(\omega), \tag{15.32}$$

one can find that the emitted optical activity FID field after passing through the sample with length L is given as

$$E_s^Y(L,\omega) = \frac{\sqrt{2}\pi\omega L}{n(\omega)c}\Delta\chi(\omega)E_s^X(L,\omega). \tag{15.33}$$

This result shows that the spectrum of the Y-component (perpendicular component) of the emitted electric field is linearly proportional to that of the X-component of the transmitted electric field and the major frequency-dependent part of the above connection formula is the optical activity (chiral) susceptibility $\Delta\chi(\omega)$. Therefore, the circular dichroism spectrum can be retrieved from the measurements of the X- and Y-components of the generated signal field $\mathbf{E}_s(\omega)$ as

$$\Delta\kappa_a(\omega) = \frac{4\pi\omega}{n(\omega)c}\mathrm{Im}[\Delta\tilde{\chi}(\omega)] = \frac{2\sqrt{2}}{L}\mathrm{Im}\left[\frac{E_s^Y(L,\omega)}{E_s^X(L,\omega)}\right]. \tag{15.34}$$

The above result is particularly useful since the X- and Y-components of the FID field can be selectively measured by using a properly chosen linear polarizer whose polarization direction is either parallel or perpendicular to the incident beam polarization direction. The electric field spectra, which are complex functions with respect to frequency, can be characterized by using heterodyne-detection method such as Fourier transform spectral interferometry based on a modified Mach-Zehnder interferometer.

EXERCISE 15.2
Derive Equations 15.30 and 15.33.

Next, from the relationship in Equation 15.33 between the optical activity susceptibility and two experimentally measured *X*- and *Y*-components of the FID field, one can obtain the circular dichroism (ΔA) and optical rotatory dispersion ($\Delta\varphi$) spectra as

$$\Delta A(\omega) = \frac{\Delta\kappa_a(\omega)L}{2.303} = \frac{2\sqrt{2}}{2.303}\mathrm{Im}\left[\frac{E_s^Y(\omega)}{E_s^X(\omega)}\right] \tag{15.35}$$

$$\Delta\varphi(\omega) = \frac{\Delta n(\omega)\omega L}{2c} = \frac{1}{\sqrt{2}}\mathrm{Re}\left[\frac{E_s^Y(\omega)}{E_s^X(\omega)}\right]. \tag{15.36}$$

Note that the optical rotation angle is defined as the half of the phase change between LCP and RCP after passing through the sample with length L.

15.3 RAMAN OPTICAL ACTIVITY

The vibrational CD is an IR analog of the electronic CD. The electronic CD is related to the magnetic dipole induced by angular motions of electrons, whereas the VCD is to that by angular oscillations associated with *nuclear* motions. Thus, the vibrational CD signal is a few orders of magnitude smaller than the electronic CD signal. The Raman analog of the vibrational CD is called the ROA.[4] LCP and RCP beams are used to induce inelastic Raman scattering processes, and the difference between the two Raman spectra obtained with LCP and RCP lights corresponds to the ROA spectrum. In Section 3.5, for a theoretical description of the coherent raman scattering (CRS) process, it was necessary to consider the first-order induced dipole given as $\boldsymbol{\mu}_{ind}(\mathbf{r},t) = \boldsymbol{\alpha}\cdot\mathbf{E}(\mathbf{r},t)$. However, such approach is valid only within the electric dipole approximation, and it ignores the magnetic dipole–magnetic field and electric quadrupole–electric field interaction-induced dipole contributions to the total first-order induced dipole. Including the latter two contributions, though they are two to three orders of magnitude smaller than $\boldsymbol{\alpha}\cdot\mathbf{E}(\mathbf{r},t)$, we have the more general first-order induced *electric* dipole operator, which is

$$\boldsymbol{\mu}_{ind}(\mathbf{r},t) = \boldsymbol{\alpha}\cdot\mathbf{E}(\mathbf{r},t) + \mathbf{G}\cdot\mathbf{B}(\mathbf{r},t) + \frac{1}{2}\mathbf{A}:\nabla\mathbf{E}(\mathbf{r},t). \tag{15.37}$$

The second term in Equation 15.37 is the electric dipole induced by the interaction between molecular magnetic dipole–ROA tensor and external magnetic field. The third is that induced by the interaction between molecular electric quadrupole–ROA tensor and gradient of external electric field.

The next step is to calculate the material polarization. In addition to the expectation value of the above induced electric dipole operator, one needs to consider the expectation values of *induced* magnetic dipole and electric quadrupole operators over the density matrix, as can be seen in Equation 15.4. The induced magnetic dipole and induced electric quadrupole operators are, respectively, given as

$$\mathbf{m}_{ind}(\mathbf{r},t) = \bar{\mathbf{G}} \cdot \mathbf{E}(\mathbf{r},t) \tag{15.38}$$

$$\mathbf{Q}_{ind}(\mathbf{r},t) = \frac{1}{2}\bar{\mathbf{A}} \cdot \mathbf{E}(\mathbf{r},t). \tag{15.39}$$

The jth vector element of the above induced electric and magnetic dipoles and the jkth tensor element of the induced quadrupole are

$$\mu_{ind}^{j}(\mathbf{r},t) = \alpha_{jk}E_k(\mathbf{r},t) + G_{jk}B_k(\mathbf{r},t) + (1/2)A_{jkl}\nabla_k E_l(\mathbf{r},t)$$

$$m_{ind}^{j}(\mathbf{r},t) = \bar{G}_{jk}E_k(\mathbf{r},t)$$

$$Q_{ind}^{jk}(\mathbf{r},t) = \frac{1}{2}\bar{A}_{jkl}E_l(\mathbf{r},t). \tag{15.40}$$

Here, $\bar{\mathbf{G}}$ and $\bar{\mathbf{A}}$ are different from **G** and **A**, but they are also magnetic dipole–ROA and electric quadrupole–ROA tensors.[8] Note that **G** and $\bar{\mathbf{G}}$ are second-rank tensors, whereas **A** and $\bar{\mathbf{A}}$ are third-rank tensors. In the far-from-electronic-resonance limit, where all the incident beams are nonresonant with any of electronic transitions of optical chromophores, these four different ROA tensor operators are defined as

$$G_{\alpha\beta}(\omega) \equiv \frac{1}{\hbar}\sum_{e\neq g}\frac{\mu_\alpha|e\rangle\langle e|m_\beta}{\omega_{eg}-\omega} + \frac{m_\beta|e\rangle\langle e|\mu_\alpha}{\omega_{eg}+\omega}$$

$$\bar{G}_{\alpha\beta}(\omega) \equiv \frac{1}{\hbar}\sum_{e\neq g}\frac{m_\alpha|e\rangle\langle e|\mu_\beta}{\omega_{eg}-\omega} + \frac{\mu_\beta|e\rangle\langle e|m_\alpha}{\omega_{eg}+\omega}$$

$$A_{\alpha\beta\gamma}(\omega) \equiv \frac{1}{\hbar}\sum_{e\neq g}\frac{\mu_\alpha|e\rangle\langle e|Q_{\beta\gamma}}{\omega_{eg}-\omega} + \frac{Q_{\beta\gamma}|e\rangle\langle e|\mu_\alpha}{\omega_{eg}+\omega}$$

$$\bar{A}_{\alpha\beta\gamma}(\omega) \equiv \frac{1}{\hbar}\sum_{e\neq g}\frac{Q_{\alpha\beta}|e\rangle\langle e|\mu_\gamma}{\omega_{eg}-\omega} + \frac{\mu_\gamma|e\rangle\langle e|Q_{\alpha\beta}}{\omega_{eg}+\omega}. \tag{15.41}$$

Now, from the generalized induced electric dipole, magnetic dipole, and electric quadrupole in Equations 15.37–15.39, the effective radiation–matter interaction

Hamiltonian is written as

$$H_{rad-mat} = -\boldsymbol{\mu}_{ind}(\mathbf{r},t)\cdot\mathbf{E}(\mathbf{r},t) - \mathbf{m}_{ind}(\mathbf{r},t)\cdot\mathbf{B}(\mathbf{r},t) - \frac{1}{2}\mathrm{Q}_{ind}(\mathbf{r},t)\cdot\nabla\mathbf{E}(\mathbf{r},t)$$

$$= -\boldsymbol{\alpha} : \mathbf{E}^2(\mathbf{r},t) - \mathbf{G} : \mathbf{E}(\mathbf{r},t)\mathbf{B}(\mathbf{r},t) - \bar{\mathbf{G}} : \mathbf{B}(\mathbf{r},t)\mathbf{E}(\mathbf{r},t)$$

$$-(1/2)\mathbf{A} \vdots \mathbf{E}(\mathbf{r},t)\nabla\mathbf{E}(\mathbf{r},t) - (1/2)\bar{\mathbf{A}} \vdots (\nabla\mathbf{E}(\mathbf{r},t))\mathbf{E}(\mathbf{r},t). \tag{15.42}$$

Note that the last four terms on the right-hand side of Equation 15.42 correspond to the fifth and sixth conjugate pairs given in Scheme 3.1.

In the present section, we focus on the time-domain coherent ROA spectroscopy utilizing ultrashort laser pulses, instead of the frequency-domain ROA. Let us consider the case that two pump pulses with center frequencies ω_1 and ω_2 and wavevectors $\mathbf{k}_1$ and $\mathbf{k}_2$ are used to create the transient grating with wavevector $\mathbf{k}_1$-$\mathbf{k}_2$ in the sample. After a finite delay time T from the first pair of pulses, the third (linearly polarized) pulse with frequency ω_3 and wavevector $\mathbf{k}_3$ is injected into the sample to stimulate a Raman scattering process. The scattering signal field with wavevector $\mathbf{k}_1$-$\mathbf{k}_2$+$\mathbf{k}_3$ is then detected. Unlike the case of the normal CRS discussed in Section 3.5, one might use LCP and RCP beams for the ω_1-pulse or use special beam polarization configuration to selectively measure the ROA of chiral molecules in solution. Conventional ROA spectroscopy uses LCP and RCP beams to measure the LCP- and RCP-Raman spectra independently, and the difference is taken as the ROA spectrum. However, there are other possibilities to measure the ROA properties by deliberately controlling the incident beam polarization directions and by selectively measuring particular polarization component of the radiated coherent Raman optical activity (CROA) signal.

The electric field used for a CROA experiment is given as

$$\mathbf{E}(\mathbf{r},t) = \mathbf{e}_1 E_1(t+T)e^{i\mathbf{k}_1\cdot\mathbf{r}-i\omega_1 t} + \mathbf{e}_2 E_2(t+T)e^{i\mathbf{k}_2\cdot\mathbf{r}-i\omega_2 t} + \mathbf{e}_3 E_3(t)e^{i\mathbf{k}_3\cdot\mathbf{r}-i\omega_3 t} + c.c.. \tag{15.43}$$

In the present case, the first two radiation–matter interactions in a CROA measurement can be effectively written as

$$H_{rad-mat} = \{-\boldsymbol{\alpha} : \mathbf{e}_2^*\mathbf{e}_1 E_2^*(t+T)E_1(t+T) - \mathbf{G} : \mathbf{e}_2^*\mathbf{b}_1 E_2^*(t+T)B_1(t+T)$$

$$-\bar{\mathbf{G}} : \mathbf{b}_2^*\mathbf{e}_1 B_2^*(t+T)E_1(t+T) - (i/2)\mathbf{A} \vdots \mathbf{e}_2^*\mathbf{k}_1\mathbf{e}_1 E_2^*(t+T)E_1(t+T)$$

$$+ (i/2)\bar{\mathbf{A}} \vdots \mathbf{k}_2\mathbf{e}_2^*\mathbf{e}_1 E_2^*(t+T)E_1(t+T)\}e^{i(\mathbf{k}_1-\mathbf{k}_2)\cdot\mathbf{r}-i(\omega_1-\omega_2)t}. \tag{15.44}$$

Equation 15.44 shows that, at least, one needs to consider five different cause operators. From Equation 15.4, the CROA polarization is then given as the sum of induced electric dipole, induced magnetic dipole, and induced quadrupole contributions as

$$\mathbf{P}_{CROA}(\mathbf{r},t) = \bar{\boldsymbol{\mu}}_{ind}(\mathbf{r},t) + \bar{\mathbf{m}}_{ind}(\mathbf{r},t)\times\hat{\mathbf{k}}_s - (i/2)\mathbf{k}_s\cdot\bar{\mathbf{Q}}_{ind}(\mathbf{r},t), \tag{15.45}$$

where, specifically for the CROA, we have

$$\boldsymbol{\mu}_{ind}(\mathbf{r},t) = \left(\boldsymbol{\alpha}\cdot\mathbf{e}_3 + \mathbf{G}\cdot\mathbf{b}_3 + \frac{i}{2}\mathbf{A}:\mathbf{k}_3\mathbf{e}_3\right)E_3(t)e^{i\mathbf{k}_3\cdot\mathbf{r}-i\omega_3 t}$$

$$\mathbf{m}_{ind}(\mathbf{r},t) = \bar{\mathbf{G}}\cdot\mathbf{e}_3E_3(t)e^{i\mathbf{k}_3\cdot\mathbf{r}-i\omega_3 t}$$

$$\mathbf{Q}_{ind}(\mathbf{r},t) = \frac{1}{2}\bar{\mathbf{A}}\cdot\mathbf{e}_3E_3(t)e^{i\mathbf{k}_3\cdot\mathbf{r}-i\omega_3 t}. \tag{15.46}$$

From the effective radiation–matter interaction Hamiltonian in Equation 15.44 and the CROA polarization in terms of induced electric and magnetic dipoles and induced quadrupole in Equation 15.45, one can find that nine cases in total should be taken into consideration to fully calculate the CROA polarization and signal. The corresponding cause opearators, conjugate external fields, and effect operators are

(1) $\hat{A} = \boldsymbol{\alpha}\cdot\mathbf{E}_1(\mathbf{r},t),\ F = \mathbf{E}_2(\mathbf{r},t),$ and $\hat{B} = \boldsymbol{\alpha}\cdot\mathbf{E}_3(\mathbf{r},t)$

(2) $\hat{A} = \mathbf{G}\cdot\mathbf{B}_1(\mathbf{r},t),\ F = \mathbf{E}_2(\mathbf{r},t),$ and $\hat{B} = \boldsymbol{\alpha}\cdot\mathbf{E}_3(\mathbf{r},t)$

(3) $\hat{A} = \bar{\mathbf{G}}\cdot\mathbf{E}_1(\mathbf{r},t),\ F = \mathbf{B}_2(\mathbf{r},t),$ and $\hat{B} = \boldsymbol{\alpha}\cdot\mathbf{E}_3(\mathbf{r},t)$

(4) $\hat{A} = (1/2)\mathbf{A}:\nabla\mathbf{E}_1(\mathbf{r},t),\ F = \mathbf{E}_2(\mathbf{r},t),$ and $\hat{B} = \boldsymbol{\alpha}\cdot\mathbf{E}_3(\mathbf{r},t)$

(5) $\hat{A} = (1/2)\bar{\mathbf{A}}\cdot\mathbf{E}_1(\mathbf{r},t),\ F = \nabla\mathbf{E}_2(\mathbf{r},t),$ and $\hat{B} = \boldsymbol{\alpha}\cdot\mathbf{E}_3(\mathbf{r},t)$

(6) $\hat{A} = \boldsymbol{\alpha}\cdot\mathbf{E}_1(\mathbf{r},t),\ F = \mathbf{E}_2(\mathbf{r},t),$ and $\hat{B} = \mathbf{G}\cdot\mathbf{B}_3(\mathbf{r},t)$

(7) $\hat{A} = \boldsymbol{\alpha}\cdot\mathbf{E}_1(\mathbf{r},t),\ F = \mathbf{E}_2(\mathbf{r},t),$ and $\hat{B} = \{\bar{\mathbf{G}}\cdot\mathbf{E}_3(\mathbf{r},t)\}\times\hat{\mathbf{k}}_s$

(8) $\hat{A} = \boldsymbol{\alpha}\cdot\mathbf{E}_1(\mathbf{r},t),\ F = \mathbf{E}_2(\mathbf{r},t),$ and $\hat{B} = (1/2)\mathbf{A}:\nabla\mathbf{E}_3(\mathbf{r},t)$

(9) $\hat{A} = \boldsymbol{\alpha}\cdot\mathbf{E}_1(\mathbf{r},t),\ F = \mathbf{E}_2(\mathbf{r},t),$ and $\hat{B} = -(1/2)\mathbf{k}_3\cdot\{\mathbf{A}\cdot\mathbf{E}_3(\mathbf{r},t)\}.$ (15.47)

The other cases that are not listed in Equation 15.47 can be ignored since they are at least second-order with respect to small quantities, such as magnetic dipole–magnetic field and electric quadrupole–electric field interactions.

Using the linear response theory with the cause-and-effect operators with conjugate fields in Equation 15.47, one can find that the expectation value of the above induced dipole, which is the CROA polarization, is given by

$$
\begin{aligned}
\mathbf{P}_{CROA}(\mathbf{r},t) = {} & \langle \alpha\mathbf{E}_3 \overset{\alpha\mathbf{E}_2^*\mathbf{E}_1}{\Longleftarrow} \rho(t_0)\rangle + \langle \alpha\mathbf{E}_3 \overset{\mathbf{G}\mathbf{E}_2^*\mathbf{B}_1}{\Longleftarrow} \rho(t_0)\rangle + \langle \alpha\mathbf{E}_3 \overset{\bar{\mathbf{G}}\mathbf{B}_2^*\mathbf{E}_1}{\Longleftarrow} \rho(t_0)\rangle \\
& + \langle \alpha\mathbf{E}_3 \overset{(1/2)\mathbf{A}\mathbf{E}_2^*\nabla\mathbf{E}_1}{\Longleftarrow} \rho(t_0)\rangle + \langle \alpha\mathbf{E}_3 \overset{(1/2)\bar{\mathbf{A}}(\nabla\mathbf{E}_2^*)\mathbf{E}_1}{\Longleftarrow} \rho(t_0)\rangle + \langle \mathbf{G}\mathbf{B}_3 \overset{\alpha\mathbf{E}_2^*\mathbf{E}_1}{\Longleftarrow} \rho(t_0)\rangle \\
& + \langle (\bar{\mathbf{G}}\mathbf{E}_3)\times\hat{\mathbf{k}}_3 \overset{\alpha\mathbf{E}_2^*\mathbf{E}_1}{\Longleftarrow} \rho(t_0)\rangle + \langle (i/2)\mathbf{A}\nabla\mathbf{E}_3 \overset{\alpha\mathbf{E}_2^*\mathbf{E}_1}{\Longleftarrow} \rho(t_0)\rangle - \langle (i/2)\mathbf{k}_s\cdot(\mathbf{A}\mathbf{E}_3) \overset{\alpha\mathbf{E}_2^*\mathbf{E}_1}{\Longleftarrow} \rho(t_0)\rangle .
\end{aligned}
\tag{15.48}
$$

The corresponding energy-level diagrams are shown in Figure 15.3. Then, the CROA polarization, which includes magnetic dipole and electric quadrupole contributions,

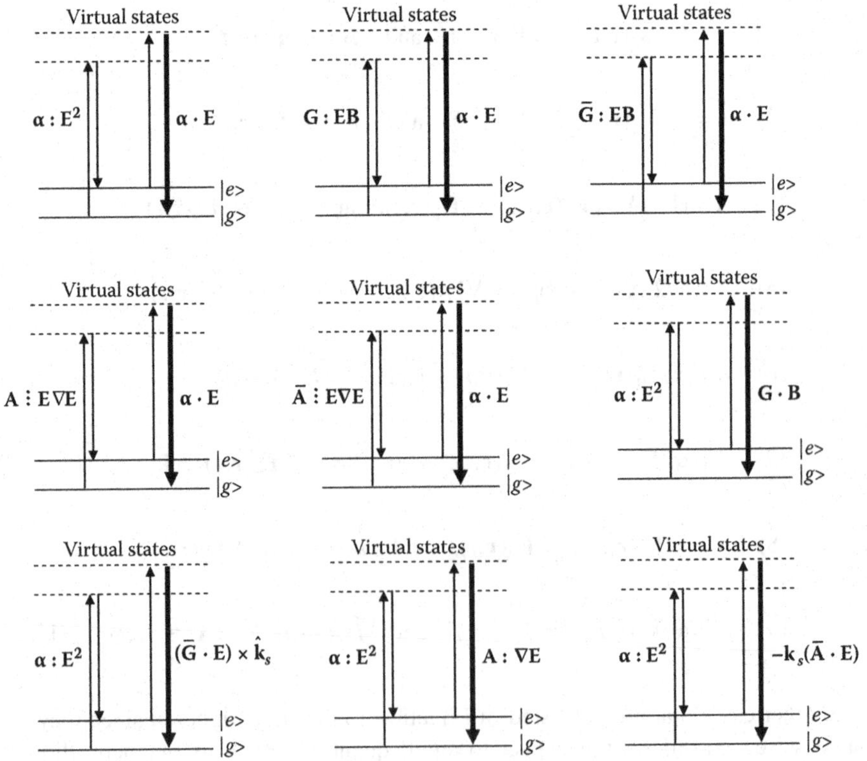

FIGURE 15.3 Nine different energy-level diagrams for polarizations contributing to the coherent Raman optical activity.

is given as

$$P_{CROA}(\mathbf{r},t) = e^{i(\mathbf{k}_1-\mathbf{k}_2+\mathbf{k}_3)\cdot\mathbf{r}-i(\omega_1-\omega_2+\omega_3)t} E_3(t)\int_0^\infty d\tau\{\phi_{\alpha\alpha}(\tau)E_2^*(t+T-\tau)E_1(t+T-\tau)$$

$$+\phi_{\alpha G}(\tau)E_2^*(t+T-\tau)B_1(t+T-\tau)+\phi_{\alpha\bar{G}}(\tau)B_2^*(t+T-\tau)E_1(t+T-\tau)$$

$$+(k_1/2)\phi_{\alpha A}(\tau)E_2^*(t+T-\tau)E_1(t+T-\tau)-(k_2/2)\phi_{\alpha\bar{A}}(\tau)E_2^*(t+T-\tau)E_1(t+T-\tau)$$

$$+\phi_{G\alpha}(\tau)E_2^*(t+T-\tau)E_1(t+T-\tau)+\phi_{\bar{G}\alpha}(\tau)E_2^*(t+T-\tau)E_1(t+T-\tau)$$

$$+(k_3/2)\phi_{A\alpha}(\tau)E_2^*(t+T-\tau)E_1(t+T-\tau)$$

$$-(k_s/2)\phi_{\bar{A}\alpha}(\tau)E_2^*(t+T-\tau)E_1(t+T-\tau)\}e^{i(\omega_1-\omega_2)\tau}. \tag{15.49}$$

The polarizability-polarizability response function in Equation 15.46 was already discussed in Section 3.5, and it is insensitive to molecular chirality at all. Now, the polarizability–magnetic dipole ROA tensor response functions $\phi_{\alpha G}(\tau), \phi_{G\alpha}(\tau)$, $\phi_{\alpha\bar{G}}(\tau)$, and $\phi_{\bar{G}\alpha}(\tau)$, the polarizability–electric quadrupole ROA tensor response function $\phi_{\alpha A}(\tau), \phi_{A\alpha}(\tau), \phi_{\alpha\bar{A}}(\tau)$, and $\phi_{\bar{A}\alpha}(\tau)$ are defined as

$$\phi_{\alpha\alpha}(\tau) \equiv \frac{i}{\hbar}\theta(\tau) < [\boldsymbol{\alpha}(\tau):\mathbf{e}_s\mathbf{e}_3, \boldsymbol{\alpha}(0):\mathbf{e}_2^*\mathbf{e}_1]\rho(-\infty) >$$

$$\phi_{\alpha G}(\tau) \equiv \frac{i}{\hbar}\theta(\tau) < [\boldsymbol{\alpha}(\tau):\mathbf{e}_s\mathbf{e}_3, \mathbf{G}(0):\mathbf{e}_2^*\mathbf{b}_1]\rho(-\infty) >$$

$$\phi_{\alpha\bar{G}}(\tau) \equiv \frac{i}{\hbar}\theta(\tau) < [\boldsymbol{\alpha}(\tau):\mathbf{e}_s\mathbf{e}_3, \bar{\mathbf{G}}(0):\mathbf{b}_2^*\mathbf{e}_1]\rho(-\infty) >$$

$$\phi_{\alpha A}(\tau) \equiv \frac{i}{\hbar}\theta(\tau) < [\boldsymbol{\alpha}(\tau):\mathbf{e}_s\mathbf{e}_3, i\mathbf{A}(0)\vdots\mathbf{e}_2^*\hat{\mathbf{k}}_1\mathbf{e}_1]\rho(-\infty) >$$

$$\phi_{\alpha\bar{A}}(\tau) \equiv \frac{i}{\hbar}\theta(\tau) < [\boldsymbol{\alpha}(\tau):\mathbf{e}_s\mathbf{e}_3, i\bar{\mathbf{A}}(0)\vdots\hat{\mathbf{k}}_2\mathbf{e}_2^*\mathbf{e}_1]\rho(-\infty) >$$

$$\phi_{G\alpha}(\tau) \equiv \frac{i}{\hbar}\theta(\tau) < [\mathbf{G}(\tau):\mathbf{e}_s\mathbf{b}_3, \boldsymbol{\alpha}(0):\mathbf{e}_2^*\mathbf{e}_1]\rho(-\infty) >$$

$$\phi_{\bar{G}\alpha}(\tau) \equiv \frac{i}{\hbar}\theta(\tau) < [\bar{\mathbf{G}}(\tau):(\hat{\mathbf{k}}_s\times\mathbf{e}_s)\mathbf{e}_3, \boldsymbol{\alpha}(0):\mathbf{e}_2^*\mathbf{e}_1]\rho(-\infty) >$$

$$\phi_{A\alpha}(\tau) \equiv \frac{i}{\hbar}\theta(\tau) < [i\mathbf{A}(\tau)\vdots\mathbf{e}_s\hat{\mathbf{k}}_3\mathbf{e}_3, \boldsymbol{\alpha}(0):\mathbf{e}_2^*\mathbf{e}_1]\rho(-\infty) >$$

$$\phi_{\bar{A}\alpha}(\tau) \equiv \frac{i}{\hbar}\theta(\tau) < [i\bar{\mathbf{A}}(\tau)\vdots\hat{\mathbf{k}}_s\mathbf{e}_s\mathbf{e}_3, \boldsymbol{\alpha}(0):\mathbf{e}_2^*\mathbf{e}_1]\rho(-\infty) >. \tag{15.50}$$

Here, $\mathbf{e}_s$ denotes the unit vector of the CROA polarization direction.

Except for the first term in Equation 15.49, the remaining eight contributions involve either magnetic dipole–magnetic field or electric quadrupole–electric field interaction. Thus, the coherent Raman spectroscopy measuring the polarizability-polarizability response function or susceptibility requires only the first term in Equation 15.49. Depending on detailed beam polarization states and detection methods, one or just a few terms in Equation 15.49 are only experimentally measured. However, the result in Equation 15.49 with definitions of relevant response functions in Equation 15.50 is quite general so that it can be used to calculate the CROA polarization and its signal electric field for any arbitrary beam polarization states and detection schemes.

One of the possible experiments for measuring the ROA signal in time domain is to use a circularly polarized pulse for one of the three incident beams to measure the LCP and RCP CRS signals. Then, the difference signal will correspond to the CROA, since the all-electric-dipole polarizability-polarizability response function contributes to the LCP and RCP signals equally and they cancel out when the difference signal is taken. Depending on which pulse among the three incident pulses is controlled to be circularly polarized, there are a series of different circularly polarized-CROA measurements.

EXERCISE 15.3

Consider the following specific beam configurations. The three beam propagation directions are parallel to one another as, $\hat{\mathbf{k}}_1 = \hat{\mathbf{k}}_2 = \hat{\mathbf{k}}_3 = \hat{Z}$. The second and third pulses are linearly polarized beams and the polarization directions are along the X-axis as $\mathbf{e}_2 = \mathbf{e}_3 = \hat{X}$. The first pulse is however either LCP or RCP, that is, $\mathbf{e}_1 = \mathbf{e}_{LCP} = (\hat{X} + i\hat{Y})/\sqrt{2}$ or $\mathbf{e}_1 = \mathbf{e}_{RCP} = (\hat{X} - i\hat{Y})/\sqrt{2}$. Now, let us assume that the X-component of the CROA polarization is detected. Then, obtain expressions for $\tilde{P}^X_{LCP-CROA}(\mathbf{r},t)$ and $\tilde{P}^X_{RCP-CROA}(\mathbf{r},t)$ and those of the corresponding electric field amplitudes $E^X_{LCP-CROA}(t)$ and $E^X_{RCP-CROA}(t)$. What determines the difference electric field defined as $\Delta E^X_{CROA}(t) \equiv E^X_{LCP-CROA}(t) - E^X_{RCP-CROA}(t)$? Suppose that the time-integrated signal field intensities $I_{LCP-CROA}(t)$ and $I_{RCP-CROA}(t)$ are measured via a homodyne-detection method. Obtain the expression for the difference signal defined as $\Delta I_{CROA}(t) = I_{RCP-CROA}(t) - I_{LCP-CROA}(t)$, which is by definition the CROA signal.

Alternative ways to measure various ROA terms in Equation 15.49 are to use specifically designed polarization-controlled measurement methods. In this case, all the incident beams and detected signal fields are assumed to be linearly polarized. Thus, the beam polarization configuration should be properly chosen to nullify the first term in Equation 15.49, which is associated with the all-electric-dipole-allowed polarizability-polarizability response function. For randomly oriented molecules in solution, the three fourth-rank tensorial isomers that are rotationally invariant are $\delta_{l_1,l_2}\delta_{l_3,l_4}$, $\delta_{l_1,l_3}\delta_{l_2,l_4}$, and $\delta_{l_1,l_4}\delta_{l_2,l_3}$, where l_j for $j = 1 \sim 4$ are Cartesian coordinates in a space-fixed frame. Therefore, the rotationally averaged tensor elements of $\phi_{\alpha\alpha}$ with even number of X, Y, or Z indices in $[\phi_{\alpha\alpha}]_{l_1l_2l_3l_4}$, such as $[\phi_{\alpha\alpha}]_{XXXX}$, $[\phi_{\alpha\alpha}]_{XYXY}$, $[\phi_{\alpha\alpha}]_{XYYX}$, and so on, do not vanish. On the other hand, those having an odd number of X, Y, and Z indexes, such as $[\phi_{\alpha\alpha}]_{XXXY}$, $[\phi_{\alpha\alpha}]_{XXYX}$, and so forth, vanish. Therefore, if one can selectively choose the incident beam polarization directions and detect an appropriate vector component of the CROA polarization, the dominant contribution from the polarizability-polarizability response can be eliminated. This is similar to the cross-polarization detection scheme designed for the linear optical activity FID measurement, which was discussed previously.

EXERCISE 15.4

Instead of using circularly polarized radiations, one can use linearly polarized beams to selectively measure the CROA signal. As an example, consider the following beam configuration. The first two pulses propagate along the Z axis, that is, $\hat{\mathbf{k}}_1 = \hat{\mathbf{k}}_2 = \hat{Z}$. They are linearly polarized as $\mathbf{e}_1 = \mathbf{e}_2 = \hat{X}$. Now, the third pulse propagates along the X-axis as $\hat{\mathbf{k}}_3 = \hat{X}$, and its polarization direction is parallel to Z-axis, that is, $\mathbf{e}_3 = \hat{Z}$. Now, placing a linear polarizer between the optical sample and the detector, only the Y-component of the CROA field is detected. That is to say, $\mathbf{e}_s = \hat{Y}$. This is one of the cross-polarization detection schemes because $\mathbf{e}_s$ is perpendicular to the other beam polarization directions, particularly to $\mathbf{e}_3$. In this case, show that the all-electric-dipole-allowed polarizability-polarizability contribution, which is an *achiral* component, to CROA polarization vanishes. Then, obtain the expressions for $\hat{P}^{Y}_{CROA}(\mathbf{r},t)$ in terms of ROA response functions in Equation 15.50. By measuring the corresponding CROA signal field $E^{Y}_{CROA}(t)$, one can determine the real and imaginary parts of the CROA susceptibility separately. Finally, obtain the expression for the time-integrated signal field intensity $I_{CROA}(t)$ in the present case of cross-polarization detection scheme and compare the result with $\Delta I_{CROA}(t)$ obtained by using a circularly polarized pulse in Exercise 15.3.

15.4 IR-RAMAN OPTICAL ACTIVITY SPECTROSCOPY

In Section 3.7, the IR-vis SFG (IV-SFG) spectroscopy was shown to be particularly useful for studying vibrational dynamics of molecules on surface or at interface, where the system has no centrosymmetry. In the case of the IV-SFG, the dipole-polarizability response function $\phi_{\alpha\mu}(t)$ is required for the calculation of the signal in time domain or the corresponding susceptibility in frequency domain. The IV-SFG experiment was usually performed by scanning the IR field frequency (ω_{IR}), and the homodyne-detected signal of the IV-SFG field was recorded with respect to ω_{IR} to obtain the surface vibrational spectrum. One can carry out a DFG experiment with two electronically nonresonant beams. If the difference of the two field frequencies, $\omega_1 - \omega_2$, is identical to one of the Raman-active mode frequencies, one can expect vibrational resonance enhancement of the DFG process, and then an electric field with frequency of $\omega_1 - \omega_2$ is emitted by the transient grating in the optical sample on surface or at interface. This Raman-IR DFG spectroscopy is similar to the CRS of molecules in an isotropic medium, except that the Raman-IR DFG is to detect the radiated coherent IR field from the Raman-excited state, whereas the CRS field is produced by Raman scattering field.

In this section, it is shown that the IV-SFG, which is an all-electric-dipole-allowed three-wave-mixing spectroscopy, is an allowed process even in the case of solution sample containing chiral molecules, if one takes into account the magnetic dipole–magnetic field and electric quadrupole–electric field interactions or the effects from the breakdown of Born–Oppenheimer approximation.[9–11] Therefore, the IV-SFG of chiral molecules dissolved in solution can be experimentally detected and is one of the optical activity measurement techniques. We shall particularly consider the far-from-resonance limit of IV-SFG, which will be called the IR-Raman spectroscopy because it involves an IR-excitation and a Raman scattering measurement. It is interesting to note that the IR optical activity such as vibrational CD is an IR-excitation + IR-detection method. On the other hand, the vibrational ROA can be classified as a Raman-excitation + Raman-detection. The present IR-Raman optical activity spectroscopy such as IV-SFG is thus a combination of IR and Raman processes. The other possible combination, Raman-IR optical activity spectroscopy, will be discussed in the following section.

In order to theoretically describe the IR-Raman optical activity, it is necessary to consider the interaction Hamiltonian between incident IR beam and matter, which is given as

$$H_{rad-mat} = -\boldsymbol{\mu}\cdot\mathbf{E}_{IR}(\mathbf{r},t) - \mathbf{m}\cdot\mathbf{B}_{IR}(\mathbf{r},t) - (1/2)\mathbf{Q}:\nabla\mathbf{E}_{IR}(\mathbf{r},t). \tag{15.51}$$

Now, the IR-Raman polarization is given as

$$\mathbf{P}_{IR-Raman}(\mathbf{r},t) = \bar{\boldsymbol{\mu}}_{ind}(\mathbf{r},t) + \bar{\mathbf{m}}_{ind}(\mathbf{r},t)\times\hat{\mathbf{k}}_s - (i/2)\mathbf{k}_s\cdot\bar{\mathbf{Q}}_{ind}(\mathbf{r},t), \tag{15.52}$$

where the wavevector of the IR-Raman signal field is denoted as $\mathbf{k}_s$ $(=\mathbf{k}_{IR}+\mathbf{k}_{vis})$ and the induced electric dipole, magnetic dipole, and electric quadrupole are

$$\boldsymbol{\mu}_{ind}(\mathbf{r},t) = \left(\boldsymbol{\alpha}\cdot\mathbf{e}_{vis} + \mathbf{G}\cdot\mathbf{b}_{vis} + \frac{i}{2}\mathbf{A}:\mathbf{k}_{vis}\mathbf{e}_{vis}\right)E_{vis}(t)e^{i\mathbf{k}_{vis}\cdot\mathbf{r}-i\omega_{vis}t}$$

$$\mathbf{m}_{ind}(\mathbf{r},t) = \bar{\mathbf{G}}\cdot\mathbf{e}_{vis}E_{vis}(t)e^{i\mathbf{k}_{vis}\cdot\mathbf{r}-i\omega_{vis}t}$$

$$\mathbf{Q}_{ind}(\mathbf{r},t) = \frac{1}{2}\bar{\mathbf{A}}\cdot\mathbf{e}_{vis}E_{vis}(t)e^{i\mathbf{k}_{vis}\cdot\mathbf{r}-i\omega_{vis}t}. \tag{15.53}$$

Then, we need to consider seven different cases of cause opearators, conjugate external fields, and effect operators, which are

(1) $\hat{A} = \boldsymbol{\mu}$, $F = \mathbf{E}_{IR}(\mathbf{r},t)$, and $\hat{B} = \boldsymbol{\alpha}\cdot\mathbf{E}_{vis}(\mathbf{r},t)$

(2) $\hat{A} = \mathbf{m}$, $F = \mathbf{B}_{IR}(\mathbf{r},t)$, and $\hat{B} = \boldsymbol{\alpha}\cdot\mathbf{E}_{vis}(\mathbf{r},t)$

(3) $\hat{A} = (1/2)\mathbf{Q}$, $F = \nabla\mathbf{E}_{IR}(\mathbf{r},t)$, and $\hat{B} = \boldsymbol{\alpha}\cdot\mathbf{E}_{vis}(\mathbf{r},t)$

(4) $\hat{A} = \boldsymbol{\mu}$, $F = \mathbf{E}_{IR}(\mathbf{r},t)$, and $\hat{B} = \mathbf{G}\cdot\mathbf{B}_{vis}(\mathbf{r},t)$

$$(5)\quad \hat{A} = \boldsymbol{\mu},\ F = \mathbf{E}_{IR}(\mathbf{r},t),\quad \text{and}\quad \hat{B} = \{\bar{\mathbf{G}} \cdot \mathbf{E}_{vis}(\mathbf{r},t)\} \times \hat{\mathbf{k}}_s$$

$$(6)\quad \hat{A} = \boldsymbol{\mu},\ F = \mathbf{E}_{IR}(\mathbf{r},t),\quad \text{and}\quad \hat{B} = (1/2)\mathbf{A} : \nabla \mathbf{E}_{vis}(\mathbf{r},t)$$

$$(7)\quad \hat{A} = \boldsymbol{\mu},\ F = \mathbf{E}_{IR}(\mathbf{r},t),\quad \text{and}\quad \hat{B} = -(1/2)\mathbf{k}_s \cdot \{\bar{\mathbf{A}} \cdot \mathbf{E}_{vis}(\mathbf{r},t)\}. \qquad (15.54)$$

Using the linear response theory with the above cause-effect combinations, one can obtain the expression for the IR-Raman polarization as

$$\mathbf{P}_{IR-Raman}(\mathbf{r},t) = <\boldsymbol{\alpha}\mathbf{E}_{vis} \overset{\boldsymbol{\mu}\mathbf{E}_{IR}}{\Longleftarrow} \rho(t_0)> + <\boldsymbol{\alpha}\mathbf{E}_{vis} \overset{\mathbf{m}\mathbf{B}_{IR}}{\Longleftarrow} \rho(t_0)> + <\boldsymbol{\alpha}\mathbf{E}_{vis} \overset{(1/2)\mathbf{Q}\nabla\mathbf{E}_{IR}}{\Longleftarrow} \rho(t_0)>$$

$$+ <\mathbf{G}\mathbf{B}_{vis} \overset{\boldsymbol{\mu}\mathbf{E}_{IR}}{\Longleftarrow} \rho(t_0)> + <\bar{\mathbf{G}}\mathbf{E}_{vis} \times \hat{\mathbf{k}}_{vis} \overset{\boldsymbol{\mu}\mathbf{E}_{IR}}{\Longleftarrow} \rho(t_0)>$$

$$+ <(i/2)\mathbf{A}\nabla\mathbf{E}_{vis} \overset{\boldsymbol{\mu}\mathbf{E}_{IR}}{\Longleftarrow} \rho(t_0)> - <(i/2)\mathbf{k}_s \cdot (\mathbf{A}\mathbf{E}_{vis}) \overset{\boldsymbol{\mu}\mathbf{E}_{IR}}{\Longleftarrow} \rho(t_0)>$$

$$= e^{i(\mathbf{k}_{IR}+\mathbf{k}_{vis})\cdot\mathbf{r} - i(\omega_{IR}+\omega_{vis})t} E_{vis}(t) \int_0^\infty d\tau \{\phi_{\alpha\mu}(\tau) E_{IR}(t+T-\tau) + \phi_{\alpha m}(\tau) B_{IR}(t+T-\tau)$$

$$+ \frac{k_{IR}}{2} \phi_{\alpha Q}(\tau) E_{IR}(t+T-\tau) + \phi_{G\mu}(\tau) E_{IR}(t+T-\tau)$$

$$+ \phi_{\bar{G}\mu}(\tau) E_{IR}(t+T-\tau) + \frac{k_{vis}}{2} \phi_{A\mu}(\tau) E_{IR}(t+T-\tau)$$

$$- \frac{k_s}{2} \phi_{\bar{A}\mu}(\tau) E_{IR}(t+T-\tau)\} e^{i\omega_1 \tau}. \qquad (15.55)$$

Here, the linear response functions in Equation 15.55 are defined as

$$\phi_{\alpha\mu}(\tau) \equiv \frac{i}{\hbar} \theta(\tau) < [\boldsymbol{\alpha}(\tau) : \mathbf{e}_s \mathbf{e}_{vis}, \boldsymbol{\mu}(0) \cdot \mathbf{e}_{IR}] \rho(-\infty) >$$

$$\phi_{\alpha m}(\tau) \equiv \frac{i}{\hbar} \theta(\tau) < [\boldsymbol{\alpha}(\tau) : \mathbf{e}_s \mathbf{e}_{vis}, \mathrm{m}(0) \cdot \mathbf{b}_{IR}] \rho(-\infty) >$$

$$\phi_{\alpha Q}(\tau) \equiv \frac{i}{\hbar} \theta(\tau) < [\boldsymbol{\alpha}(\tau) : \mathbf{e}_s \mathbf{e}_{vis}, i\mathrm{Q}(0) : \hat{\mathbf{k}}_{IR} \mathbf{e}_{IR}] \rho(-\infty) >$$

$$\phi_{G\mu}(\tau) \equiv \frac{i}{\hbar}\theta(\tau) < [\mathbf{G}(\tau) : \mathbf{e}_s \mathbf{b}_{vis}, \boldsymbol{\mu}(0) \cdot \mathbf{e}_{IR}]\rho(-\infty) >$$

$$\phi_{\bar{G}\mu}(\tau) \equiv \frac{i}{\hbar}\theta(\tau) < [\bar{\mathbf{G}}(\tau) : (\hat{\mathbf{k}}_s \times \mathbf{e}_s)\mathbf{e}_{vis}, \boldsymbol{\mu}(0) \cdot \mathbf{e}_{IR}]\rho(-\infty) >$$

$$\phi_{A\mu}(\tau) \equiv \frac{i}{\hbar}\theta(\tau) < [i\mathbf{A}(\tau) \vdots \mathbf{e}_s \hat{\mathbf{k}}_{vis} \mathbf{e}_{vis}, \boldsymbol{\mu}(0) \cdot \mathbf{e}_{IR}]\rho(-\infty) >$$

$$\phi_{\bar{A}\mu}(\tau) \equiv \frac{i}{\hbar}\theta(\tau) < [i\bar{\mathbf{A}}(\tau) \vdots \hat{\mathbf{k}}_s \mathbf{e}_s \mathbf{e}_{vis}, \boldsymbol{\mu}(0) \cdot \mathbf{e}_{IR}]\rho(-\infty) >. \quad (15.56)$$

The energy-level diagrams corresponding to the seven terms in Equation 15.55 are shown in Figure 15.4. In Section 3.7, only the first term, which is an all-electric-dipole-allowed term, was considered, because it is the dominant term for any anisotropic molecular system on surface or at interface. However, since we are interested in the case that chiral molecules are dissolved in an isotropic medium like solutions, it is necessary to take the rotational average $\mathbf{P}_{IR-Raman}(t)$ for randomly oriented molecules, and then only certain tensor elements do not vanish. Equation 15.55, which contains terms that are linearly proportional to magnetic dipoles or electric quadrupoles associated with vibrational (nuclear) or electronic motions, is a quite general expression valid for any arbitrary beam configurations, polarization states of radiations, and temporal profiles of incident pulses.

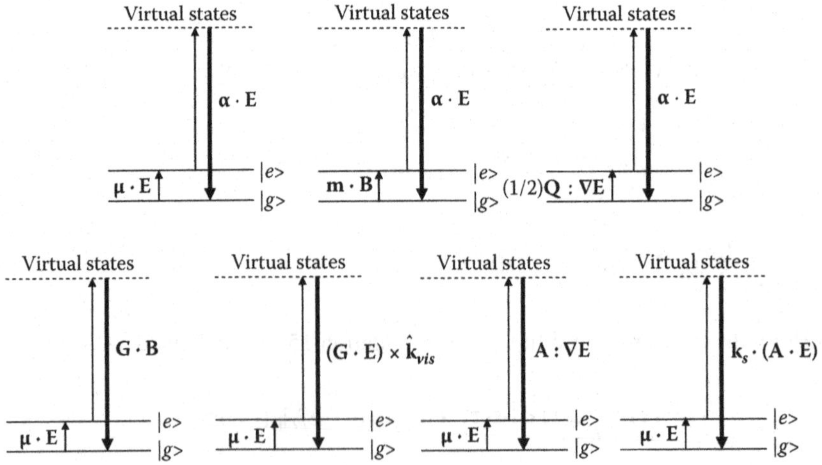

FIGURE 15.4 Seven different energy-level diagrams associated with IR-Raman optical activity spectroscopy.

Orthogonal beam configuration (ZYX-measurement). Since the only rotationally invariant third-rank tensor is the Levi–Civita epsilon, without loss of generality we will consider the case when the Z-component of the $\mathbf{P}_{IR-Raman}(t)$ vector is detected and the incident IR and visible beam polarization directions are parallel to $\hat{X}$ and $\hat{Y}$, respectively, that is,

$$\mathbf{e}_{IR} = \hat{X} \quad \text{and} \quad \mathbf{b}_{IR} = (\hat{\mathbf{k}}_{IR} \times \mathbf{e}_{IR}) = -\hat{Z}$$

$$\mathbf{e}_{vis} = \hat{Y}$$

$$\mathbf{P}_{IR-Raman}(t)/|\mathbf{P}_{IR-Raman}(t)| = \hat{Z}. \tag{15.57}$$

This is the case when the polarization directions of IR, visible, and emitted signal field are mutually perpendicular to one another. Since the Z-component of $\mathbf{P}_{IR-Raman}(t)$ is detected with $\hat{Y}$-polarized visible beam and $\hat{X}$-polarized IR beam, we shall call this particular beam configuration as the ZYX-measurement. For this mutually perpendicular beam configuration, the rotationally averaged $\mathbf{P}_{IR-Raman}(t)$ is determined solely by the first term in Equation 15.55, which is the dipole-polarizability response function, as

$$[\widehat{\mathbf{P}}_{IR-Raman}(t)]_Z = E_{vis}(t)\int_0^\infty d\tau [\phi_{\alpha\mu}(\tau)]_{ZYX} E_{IR}(t+T-\tau) e^{i\omega_1\tau}. \tag{15.58}$$

Interestingly, all the other terms in Equation 15.55 vanish after rotational averaging. From Equation 3.71, we have

$$[\phi_{\alpha\mu}(t)]_{ZYX} = -\frac{1}{6}\sum_{m_1,m_2,m_3} \varepsilon_{m_1m_2m_3}[\phi_{\alpha\mu}(t)]_{m_1m_2m_3} = -\frac{1}{6}\{[\phi_{\alpha\mu}(t)]_{xyz} - [\phi_{\alpha\mu}(t)]_{yxz}$$

$$+[\phi_{\alpha\mu}(t)]_{yzx} - [\phi_{\alpha\mu}(t)]_{zyx} + [\phi_{\alpha\mu}(t)]_{zxy} - [\phi_{\alpha\mu}(t)]_{xzy}\} \tag{15.59}$$

where x, y, and z are the Cartesian coordinates in a molecule-fixed frame. From the definition of the dipole-polarizability response function, Equation 15.59 can rewritten as, for a 2LS for example,

$$[\phi_{\alpha\mu}(t)]_{ZYX} = -\frac{i}{6\hbar}\theta(t)\{([\alpha_{ge}]_{xy} - [\alpha_{ge}]_{yx})[\mu_{eg}]_z + ([\alpha_{ge}]_{yz} - [\alpha_{ge}]_{zy})[\mu_{eg}]_x$$

$$+([\alpha_{ge}]_{zx} - [\alpha_{ge}]_{xz})[\mu_{eg}]_y\}\{e^{-i\bar{\omega}_{eg}t-g(t)} - e^{i\bar{\omega}_{eg}t-g^*(t)}\}. \tag{15.60}$$

Within the Born–Oppenheimer approximation, we have

$$[\alpha_{ge}]_{m_1m_2} = [\alpha_{ge}]_{m_2m_1} \quad \text{for} \quad m_1 \neq m_2. \tag{15.61}$$

Thus, Equation 15.60 vanishes within the Born–Oppenheimer approximation. However, due to the breakdown of the Born–Oppenheimer approximation, it was found that the antisymmetric Raman tensor elements are finite, that is, $[\alpha_{ge}]_{m_1m_2} - [\alpha_{ge}]_{m_2m_1} \neq 0$ for $m_1 \neq m_2$ and their magnitudes are dependent on molecular chirality. Consequently, the ZYX-measurement of IR-Raman signal can be of use to distinguish two different chiral molecules in solutions.

Circularly polarized IR-Raman. In the above, the ZYX-measurement scheme was shown to be useful to selectively measure the chiral dipole-polarizability response function (or susceptibility), which is all-electric-dipole-allowed contribution to the IR-Raman polarization. One can, however, selectively measure the other terms in Equation 15.55 by controlling the polarization state of incident IR or visible beam to be LCP and RCP and by measuring the difference signal.[10, 12]

EXERCISE 15.5

To carry out an IR-Raman OA measurement, one can use circularly polarized IR or circularly polarized–vis beam. Firstly, assume that the IR beam propagation direction is along the Z-axis in a space-fixed frame, that is, $\hat{\mathbf{k}}_{IR} = \hat{Z}$, and its polarization is modulated to be LCP and RCP, that is, $\mathbf{e}_{LCP} = (\hat{X} + i\hat{Y})/\sqrt{2}$ or $\mathbf{e}_{RCP} = (\hat{X} - i\hat{Y})/\sqrt{2}$. The visible beam crosses with the IR beam at the center of the optical sample containing chiral molecules, where the beam crossing angle is θ. Furthermore, it is assumed that $\hat{\mathbf{k}}_{vis} = \hat{Z}\cos\theta + \hat{Y}\sin\theta$. Note that the visible beam polarization plane is assumed to be on the Y–Z plane in a space-fixed frame. In this particular case, what are the LCP and RCP IR-Raman polarizations? Obtain the circular IR-Raman intensity difference defined as $\Delta I_{IR-Raman}(t) = I_{LCP-IR-Raman}(t) - I_{RCP-IR-Raman}(t)$. Secondly, consider the case when the visible beam is circularly polarized and the IR beam is linearly polarized. For the same beam configuration, obtain the circular IR-Raman intensity difference in this second case, and compare the result with the above case using the circularly polarized IR beam.

15.5 RAMAN-IR OPTICAL ACTIVITY SPECTROSCOPY

The IR-Raman OA spectroscopy based on an SFG scheme was shown to be useful in studying chiro-optical properties of molecules in an isotropic medium. The surface-specific Raman-IR spectroscopy dicussed in Section 3.8 is also a potentially useful optical activity measurement tool for chiral molecules in solution. Due to the breakdown of Born–Oppenheimer approximation, the all-electric-dipole-allowed contribution to the Raman-IR signal becomes nonzero because of the nonzero antisymmetric Raman tensor elements. In addition, properly controlling the incident beam polarization states and taking into account the magentic dipole–magnetic field and electric quadrupole–electric field interactions, one can selectively measure different chiral components of the Raman-IR polarization.

The Raman-IR optical activity spectroscopy requires three distinctively different radiation–matter interactions including that between oscillating dipoles associated with Raman- and ROA-active vibrations and vacuum field. The first visible beam, which is in nonresonance with electronic transitions, induces an excitation of the molecular system, and the second radiation–matter interaction with another visible field propagating in the direction of -$\mathbf{k}_2$ produces a vibrational coherence on the electronically ground state. Therefore, within the electric dipole approximation, the first two radiation–matter interactions correspond to a Raman excitation of a given vibrational mode whose frequency is close to the difference frequency $\omega_1 - \omega_2$. Thus created vibrational transient grating can radiate an IR field with wavevector $\mathbf{k}_1 - \mathbf{k}_2$. Note that unlike the case of the Raman-IR spectroscopy discussed in Section 3.8, we consider a *solution* sample containing chiral molecules.

The effective radiation–matter interaction Hamiltonian that should be considered to theoretically describe the Raman-IR optical activity is

$$H_{rad-mat} = \{-\boldsymbol{\alpha} : \mathbf{e}_2\mathbf{e}_1 E_2^*(t)E_1(t) - \mathbf{G} : \mathbf{e}_2\mathbf{b}_1 E_2^*(t)B_1(t) - \bar{\mathbf{G}} : \mathbf{b}_2^*\mathbf{e}_1 B_2^*(t)E_1(t)$$

$$-(i/2)\mathbf{A} \vdots \mathbf{e}_2^*\mathbf{k}_1\mathbf{e}_1 E_2^*(t)E_1(t) + (i/2)\bar{\mathbf{A}} \vdots \mathbf{k}_2\mathbf{e}_2^*\mathbf{e}_1 E_2^*(t)E_1(t)\} e^{i(\mathbf{k}_1-\mathbf{k}_2)\cdot\mathbf{r} - i(\omega_1-\omega_2)t}. \quad (15.62)$$

The first term on the right-hand side of this equation is responsible for Raman excitation of a vibrational mode; the second and third terms involve interactions between magnetic dipole–ROA tensors and external electromagnetic field; and the fourth and fifth ones represent the interactions between electric quadrupole–ROA tensors and external field.

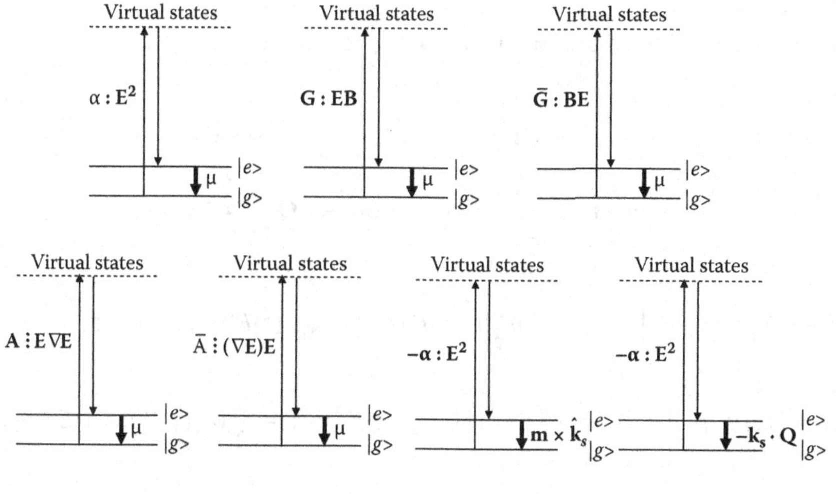

FIGURE 15.5 Seven different energy-level diagrams associated with Raman-IR optical activity spectroscopy.

In this case of the Raman-IR optical activity spectroscopy, the following seven cases are to be considered:

$$(1)\quad \hat{A} = \boldsymbol{\alpha}\cdot\mathbf{E}_1(\mathbf{r},t),\ F = \mathbf{E}_2(\mathbf{r},t),\quad \text{and}\quad \hat{B} = \boldsymbol{\mu}$$

$$(2)\quad \hat{A} = \mathbf{G}\cdot\mathbf{B}_1(\mathbf{r},t),\ F = \mathbf{E}_2(\mathbf{r},t)\quad \text{and}\quad \hat{B} = \boldsymbol{\mu}$$

$$(3)\quad \hat{A} = \bar{\mathbf{G}}\cdot\mathbf{E}_1(\mathbf{r},t),\ F = \mathbf{B}_2(\mathbf{r},t)\quad \text{and}\quad \hat{B} = \boldsymbol{\mu}$$

$$(4)\quad \hat{A} = (1/2)\mathbf{A}:\nabla\mathbf{E}_1(\mathbf{r},t),\ F = \mathbf{E}_2(\mathrm{r},t),\quad \text{and}\quad \hat{B} = \boldsymbol{\mu}$$

$$(5)\quad \hat{A} = (1/2)\bar{\mathbf{A}}\cdot\mathbf{E}_1(\mathbf{r},t),\ F = \nabla\mathbf{E}_2(\mathbf{r},t),\quad \text{and}\quad \hat{B} = \boldsymbol{\mu}$$

$$(6)\quad \hat{A} = \boldsymbol{\alpha}\cdot\mathbf{E}_1(\mathbf{r},t),\ F = \mathrm{E}_2(\mathbf{r},t),\quad \text{and}\quad \hat{B} = \mathbf{m}\times\hat{\mathbf{k}}_s$$

$$(7)\quad \hat{A} = \boldsymbol{\alpha}\cdot\mathbf{E}_1(\mathbf{r},t),\ F = \mathbf{E}_2(\mathbf{r},t),\quad \text{and}\quad \hat{B} = -(i/2)\mathbf{k}_s\cdot\mathbf{Q}. \qquad (15.63)$$

From the linear response theory, one can find that the Raman-IR polarization is given as

$$\mathbf{P}_{Raman-IR}(\mathbf{r},t) = \langle \boldsymbol{\mu} \overset{\boldsymbol{\alpha}\mathbf{E}_2^*\mathbf{E}_1}{\Longleftarrow} \rho(t_0)\rangle + \langle \boldsymbol{\mu} \overset{\mathbf{G}\mathbf{E}_2^*\mathbf{B}_1}{\Longleftarrow} \rho(t_0)\rangle + \langle \boldsymbol{\mu} \overset{\bar{\mathbf{G}}\mathbf{B}_2^*\mathbf{E}_1}{\Longleftarrow} \rho(t_0)\rangle$$

$$+ \langle \boldsymbol{\mu} \overset{(1/2)\mathbf{A}\mathbf{E}_2^*\nabla\mathbf{E}_1}{\Longleftarrow} \rho(t_0)\rangle + \langle \boldsymbol{\mu} \overset{(1/2)\mathbf{A}(\nabla\mathbf{E}_2^*)\mathbf{E}_1}{\Longleftarrow} \rho(t_0)\rangle$$

$$+ \langle \mathbf{m}\times\hat{\mathbf{k}}_s \overset{\boldsymbol{\alpha}\mathbf{E}_2^*\mathbf{E}_1}{\Longleftarrow} \rho(t_0)\rangle - \langle (i/2)\mathbf{k}_s\cdot\mathbf{Q} \overset{\boldsymbol{\alpha}\mathbf{E}_2^*\mathbf{E}_1}{\Longleftarrow} \rho(t_0)\rangle$$

$$= e^{i(\mathbf{k}_1-\mathbf{k}_2)\cdot\mathbf{r}-i(\omega_1-\omega_2)t}\int_0^\infty d\tau\{\phi_{\mu\alpha}(\tau)E_2^*(t-\tau)E_1(t-\tau) + \phi_{\mu G}(\tau)E_2^*(t-\tau)B_1(t-\tau)$$

$$+ \phi_{\mu\bar{G}}(\tau)B_2^*(t-\tau)E_1(t-\tau) + \frac{k_1}{2}\phi_{\mu A}(\tau)E_2^*(t-\tau)E_1(t-\tau) - \frac{k_2}{2}\phi_{\mu\bar{A}}(\tau)E_2^*(t-\tau)E_1(t-\tau)$$

$$+ \phi_{m\alpha}(\tau)E_2^*(t-\tau)E_1(t-\tau) - \frac{k_s}{2}\phi_{Q\alpha}(\tau)E_2^*(t-\tau)E_1(t-\tau)\}e^{i(\omega_1-\omega_2)\tau}. \qquad (15.64)$$

Here, the polarizability-dipole response function $\phi_{\mu\alpha}(\tau)$ was defined in Equation 3.145, and the other relevant linear response functions in Equation 15.64 are

$$\phi_{\mu\alpha}(\tau) \equiv \frac{i}{\hbar}\theta(\tau) < [\boldsymbol{\mu}(\tau)\cdot \mathbf{e}_s, \boldsymbol{\alpha}(0) : \mathbf{e}_2^*\mathbf{e}_1]\rho(-\infty) >$$

$$\phi_{\mu G}(\tau) \equiv \frac{i}{\hbar}\theta(\tau) < [\boldsymbol{\mu}(\tau)\cdot \mathbf{e}_s, \mathbf{G}(0) : \mathbf{e}_2^*\mathbf{b}_1]\rho(-\infty) >$$

$$\phi_{\mu \bar{G}}(\tau) \equiv \frac{i}{\hbar}\theta(\tau) < [\boldsymbol{\mu}(\tau)\cdot \mathbf{e}_s, \bar{\mathbf{G}}(0) : \mathbf{b}_2^*\mathbf{e}_1]\rho(-\infty) >$$

$$\phi_{\mu A}(\tau) \equiv \frac{i}{\hbar}\theta(\tau) < [\boldsymbol{\mu}(\tau)\cdot \mathbf{e}_s, i\mathbf{A}(0) \vdots \mathbf{e}_2^*\hat{\mathbf{k}}_1\mathbf{e}_1]\rho(-\infty) >$$

$$\phi_{\mu \bar{A}}(\tau) \equiv \frac{i}{\hbar}\theta(\tau) < [\boldsymbol{\mu}(\tau)\cdot \mathbf{e}_s, i\bar{\mathbf{A}}(0) \vdots \hat{\mathbf{k}}_2\mathbf{e}_2^*\mathbf{e}_1]\rho(-\infty) >$$

$$\phi_{m\alpha}(\tau) \equiv \frac{i}{\hbar}\theta(\tau) < [\mathbf{m}(\tau)\cdot (\hat{\mathbf{k}}_s \times \mathbf{e}_s), \boldsymbol{\alpha}(0) : \mathbf{e}_2^*\mathbf{e}_1]\rho(-\infty) >$$

$$\phi_{Q\alpha}(\tau) \equiv \frac{i}{\hbar}\theta(\tau) < [i\mathbf{Q}(\tau) : \hat{\mathbf{k}}_s\mathbf{e}_s, \boldsymbol{\alpha}(0) : \mathbf{e}_2^*\mathbf{e}_1]\rho(-\infty) > . \quad (15.65)$$

The unit vector of the Raman-IR polarization was denoted as $\mathbf{e}_s$ in Equation 15.65. The energy-level diagrams associated with the seven terms in Equation 15.41 are shown in Figure 15.5.

Similar to the IR-ROA spectroscopy, the *ZYX*-measurement scheme can be used to selectively measure the first term in Equation 15.64. As an example, if the beam configuration is specified as $\mathbf{e}_1 = \hat{X}$, $\hat{\mathbf{k}}_1 = \hat{Z}$, $\mathbf{e}_2 = \hat{Y}$, $\hat{\mathbf{k}}_2 = \hat{X}$, and $\mathbf{P}_{Raman-IR}(t)/|\mathbf{P}_{Raman-IR}(t)| = \hat{Z}$, one can show that the rotationally averaged $\mathbf{P}_{Raman-IR}(t)$ is determined by the polarizability-dipole response function, as

$$[\mathbf{P}_{Raman-IR}(t)]_Z = \int_0^\infty d\tau [\phi_{\mu\alpha}(\tau)]_{ZYX} E_2^*(t-\tau)E_1(t-\tau)e^{i(\omega_1-\omega_2)\tau}. \quad (15.66)$$

From Equation 3.71, we have

$$[\phi_{\mu\alpha}(t)]_{ZYX} = -\frac{1}{6}\{[\phi_{\mu\alpha}(t)]_{xyz} - [\phi_{\mu\alpha}(t)]_{yxz} + [\phi_{\mu\alpha}(t)]_{yzx}$$
$$-[\phi_{\mu\alpha}(t)]_{ZYX} + [\phi_{\mu\alpha}(t)]_{zxy} - [\phi_{\mu\alpha}(t)]_{xzy}\}. \quad (15.67)$$

Due to the breakdown of the Born–Oppenheimer approximation, the antisymmetric Raman tensor elements are finite, that is, $[\alpha_{ge}]_{m_1m_2} - [\alpha_{ge}]_{m_2m_1} \neq 0$ for $m_1 \neq m_2$ so that the *ZYX*-measurement of the Raman-IR optical activity signal can be measurably large and would provide information on molecular chirality and its dynamics with a time-resolved Raman-IR measurement.

EXERCISE 15.6

To carry out an Raman-IR optical activity measurement, one can use circularly polarized–visible-1 or circularly polarized–visible-2 beam (note that the first two beams are visible fields whose frequencies are far from any of electronic transition frequencies). Now, assume that the first visible beam propagation direction is along the Z-axis in a space-fixed frame, that is, $\hat{\mathbf{k}}_1 = \hat{Z}$, and its polarization is modulated to be LCP and RCP, that is, $\mathbf{e}_{LCP} = (\hat{X} + i\hat{Y})/\sqrt{2}$ or $\mathbf{e}_{RCP} = (\hat{X} - i\hat{Y})/\sqrt{2}$. The second visible beam crosses with the first one at the center of optical sample containing chiral molecules, where the beam crossing angle is θ. Furthermore, it is assumed that $\hat{\mathbf{k}}_2 = \hat{Z}\cos\theta + \hat{Y}\sin\theta$. The second visible beam polarization plane is assumed to be on the Y–Z plane in a space-fixed frame. In this particular case, what are the LCP and RCP Raman-IR polarizations? Obtain the circular Raman-IR intensity difference defined as $\Delta I_{Raman-IR}(t) = I_{LCP-Raman-IR}(t) - I_{RCP-Raman-IR}(t)$. Compare the results with the cases of circularly polarized IR-Raman measurements in Exercise 15.5.

REFERENCES

1. Berova, N.; Nakanishi, K.; Woody, R. W., *Circular dichroism: principles and applications*. Wiley-VCH: New York, 2000.
2. Keiderling, T. A., Peptide and protein conformational studies with vibrational Circular dichroism and relgted spectroscopies. In *Circular dichroism: principles and applications*. Wiley-VCH: New York, 2000; 621–666.
3. Nafie, L. A., Infrared and Raman vibrational optical activity: Theoretical and experimental aspects. *Annual Review of Physical Chemistry* 1997, 48, 357–386.
4. Barron, L. D.; Bogaard, M. P.; Buckingham, A.D., Raman-scattering of circularly polarized-light by optically-active molecules. *Journal of the American Chemical Society* 1973, 95, 603–605.
5. Barron, L. D.; Hecht, L.; Blanch, E. W.; Bell, A. F., Solution structure and dynamics of biomolecules from Raman optical activity. *Progress in Biophysics and Molecular Biology* 2000, 73, 1–49.
6. Craig, D. P.; Thirunamachandran, T., *Molecular quantum electrodyanmics: An introduction to radiation molecule interactions*. Dover Publications, Inc.: New York, 1998.
7. Rhee, H.; Ha, J.-H.; Jeon, S.-J.; Cho, M., Femtosecond spectral interferometry of optical activity: Theory. *Journal of Chemical Physics* 2008, 129, 094507.
8. Nafie, L. A., Theory of Raman scattering and Raman optical activity: near resonance theory and levels of approximation. *Theoretical Chemistry Accounts* 2008, 119, 39–55.
9. Belkin, M. A.; Kulakov, T. A.; Ernst, K.-H.; Yan, L.; Shen, Y. R., Sum frequency vibrational spectroscopy on chiral liquids: A novel technique to probe molecular chirality. *Physical Review Letters* 2000, 85, 4474.
10. Cho, M., Time-resolved vibrational optical activity measurement by the infrared-visible sum frequency-generation with circularly polarized infrared light. *Journal of Chemical Physics* 2002, 116, 1562–1570.
11. Belkin, M. A.; Shen, Y.-R.; Harris, R. A., Sum frequency vibrational spectroscopy of chiral liquids off and close to electronic resonance and the antisymmetric Raman tensor. *Journal of Chemical Physics* 2004, 120, 10118–10126.
12. Cheon, S.; Cho, M., Circularly polarized infrared and visible sum frequency-generation spectroscopy: Vibrational optical activity measurement. *Physical Review A* 2005, 71, 013808.

16 Nonlinear Optical Activity Spectroscopy

In the previous chapter, optical activity spectroscopic methods based on linear response measurements such as circular dichroism (CD), optical rotatory dispersion, Raman optical activity (ROA), and so forth were discussed. They have been used to determine absolute configurations of chiral molecules including natural products, drugs, proteins, and other biomolecules. For instance, let us consider the circular dichroism whose intensity is determined by the so-called rotatory strength, $\mathrm{Im}\,[\boldsymbol{\mu}_{ge} \cdot \mathbf{m}_{eg}]$. It turned out that the sign of $\mathrm{Im}\,[\boldsymbol{\mu}_{ge} \cdot \mathbf{m}_{eg}]$ depends on the absolute configuration of a given chiral molecule so that the CD spectrum of *R*-form molecule exhibits spectral pattern opposite in sign to its mirror image *S*-form molecule.[1] This renders the CD or any other optical activity spectroscopy extremely useful for studying molecular chirality and 3D configuration. Nevertheless, these linear optical activity measurement methods, even though they are superior in frequency-resolution to the other linear spectroscopic methods, are a 1D technique.

A clear advantage of 2D optical spectroscopy is that the two-dimensionally displayed electronic or vibrational spectrum has significantly increased information density.[2] Furthermore, it enables us to determine comparatively weak secondary spectroscopic properties of complex molecules. However, the 2D spectroscopy based on photon echo or pump–probe methods cannot be used to distinguish two different chiral structures, because the 2D optical transition amplitude is determined by products of transition electric dipole moments, which are not sensitive to molecular chirality. Thus, it is highly desired to develop potentially useful 2D optical activity measurement techniques, which combine both advantages of optical activity and 2D spectroscopy.

There have been a few attempts to carry out time-resolved nonlinear optical activity measurements for chiral molecules by employing the pump–probe method with circularly polarized pump beams.[3,4] Employing a polarization modulation technique, one can control the polarization state of pump pulse and generate a train of alternating LCP and RCP pulses. Then, the difference between the measured LCP and RCP pump–probe signals provides information on the time evolution of electronic and magnetic properties of chiral molecules. In this chapter, theoretical descriptions of 2D optical activity spectroscopic techniques will be discussed.

16.1 NONLINEAR OPTICAL ACTIVITY MEASUREMENT METHODS

It is noted again that the optical activity is, by definition, related to the *differential interaction of a chiral molecule with LCP and RCP radiation*. Therefore, the optical activity signal, denoted as ΔS, can always be defined as the difference between two signals obtained with LCP and RCP beams as

$$\Delta S = S_L - S_R. \tag{16.1}$$

Here, the subscripts L and R mean that the polarization state of an injected beam is LCP or RCP, respectively. Instead of LCP and RCP lights to measure optical activity properties of chiral molecule, one can use left- and right-elliptically polarized lights or purely linearly polarized light, depending on the optical activity property of interest and measurement method. For instance, the CD signal is the differential absorbance, that is, $\Delta A = A_L - A_R$. Optical rotatory dispersion is to measure the rotation angle of the transmitted polarization direction with respect to the incident beam polarization direction. However, regardless of beam polarization state or detection method, the underlying physics behind all these optical activity properties is the same as defined above in Equation 16.1.

Furthermore, the definition of optical activity signal in Equation 16.1 is valid even for nonlinear optical activity measurement experiments. For example, the circularly polarized pump–probe (CP–PP) is one of the 2D optical activity measurement methods, and its signal is defined as the difference between the pump–probe signal with LCP-pump and that with RCP-pump.[5] The 2D circularly polarized photon echo experiment is also a straightforward extension of 2D photon echo by replacing one of the linearly polarized incident pulses with a circularly polarized one.[6–8] Thus, the optical activity spectroscopies using the definition in Equation 16.1 will be referred to as *differential* optical activity measurement techniques.[8]

Instead of the differential measurement scheme in Equation 16.1, one can carry out linear or nonlinear optical activity experiments by selectively measuring the spectroscopic response functions that are not rotationally invariant within the electric dipole approximation, for example, S_{XXXY}. As shown in the previous chapter, the linear optical activity, such as CD and ORD, can be studied by measuring the YX-tensor element of the generalized linear response function including both magnetic dipole and electric quadrupole terms (see Section 15.2). Note that the rotationally invariant tensor elements of electric dipole–dipole response function are XX, YY, and ZZ, because the only rotationally invariant second-rank tensor in 3D space is the Kronecker delta. Thus, all the other tensor elements except for these three should vanish if only the electric dipole response is considered. However, since the magnetic field vector is orthogonal to the electric field, the YX tensor element of the magnetic dipole–electric dipole response function, where Y and X particularly denote the *electric* field vector elements, does not vanish and contains information of the handedness of chiral molecules.

The same argument can be applied to nonlinear response measurements. In the case of all-electric-dipole-allowed four-wave-mixing spectroscopy, the elements of the fourth-rank tensorial response function, which contain rotationally invariant isomers like $\delta_{l_1l_2}\delta_{l_3l_4}$, $\delta_{l_1l_3}\delta_{l_2l_4}$ and $\delta_{l_1l_4}\delta_{l_2l_3}$, can be experimentally measured. For example, the parallel-polarization and perpendicular-polarization photon echo signals, denoted as E_{PE}^{ZZZZ} and E_{PE}^{ZYYZ}, are to measure the $ZZZZ$- and $ZYYZ$-tensor elements of the photon echo response function, respectively, when the incident beams and emitted photon echo field propagate along the X-axis in a space-fixed frame. Thus, for example the

ZZZY-tensor element of the all-electric-dipole third-order response function vanishes. However, the same *ZZZY*-tensor element of the generalized response function beyond the electric dipole approximation (or long wavelength limit) does not vanish for chiral molecules, because the magnetic dipole and electric quadrupole contributions are finite in such cases.[8–11] This can also be understood from the fact that the magnetic field vector is orthogonal to the electric field vector in a given electromagnetic field. If the first electric field is Y-polarized for the *ZZZY*-measurement, its magnetic field vector is parallel to the Z-axis so that there is a third-order response function component $[\boldsymbol{\mu\mu\mu m}]_{ZZZZ}$ that is rotationally invariant. Although the *ZZZY*-measurement for example involves linearly polarized beams only, one of the linearly polarized beams should be perpendicular to the other polarization directions. Thus, as shown in Section 15.2, it requires a cross-polarization detection method where the incident beam polarization directions are perpendicular to the polarization direction of the emitted signal electric field. From now on, this scheme will be referred to as *cross-polarization* optical activity measurements.

In summary, we have discussed two different measurement schemes, differential and cross-polarization optical activity measurements, which are different from each other by the beam polarization states. The former requires LCP and RCP (or sometimes left- and right-elliptically polarized) beams to carry out an optical activity measurement, whereas the latter requires linearly polarized beams with a properly designed cross-polarization detection instrument. Although these two methods appear to be different from each other, the measured quantities are essentially identical.[7] This will be proved in the following section. Then, a few examples of 2D optical activity measurement methods will be discussed later.

16.2 ROTATIONAL AVERAGING OF HIGHER-RANK TENSORS

As emphasized throughout the book, the $(n-1)$th-order spectroscopic signal with respect to the electric dipole–electric field interaction can be conveniently expressed in terms of the corresponding nth rank tensorial all-electric-dipole response function, $R^{(n)}(t_1,t_2,\cdots t_n)$. Controlling the polarization states of incident beams and measuring a particular vector element of detected signal field, one can selectively measure one or multiple tensor elements of the nonlinear response function. Now, let us denote $S^{(n)}_{l_1,l_2,\cdots,l_n}$ the observable (signal) that is linearly proportional to the $[l_1,l_2,\cdots l_n]$ tensor element of $R^{(n)}(t_1,t_2,\cdots t_n)$, where l_j is one of the Cartesian coordinates in a space-fixed frame. The polarization direction of the jth *electric* field involved in the jth field-matter interaction is specified by l_j.

When the optically active system (molecule) is randomly oriented in condensed phases, only the rotationally invariant tensor elements of $R^{(n)}(t_1,t_2,\cdots t_n)$ do not vanish. Let us denote as $\Phi^{(n)}$ the set of those rotationally invariant tensor elements within the electric dipole approximation. For example, for a second-rank tensorial response function, $\Phi^{(2)}$ consists of $[x,x]$, $[y,y]$, and $[z,z]$. Then, we have, for any arbitrary nth-rank tensors,

$$S^{(n)}_{l_1,l_2,\cdots,l_n} \neq 0 \quad \text{when} \quad [l_1,l_2,\cdots,l_n] \in \Phi^{(n)} \tag{16.2}$$

and

$$S^{(n)}_{l_1,l_2,\cdots,l_n} = \sum_{m_1,m_2,\cdots,m_n} \Gamma^{(n)}_{\{l_1,l_2,\cdots,l_n\}\{m_1,m_2,\cdots,m_n\}} S^{(n)}_{m_1,m_2,\cdots,m_n}. \tag{16.3}$$

Here, m_j (for j=1~n) is one of the Cartesian coordinates in a molecule-fixed frame, and $\Gamma^{(n)}_{\{l_1,l_2,\cdots,l_n\}\{m_1,m_2,\cdots,m_n\}}$ are the expansion coefficients that were discussed in Section 3.3. $S^{(n)}_{m_1,m_2,\cdots,m_n}$ is the molecular property determined by the $[m_1,m_2,\cdots,m_n]$ tensor element of $R^{(n)}(t_1,t_2,\cdots t_n)$ in a molecule-fixed frame. In order to obtain Equation 16.3, we used the Weyl's theorem.

It is well known that a rotationally invariant tensor can be expressed as a linear combination of isotropic tensors. In 3D space, there are two fundamental isotropic tensors, which are Kronecker delta, δ_{ij}, and Levi–Civita epsilon ε_{ijk}. Note that all higher rank isotropic tensors can be expressed in terms of Kronecker deltas and Levi–Civita epsilons. These possible products are called isomers. As mentioned in Section 3.3, when $n = 4$, the isotropic tensors are products of two Kronecker deltas such as $\delta_{ij}\delta_{kl}$, $\delta_{ik}\delta_{jl}$, and $\delta_{il}\delta_{jk}$. Denoting the rth (sth) member of the set of isomers of rank n in a space-fixed (molecule-fixed) frame as $\sigma^{(n)}_{r,\{l_1,l_2,\cdots,l_n\}}$ ($\mu^{(n)}_{s,\{m_1,m_2,\cdots,m_n\}}$), we have

$$S^{(n)}_{l_1,l_2,\cdots,l_n} = \sum_{m_1,m_2,\cdots,m_n} \sum_{r,s} \sigma^{(n)}_{r,\{l_1,l_2,\cdots,l_n\}} \mu^{(n)}_{s,\{m_1,m_2,\cdots,m_n\}} S^{(n)}_{m_1,m_2,\cdots,m_n}. \tag{16.4}$$

From Equations 16.3 and 16.4, we find that

$$\Gamma^{(n)}_{\{l_1,l_2,\cdots,l_n\}\{m_1,m_2,\cdots,m_n\}} = \sum_{r,s} \sigma^{(n)}_{r,\{l_1,l_2,\cdots,l_n\}} \mu^{(n)}_{s,\{m_1,m_2,\cdots,m_n\}}. \tag{16.5}$$

For $n = 2$, there is only one isomer, that is,

$$\sigma^{(2)}_{\{l_1,l_2\}} = \delta_{l_1,l_2}. \tag{16.6}$$

For $n = 3$, there is also one isomer,

$$\sigma^{(3)}_{\{l_1,l_2,l_3\}} = \varepsilon_{l_1,l_2,l_3}. \tag{16.7}$$

For $n = 4$, there are three isomers, that is,

$$\sigma^{(4)}_{1,\{l_1,l_2,l_3,l_4\}} = \delta_{l_1,l_2}\delta_{l_3,l_4}, \sigma^{(4)}_{2,\{l_1,l_2,l_3,l_4\}} = \delta_{l_1,l_3}\delta_{l_2,l_4}, \text{ and } \sigma^{(4)}_{3,\{l_1,l_2,l_3,l_4\}} = \delta_{l_1,l_4}\delta_{l_2,l_3}. \tag{16.8}$$

For $n = 5$, there are six independent isomers, and so on. Similarly, the isomers of rank n in a molecule-fixed frame, $\mu^{(n)}_{s,\{m_1,m_2,\cdots,m_n\}}$, can be obtained by replacing the indexes of the space-fixed frame in Equations 16.6–16.8 with those of the molecule-fixed frame.

Now, let us consider a general optical activity measurement spectroscopy. The jth radiation is assumed to be either LCP or RCP radiation, whereas all the other radiations are linearly polarized. The measured signals using these circularly polarized radiations will be denoted as $S^{(n)}_{l_1,l_2,\cdots,l_{j-1},L,l_{j+1},\cdots,l_n}$ and $S^{(n)}_{l_1,l_2,\cdots,l_{j-1},R,l_{j+1},\cdots,l_n}$, respectively (note that the jth index in the subscripts is either L or R to indicate that the jth beam polarization state is LCP or RCP, respectively). The nth-order optical activity signal is defined as the difference between these two signals so that the differential optical activity in such an nth-order spectroscopy is given as

$$\Delta S^{(n)}_{l_1,l_2,\cdots,l_{j-1},C,l_{j+1},\cdots,l_n} \equiv S^{(n)}_{l_1,l_2,\cdots,l_{j-1},L,l_{j+1},\cdots,l_n} - S^{(n)}_{l_1,l_2,\cdots,l_{j-1},R,l_{j+1},\cdots,l_n}. \tag{16.9}$$

This signal $\Delta S^{(n)}_{l_1,l_2,\cdots,l_{j-1},C,l_{j+1},\cdots,l_n}$ will be called the nth-order differential optical activity signal.

In order to rewrite Equation 16.9, we need to consider the nature of circularly polarized radiation more in detail. The LCP and RCP radiations can be written as linear combinations of two linearly polarized radiations, that is,

$$\mathbf{e}^{(L)} = (\mathbf{x} + i\mathbf{y})/\sqrt{2} \quad \text{and} \quad \mathbf{e}^{(R)} = (\mathbf{x} - i\mathbf{y})/\sqrt{2} \tag{16.10}$$

or

$$\mathbf{e}^{(L)*} = (\mathbf{x} - i\mathbf{y})/\sqrt{2} \quad \text{and} \quad \mathbf{e}^{(R)*} = (\mathbf{x} + i\mathbf{y})/\sqrt{2}. \tag{16.11}$$

The LCP and RCP polarized transverse electric fields are given as

$$\mathbf{E}_{LCP}(\mathbf{r},t) = \mathbf{e}^{(L)}E(t)\mathrm{e}^{i\mathbf{k}\cdot\mathbf{r}-i\omega t} + \mathbf{e}^{(L)*}E^*(t)\mathrm{e}^{-i\mathbf{k}\cdot\mathbf{r}+i\omega t} \tag{16.12}$$

$$\mathbf{E}_{RCP}(\mathbf{r},t) = \mathbf{e}^{(R)}E(t)\mathrm{e}^{i\mathbf{k}\cdot\mathbf{r}-i\omega t} + \mathbf{e}^{(R)*}E^*(t)\mathrm{e}^{-i\mathbf{k}\cdot\mathbf{r}+i\omega t}. \tag{16.13}$$

The first term describing the traveling field in the direction of $\mathbf{k}$ is involved in an absorptive radiation–matter interaction, whereas the second is in a stimulated emissive interaction. Therefore, depending on a specific nonlinear optical transition pathway, one should carefully consider either $\mathbf{e}^{(L)}$ or $\mathbf{e}^{(L)*}$. A few examples will be discussed in detail later in this chapter.

Here, without loss of generality, the beam propagation direction is assumed to be along the z-axis in a space-fixed frame. Now, the choice of the x-axis in a space-fixed frame is arbitrary. We will assume that the x-axis is chosen in such a way that $[l_1, l_2, \cdots, l_{j-1}, x, l_{j+1}, \cdots, l_n] \in \Phi^{(n)}$. This means that $S^{(n)}_{l_1,l_2,\cdots,l_{j-1},x,l_{j+1},\cdots,l_n}$ is rotationally invariant signal within the electric dipole approximation. Then, the nth-order differential optical activity signal can be rewritten as

$$\begin{aligned}\Delta S^{(n)}_{l_1,l_2,\cdots,l_{j-1},C,l_{j+1},\cdots,l_n} &= \frac{1}{\sqrt{2}}\left(S^{(n)}_{l_1,l_2,\cdots,l_{j-1},x,l_{j+1},\cdots,l_n} \pm iS^{(n)}_{l_1,l_2,\cdots,l_{j-1},y,l_{j+1},\cdots,l_n}\right) \\ &\quad - \frac{1}{\sqrt{2}}\left(S^{(n)}_{l_1,l_2,\cdots,l_{j-1},x,l_{j+1},\cdots,l_n} \mp iS^{(n)}_{l_1,l_2,\cdots,l_{j-1},y,l_{j+1},\cdots,l_n}\right) \\ &= \pm\sqrt{2}iS^{(n)}_{l_1,l_2,\cdots,l_{j-1},y,l_{j+1},\cdots,l_n}.\end{aligned} \tag{16.14}$$

Here, the upper signs should be chosen when the LCP and RCP beam states are given by Equation 16.10, whereas the lower signs correspond to the case of Equation 16.11.

Note that the rotationally invariant terms $S^{(n)}_{l_1,l_2,\cdots,l_{j-1},x,l_{j+1},\cdots,l_n}$ on the right-hand side of Equation 16.14 cancel out and do not contribute to $\Delta S^{(n)}_{l_1,l_2,\cdots,l_{j-1},C,l_{j+1},\cdots,l_n}$. Now, the next step is to show that $S^{(n)}_{l_1,l_2,\cdots,l_{j-1},y,l_{j+1},\cdots,l_n}$ is not rotationally invariant within the electric dipole approximation. In order to prove this, we need to consider two different cases separately. The first group consists of the cases when the l_j index is found in a Kronecker delta, e.g., $\delta_{l_j l_k} = \delta_{x l_k}$. Since $[l_1,l_2,\cdots,l_{j-1},x,l_{j+1},\cdots,l_n] \in \Phi^{(n)}$, we find that l_k (for $k \neq j$) should be x. Consequently, if l_j is replaced with y, $[l_1,l_2,\cdots,l_{j-1},y,l_{j+1},\cdots,l_n] \notin \Phi^{(n)}$ due to $\delta_{xy} = 0$. The second group consists of the cases when the l_j index is found in a Levi–Civita epsilon such as $\varepsilon_{l_j l_k l_m} = \varepsilon_{x l_k l_m}$. Again, because $[l_1,l_2,\cdots,l_{j-1},x,l_{j+1},\cdots,l_n] \in \Phi^{(n)}$, the other two indexes l_k and l_m (for $k \neq j$ and $m \neq j$) and x should be different from one another, that is, $\varepsilon_{x,y,z} = \varepsilon_{z,x,y} = \varepsilon_{y,z,x} = 1$ or $\varepsilon_{x,z,y} = \varepsilon_{z,y,x} = \varepsilon_{y,x,z} = -1$. Therefore, if l_j is replaced with y in these cases belonging to the second group, the Levi–Civita tensor element vanishes, e.g., $\varepsilon_{y,y,z} = 0$. Therefore, we proved that $[l_1,l_2,\cdots,l_{j-1},y,l_{j+1},\cdots,l_n] \notin \Phi^{(n)}$.

Now, we will apply this theorem to a few specific cases. For n=2, we have

$$\Delta S^{(2)}_{x,C} = S^{(2)}_{x,L} - S^{(2)}_{x,R} = \pm\sqrt{2}iS^{(2)}_{x,y}$$

$$\Delta S^{(2)}_{C,x} = S^{(2)}_{L,x} - S^{(2)}_{R,x} = \pm\sqrt{2}iS^{(2)}_{y,x}. \tag{16.15}$$

Again, the upper signs should be chosen when the LCP and RCP beam states are given by Equation 16.10, whereas the lower signs correspond to the case of Equation 16.11. The results in Equation 16.15 show that the circular dichroism signal is related to the measurement of [x,y] or [y,x] tensor element of the linear response function beyond the electric dipole approximation. In the case of $\Delta S^{(2)}_{x,C}$, the first field-matter interaction is with the linearly polarized radiation with polarization direction parallel to the x-axis in a space-fixed frame, and the observable is the circular polarization component of the radiated signal field. On the other hand, the measurement of $\Delta S^{(2)}_{C,x}$ means that the initial field-matter interaction is with LCP or RCP light, and the x-polarized signal field is detected. The previous chapter showed that the cross-polarization detection of the $S^{(2)}_{y,x}$ signal can provide information on the complex optical activity (chiral) susceptibility, where the real and imaginary parts of the chiral susceptibility correspond to the CD and ORD spectra, respectively.

For n=3, we have

$$\Delta S^{(3)}_{x,y,C} = S^{(3)}_{x,y,L} - S^{(3)}_{x,y,R} = \pm\sqrt{2}iS^{(2)}_{x,y,y}$$

$$\Delta S^{(3)}_{x,C,y} = S^{(3)}_{x,L,y} - S^{(3)}_{x,L,y} = \pm\sqrt{2}iS^{(2)}_{x,y,y}$$

$$\Delta S^{(3)}_{C,x,y} = S^{(3)}_{L,x,y} - S^{(3)}_{R,x,y} = \pm\sqrt{2}iS^{(2)}_{y,x,y}. \tag{16.16}$$

The first case in Equation 16.16 corresponds to the measurement that the first two field-matter interactions are with x- and y-polarized radiations and the circular polarization component of the signal is detected. The second case is to use LCP and RCP light for the second field-matter interaction. The third case is to use the circularly polarized radiation for the first field-matter interaction. In Exercise 15.5, the IV-SFG (or IR-Raman) spectroscopy of chiral molecules in solution was considered. In particular, the incident IR beam was controlled to be either LCP or RCP. The LCP and RCP IR-Raman signals were measured separately. Then, it was shown that the difference signal can provide information on chiro-optical properties of chiral molecules. By using Equation 16.16, it is now possible to establish a relationship between that experimental observable and the cross-polarization-detected third-rank tensorial observable. This will be left for the readers.

It is now natural to extend the 2D four-wave-mixing spectroscopy to 2D optical activity measurement. The associated response function is a fourth-rank tensor so that the case when $n = 4$ should be considered in detail. From Equation 16.14, assuming that the propagation direction of the circularly polarized beam is along the Z-axis in a space-fixed frame and that the unit vectors of the circularly polarized beam are given as Equations 16.10 and 16.11, we find the following relationships:

$$\Delta S^{(4)}_{l_1,l_2,l_3,C} = S^{(4)}_{l_1,l_2,l_3,L} - S^{(4)}_{l_1,l_2,l_3,R} = \pm\sqrt{2}iS^{(4)}_{l_1,l_2,l_3,y} \tag{16.17}$$

$$\Delta S^{(4)}_{l_1,l_2,C,l_3} = S^{(4)}_{l_1,l_2,L,l_3} - S^{(4)}_{l_1,l_2,R,l_3} = \pm\sqrt{2}iS^{(4)}_{l_1,l_2,y,l_3} \tag{16.18}$$

$$\Delta S^{(4)}_{l_1,C,l_2,l_3} = S^{(4)}_{l_1,L,l_2,l_3} - S^{(4)}_{l_1,R,l_2,l_3} = \pm\sqrt{2}iS^{(4)}_{l_1,y,l_2,l_3} \tag{16.19}$$

$$\Delta S^{(4)}_{C,l_1,l_2,l_3} = S^{(4)}_{L,l_1,l_2,l_3} - S^{(4)}_{R,l_1,l_2,l_3} = \pm\sqrt{2}iS^{(4)}_{y,l_1,l_2,l_3}. \tag{16.20}$$

For any arbitrary beam configurations, once the circularly polarized beam wavevector direction is chosen as the Z-axis in a space-fixed frame, the differential optical activity signal can be written as a linear combination of terms on the right-hand side of Equations 16.17–16.20. Furthermore, the above relationships in Equations 16.17–16.20 show that a particular cross-polarization optical activity measurement is inversely related to specific differential optical activity measurement. For instance, the circularly polarized pump–probe (CP–PP) spectroscopy, where the pump–pulse is circularly polarized, can be related to a particular combination of two cross-polarization optical activity signals. Denoting the heterodyne-detected circularly polarized pump–probe signal as $\Delta S^{(CP-PP)}$, from the relations in Equations 16.19 and 16.20 we find that when the pump– and probe–pulses are collinear,

$$\Delta S^{(CP-PP)} = S^{(4)}_{L,x,x,x} - S^{(4)}_{R,x,x,x} + S^{(4)}_{x,L,x,x} - S^{(4)}_{x,R,x,x} = \sqrt{2}i\left(S^{(4)}_{y,x,x,x} - S^{(4)}_{x,y,x,x}\right). \tag{16.21}$$

Here, the reason why the second term in the last equation has a negative sign is that the second radiation–matter interaction is between molecular dipole and $\mathbf{e}^{(L)*}E^*(t)e^{-i\mathbf{k}\cdot\mathbf{r}+i\omega t}$ ($\mathbf{e}^{(R)*}E^*(t)e^{-i\mathbf{k}\cdot\mathbf{r}+i\omega t}$) for the LCP (RCP) pump pulse.

Using the theoretical results established in this section, one can always find relationships between differential and cross-polarization-detected optical activity measurements. Since, by definition, optical activity of a chiral molecule is induced by the differential interaction of a chiral molecule with LCP and RCP radiation during quantum excitation, we will follow this conventional definition of optical activity to develop theoretical descriptions of a few 2D optical activity spectroscopies in the following sections.

16.3 TWO-DIMENSIONAL OPTICAL ACTIVITY PUMP–PROBE: TWO-LEVEL SYSTEM

The 2D pump–probe spectroscopy within the electric dipole approximation was already discussed in Chapter 6. Generally, transient grating, dichroism, and birefringence spectroscopies have been used to study wavepacket (particle and hole) evolutions on the excited and ground potential-energy surfaces, ultrafast chemical reaction dynamics, and lifetimes of the excited states. A single pulse or a pair of pulses is used to perturb the molecular system and to create either population or coherences on excited or ground state. An incident probe laser field that is delayed in time interacts with the same molecular system, the corresponding third-order polarization is created, and then the coherent signal field is detected. The transient grating, dichroism, and birefringence measurements differ from one another by how the signal field is experimentally detected. They, in fact, correspond to the intensity, imaginary ($\pi/2$ phase different) part, and real (in-phase) part of the third-order material polarization (with respect to the phase of local oscillator field), respectively.

For a 2LS, the previous description of the 2D pump–probe spectroscopy was based on the electric dipole approximation so that its signal is insensitive to molecular chirality. However, if one of the incident beams is controlled to be circularly polarized and if the difference between the LCP and RCP pump–probe signals is detected, the all-electric-dipole-allowed pump–probe signal vanishes. Therefore, instead of the lowest-order radiation–matter interaction Hamiltonian, $-\boldsymbol{\mu}\cdot\mathbf{E}(\mathbf{r},t)$, the generalized one including both magnetic dipole–magnetic field and electric quadrupole–electric field interactions should be considered, which is

$$H_{rad-mat} = -\{\boldsymbol{\mu}+(\mathbf{m}\times\hat{\mathbf{k}})+(i/2)\mathbf{k}\cdot\mathbf{Q}\}\cdot\mathbf{e}E(t)e^{i\mathbf{k}\cdot\mathbf{r}-i\omega t}$$
$$-\{\boldsymbol{\mu}+(\mathbf{m}\times\hat{\mathbf{k}})-(i/2)\mathbf{k}\cdot\mathbf{Q}\}\cdot\mathbf{e}^{*}E^{*}(t)e^{-i\mathbf{k}\cdot\mathbf{r}+i\omega t}. \quad (16.22)$$

Due to these two additional radiation–matter interactions, the pump–probe polarization can be expanded in a power series of **m** and **Q** as

$$\mathbf{P}_{PP}(t) = \mathbf{P}_{PP}^{(0)}(t) + \mathbf{P}_{PP}^{(1)}(t;m) + \mathbf{P}_{PP}^{(1)}(t;Q) + \cdots. \quad (16.23)$$

The higher order terms in the above series expansion are the pump–probe polarizations that are proportional to m^2, mQ, Q^2, and so on.[5] Thus, they are again two to three orders of magnitude smaller than the second and third terms in Equation 16.23 in general, that is,

$$|\mathbf{P}_{PP}^{(0)}(t)| \gg |\mathbf{P}_{PP}^{(1)}(t;m)| \approx |\mathbf{P}_{PP}^{(1)}(t;Q)| \gg |\mathbf{P}_{PP}^{(2)}| \gg |\mathbf{P}_{PP}^{(3)}|. \quad (16.24)$$

Although there are a variety of different ways to measure the above pump–probe polarization in Equation 16.23, we shall specifically consider the self-heterodyne-detected transient dichroism (see Section 6.2) signal defined as

$$S_{TD}(\omega_{pu},\omega_{pr};T) = \text{Im}\left[\int_{-\infty}^{\infty} dt\, \mathbf{E}_{pr}^*(t)\cdot \mathbf{P}_{PP}(t)\right]. \tag{16.25}$$

Inserting Equation 16.23 into 16.25, we have

$$S_{TD}(\omega_{pu},\omega_{pr};T) \cong S_{TD}^{(0)}(\omega_{pu},\omega_{pr};T) + S_{TD}^{(1)}(\omega_{pu},\omega_{pr};T;m) + S_{TD}^{(1)}(\omega_{pu},\omega_{pr};T;Q). \tag{16.26}$$

In was previously shown that the all-electric-dipole-allowed transient dichroism spectrum $S_{TD}^{(0)}(\omega_{pu},\omega_{pr};T)$ is approximately given as, for a 2LS,

$$S_{TD}^{(0)}(\omega_{pu},\omega_{pr};T) \propto [\boldsymbol{\mu}_{ge}\boldsymbol{\mu}_{eg}\boldsymbol{\mu}_{ge}\boldsymbol{\mu}_{eg}] \otimes \mathbf{e}_{pr}^*\mathbf{e}_{pr}\mathbf{e}_{pu}^*\mathbf{e}_{pu}\Gamma_{TD}^{2LS}(\omega_{pu},\omega_{pr};T) \tag{16.27}$$

where the normalized 2D Gaussian peak shape function for this 2D pump–probe spectrum is defined as

$$\Gamma_{TD}^{2LS}(\omega_{pu},\omega_{pr};T) = \frac{-\pi \exp(-X^2)}{(\Omega^2 + w^2)^{1/2}\left(\Omega^2 + \overline{w}^2 - \frac{H^2(T)}{\Omega^2 + w^2}\right)^{1/2}}\{\exp(-Y^2(T)) + \exp(-Z^2(T))\}. \tag{16.28}$$

The auxiliary functions such as X, $Y(T)$, $Z(T)$, and $H(T)$ were defined in Equations 6.8 and 5.51. In Equation 16.27 above, we specifically emphasize the complex nature of the unit vectors of beam polarization directions. In the previous chapters, the cases when the incident beams and detected signal field are always linearly polarized were discussed so that the unit vector e is always real. However, circularly polarized beams are considered in this chapter and their unit vectors are complex, as shown in Equations 16.10 and 16.11. One should therefore be careful about such complex natures of e's hereafter.

The next step is to calculate the transient dichroism spectra that are linear with respect to either m or Q. First of all, let us consider $S_{TD}^{(1)}(\omega_{pu},\omega_{pr};T;m)$, which is associated with the third-order polarization created by two electric dipole–electric field interactions and one magnetic dipole–magnetic field interaction. Since one of the three radiation–matter interactions should be replaced with magnetic dipole–magnetic field interaction, there are twelve ($= 4 \times 3$) diagrams. For example, one of them is

$$\langle \boldsymbol{\mu}_B \xleftarrow[g\,\zeta e\,\zeta]{\substack{\mathbf{mB}_{pu} \\ e\,\zeta}} |g\rangle\langle g|. \tag{16.29}$$

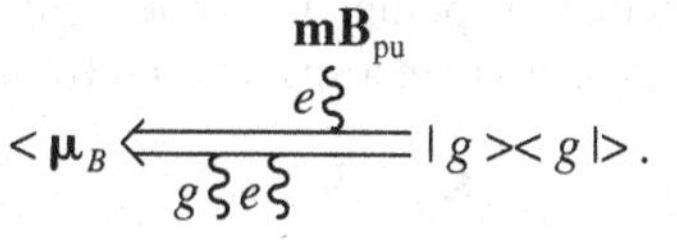

In addition to those twelve diagrams, there are four additional diagrams representing the magnetic dipole contribution to the third-order polarization. One of these four diagrams is

$$<\mathbf{m}\times\mathbf{k}_{pr} \xleftarrow[g\xi\, e\xi]{e\xi} |g><g|>. \tag{16.30}$$

EXERCISE 16.1

What are the other fourteen diagrams, in addition to the two in Equations 16.29 and 16.30?

Taking into account all these sixteen contributions to $S_{TD}^{(1)}(\omega_{pu},\omega_{pr};T;m)$, which are all linear in m, one can obtain the expression for $S_{TD}^{(1)}(\omega_{pu},\omega_{pr};T;m)$ as

$$S_{TD}^{(1)}(\omega_{pu},\omega_{pr};T;m) \propto \{[\boldsymbol{\mu}_{ge}\boldsymbol{\mu}_{eg}\boldsymbol{\mu}_{ge}(\mathbf{m}_{eg}\times\hat{\mathbf{k}}_{pu})]+[\boldsymbol{\mu}_{ge}\boldsymbol{\mu}_{eg}(\mathbf{m}_{ge}\times\hat{\mathbf{k}}_{pu})\boldsymbol{\mu}_{eg}]$$

$$+[\boldsymbol{\mu}_{ge}(\mathbf{m}_{eg}\times\hat{\mathbf{k}}_{pr})\boldsymbol{\mu}_{ge}\boldsymbol{\mu}_{eg}]+[(\mathbf{m}_{ge}\times\hat{\mathbf{k}}_{pr})\boldsymbol{\mu}_{eg}\boldsymbol{\mu}_{ge}\boldsymbol{\mu}_{eg}]\}\otimes \mathbf{e}_{pr}^{*}\mathbf{e}_{pr}\mathbf{e}_{pu}^{*}\mathbf{e}_{pu}\Gamma_{TD}^{2LS}(\omega_{pu},\omega_{pr};T). \tag{16.31}$$

By following the same procedure and simply replacing the operator $(\mathbf{m}\times\hat{\mathbf{k}})$ with $(i/2)\mathbf{k}\cdot\mathbf{Q}$ operator, one can find that the quadrupole contribution to the 2D transient dichroism (TD) spectrum, $S_{TD}^{(1)}(\omega_{pu},\omega_{pr};T;Q)$, is expressed as

$$S_{TD}^{(1)}(\omega_{pu},\omega_{pr};T;Q) \propto (i/2)\{[\boldsymbol{\mu}_{ge}\boldsymbol{\mu}_{eg}\boldsymbol{\mu}_{ge}(\mathbf{k}_{pu}\cdot\mathbf{Q}_{eg})]-[\boldsymbol{\mu}_{ge}\boldsymbol{\mu}_{eg}(\mathbf{k}_{pu}\cdot\mathbf{Q}_{eg})\boldsymbol{\mu}_{ge}]\}$$

$$+[\boldsymbol{\mu}_{ge}(\mathbf{k}_{pr}\cdot\mathbf{Q}_{eg})\boldsymbol{\mu}_{ge}\boldsymbol{\mu}_{eg}-[(\mathbf{k}_{pr}\cdot\mathbf{Q}_{ge})\boldsymbol{\mu}_{eg}\boldsymbol{\mu}_{ge}\boldsymbol{\mu}_{eg}]\}\otimes\mathbf{e}_{pr}^{*}\mathbf{e}_{pr}\mathbf{e}_{pu}^{*}\mathbf{e}_{pu}\Gamma_{TD}^{2LS}(\omega_{pu},\omega_{pr};T). \tag{16.32}$$

Thus, the expanded 2D TD spectrum up to the first order in m or Q is finally given as

$$S_{TD}(\omega_{pu},\omega_{pr};T) \propto ([\boldsymbol{\mu}_{ge}\boldsymbol{\mu}_{eg}\boldsymbol{\mu}_{ge}\boldsymbol{\mu}_{eg}]+\{[\boldsymbol{\mu}_{ge}\boldsymbol{\mu}_{eg}\boldsymbol{\mu}_{ge}(\mathbf{m}_{eg}\times\hat{\mathbf{k}}_{pu})]$$

$$+[\boldsymbol{\mu}_{ge}\boldsymbol{\mu}_{eg}(\mathbf{m}_{ge}\times\hat{\mathbf{k}}_{pu})\boldsymbol{\mu}_{eg}]+[\boldsymbol{\mu}_{ge}(\mathbf{m}_{eg}\times\hat{\mathbf{k}}_{pr})\boldsymbol{\mu}_{ge}\boldsymbol{\mu}_{eg}]+[(\mathbf{m}_{ge}\times\hat{\mathbf{k}}_{pr})\boldsymbol{\mu}_{eg}\boldsymbol{\mu}_{ge}\boldsymbol{\mu}_{eg}]\}$$

$$+(i/2)\{[\boldsymbol{\mu}_{ge}\boldsymbol{\mu}_{eg}\boldsymbol{\mu}_{ge}(\mathbf{k}_{pu}\cdot\mathbf{Q}_{eg})]-[\boldsymbol{\mu}_{ge}\boldsymbol{\mu}_{eg}(\mathbf{k}_{pu}\cdot\mathbf{Q}_{ge})\boldsymbol{\mu}_{eg}]+[\boldsymbol{\mu}_{ge}(\mathbf{k}_{pr}\cdot\mathbf{Q}_{eg})\boldsymbol{\mu}_{ge}\boldsymbol{\mu}_{eg}]$$

$$-[(\mathbf{k}_{pr}\cdot\mathbf{Q}_{ge})\boldsymbol{\mu}_{eg}\boldsymbol{\mu}_{ge}\boldsymbol{\mu}_{eg}]\}\otimes\mathbf{e}_{pr}^{*}\mathbf{e}_{pr}\mathbf{e}_{pu}^{*}\mathbf{e}_{pu}\Gamma_{TD}^{2LS}(\omega_{pu},\omega_{pr};T). \tag{16.33}$$

This result is quite general for any arbitrary beam configuration. Usually, the pump and probe beam propagation directions are not collinear so that the angle between them is another experimentally controllable variable.

Hereafter, it is assumed that the pump and probe beam propagation directions are approximately parallel to the Z-axis in a space-fixed frame, that is,

$$\hat{\mathbf{k}}_{pu} = \hat{\mathbf{k}}_{pr} = \hat{Z}. \tag{16.34}$$

The polarization direction of the linearly polarized probe (and local oscillator) beam is parallel to the X-axis, as $\mathbf{e}_{pr} = \hat{X}$. The differential signal $\Delta S_{TD}(\omega_{pu},\omega_{pr};T)$ is then defined as

$$\Delta S_{TD}(\omega_{pu},\omega_{pr};T) = S_{TD}^{LCP-pump}(\omega_{pu},\omega_{pr};T) - S_{TD}^{RCP-pump}(\omega_{pu},\omega_{pr};T). \tag{16.35}$$

For further theoretical considerations, we instead use the relationship in Equation 16.21 to rewrite Equation 16.35 as

$$\Delta S_{TD}(\omega_{pu},\omega_{pr};T) = \sqrt{2}i\{S_{TD}^{XXXY}(\omega_{pu},\omega_{pr};T) - S_{TD}^{XXYX}(\omega_{pu},\omega_{pr};T)\}, \tag{16.36}$$

where the superscripts $XXXY$ and $XXYX$ mean that the $XXXY$ and $XXYX$ elements of all the four-rank tensors in Equation 16.33 should be taken into account. Now, let us consider the $XXXY$ and $XXYX$ elements of relevant fourth-rank tensors for a *multilevel* system first, and then apply the results to the present specific case of a 2LS. Now, the fourth- or fifth-rank tensors needed to be considered for a multilevel system are $[\boldsymbol{\mu}_4\boldsymbol{\mu}_3\boldsymbol{\mu}_2\boldsymbol{\mu}_1]$, $[\boldsymbol{\mu}_4\boldsymbol{\mu}_3\boldsymbol{\mu}_2(\mathbf{m}_1\times\hat{\mathbf{k}}_1)]$, $[\boldsymbol{\mu}_4\boldsymbol{\mu}_3(\mathbf{m}_2\times\hat{\mathbf{k}}_2)\boldsymbol{\mu}_1]$, $[\boldsymbol{\mu}_4(\mathbf{m}_3\times\hat{\mathbf{k}}_3)\boldsymbol{\mu}_2\boldsymbol{\mu}_1]$, $[(\mathbf{m}_4\times\hat{\mathbf{k}}_4)\boldsymbol{\mu}_3\boldsymbol{\mu}_2\boldsymbol{\mu}_1]$, $[\boldsymbol{\mu}_4\boldsymbol{\mu}_3\boldsymbol{\mu}_2(\mathbf{k}_1\cdot\mathbf{Q}_1)]$, $[\boldsymbol{\mu}_4\boldsymbol{\mu}_3(\mathbf{k}_2\cdot\mathbf{Q}_2)\boldsymbol{\mu}_1]$, $[\boldsymbol{\mu}_4(\mathbf{k}_3\cdot\mathbf{Q}_3)\boldsymbol{\mu}_2\boldsymbol{\mu}_1]$, and $[(\mathbf{k}_4\cdot\mathbf{Q}_4)\boldsymbol{\mu}_3\boldsymbol{\mu}_2\boldsymbol{\mu}_1]$. Here, the subscripts 1–4 represent different transitions. As an example, if $1 = eg$, $\boldsymbol{\mu}_1$ corresponds to $\boldsymbol{\mu}_g$ that is the transition dipole matrix element between g to e.

First of all, one can easily show that $[\boldsymbol{\mu}_4\boldsymbol{\mu}_3\boldsymbol{\mu}_2\boldsymbol{\mu}_1]_{XXXY}$ and $[\boldsymbol{\mu}_4\boldsymbol{\mu}_3\boldsymbol{\mu}_2\boldsymbol{\mu}_1]_{XXYX}$ vanish, since the isomers of fourth-rank tensors that are rotationally invariant are $\delta_{l_1l_2}\delta_{l_3l_4}$, $\delta_{l_1l_3}\delta_{l_2l_4}$, and $\delta_{l_1l_4}\delta_{l_2l_3}$. This suggests that the all-electric-dipole term $[\boldsymbol{\mu}_4\boldsymbol{\mu}_3\boldsymbol{\mu}_2\boldsymbol{\mu}_1]$ does not contribute to the present nonlinear optical activity signal, as expected. We next consider the magnetic dipole contribution to ΔS_{TD}, which is the sum of four terms from the second one in Equation 16.33. Note that the X and Y components of $\mathbf{m}\times\hat{\mathbf{k}}_{pu}(=\mathbf{m}\times\hat{Z})$ vector are m_y and $-m_X$, that is,

$$\mathbf{m}\times\hat{\mathbf{k}}_{pu} = m_Y\hat{X} - m_X\hat{Y}. \tag{16.37}$$

Hereafter, for later uses, let us define two auxiliary functions f_{XXXY}^{m} and f_{XXYX}^{m} as

$$\begin{aligned} f_{XXXY}^{m}(4,3,2,1) = {} & [\boldsymbol{\mu}_4\boldsymbol{\mu}_3\boldsymbol{\mu}_2(\mathbf{m}_1\times\hat{\mathbf{k}}_1)]_{XXXY} + [\boldsymbol{\mu}_4\boldsymbol{\mu}_3(\mathbf{m}_2\times\hat{\mathbf{k}}_2)\boldsymbol{\mu}_1]_{XXXY} \\ & + [\boldsymbol{\mu}_4(\mathbf{m}_3\times\hat{\mathbf{k}}_3)\boldsymbol{\mu}_2\boldsymbol{\mu}_1]_{XXXY} + [(\mathbf{m}_4\times\hat{\mathbf{k}}_4)\boldsymbol{\mu}_3\boldsymbol{\mu}_2\boldsymbol{\mu}_1]_{XXXY} \end{aligned} \tag{16.38}$$

$$\begin{aligned} f_{XXYX}^{m}(4,3,2,1) = {} & [\boldsymbol{\mu}_4\boldsymbol{\mu}_3\boldsymbol{\mu}_2(\mathbf{m}_1\times\hat{\mathbf{k}}_1)]_{XXYX} + [\boldsymbol{\mu}_4\boldsymbol{\mu}_3(\mathbf{m}_2\times\hat{\mathbf{k}}_2)\boldsymbol{\mu}_1]_{XXYX} \\ & + [\boldsymbol{\mu}_4(\mathbf{m}_3\times\hat{\mathbf{k}}_3)\boldsymbol{\mu}_2\boldsymbol{\mu}_1]_{XXYX} + [(\mathbf{m}_4\times\hat{\mathbf{k}}_4)\boldsymbol{\mu}_3\boldsymbol{\mu}_2\boldsymbol{\mu}_1]_{XXYX}. \end{aligned} \tag{16.39}$$

The numbers in $f_{XXXY}^{m}(4,3,2,1)$ and $f_{XXYX}^{m}(4,3,2,1)$ represent specific quantum transition. For example, $f_{XXXY}^{m}(ge,eg,ge,eg)$ means that the four transitions are between g and e states. In Equations 16.38 and 16.39, the wavevector of the radiation involved in the jth radiation–matter interaction is denoted as $\mathbf{k}_j$.

In the present case, $\hat{\mathbf{k}}_1 = \hat{\mathbf{k}}_2 = \hat{\mathbf{k}}_{pu}$ and $\hat{\mathbf{k}}_3 = \hat{\mathbf{k}}_4 = \hat{\mathbf{k}}_{pr}$. Then, one can find that the tensor elements $[\boldsymbol{\mu}_4\boldsymbol{\mu}_3\boldsymbol{\mu}_2(\mathbf{m}_1\times\hat{\mathbf{k}}_{pu})]_{XXXY}$, $[\boldsymbol{\mu}_4\boldsymbol{\mu}_3(\mathbf{m}_2\times\hat{\mathbf{k}}_{pu})\boldsymbol{\mu}_1]_{XXXY}$, $[\boldsymbol{\mu}_4(\mathbf{m}_3\times\hat{\mathbf{k}}_{pu})\boldsymbol{\mu}_2\boldsymbol{\mu}_1]_{XXXY}$, and $[(\mathbf{m}_4 \times \hat{\mathbf{k}}_{pu})\boldsymbol{\mu}_3\boldsymbol{\mu}_2\boldsymbol{\mu}_1]_{XXXY}$ are

$$[\boldsymbol{\mu}_4\boldsymbol{\mu}_3\boldsymbol{\mu}_2(\mathbf{m}_1 \times \hat{\mathbf{k}}_{pu})]_{XXXY} = -i[\boldsymbol{\mu}_4\boldsymbol{\mu}_3\boldsymbol{\mu}_2\mathbf{M}_1]_{XXXX}$$

$$= -\frac{i}{30}\sum_{m_1,m_2,m_3,m_4=x,y,z}\{2\delta_{m_1m_2}\delta_{m_3m_4} + 2\delta_{m_1m_3}\delta_{m_2m_4} + 2\delta_{m_1m_4}\delta_{m_2m_3}\}[\boldsymbol{\mu}_4\boldsymbol{\mu}_3\boldsymbol{\mu}_2\mathbf{M}_1]^M_{m_1m_2m_3m_4}$$

$$= -\frac{i}{30}\{2(\boldsymbol{\mu}_4\cdot\boldsymbol{\mu}_3)^M(\boldsymbol{\mu}_2\cdot\mathbf{M}_1)^M + 2(\boldsymbol{\mu}_4\cdot\boldsymbol{\mu}_2)^M(\boldsymbol{\mu}_3\cdot\mathbf{M}_1)^M + 2(\boldsymbol{\mu}_4\cdot\mathbf{M}_1)^M(\boldsymbol{\mu}_3\cdot\boldsymbol{\mu}_2)^M\}$$

$$[\boldsymbol{\mu}_4\boldsymbol{\mu}_3(\mathbf{m}_2 \times \hat{\mathbf{k}}_{pu})\boldsymbol{\mu}_1]_{XXXY} = i[\boldsymbol{\mu}_4\boldsymbol{\mu}_3\mathbf{M}_2\boldsymbol{\mu}_1]_{XXYY}$$

$$= \frac{i}{30}\sum_{m_1,m_2,m_3,m_4=x,y,z}\{4\delta_{m_1m_2}\delta_{m_3m_4} - \delta_{m_1m_3}\delta_{m_2m_4} - \delta_{m_1m_4}\delta_{m_2m_3}\}[\boldsymbol{\mu}_4\boldsymbol{\mu}_3\mathbf{M}_2\boldsymbol{\mu}_1]^M_{m_1m_2m_3m_4}$$

$$= \frac{i}{30}\{4(\boldsymbol{\mu}_4\cdot\boldsymbol{\mu}_3)^M(\mathbf{M}_2\cdot\boldsymbol{\mu}_1)^M - (\boldsymbol{\mu}_4\cdot\mathbf{M}_2)^M(\boldsymbol{\mu}_3\cdot\boldsymbol{\mu}_1)^M - (\boldsymbol{\mu}_4\cdot\boldsymbol{\mu}_1)^M(\boldsymbol{\mu}_3\cdot\mathbf{M}_2)^M\}$$

$$[\boldsymbol{\mu}_4(\mathbf{m}_3 \times \hat{\mathbf{k}}_{pu})\boldsymbol{\mu}_2\boldsymbol{\mu}_1]_{XXXY} = i[\boldsymbol{\mu}_4\mathbf{M}_3\boldsymbol{\mu}_2\boldsymbol{\mu}_1]_{XYXY} = \frac{i}{30}\{-(\boldsymbol{\mu}_4\cdot\mathbf{M}_3)^M(\boldsymbol{\mu}_2\cdot\boldsymbol{\mu}_1)^M$$

$$+ 4(\boldsymbol{\mu}_4\cdot\boldsymbol{\mu}_2)^M(\mathbf{M}_3\cdot\boldsymbol{\mu}_1)^M - (\boldsymbol{\mu}_4\cdot\boldsymbol{\mu}_1)^M(\mathbf{M}_3\cdot\boldsymbol{\mu}_2)^M\}$$

$$[(\mathbf{m}_4 \times \hat{\mathbf{k}}_{pu})\boldsymbol{\mu}_3\boldsymbol{\mu}_2\boldsymbol{\mu}_1]_{XXXY} = i[\mathbf{M}_4\boldsymbol{\mu}_3\boldsymbol{\mu}_2\boldsymbol{\mu}_1]_{YXXY} = \frac{i}{30}\{-(\mathbf{M}_4\cdot\boldsymbol{\mu}_3)^M(\boldsymbol{\mu}_2\cdot\boldsymbol{\mu}_1)^M$$

$$- (\mathbf{M}_4\cdot\boldsymbol{\mu}_2)^M(\boldsymbol{\mu}_3\cdot\boldsymbol{\mu}_1)^M + 4(\mathbf{M}_4\cdot\boldsymbol{\mu}_1)^M(\boldsymbol{\mu}_3\cdot\boldsymbol{\mu}_2)^M\}. \tag{16.40}$$

Similarly, those tensor elements $[\boldsymbol{\mu}_4\boldsymbol{\mu}_3\boldsymbol{\mu}_2(\mathbf{m}_1 \times \hat{\mathbf{k}}_{pu})]_{XXYX}$, $[\boldsymbol{\mu}_4\boldsymbol{\mu}_3(\mathbf{m}_2 \times \hat{\mathbf{k}}_{pu})\boldsymbol{\mu}_1]_{XXYX}$, $[\boldsymbol{\mu}_4(\mathbf{m}_3 \times \hat{\mathbf{k}}_{pu})\boldsymbol{\mu}_2\boldsymbol{\mu}_1]_{XXYX}$, and $[(\mathbf{m}_4 \times \hat{\mathbf{k}}_{pu})\boldsymbol{\mu}_3\boldsymbol{\mu}_2\boldsymbol{\mu}_1]_{XXYX}$ are

$$[\boldsymbol{\mu}_4\boldsymbol{\mu}_3\boldsymbol{\mu}_2(\mathbf{m}_1 \times \hat{\mathbf{k}}_{pu})]_{XXYX} = i[\boldsymbol{\mu}_4\boldsymbol{\mu}_3\boldsymbol{\mu}_2\mathbf{M}_1]_{XXYY}$$

$$= \frac{i}{30}\sum_{m_1,m_2,m_3,m_4=x,y,z}\{4\delta_{m_1m_2}\delta_{m_3m_4} - \delta_{m_1m_3}\delta_{m_2m_4} - \delta_{m_1m_4}\delta_{m_2m_3}\}[\boldsymbol{\mu}_4\boldsymbol{\mu}_3\boldsymbol{\mu}_2\mathbf{M}_1]^M_{m_1m_2m_3m_4}$$

$$= \frac{i}{30}\{4(\boldsymbol{\mu}_4\cdot\boldsymbol{\mu}_3)^M(\boldsymbol{\mu}_2\cdot\mathbf{M}_1)^M - (\boldsymbol{\mu}_4\cdot\boldsymbol{\mu}_2)^M(\boldsymbol{\mu}_3\cdot\mathbf{M}_1)^M - (\boldsymbol{\mu}_4\cdot\mathbf{M}_1)^M(\boldsymbol{\mu}_3\cdot\boldsymbol{\mu}_2)^M\}$$

$$[\boldsymbol{\mu}_4\boldsymbol{\mu}_3(\mathbf{m}_2 \times \hat{\mathbf{k}}_{pu})\boldsymbol{\mu}_1]_{XXYX} = -i[\boldsymbol{\mu}_4\boldsymbol{\mu}_3\mathbf{M}_2\boldsymbol{\mu}_1]_{XXXX}$$

$$= \frac{-i}{30}\{2(\boldsymbol{\mu}_4\cdot\boldsymbol{\mu}_3)^M(\mathbf{M}_2\cdot\boldsymbol{\mu}_1)^M + 2(\boldsymbol{\mu}_4\cdot\mathbf{M}_2)^M(\boldsymbol{\mu}_3\cdot\boldsymbol{\mu}_1)^M + 2(\boldsymbol{\mu}_4\cdot\boldsymbol{\mu}_1)^M(\boldsymbol{\mu}_3\cdot\mathbf{M}_2)^M\}$$

$$[\boldsymbol{\mu}_4(\mathbf{m}_3 \times \hat{\mathbf{k}}_{pu})\boldsymbol{\mu}_2\boldsymbol{\mu}_1]_{XXYX} = i[\boldsymbol{\mu}_4\mathbf{M}_3\boldsymbol{\mu}_2\boldsymbol{\mu}_1]_{XYYX}$$

$$= \frac{i}{30}\{-(\boldsymbol{\mu}_4\cdot\mathbf{M}_3)^M(\boldsymbol{\mu}_2\cdot\boldsymbol{\mu}_1)^M - (\boldsymbol{\mu}_4\cdot\boldsymbol{\mu}_2)^M(\mathbf{M}_3\cdot\boldsymbol{\mu}_1)^M + 4(\boldsymbol{\mu}_4\cdot\boldsymbol{\mu}_1)^M(\mathbf{M}_3\cdot\boldsymbol{\mu}_2)^M\}$$

$$[(\mathbf{m}_4 \times \hat{\mathbf{k}}_{pu})\boldsymbol{\mu}_3\boldsymbol{\mu}_2\boldsymbol{\mu}_1]_{XXYX} = i[\mathbf{M}_4\boldsymbol{\mu}_3\boldsymbol{\mu}_2\boldsymbol{\mu}_1]_{YXYX}$$
$$= \frac{i}{30}\left\{-(\mathbf{M}_4\cdot\boldsymbol{\mu}_3)^M(\boldsymbol{\mu}_2\cdot\boldsymbol{\mu}_1)^M + 4(\mathbf{M}_4\cdot\boldsymbol{\mu}_2)^M(\boldsymbol{\mu}_3\cdot\boldsymbol{\mu}_1)^M - (\mathbf{M}_4\cdot\boldsymbol{\mu}_1)^M(\boldsymbol{\mu}_3\cdot\boldsymbol{\mu}_2)^M\right\}. \tag{16.41}$$

It should be noted that the transition magnetic dipole matrix elements are purely imaginary for real wavefunctions so that we used the notation $\mathbf{m}_1 = i\mathbf{M}_1$, where $\mathbf{M}_1$ is purely real.

The next step is to consider the electric quadrupole contributions. Similar to Equations 16.38 and 16.39, we define two auxiliary functions as

$$f^Q_{XXXY}(4,3,2,1) = [\boldsymbol{\mu}_4\boldsymbol{\mu}_3\boldsymbol{\mu}_2(\pm\mathbf{k}_1\cdot\mathbf{Q}_1)]_{XXXY} + [\boldsymbol{\mu}_4\boldsymbol{\mu}_3(\pm\mathbf{k}_2\cdot\mathbf{Q}_2)\boldsymbol{\mu}_1]_{XXXY}$$
$$+ [\boldsymbol{\mu}_4(\pm\mathbf{k}_3\cdot\mathbf{Q}_3)\boldsymbol{\mu}_2\boldsymbol{\mu}_1]_{XXXY} - [(\mathbf{k}_4\cdot\mathbf{Q}_4)\boldsymbol{\mu}_3\boldsymbol{\mu}_2\boldsymbol{\mu}_1]_{XXXY} \tag{16.42}$$

$$f^Q_{XXYX}(4,3,2,1) = [\boldsymbol{\mu}_4\boldsymbol{\mu}_3\boldsymbol{\mu}_2(\pm\mathbf{k}_1\cdot\mathbf{Q}_1)]_{XXYX} + [\boldsymbol{\mu}_4\boldsymbol{\mu}_3(\pm\mathbf{k}_2\cdot\mathbf{Q}_2)\boldsymbol{\mu}_1]_{XXYX}$$
$$+ [\boldsymbol{\mu}_4(\pm\mathbf{k}_3\cdot\mathbf{Q}_3)\boldsymbol{\mu}_2\boldsymbol{\mu}_1]_{XXYX} - [(\mathbf{k}_4\cdot\mathbf{Q}_4)\boldsymbol{\mu}_3\boldsymbol{\mu}_2\boldsymbol{\mu}_1]_{XXYX}. \tag{16.43}$$

The upper or lower signs in each term are determined by the phase-matching condition. For example, in the present case of pump–probe, the phase-matching condition is $+\mathbf{k}_1 - \mathbf{k}_2 + \mathbf{k}_3$ with $\mathbf{k}_1 = \mathbf{k}_2 = \mathbf{k}_{pu}$ and $\mathbf{k}_3 = \mathbf{k}_{\mathrm{pu}}$. Thus, one should choose +, −, and + signs for the first three terms in the above equations. The tensor elements $[\boldsymbol{\mu}_4\boldsymbol{\mu}_3\boldsymbol{\mu}_2(\mathbf{k}_{pu}\cdot\mathbf{Q}_1)]_{XXXY}$, $[\boldsymbol{\mu}_4\boldsymbol{\mu}_3(\mathbf{k}_{pu}\cdot\mathbf{Q}_2)\boldsymbol{\mu}_1]_{XXXY}$, $[\boldsymbol{\mu}_4(\mathbf{k}_{pr}\cdot\mathbf{Q}_3)\boldsymbol{\mu}_2\boldsymbol{\mu}_1]_{XXXY}$, and $[(\mathbf{k}_{pr}\cdot\mathbf{Q}_4)\boldsymbol{\mu}_3\boldsymbol{\mu}_2\boldsymbol{\mu}_1]_{XXXY}$ are found to be

$$[\boldsymbol{\mu}_4\boldsymbol{\mu}_3\boldsymbol{\mu}_2(\mathbf{k}_1\cdot\mathbf{Q}_1)]_{XXXY} = k_1[\boldsymbol{\mu}_4\boldsymbol{\mu}_3\boldsymbol{\mu}_2\mathbf{Q}_1]_{XXXZY}$$
$$= \frac{k_1}{30}\sum_{m_1,m_2,m_3,m_4,m_5=x,y,z}\{-\varepsilon_{m_1m_4m_5}\delta_{m_2m_3} - \varepsilon_{m_2m_4m_5}\delta_{m_1m_3} - \varepsilon_{m_3m_4m_5}\delta_{m_1m_2}\}$$
$$\times[\boldsymbol{\mu}_4\boldsymbol{\mu}_3\boldsymbol{\mu}_2\mathbf{Q}_1]^M_{m_1m_2m_3m_4m_5} = 0$$

$$[\boldsymbol{\mu}_4\boldsymbol{\mu}_3(\mathbf{k}_2\cdot\mathbf{Q}_2)\boldsymbol{\mu}_1]_{XXXY} = k_2[\boldsymbol{\mu}_4\boldsymbol{\mu}_3\mathbf{Q}_2\boldsymbol{\mu}_1]_{XXZXY}$$
$$= \frac{k_2}{30}\sum_{m_1,m_2,m_3,m_4,m_5=x,y,z}\{-\varepsilon_{m_1m_3m_5}\delta_{m_2m_4} - \varepsilon_{m_2m_3m_5}\delta_{m_1m_4} + \varepsilon_{m_3m_4m_5}\delta_{m_1m_2}\}[\boldsymbol{\mu}_4\boldsymbol{\mu}_3\mathbf{Q}_2\boldsymbol{\mu}_1]^M_{m_1m_2m_3m_4m_5}$$
$$= \frac{k_2}{30}\left\{[\boldsymbol{\mu}_4\cdot\{\boldsymbol{\mu}_1\times(\mathbf{Q}_2\cdot\boldsymbol{\mu}_3)\}]^M + [\boldsymbol{\mu}_3\cdot\{\boldsymbol{\mu}_1\times(\mathbf{Q}_2\cdot\boldsymbol{\mu}_4)\}]^M\right\}$$

$$[\boldsymbol{\mu}_4(\mathbf{k}_3\cdot\mathbf{Q}_3)\boldsymbol{\mu}_2\boldsymbol{\mu}_1]_{XXXY} = k_3[\boldsymbol{\mu}_4\mathbf{Q}_3\boldsymbol{\mu}_2\boldsymbol{\mu}_1]_{XZXXY}$$
$$= \frac{k_3}{30}\sum_{m_1,m_2,m_3,m_4,m_5=x,y,z}\{-\varepsilon_{m_1m_2m_5}\delta_{m_3m_4} + \varepsilon_{m_2m_3m_5}\delta_{m_1m_4} + \varepsilon_{m_2m_4m_5}\delta_{m_1m_3}\}[\boldsymbol{\mu}_4\mathbf{Q}_3\boldsymbol{\mu}_2\boldsymbol{\mu}_1]^M_{m_1m_2m_3m_4m_5}$$
$$= \frac{k_3}{30}\left\{[\boldsymbol{\mu}_4\cdot\{\boldsymbol{\mu}_1\times(\mathbf{Q}_3\cdot\boldsymbol{\mu}_2)\}]^M + [(\mathbf{Q}_3\cdot\boldsymbol{\mu}_4)\cdot\{\boldsymbol{\mu}_2\times\boldsymbol{\mu}_1\}]^M\right\}$$

$$[(\mathbf{k}_4\cdot\mathbf{Q}_4)\boldsymbol{\mu}_3\boldsymbol{\mu}_2\boldsymbol{\mu}_1]_{XXXY} = k_4[\mathbf{Q}_4\boldsymbol{\mu}_3\boldsymbol{\mu}_2\boldsymbol{\mu}_1]_{ZXXXY}$$

$$= \frac{k_4}{30}\sum_{m_1,m_2,m_3,m_4,m_5=x,y,z}\{\varepsilon_{m_1m_2m_5}\delta_{m_3m_4} + \varepsilon_{m_1m_3m_5}\delta_{m_2m_4} + \varepsilon_{m_1m_4m_5}\delta_{m_2m_3}\}[\mathbf{Q}_4\boldsymbol{\mu}_3\boldsymbol{\mu}_2\boldsymbol{\mu}_1]^M_{m_1m_2m_3m_4m_5}$$

$$= \frac{k_4}{30}\left\{[(\mathbf{Q}_4\cdot\boldsymbol{\mu}_2)\cdot\{\boldsymbol{\mu}_3\times\boldsymbol{\mu}_1\}]^M + (\mathbf{Q}_4\cdot\boldsymbol{\mu}_3)\cdot\{\boldsymbol{\mu}_2\times\boldsymbol{\mu}_1\}]^M\right\}. \quad (16.44)$$

The remaining tensor elements $[\boldsymbol{\mu}_4\boldsymbol{\mu}_3\boldsymbol{\mu}_2(\mathbf{k}_1\cdot\mathbf{Q}_1)]_{XXYX}$, $[\boldsymbol{\mu}_4\boldsymbol{\mu}_3(\mathbf{k}_2\cdot\mathbf{Q}_2)\boldsymbol{\mu}_1]_{XXYX}$, $[\boldsymbol{\mu}_4(\mathbf{k}_3\cdot\mathbf{Q}_3)\boldsymbol{\mu}_2\boldsymbol{\mu}_1]_{XXYX}$, and $[(\mathbf{k}_4\cdot\mathbf{Q}_4)\boldsymbol{\mu}_3\boldsymbol{\mu}_2\boldsymbol{\mu}_1]_{XXYX}$ are given as

$$[\boldsymbol{\mu}_4\boldsymbol{\mu}_3\boldsymbol{\mu}_2(\mathbf{k}_1\cdot\mathbf{Q}_1)]_{XXYX} = k_1[\boldsymbol{\mu}_4\boldsymbol{\mu}_3\boldsymbol{\mu}_2\mathbf{Q}_1]_{XXYZX}$$

$$= \frac{k_1}{30}\sum_{m_1,m_2,m_3,m_4,m_5=x,y,z}\{\varepsilon_{m_1m_3m_4}\delta_{m_2m_5} + \varepsilon_{m_2m_3m_4}\delta_{m_1m_5} + \varepsilon_{m_3m_4m_5}\delta_{m_1m_2}\}[\boldsymbol{\mu}_4\boldsymbol{\mu}_3\boldsymbol{\mu}_2\mathbf{Q}_1]^M_{m_1m_2m_3m_4m_5}$$

$$= \frac{k_1}{30}\left\{[\boldsymbol{\mu}_4\cdot\{\boldsymbol{\mu}_2\times(\mathbf{Q}_1\cdot\boldsymbol{\mu}_3)\}]^M + [\boldsymbol{\mu}_3\cdot\{\boldsymbol{\mu}_2\times(\mathbf{Q}_1\cdot\boldsymbol{\mu}_4)\}]^M\right\}$$

$$[\boldsymbol{\mu}_4\boldsymbol{\mu}_3(\mathbf{k}_2\cdot\mathbf{Q}_2)\boldsymbol{\mu}_1]_{XXYX} = k_2[\boldsymbol{\mu}_4\boldsymbol{\mu}_3\mathbf{Q}_2\boldsymbol{\mu}_1]_{XXZYX}$$

$$= \frac{k_2}{30}\sum_{m_1,m_2,m_3,m_4,m_5=x,y,z}\{-\varepsilon_{m_1m_3m_4}\delta_{m_2m_5} - \varepsilon_{m_2m_3m_4}\delta_{m_1m_4} - \varepsilon_{m_3m_4m_5}\delta_{m_1m_2}\}$$

$$\times[\boldsymbol{\mu}_4\boldsymbol{\mu}_3\mathbf{Q}_2\boldsymbol{\mu}_1]^M_{m_1m_2m_3m_4m_5} = 0$$

$$[\boldsymbol{\mu}_4(\mathbf{k}_3\cdot\mathbf{Q}_3)\boldsymbol{\mu}_2\boldsymbol{\mu}_1]_{XXYX} = k_3[\boldsymbol{\mu}_4\mathbf{Q}_3\boldsymbol{\mu}_2\boldsymbol{\mu}_1]_{XZXYX}$$

$$= \frac{k_3}{30}\sum_{m_1,m_2,m_3,m_4,m_5=x,y,z}\{-\varepsilon_{m_1m_2m_4}\delta_{m_3m_5} + \varepsilon_{m_2m_3m_4}\delta_{m_1m_5} - \varepsilon_{m_2m_4m_5}\delta_{m_1m_3}\}[\boldsymbol{\mu}_4\mathbf{Q}_3\boldsymbol{\mu}_2\boldsymbol{\mu}_1]^M_{m_1m_2m_3m_4m_5}$$

$$= \frac{k_3}{30}\left\{[\boldsymbol{\mu}_4\cdot\{\boldsymbol{\mu}_2\times(\mathbf{Q}_3\cdot\boldsymbol{\mu}_1)\}]^M + [(\mathbf{Q}_3\cdot\boldsymbol{\mu}_4)\cdot\{\boldsymbol{\mu}_1\times\boldsymbol{\mu}_2\}]^M\right\}$$

$$[(\mathbf{k}_4\cdot\mathbf{Q}_4)\boldsymbol{\mu}_3\boldsymbol{\mu}_2\boldsymbol{\mu}_1]_{XXYX} = k_4[\mathbf{Q}_4\boldsymbol{\mu}_3\boldsymbol{\mu}_2\boldsymbol{\mu}_1]_{ZXXYX}$$

$$= \frac{k_4}{30}\sum_{m_1,m_2,m_3,m_4,m_5=x,y,z}\{\varepsilon_{m_1m_2m_4}\delta_{m_3m_5} + \varepsilon_{m_1m_3m_4}\delta_{m_2m_5} - \varepsilon_{m_1m_4m_5}\delta_{m_2m_3}\}[\mathbf{Q}_4\boldsymbol{\mu}_3\boldsymbol{\mu}_2\boldsymbol{\mu}_1]^M_{m_1m_2m_3m_4m_5}$$

$$= \frac{k_4}{30}\left\{[(\mathbf{Q}_4\cdot\boldsymbol{\mu}_1)\cdot\{\boldsymbol{\mu}_3\times\boldsymbol{\mu}_2\}]^M + (\mathbf{Q}_4\cdot\boldsymbol{\mu}_3)\cdot\{\boldsymbol{\mu}_1\times\boldsymbol{\mu}_2\}]^M\right\}. \quad (16.45)$$

It is again noted that the **Q** matrix is symmetric with respect to two indexes, for example, $Q_{m_1m_2} = Q_{m_2m_1}$; but the Levi–Civita tensor is antisymmetric, for example, $\varepsilon_{m_1m_2m_3} = -\varepsilon_{m_1m_3m_2}$. Thus, in the summations of Equation 16.45, there are terms that vanish due to rotational averaging.

Using the above general results for multilevel systems and from Equation 16.36, one can obtain the differential signal, $\Delta S_{TD}(\omega_{pu},\omega_{pr};T)$, for a 2LS. The first term in

Equation 16.33, which is $\sqrt{2}iS_{TD}^{XXXY}(\omega_{pu},\omega_{pr};T;m)$, is found to be

$$\sqrt{2}if_{XXXY}^{m}(ge,eg,ge,eg) = \sqrt{2}i\{[\boldsymbol{\mu}_{ge}\boldsymbol{\mu}_{eg}\boldsymbol{\mu}_{ge}(\mathbf{m}_{eg}\times\hat{\mathbf{k}}_{pu})]_{XXXY} + [\boldsymbol{\mu}_{ge}\boldsymbol{\mu}_{eg}(\mathbf{m}_{ge}\times\hat{\mathbf{k}}_{pu})\boldsymbol{\mu}_{eg}]_{XXXY}$$
$$+[\boldsymbol{\mu}_{ge}(\mathbf{m}_{eg}\times\hat{\mathbf{k}}_{pu})\boldsymbol{\mu}_{ge}\boldsymbol{\mu}_{eg}]_{XXXY} + [(\mathbf{m}_{ge}\times\hat{\mathbf{k}}_{pu})\boldsymbol{\mu}_{eg}\boldsymbol{\mu}_{ge}\boldsymbol{\mu}_{eg}]_{XXXY}\}$$
$$= \frac{4\sqrt{2}}{15}(\boldsymbol{\mu}_{ge}\cdot\boldsymbol{\mu}_{eg})^{M}(\boldsymbol{\mu}_{ge}\cdot\mathbf{M}_{eg})^{M}. \tag{16.46}$$

Similarly, $\sqrt{2}iS_{TD}^{XXYX}(\omega_{pu},\omega_{pr};T;m)$ is given as

$$\sqrt{2}if_{XXYX}^{m}(ge,eg,ge,eg) = \sqrt{2}i\{[\boldsymbol{\mu}_{ge}\boldsymbol{\mu}_{eg}\boldsymbol{\mu}_{ge}(\mathbf{m}_{eg}\times\hat{\mathbf{k}}_{pu})]_{XXYX} + [\boldsymbol{\mu}_{ge}\boldsymbol{\mu}_{eg}(\mathbf{m}_{ge}\times\hat{\mathbf{k}}_{pu})\boldsymbol{\mu}_{eg}]_{XXYX}$$
$$+[\boldsymbol{\mu}_{ge}(\mathbf{m}_{eg}\times\hat{\mathbf{k}}_{pu})\boldsymbol{\mu}_{ge}\boldsymbol{\mu}_{eg}]_{XXYX} + [(\mathbf{m}_{ge}\times\hat{\mathbf{k}}_{pu})\boldsymbol{\mu}_{eg}\boldsymbol{\mu}_{ge}\boldsymbol{\mu}_{eg}]_{XXYX}\}$$
$$= -\frac{4\sqrt{2}}{15}(\boldsymbol{\mu}_{ge}\cdot\boldsymbol{\mu}_{eg})^{M}(\boldsymbol{\mu}_{ge}\cdot\mathbf{M}_{eg})^{M}. \tag{16.47}$$

Here, $\mathbf{m}_{eg}$ and $\mathbf{m}_{ge}$ are purely imaginary as mentioned above so that $\mathbf{m}_{eg} = i\mathbf{M}_{eg}$. Furthermore, we have

$$\mathbf{m}_{ge} = \mathbf{m}_{eg}^{*} = -i\mathbf{M}_{eg} = i\mathbf{M}_{ge}. \tag{16.48}$$

The transition electric dipole matrix elements are purely real and $\boldsymbol{\mu}_{ge} = \boldsymbol{\mu}_{eg}$. Also, it is noted that $\hat{\boldsymbol{\mu}}$ is not commute with $\hat{\mathbf{m}}$ and that $\hat{\boldsymbol{\mu}}\cdot\hat{\mathbf{m}}$ is a Hermitian operator.

EXERCISE 16.2

Show that $\mathbf{m}_{ge} = \mathbf{m}_{eg}^{*}$ by using the integration by part method. Note that for a single electron system the magnetic dipole operator is $\mathbf{m} = (e/2mc)(\hat{\mathbf{r}}\times\hat{\mathbf{p}})$. Also, prove that the sum of the rotatory strengths for all states vanishes.

The transition electric and magnetic dipole matrix elements inside the brackets $[\cdots]^{M}$ or $(\cdots)^{M}$ are those in a molecule-fixed frame. Now, we introduce generalized definitions of dipole and rotatory strengths,

$$D_{ee}^{g} \equiv [\boldsymbol{\mu}_{ge}\cdot\boldsymbol{\mu}_{eg}]^{M}$$
$$R_{ee}^{g} \equiv \mathrm{Im}[\boldsymbol{\mu}_{ge}\cdot\mathbf{m}_{eg}]^{M}. \tag{16.49}$$

Here, the dipole and rotatory strengths in Equation 16.49 are those of ground-state properties, and they determine the all-electric-dipole-induced transition probability and electric dipole/magnetic dipole–induced transition probability from g to e states, respectively. In the cases of nonlinear optical spectroscopy, not only the transitions between g and e but also those between e and other higher-lying (doubly) excited states should be taken into account. Then, the dipole and rotatory strengths of excited states become important in quantitative descriptions of nonlinear optical activity. Thus, instead of conventional notations for the dipole and rotatory strengths used for linear optical activity, we shall use the new notations given in Equation 16.49.

Then, one can find that the magnetic dipole contribution to the 2D transient dichroism spectrum, $\Delta S_{TD}(\omega_{pu},\omega_{pr};T)$, is given as

$$\Delta S_{TD}(\omega_{pu},\omega_{pr};T;m)=\frac{8\sqrt{2}}{15}D_{ee}^{g}R_{ee}^{g}\Gamma_{TD}^{2LS}(\omega_{pu},\omega_{pr};T). \tag{16.50}$$

It is interesting to note that the entire transition strength is determined by the product of dipole strength and rotatory strength. Therefore, the sign of the 2D optical activity TD peak is determined by the rotatory strength, which can be either positive or negative.

In addition to the above magnetic dipole contribution, it is necessary to include the electric quadrupole contribution. For this specific case of 2LS, due to the following equalities

$$\vec{a}\cdot\{\vec{b}\times\vec{a}\}=-\vec{a}\cdot\{\vec{a}\times\vec{b}\}=\vec{b}\cdot\{\vec{a}\times\vec{a}\}=0, \tag{16.51}$$

one can show that the quadrupole contribution to the 2D optical activity TD spectrum vanishes for any 2LSs, that is,

$$\Delta S_{TD}(\omega_{pu},\omega_{pr};T;Q)=0 \quad \text{(for 2LS)}. \tag{16.52}$$

From Equations 16.50 and 16.52, the 2D optical activity TD spectrum is finally given as

$$\Delta S_{TD}(\omega_{pu},\omega_{pr};T)=\frac{8\sqrt{2}}{15}D_{ee}^{g}R_{ee}^{g}\Gamma_{TD}^{2LS}(\omega_{pu},\omega_{pr};T) \quad \text{(for 2LS)}. \tag{16.53}$$

One can also obtain a similar expression for the 2D optical activity transient birefringence spectrum by simply replacing the 2D peak shape function $\Gamma_{TD}^{2LS}(\omega_{pu},\omega_{pr};T)$ in Equation 16.53 with $\Gamma_{TB}^{2LS}(\omega_{pu},\omega_{pr};T)$. Here, it should be emphasized that such a vanishing quadrupole contribution to the 2D optical activity TD spectroscopy is valid only for the case of 2LS.

EXERCISE 16.3

The 2D transient dichroism and birefringence spectra of a weakly anharmonic oscillator were considered in Section 6.3 in detail. Considering the low-lying three vibrational states, |0>, |1>, and |2>, and assuming $\boldsymbol{\mu}_{21}=\sqrt{2}\boldsymbol{\mu}_{10}$, obtain the corresponding expression for $\Delta S_{TD}(\omega_{pu},\omega_{pr};T)$ and show its relationship to Equation 16.53.

In this section we focused on the 2D circularly polarized pump–probe spectroscopy of a 2LS. The rotational averages of fourth- and fifth-rank tensors involving magnetic dipole and electric quadrupole transition matrix elements were discussed in detail. Although one can generalize the 2D circularly polarized pump–probe spectroscopy for coupled multi-chromophore systems, such extensions will be left for the readers. Instead, we next consider 2D circularly polarized photon echo spectroscopy, because the photon echo method is the direct analog of 2D COSY (correlation spectroscopy) NMR and has been found to be useful in obtaining various 2D vibrational or electronic spectra of complex molecules.

16.4 TWO-DIMENSIONAL OPTICAL ACTIVITY PHOTON ECHO: TWO-LEVEL SYSTEM

A detailed description on the 2D photon echo spectroscopy of 2LS and anharmonic oscillator was already presented and discussed in Chapter 7. Interesting 2D peak shapes and transient behaviors of diagonally elongated peak shape were also discussed. However, only the electric-dipole-allowed transitions were considered to describe the photon echo phenomenon, and that is quantitatively acceptable because the magnetic dipole–magnetic field and electric quadrupole–electric field interactions are quite small. Note that the incident beams used for typical 2D photon echo measurements are all linearly polarized and the rotationally invariant elements of the fourth-rank tensorial response function were only considered, for example, S_{ZZZZ}, S_{ZYYZ}, and so forth. However, if one of the incident beams is circularly polarized and the LCP and RCP photon echo signals are obtained, the difference signal will be critically dependent on molecular chirality.[8, 12]

Depending on which of the three incident pulses is controlled to be circularly polarized, there exist several different ways to carry out circularly polarized photon echo measurements. In this chapter, the case when the first incident pulse is circularly polarized will be mainly considered in detail. By following the same arguments presented in the previous section, one can generally expand the 2D photon echo spectrum as a power series with respect to magnetic dipole and electric quadrupole matrix elements, that is,

$$\tilde{E}_{PE}(\omega_t,T,\omega_\tau)=\tilde{E}_{PE}^{(0)}(\omega_t,T,\omega_\tau)+\tilde{E}_{PE}^{(1)}(\omega_t,T,\omega_\tau;m)+\tilde{E}_{PE}^{(1)}(\omega_t,T,\omega_\tau;Q)+\cdots. \tag{16.54}$$

This equation is analogous to Equation 16.26 for the 2D TD spectrum up to the first order with respect to m and Q. The first term in Equation 16.54 is the usual 2D photon echo spectrum within the electric dipole approximation. The second and third terms are then linearly proportional to the magnetic dipole and electric quadrupole, respectively.

For a 2LS, it was shown that the all-electric-dipole-allowed photon echo spectrum, $\tilde{E}_{PE}^{(0)}(\omega_t,T,\omega_\tau)$, is given as

$$\tilde{E}_{PE}^{(0)}(\omega_t,T,\omega_\tau)=2[\boldsymbol{\mu}_{ge}\boldsymbol{\mu}_{eg}\boldsymbol{\mu}_{eg}\boldsymbol{\mu}_{ge}]\otimes\,\mathbf{e}_s^*\mathbf{e}_3\mathbf{e}_2\mathbf{e}_1^*\Gamma(\bar{\omega}_{eg},\Omega^2,\bar{\omega}_{eg},\Omega^2), \tag{16.55}$$

where only the two resphasing diagrams were taken into consideration.

In order to obtain the first-order magnetic dipole correction term, which is $\tilde{E}_{PE}^{(1)}(\omega_t, T, \omega_\tau; m)$ in Equation 16.54, we need to consider diagrams like

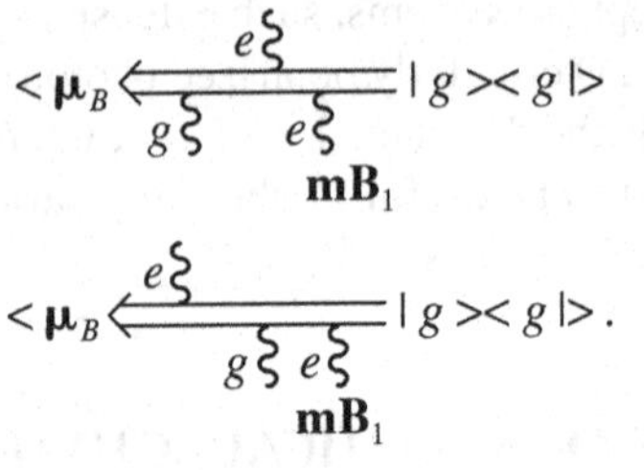

(16.56)

The first is the stimulated emission diagram, where the first coherence is generated by the magnetic dipole–magnetic field interaction. The second diagram corresponds to the ground-state bleaching. Because only the first incident beam is assumed to be either LCP or RCP, other diagrams with different time-orderings are not included. Then, the magnetic dipole correction term $\tilde{E}_{PE}^{(1)}(\omega_t, T, \omega_\tau; m)$ is found to be

$$\begin{aligned}\tilde{E}_{PE}^{(1)}(\omega_t, T, \omega_\tau; m) = 2\{&[\boldsymbol{\mu}_{ge}\boldsymbol{\mu}_{eg}\boldsymbol{\mu}_{eg}(\mathbf{m}_{ge} \times \hat{\mathbf{k}}_1)] \\ &+[\boldsymbol{\mu}_{ge}\boldsymbol{\mu}_{eg}(\mathbf{m}_{eg} \times \hat{\mathbf{k}}_2)\boldsymbol{\mu}_{ge}] + [\boldsymbol{\mu}_{ge}(\mathbf{m}_{eg} \times \hat{\mathbf{k}}_3)\boldsymbol{\mu}_{eg}\boldsymbol{\mu}_{ge}] \\ &+[(\mathbf{m}_{ge} \times \hat{\mathbf{k}}_s)\boldsymbol{\mu}_{eg}\boldsymbol{\mu}_{eg}\boldsymbol{\mu}_{ge}]\} \otimes \mathbf{e}_s^*\mathbf{e}_3\mathbf{e}_2\mathbf{e}_1^*\Gamma\left(\bar{\omega}_{eg}, \Omega^2, \bar{\omega}_{eg}, \Omega^2\right). \quad (16.57)\end{aligned}$$

The first-order electric quadrupole correction term to the 2D optical activity photon echo, $\tilde{E}_{PE}^{(1)}(\omega_t, T, \omega_\tau; Q)$, is then given as

$$\begin{aligned}\tilde{E}_{PE}^{(1)}(\omega_t, T, \omega_\tau; Q) = i\{&-[\boldsymbol{\mu}_{ge}\boldsymbol{\mu}_{eg}\boldsymbol{\mu}_{eg}(\mathbf{k}_1 \cdot \mathbf{Q}_{ge})] \\ &+[\boldsymbol{\mu}_{ge}\boldsymbol{\mu}_{eg}(\mathbf{k}_2 \cdot \mathbf{Q}_{eg})\boldsymbol{\mu}_{ge}] + [\boldsymbol{\mu}_{ge}(\mathbf{k}_3 \cdot \mathbf{Q}_{eg})\boldsymbol{\mu}_{eg}\boldsymbol{\mu}_{ge}] \\ &-[(\mathbf{k}_s \cdot \mathbf{Q}_{ge})\boldsymbol{\mu}_{eg}\boldsymbol{\mu}_{eg}\boldsymbol{\mu}_{ge}]\} \otimes \mathbf{e}_s^*\mathbf{e}_3\mathbf{e}_2\mathbf{e}_1^*\Gamma\left(\bar{\omega}_{eg}, \Omega^2, \bar{\omega}_{eg}, \Omega^2\right). \quad (16.58)\end{aligned}$$

Combining Equations 16.55, 16.57, and 16.58, we have the general expression for the 2D optical activity photon echo spectrum for a 2LS, which is valid for any arbitrary beam configurations.

Now, for the sake of simplicity, it is assumed that the three incident beam propagation directions are almost collinear, so that $\mathbf{k}_j = \hat{Z}$ for all j. Let us assume that, except for the first pulse, the polarization directions of the second, third, and echo fields are all parallel to the X-axis in a space-fixed frame. The differential 2D photon echo spectrum is defined as

$$\Delta\tilde{E}_{PE}(\omega_t, T, \omega_\tau) = \tilde{E}_{PE}^{LCP}(\omega_t, T, \omega_\tau) - \tilde{E}_{PE}^{RCP}(\omega_t, T, \omega_\tau). \quad (16.59)$$

To obtain $\Delta\tilde{E}_{PE}(\omega_t, T, \omega_\tau)$, one can derive proper expressions for both terms on the right-hand side of Equation 16.59 separately and take the difference. However, alternatively, one can use the relationship in Equation 16.20 and find that $\Delta\tilde{E}_{PE}(\omega_t, T, \omega_\tau)$

is given as

$$\Delta\tilde{E}_{PE}(\omega_t,T,\omega_\tau) = -\sqrt{2}i\tilde{E}_{PE}^{XXXY}(\omega_t,T,\omega_\tau). \tag{16.60}$$

Here, $\tilde{E}_{PE}^{XXXY}(\omega_t,T,\omega_\tau)$ is the 2D photon echo spectrum obtained by using Y-polarized beam 1 and X-polarized beams 2 and 3, and by detecting the X-component of the radiated echo field vector. The negative sign in Equation 16.60 was chosen because the first radiation–matter interaction is between the molecular dipole and $\mathbf{e}_1^*$-component of the first beam. In order to calculate the $XXXY$ elements of the three tensors in Equations 16.57 and 16.58, one can use the results in the previous section, particularly, Equations 16.46 and 16.52. We thus have

$$\Delta\tilde{E}_{PE}^{(1)}(\omega_t,T,\omega_\tau;m) = \frac{8\sqrt{2}}{15}D_{ee}^{g}R_{ee}^{g}\Gamma\left(\bar{\omega}_{eg},\Omega^2,\bar{\omega}_{eg},\Omega^2\right) \tag{16.61}$$

$$\Delta\tilde{E}_{PE}^{(1)}(\omega_t,T,\omega_\tau;Q) = 0. \tag{16.62}$$

Therefore, the 2D optical activity photon echo spectrum of a 2LS is found to be solely determined by the first-order magnetic dipole correction term as

$$\Delta\tilde{E}_{PE}(\omega_t,T,\omega_\tau) = \frac{8\sqrt{2}}{15}D_{ee}^{g}R_{ee}^{g}\Gamma\left(\bar{\omega}_{eg},\Omega^2,\bar{\omega}_{eg},\Omega^2\right). \tag{16.63}$$

Similarly, for a weakly anharmonic oscillator system, other than an additional peak from the excited-state absorption, the overall amplitude and sign of the 2D photon echo peak is determined by the product of dipole strength and rotatory strength of the oscillator.

16.5 TWO-DIMENSIONAL OPTICAL ACTIVITY PHOTON ECHO OF COUPLED TWO-LEVEL SYSTEM DIMER

One of the interesting model systems that can be studied by using this 2D optical activity photon echo method is a coupled 2LS dimer, where each monomer is modeled as a 2LS. Detailed theoretical descriptions of 2D photon echo spectra of such a coupled dimer were presented in Chapter 9, where short-time quantum beats, long-time population transfers, and physical meanings of cross-peak amplitudes were discussed. In this section, we will consider the 2D optical activity photon echo of the same dimer having one ground state (g), two singly excited states (e_1 and e_2), and one doubly excited state (f). Depending on the waiting time T, there are three different regimes. At very short time ($T < \tau_{decoherence}$), the coherence evolution appearing as oscillating peak amplitudes can be observed in a series of 2D spectra recorded with respect to T. At long time T, the diagonal and cross-peak amplitudes change in time due to the population transfers between two singly excited states. However, just for the sake of simplicity, we will only focus on the intermediate time regime, that is, $\tau_{decoherence} < T < \tau_{pop}$. In this case, the diagonal and cross-peak shapes were found to be, within the electric dipole approximation,

$$\tilde{E}_{D1}^{(0)}(\omega_t,T,\omega_\tau)=2[\boldsymbol{\mu}_{ge_1}\boldsymbol{\mu}_{e_1g}\boldsymbol{\mu}_{ge_1}\boldsymbol{\mu}_{e_1g}]\otimes\mathbf{e}_s^*\mathbf{e}_3\mathbf{e}_2\mathbf{e}_1^*\Gamma\left(\bar{\omega}_{e_1g},<\delta\Omega_1^2>,\bar{\omega}_{e_1g},<\delta\Omega_1^2>\right)$$

$$\tilde{E}_{D2}^{(0)}(\omega_t,T,\omega_\tau)=2[\boldsymbol{\mu}_{ge_2}\boldsymbol{\mu}_{e_2g}\boldsymbol{\mu}_{ge_2}\boldsymbol{\mu}_{e_2g}]\otimes\mathbf{e}_s^*\mathbf{e}_3\mathbf{e}_2\mathbf{e}_1^*\Gamma\left(\bar{\omega}_{e_2g},<\delta\Omega_2^2>,\bar{\omega}_{e_2g},<\delta\Omega_2^2>\right)$$

$$\tilde{E}_{C12}^{(0)}(\omega_t,T,\omega_\tau)=[\boldsymbol{\mu}_{ge_2}\boldsymbol{\mu}_{e_2g}\boldsymbol{\mu}_{e_1g}\boldsymbol{\mu}_{ge_1}]\otimes\mathbf{e}_s^*\mathbf{e}_3\mathbf{e}_2\mathbf{e}_1^*\Gamma\left(\bar{\omega}_{e_2g},<\delta\Omega_2^2>,\bar{\omega}_{e_1g},<\delta\Omega_1^2>\right)$$

$$-[\boldsymbol{\mu}_{e_2f}\boldsymbol{\mu}_{fe_2}\boldsymbol{\mu}_{e_2g}\boldsymbol{\mu}_{ge_2}]\otimes\mathbf{e}_s^*\mathbf{e}_3\mathbf{e}_2\mathbf{e}_1^*\Gamma\left(\bar{\omega}_{fe_1},<\delta\Omega_2^2>,\bar{\omega}_{e_1g},<\delta\Omega_1^2>\right)$$

$$\tilde{E}_{C21}^{(0)}(\omega_t,T,\omega_\tau)=[\boldsymbol{\mu}_{ge_1}\boldsymbol{\mu}_{e_1g}\boldsymbol{\mu}_{e_2g}\boldsymbol{\mu}_{ge_2}]\otimes\mathbf{e}_s^*\mathbf{e}_3\mathbf{e}_2\mathbf{e}_1^*\Gamma\left(\bar{\omega}_{e_1g},<\delta\Omega_1^2>,\bar{\omega}_{e_2g},<\delta\Omega_2^2>\right)$$

$$-[\boldsymbol{\mu}_{e_2f}\boldsymbol{\mu}_{fe_2}\boldsymbol{\mu}_{e_2g}\boldsymbol{\mu}_{ge_2}]\otimes\mathbf{e}_s^*\mathbf{e}_3\mathbf{e}_2\mathbf{e}_1^*\Gamma\left(\bar{\omega}_{fe_2},<\delta\Omega_1^2>,\bar{\omega}_{e_2g},<\delta\Omega_2^2>\right).\quad(16.64)$$

Again, let us consider the specific case when the first beam is circularly polarized and when the difference signal is taken to be the 2D optical activity photon echo. Thus, the relationship $\Delta\tilde{E}_{PE}(\omega_t,T,\omega_\tau)=-\sqrt{2}i\tilde{E}_{PE}^{XXXY}(\omega_t,T,\omega_\tau)$ between the differential measurement signal and cross-polarization-detected *XXXY*-signal can be used. By following the same procedure used to obtain the 2D optical activity TD spectrum for a 2LS, one can find that the two diagonal peaks in the 2D optical activity photon echo spectrum are given as

$$\Delta\tilde{E}_{D1}(\omega_t,T,\omega_\tau)=\frac{8\sqrt{2}}{15}D_{e_1e_1}^{g}R_{e_1e_1}^{g}\Gamma\left(\bar{\omega}_{e_1g},<\delta\Omega_1^2>,\bar{\omega}_{e_1g},<\delta\Omega_1^2>\right)$$

$$\Delta\tilde{E}_{D2}(\omega_t,T,\omega_\tau)=\frac{8\sqrt{2}}{15}D_{e_2e_2}^{g}R_{e_2e_2}^{g}\Gamma\left(\bar{\omega}_{e_2g},<\delta\Omega_2^2>,\bar{\omega}_{e_2g},<\delta\Omega_2^2>\right).\quad(16.65)$$

Here, the electric quadrupole contributions to these two *diagonal* peaks vanish (see Equation 16.62). The cross-peaks in the 2D optical activity photon echo spectrum, which originate from the first-order magnetic dipole corrections, are

$$\Delta\tilde{E}_{C12}(\omega_t,T,\omega_\tau;m)=-\sqrt{2}if_{XXXY}^{m}(ge_2,e_2g,e_1g,ge_1)\Gamma\left(\bar{\omega}_{e_2g},<\delta\Omega_2^2>,\bar{\omega}_{e_1g},<\delta\Omega_1^2>\right)$$

$$+\sqrt{2}if_{XXXY}^{m}(e_1f,fe_1,e_1g,ge_1)\Gamma\left(\bar{\omega}_{fe_1},<\delta\Omega_2^2>,\bar{\omega}_{e_1g},<\delta\Omega_1^2>\right)$$

$$\Delta\tilde{E}_{C21}(\omega_t,T,\omega_\tau;m)=-\sqrt{2}if_{XXXY}^{m}(ge_1,e_1g,e_2g,ge_2)\Gamma\left(\bar{\omega}_{e_1g},<\delta\Omega_1^2>,\bar{\omega}_{e_2g},<\delta\Omega_2^2>\right)$$

$$+\sqrt{2}if_{XXXY}^{m}(e_2f,fe_2,e_2g,ge_2)\Gamma\left(\bar{\omega}_{fe_2},<\delta\Omega_1^2>,\bar{\omega}_{e_2g},<\delta\Omega_2^2>\right).\quad(16.66)$$

Similarly, the first-order electric quadrupole corrections to these cross-peaks are

$$\Delta\tilde{E}_{C12}(\omega_t,T,\omega_\tau;Q)=(1/\sqrt{2})f^{Q}_{XXXY}(ge_2,e_2g,e_1g,ge_1)\Gamma\left(\bar{\omega}_{e_2g},<\delta\Omega_2^2>,\bar{\omega}_{e_1g},<\delta\Omega_1^2>\right)$$
$$-(1/\sqrt{2})f^{Q}_{XXXY}(e_1f,fe_1,e_1g,ge_1)\Gamma\left(\bar{\omega}_{fe_1},<\delta\Omega_2^2>,\bar{\omega}_{e_1g},<\delta\Omega_1^2>\right)$$
$$\Delta\tilde{E}_{C21}(\omega_t,T,\omega_\tau;Q)=(1/\sqrt{2})f^{Q}_{XXXY}(ge_1,e_1g,e_2g,ge_2)\Gamma\left(\bar{\omega}_{e_1g},<\delta\Omega_1^2>,\bar{\omega}_{e_2g},<\delta\Omega_2^2>\right)$$
$$-(1/\sqrt{2})f^{Q}_{XXXY}(e_2f,fe_2,e_2g,ge_2)\Gamma\left(\bar{\omega}_{fe_2},<\delta\Omega_1^2>,\bar{\omega}_{e_2g},<\delta\Omega_2^2>\right). \quad (16.67)$$

From the definitions of the auxiliary functions f^{m}_{XXXY} and f^{Q}_{XXXY} in Equations 16.38 and 16.42, one can find that the magnetic dipole contributions to the two cross-peaks are

$$\Delta\tilde{E}_{C12}(\omega_t,T,\omega_\tau;m)=\frac{\sqrt{2}}{30}\left\{6D^{g}_{e_2e_2}R^{g}_{e_1e_1}+2D^{g}_{e_2e_1}R^{g}_{e_2e_1}\right\}$$
$$\times\Gamma\left(\bar{\omega}_{e_2g},<\delta\Omega_2^2>,\bar{\omega}_{e_1g},<\delta\Omega_1^2>\right)$$
$$-\frac{\sqrt{2}}{30}\left\{6D^{e_1}_{ff}R^{g}_{e_1e_1}+2[\boldsymbol{\mu}_{fe_1}\cdot\boldsymbol{\mu}_{e_1g}]^{M}\,\mathrm{Im}[\boldsymbol{\mu}_{fe_1}\cdot\mathbf{m}_{e_1g}]^{M}\right\}$$
$$\times\Gamma\left(\bar{\omega}_{fe_1},<\delta\Omega_2^2>,\bar{\omega}_{e_1g},<\delta\Omega_1^2>\right)$$
$$\Delta\tilde{E}_{C21}(\omega_t,T,\omega_\tau;m)=\frac{\sqrt{2}}{30}\left\{6D^{g}_{e_1e_1}R^{g}_{e_2e_2}+2D^{g}_{e_1e_2}R^{g}_{e_1e_2}\right\}$$
$$\times\Gamma\left(\bar{\omega}_{e_1g},<\delta\Omega_1^2>,\bar{\omega}_{e_2g},<\delta\Omega_2^2>\right)$$
$$-\frac{\sqrt{2}}{30}\left\{6D^{e_2}_{ff}R^{g}_{e_2e_2}+2[\boldsymbol{\mu}_{fe_2}\cdot\boldsymbol{\mu}_{e_2g}]^{M}\,\mathrm{Im}[\boldsymbol{\mu}_{fe_2}\cdot\mathbf{m}_{e_2g}]^{M}\right\}$$
$$\times\Gamma\left(\bar{\omega}_{fe_2},<\delta\Omega_1^2>,\bar{\omega}_{e_2g},<\delta\Omega_2^2>\right). \quad (16.68)$$

The dipole and rotatory strengths in Equation 16.68 are newly defined as

$$D^{g}_{e_je_k}\equiv[\boldsymbol{\mu}_{e_jg}\cdot\boldsymbol{\mu}_{e_kg}]^{M}$$
$$R^{g}_{e_je_k}\equiv\mathrm{Im}[\boldsymbol{\mu}_{e_jg}\cdot\mathbf{m}_{e_kg}]^{M}$$
$$D^{e_j}_{ff}\equiv[\boldsymbol{\mu}_{fe_j}\cdot\boldsymbol{\mu}_{fe_j}]^{M}. \quad (16.69)$$

The dipole strength $D^{g}_{e_je_k}$ for $j\neq k$ represents the transition strength associated with the creation of excited-state coherence $\rho^{(2)}_{e_je_k}$ via two electric dipole–electric field interactions, whereas $D^{g}_{e_je_k}$ does the same strength via both electric dipole–electric field and magnetic dipole–magnetic field interactions. Note that they should not be considered transition probability because the product state is not a population but a coherence. The dipole strength $D_{ff}^{e_j}$ is, however, the transition probability of finding the population on the fth doubly excited state when the system was initially the population on the jth singly excited state.

The electric quadrupole contributions to the cross-peaks are found to be

$$\Delta\tilde{E}_{C12}(\omega_t,T,\omega_\tau;Q)=\frac{\sqrt{2}k}{30}[\boldsymbol{\mu}_{ge_2}\cdot\{\boldsymbol{\mu}_{ge_1}\times(\mathbf{Q}_{e_1g}\cdot\boldsymbol{\mu}_{e_2g})\}]^M\,\Gamma\left(\bar{\omega}_{e_2g},<\delta\Omega_2^2>,\bar{\omega}_{e_1g},<\delta\Omega_1^2>\right)$$

$$-\frac{\sqrt{2}k}{30}[\boldsymbol{\mu}_{e_1f}\cdot\{\boldsymbol{\mu}_{ge_1}\times(\mathbf{Q}_{e_1g}\cdot\boldsymbol{\mu}_{fe_1})\}]^M\,\Gamma\left(\bar{\omega}_{fe_1},<\delta\Omega_2^2>,\bar{\omega}_{e_1g},<\delta\Omega_1^2>\right)$$

$$\Delta\tilde{E}_{C21}(\omega_t,T,\omega_\tau;Q)=\frac{\sqrt{2}k}{30}[\boldsymbol{\mu}_{ge_1}\cdot\{\boldsymbol{\mu}_{ge_2}\times(\mathbf{Q}_{e_2g}\cdot\boldsymbol{\mu}_{e_1g})\}]^M\,\Gamma\left(\bar{\omega}_{e_1g},<\delta\Omega_1^2>,\bar{\omega}_{e_2g},<\delta\Omega_2^2>\right)$$

$$-\frac{\sqrt{2}k}{30}[\boldsymbol{\mu}_{e_2f}\cdot\{\boldsymbol{\mu}_{ge_2}\times(\mathbf{Q}_{e_2g}\cdot\boldsymbol{\mu}_{fe_2})\}]^M\,\Gamma\left(\bar{\omega}_{fe_2},<\delta\Omega_1^2>,\bar{\omega}_{e_2g},<\delta\Omega_2^2>\right), \tag{16.70}$$

where $k=|\mathbf{k}_1|$.

Combining the magnetic dipole and electric quadrupole contributions to the diagonal and cross-peaks, one can obtain the final result (Equations 16.65, 16.68, and 16.70) for the 2D optical activity photon echo spectroscopy of coupled dimer systems. One can easily generalize the above results for coupled multi-chromophore systems as[8, 12]

$$\Delta\tilde{E}(\omega_t,T,\omega_\tau)=\frac{\sqrt{2}}{30}\sum_{j,k}\left\{6D_{e_ke_k}^{g}R_{e_je_j}^{g}+2D_{e_ke_j}^{g}R_{e_ke_j}^{g}\right\}\Gamma\left(\bar{\omega}_{e_kg},<\delta\Omega_{e_kg}^2>,\bar{\omega}_{e_jg},<\delta\Omega_{e_jg}^2>\right)$$

$$-\sum_{j,k}\left\{6D_{f_kf_k}^{e_j}R_{e_je_j}^{g}+2[\boldsymbol{\mu}_{f_ke_j}\cdot\boldsymbol{\mu}_{e_jg}]^M\,\mathrm{Im}[\boldsymbol{\mu}_{f_ke_j}\cdot\mathbf{m}_{e_jg}]^M\right\}$$

$$\times\Gamma\left(\bar{\omega}_{f_ke_j},<\delta\Omega_{f_ke_j}^2>,\bar{\omega}_{e_jg},<\delta\Omega_{e_jg}^2>\right)$$

$$+k\sum_{j,k\neq j}[\boldsymbol{\mu}_{ge_k}\cdot\{\boldsymbol{\mu}_{ge_j}\times(\mathbf{Q}_{e_jg}\cdot\boldsymbol{\mu}_{e_kg})]^M\,\Gamma\left(\bar{\omega}_{e_kg},<\delta\Omega_{e_kg}^2>,\bar{\omega}_{e_jg},<\delta\Omega_{e_jg}^2>\right)$$

$$-k\sum_{j,k}[\boldsymbol{\mu}_{e_jf_k}\cdot\{\boldsymbol{\mu}_{ge_j}\times(\mathbf{Q}_{e_jg}\cdot\boldsymbol{\mu}_{f_ke_j})\}]^M\,\Gamma\left(\bar{\omega}_{f_ke_j},<\delta\Omega_{f_ke_j}^2>,\bar{\omega}_{e_jg},<\delta\Omega_{e_jg}^2>\right). \tag{16.69}$$

The above theoretical expression for 2D optical activity photon echo is valid within a few approximations used. Here, the short-time quantum beat contributions, which originate from coherences created on the singly excited-state manifold, and the slow population relaxations were ignored. However, one can easily incorporate such contributions by considering the general theory of 2D photon echo spectroscopy discussed in Chapters 9 to 11 and by properly taking into consideration the rotational averages for magnetic dipole and electric quadrupole terms in the expanded nonlinear response functions with respect to m and Q.

REFERENCES

1. Berova, N.; Nakanishi, K.; Woody, R. W., *Circular dichroism: Principles and applications*. Wiley-VCH: New York, 2000.
2. Cho, M., Coherent two-dimensional optical spectroscopy. *Chemical Reviews* 2008, 108, 1331–1418.
3. Xie, X. L.; Simon, J. D., Picosecond time-resolved circular dichroism study of protein relaxation in myoglobin following photodissociation of CO. *Journal of the American Chemical Society* 1990, 112, 7802–7803.
4. Fischer, P.; Hache, F., Nonlinear optical spectroscopy of chiral molecules. *Chirality* 2005, 17, 421–437.
5. Cho, M., Two-dimensional circularly polarized pump–probe spectroscopy. *Journal of Chemical Physics* 2003, 119, 7003–7016.
6. Choi, J. H.; Cho, M., Two-dimensional circularly polarized IR photon echo spectroscopy of polypeptides: Four-wave-mixing optical activity measurement. *Journal of Physical Chemistry A* 2007, 111, 5176–5184.
7. Choi, J. H.; Cho, M. H., Quadrupole contribution to the third-order optical activity spectroscopy. *Journal of Chemical Physics* 2007, 127, 024507.
8. Choi, J. H.; Cheon, S.; Lee, H.; Cho, M., Two-dimensional nonlinear optical activity spectroscopy of coupled multi-chromophore system. *Physical Chemistry Chemical Physics* 2008, 10, 3839–3856.
9. Abramavicius, D.; Mukamel, S., Coherent third-order spectroscopic probes of molecular chirality. *Journal of Chemical Physics* 2005, 122, 134305.
10. Abramavicius, D.; Mukamel, S., Chirality-induced signals in coherent multidimensional spectroscopy of excitons. *Journal of Chemical Physics* 2006, 124, 034113.
11. Voronine, D. V.; Abramavicius, D.; Mukamel, S., Coherent control of cross-peaks in chirality-induced two-dimensional optical signals of excitons. *Journal of Chemical Physics* 2006, 125, 224504.
12. Choi, J.-H., Cho, M., Nonlinear optical activity measurement spectroscopy of coupled multi-chromophore system. *Chemical Physics* 2007, 341, 57–70.

Index

A

C

R

S

T

V

Printed in the United States
by Baker & Taylor Publisher Services